Tumors of the Mammary Gland

AFIP Atlas of Tumor Pathology

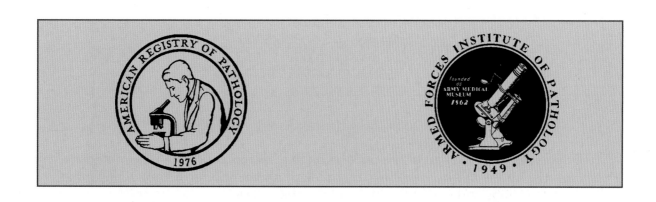

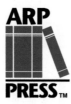

ARP PRESS™

Silver Spring, Maryland

Editorial & Production Manager: Mirlinda Q. Caton
Production Editor: Dian S. Thomas
Editorial Assistant: Melanie J. De Boer
Editorial Assistant: Magdalena C. Silva
Copyeditor: Audrey Kahn

Available from the American Registry of Pathology
Armed Forces Institute of Pathology
Washington, DC 20306-6000
www.afip.org
ISBN 1-933477-05-9
978-1-933477-05-3

AFIP ATLAS OF TUMOR PATHOLOGY

Fourth Series
Fascicle 10

TUMORS OF THE MAMMARY GLAND

by

Fattaneh A. Tavassoli, MD
Director, Women's Health Program
Gynecology and Breast Pathology
Yale University School of Medicine
New Haven, Connecticut

Vincenzo Eusebi, MD
Director and Professor of Anatomic and Cytopathology
Section of Pathology "M. Malpighi"
University of Bologna
Bologna, Italy

Published by the
American Registry of Pathology
Washington, DC
in collaboration with the
Armed Forces Institute of Pathology
Washington, DC
2009

AFIP ATLAS OF TUMOR PATHOLOGY

EDITOR
Steven G. Silverberg, MD
Department of Pathology
University of Maryland School of Medicine
Baltimore, Maryland

Manuscript Reviewed by:
Robert E. Fechner, MD
Noel Weidner, MD

EDITORS' NOTE

The Atlas of Tumor Pathology has a long and distinguished history. It was first conceived at a Cancer Research Meeting held in St. Louis in September 1947 as an attempt to standardize the nomenclature of neoplastic diseases. The first series was sponsored by the National Academy of Sciences-National Research Council. The organization of this Sisyphean effort was entrusted to the Subcommittee on Oncology of the Committee on Pathology, and Dr. Arthur Purdy Stout was the first editor-in-chief. Many of the illustrations were provided by the Medical Illustration Service of the Armed Forces Institute of Pathology (AFIP), the type was set by the Government Printing Office, and the final printing was done at the Armed Forces Institute of Pathology (hence the colloquial appellation "AFIP Fascicles"). The American Registry of Pathology (ARP) purchased the Fascicles from the Government Printing Office and sold them virtually at cost. Over a period of 20 years, approximately 15,000 copies each of nearly 40 Fascicles were produced. The worldwide impact of these publications over the years has largely surpassed the original goal. They quickly became among the most influential publications on tumor pathology, primarily because of their overall high quality but also because their low cost made them easily accessible the world over to pathologists and other students of oncology.

Upon completion of the first series, the National Academy of Sciences-National Research Council handed further pursuit of the project over to the newly created Universities Associated for Research and Education in Pathology (UAREP). A second series was started, generously supported by grants from the AFIP, the National Cancer Institute, and the American Cancer Society. Dr. Harlan I. Firminger became the editor-in-chief and was succeeded by Dr. William H. Hartmann. The second series' Fascicles were produced as bound volumes instead of loose leaflets. They featured a more comprehensive coverage of the subjects, to the extent that the Fascicles could no longer be regarded as "atlases" but rather as monographs describing and illustrating in detail the tumors and tumor-like conditions of the various organs and systems.

Once the second series was completed, with a success that matched that of the first, ARP, UAREP, and AFIP decided to embark on a third series. Dr. Juan Rosai was appointed as editor-in-chief, and Dr. Leslie H. Sobin became associate editor. A distinguished Editorial Advisory Board was also convened, and these outstanding pathologists and educators played a major role in the success of this series, the first publication of which appeared in 1991 and the last (number 32) in 2003.

The same organizational framework will apply to the current fourth series, but with UAREP no longer in existence, ARP will play the major role. New features will include a hardbound cover, illustrations almost exclusively in color, and an accompanying electronic version of each Fascicle. There will also be increased emphasis (wherever appropriate) on the cytopathologic (intraoperative, exfoliative, and/or fine needle aspiration) and molecular features that are important in diagnosis and prognosis. What will not change from the three previous series, however, is the goal of providing the practicing pathologist with thorough, concise, and up-to-date information on the nomenclature and classification; epidemiologic, clinical, and pathogenetic features; and, most importantly, guidance in the diagnosis of the tumors and tumor-like lesions of all major organ systems and body sites.

As in the third series, a continuous attempt will be made to correlate, whenever possible, the nomenclature used in the Fascicles with that proposed by the World Health Organization's Classification of Tumors, as well as to ensure a consistency of style throughout the series. Close cooperation between the various authors and their respective liaisons from the Editorial Board will continue to be emphasized in order to minimize unnecessary repetition and discrepancies in the text and illustrations.

Particular thanks are due to the members of the Editorial Advisory Board, the reviewers (at least two for each Fascicle), the editorial and production staff, and—first and foremost—the individual Fascicle authors for their ongoing efforts to ensure that this series is a worthy successor to the previous three.

Steven G. Silverberg, MD
Leslie H. Sobin, MD

ACKNOWLEDGEMENTS

The authors are grateful to those who have contributed to the completion of this work either by reviewing the chapters or by their words of encouragement. Both authors wish to thank Professor J. G. Azzopardi for being an inspiration and a mentor (directly and indirectly) during our formative years in this discipline and more recently for his generous encouragement and review of some of the chapters. We wish to thank the late Dr. J. L. Peterse, who read some of the chapters; Dr. Luisa Losi, who helped with references; and Dr. Maria P. Foschini for her constant enthusiasm and help with the whole mounts.

The outstanding assistance of Robin Anne Ferres and Douglas Landry, who provided their skills in photography and digitalization of the many images that were taken in the Armed Forces Institute of Pathology while one of us (F. Tavassoli) was working there, is acknowledged with thanks.

We wish to thank Drs. Steven Silverberg and Ronald DeLellis, the series editor and our facilitator, respectively, for their patience and the two anonymous reviewers for their many helpful suggestions and recommendations that have been incorporated in the final product.

Finally, we wish to express our gratitude to the numerous colleagues who over the years have shared with us their most challenging and intriguing cases; this atlas is our thanks to all of you.

Fattaneh A. Tavassoli, MD
Vincenzo Eusebi, MD

DEDICATIONS

To my husband, Dr. Bahman Jabbari, for his constant encouragement and patience; to my 12 brothers and sisters for the abundance of joyful times; and to my parents, Homa and Gholam-Hossein Tavassoli, who nurtured the inquisitive minds of their children.

F. A. Tavassoli

To my family: my wife Dr. Christine Betts and my son Dr. Leonardo Eusebi.

Vincenzo Eusebi

CONTENTS

NORMAL ANATOMY

"All notions that constitute anatomic pathology"—to use Pierre Masson's words—"are the result of a comparison between the features of the organism in good health and those of the diseased organism. The differences that accompany a given disease are defined as lesions" (47). The consequence is that, to be able to recognize a lesion, it is necessary to understand normal anatomy. The normal structure of the breast directly related to the understanding of various lesions is reviewed in this chapter.

MICROANATOMY AND STRUCTURE OF ADULT BREAST

Nipple-Areolar Complex

The nipple bud, recognizable in a 9-week embryo, appears as a small mass of basaloid cells separated from the surrounding mesenchyme by a thick basal lamina. Toward the end of the 3rd month of embryonic life, a larger core is obtained through invasion of the nipple bud by squamous cells of the epidermis. The squamous cells undergo keratinization and desquamate to form a hollow (nipple) pouch, while the basaloid cells sprout downward to form mammary buds, which are the precursors of the primitive ducts (25).

The nipple is covered by stratified squamous epithelium, which is in continuity with that of the surrounding areola and skin. It is unpigmented before menarche. Melanin pigmentation increases after the first menstrual cycles and is the most pronounced during pregnancy. The nipple and the areola enlarge during adolescence, parallel to the growth of the female breast.

While the squamous cells are indistinguishable from those of ordinary skin, two types of clear cells are seen in the nipple. The type most commonly seen, in about 30 percent of women, has clear cytoplasm and a semilunar nucleus compressed to the periphery (fig. 1-1). The empty cytoplasm does not stain for mucins; with antibodies against cytokeratins, epithelial

membrane antigen (EMA), and carcinoembryonic antigen (CEA); and viral antigens against Epstein-Barr virus (EBV) and human papilloma virus (HPV). The clear cytoplasm is probably the result of hydropic changes, which for unknown reasons, affect keratinocytes located, like those of the nipple, in sites close to mucosal surfaces such as the vulva, lip, and eyelids. These clear cells may be rare and scattered, or numerous enough to affect several layers of the epidermis. They may be present also in the areolar skin. They have been described by Tavassoli (76) who warned of the close mimicry with signet ring cells of Paget's carcinoma.

An even closer simulator of Paget neoplastic cells are Toker cells (TCs), the second type of clear cell. These were described in detail by Toker in 1970 (80a), although they were previously noted by Orr and Parish (57). TCs are smaller than typical Paget cells (PCs), but larger than their squamous neighbors (80a). They have a rounded, bland nucleus and cytoplasm paler than the surrounding keratinocytes (fig. 1-2). Melanin granules may be present in the cytoplasm while intermediate filaments are abundant at the ultrastructural level (45).

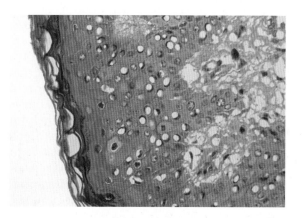

Figure 1-1

EPIDERMAL CLEAR CELLS

The cytoplasm is empty and the nuclei are dislodged to the periphery of the cell.

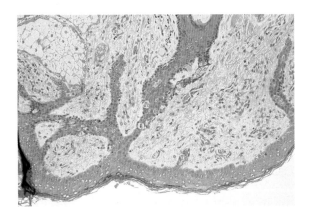
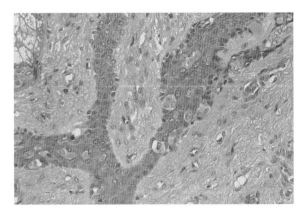

Figure 1-2

TOKER CELLS

Left: Toker cells are occasionally visible along the epidermis. Some are close to the sebaceous glands. These cells are scattered near the basal layer. The cytoplasm is more abundant but paler than the surrounding keratinocytes.

Right: The nuclei are round and bland.

TCs are common at the summit of the nipple although the lateral walls as well as the areolar skin also harbor them. TCs are most numerous immediately above the openings of lactiferous sinuses (44). They are generally aggregated in solid groups of three to four cells but single cells or tubular structures occur. They are most common near the basal layer (44), but migration to more superficial layers may also be seen.

TCs are a diagnostic problem because they are difficult to distinguish from PCs, especially when numerous and associated with a nipple duct adenoma (92). Immunohistochemistry is not helpful since TCs and PCs share the same antigenic properties, such as immunopositivity for cytokeratin (CK) 7 (fig. 1-3, left), CAM5.2, and EMA, while CK20, and S-100 protein are consistently negative (44). With CK7 stains, TCs occasionally show a dendritic shape (fig. 1-3, right). Gross cystic disease fluid protein (GCDFP)-15 is seen occasionally in PCs but is negative in TCs (44). Probably the only helpful immunostain for distinguishing the two cell types is c-erbB-2 antibody which is negative in TCs (92) but positive in PCs (39,44). As repeatedly stressed by Toker (80a), the differential diagnosis resides on the absence of the cytologic stigmata of malignancy and the absence of a carcinoma in the lactiferous ducts.

The prevalence of TCs varies. Of 190 nipple specimens from 101 patients that were stained with hematoxylin and eosin (H&E), TC was present in 23 nipples (18 patients) (80a). Only 1 of the 18 patients had mammary carcinoma; 8 patients were male. If a CK7 antibody is used, TCs are seen in 83 percent of patients (15 of 18 nipples from 10 patients in a series of non-neoplastic lesions seen at autopsy) (44). Therefore, TCs should be regarded not as neoplastic elements but as cellular extensions from the epithelium of the ducts or as remnants of embryonic tissue (76), of which the nipple bud is a strong candidate.

Smooth muscle fibers are abundant in the nipple and are confined to the dermis. They extend to the areola in a flat fashion. The deep margin of the muscles may be marked by a straight line which indicates an ideal boundary between the dermis and the breast tissue.

Apoeccrine sweat glands are present predominantly in the dermis of the areola but are also occasionally seen in the nipple. They differ from ordinary apocrine sweat glands because their ducts open directly to the epidermis and not to hair follicles (81). These glands can be distinguished from breast lobules showing apocrine change since their excretory ducts lack the myoepithelial cells present along the whole mammary glandular tree (24).

Lobules are located in 17 percent of nipples routinely examined for breast carcinoma (67). Eccrine sweat glands are observed in the mid-dermis of the areola and occasionally appear deep in the breast tissue. Sebaceous glands open directly to the epidermis and are frequently

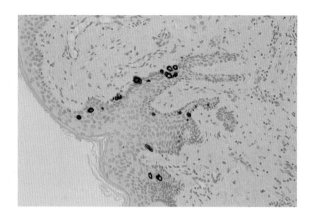
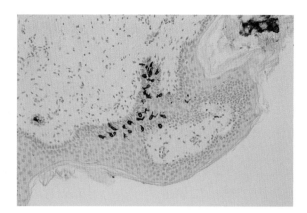

Figure 1-3

TOKER CELLS

Cytokeratin (CK) 7 stains the Toker cells (left), which in this case of nipple duct adenoma appear numerous and dendritic (right).

seen at the tip of the nipple. Sebaceous glands undergo atrophy with age.

In the areola, there are small, rounded elevations known as tubercles of Morgagni-Montgomery. G.B. Morgagni was an anatomist working in Bologna and Padua in the 18th century (before the use of the microscope) and W.F. Montgomery was a Dublin obstetrician of the 19th century. They both described tiny papules (10 to 15) in the areola but no histologic description was provided. It is, therefore, no coincidence that in the literature there is no consensus on the histology of the tubercles and opinions vary from sebaceous glands to sweat glands, to modified mammary glands, and to sebaceous glands with galactophores opening into them. Since Morgagni-Montgomery tubercles are located in the areola where sebaceous glands are less numerous, the matter remains unresolved.

The thickness of the dermis of the areola and the skin overlying the breast varies from 1.5 to 8.0 mm (mean, 3.8 mm), as seen in 10 randomly selected patients ranging from 38 to 59 years (mean, 51 years) (author's observation). It is thinner in older patients (range, 1.8 to 5.0 mm; mean, 2.6 mm), as seen in 18 patients of a mean age of 72 years (range, 60 to 79 years). The dermis is better appreciated when the breast is studied with the help of macrosections (whole mounts). The breast connective tissue is separated from the overlying dermis by a thin rim of loose connective tissue (fig. 1-4). Accordingly, all nipple connective tissue appears to be part

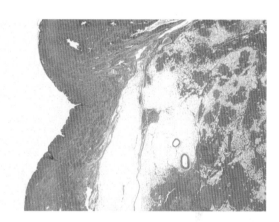

Figure 1-4

NIPPLE AND DERMIS

The dermis is readily apparent.

of the dermis but, at variance with the dermis of the rest of the skin, it is not easily separated from the stroma of the breast parenchyma since the duct entering into the nipple makes it impossible to distinguish between the periductal fibrous tissue and that of the dermis (fig. 1-5). Since extension of the tumor to the dermis is important in staging, where a decision on invasion of the skin has to be made, we feel that the use of whole mounts is very helpful.

STRUCTURE OF THE GLANDULAR TREE

The nomenclature of the different parts of the glandular tree that forms a breast lobe has not achieved universal acceptance. As pointed

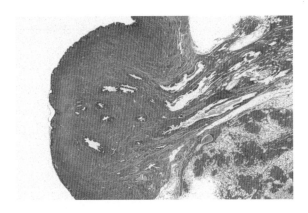

Figure 1-5

NIPPLE AND DERMIS

The periductal fibrous tissue merges with the connective tissue of the dermis.

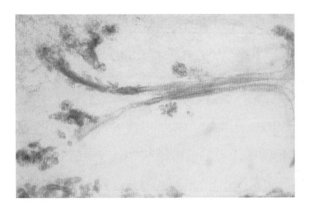

Figure 1-6

SUBSEGMENTAL DUCTS

Subsegmental ducts depart from a segmental duct in a dichotomous fashion.

out by Azzopardi et al. (3), the term "terminal duct" is attributed, according to different authors, to the smallest branch present in the lobule or to the largest duct near the nipple, depending on the perspective of the observer, whether looking at the tree from the nipple or the lobules. Azzopardi et al. also stated that it was not "entirely clear whether terminal duct should be applied to the largest or smallest duct." For practical purposes, the terminology used by Azzopardi et al. is retained. Accordingly, the term collecting ducts applies to the major ducts of the nipple region; lactiferous sinuses are those located between the collecting ducts and large (segmental) ducts, which are followed by smaller (subsegmental) ducts branching in a dichotomous fashion. From the latter, smaller ductules further branch dichotomously (fig. 1-6). This is best seen in three-dimensional (3D) sections (68,71,89).

The ductules further splay into a cluster forming, numerous finger-like minute glands that are part of the lobule. The number of ductules (acini) varies from 8 to 200 per lobule (42,68) depending on parity. The least numerous acini are mainly seen in nulliparous women, a higher number are present in parous individuals, while in pregnancy their number can range up to 400 (Dr. Tibor Tot, Sweden, personal communication, 2006). Nevertheless, lobules containing few acini can be seen in parous women, indicating that part of the breast tree has failed to respond to the influence of pregnancy and lactation.

Terminal duct lobular units (TDLUs), as defined by Wellings and Jensen (88), are extralobular ducts that subdivide into the several intralobular ductules (acini). These constitute the secretory part of the glandular tree. This region is also the most active proliferating zone of the entire lobe, as determined by the thymidine labeling index (68). Here, a lobule is defined as a functional unit formed by acini immersed in "specialized" stroma (3). These functional units develop within 6 months to 2 years from the first menstrual period (25,68). Their development is not genetically programmed and depends entirely on hormonal supply. This is clearly demonstrable in male to female transsexuals who develop lobular structures if progestational chemical castration is combined with feminizing estrogen therapy (34). The number of lobules within a lobe varies, as seen with 3D visualization, from inconspicuous at the level of the nipple up to 15,000 close to the fascia in fertile women (Dr. Tibor Tot, personal communication, 2006). The extralobular ductules supplying the lobules close to the nipple are short, and depart directly from the collecting duct. Those at the end farthest from the nipple depart from the subsegmental ducts and are generally narrow and elongated (fig. 1-7).

Three dimensionally, the breast lobe can be depicted as a cone with the apex close to the nipple and the base (where most of the lobules are located) facing the deep fascia. In one study, 15 to 25 collecting ducts drained an equivalent

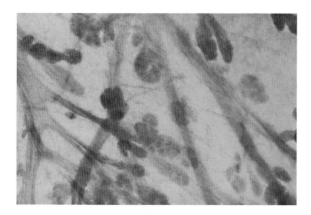

Figure 1-7

SUBSEGMENTAL DUCTS

The subsegmental ducts far from the nipple are narrow and elongated. (Courtesy of Dr. T. Tot, Falun, Sweden.)

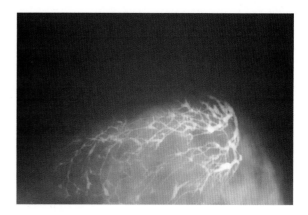

Figure 1-8

SUBSEGMENTAL DUCTS

Galactography shows that the contrast medium, which was injected into only one collecting duct, visualizes subsegmental ducts spread over more than one quadrant.

number of lobes (25). A recent 3D reconstruction of mastectomy nipples contained 11 to 48 central ducts (median, 27) (26).

Lobes cannot be macroscopically separated from one another because the branches of the tree intermingle with those of adjacent lobes. This has been illustrated by Cooper (36) and is common knowledge among radiologists. Positive subsegmental ducts frequently spread over more than one quadrant, as seen with galactographies in which contrast medium is injected into one collecting duct (fig. 1-8). Ohtake et al. (56), in a computerized 3D reconstruction of the mammary lobes, even suggested the existence of branching anastomoses between different lobes of the breast.

This finding is very important if confirmed, especially for the possibility of intraductal carcinomas extending to contiguous lobes. Radiologists are skeptical about this finding, however, since no single case of anastomosis has been revealed by galactographic procedures (Dr. L. Tabar, Sweden, personal communication, 2005). If anastomoses were present, retrograde spreading of the contrast medium into branches from different lobes would be observed, a phenomenon not seen so far. No anastomoses were found by Going and Moffat (26), who also found that 75 percent of the breast volume was drained by the largest six lobes while the eight small lobes together accounted for only 1.6 percent of breast volume.

The whole glandular tree is supported by dense collagen. A cuff of loose specialized stroma surrounds the ducts and envelops the acini (3). This differs from the interlobar stroma by being more cellular and vascularized (25). The specialized stroma is more abundant around the acini. It constitutes the bulk of each lobule and contains, in the late progestational phase, abundant acidic mucosubstances, easily revealed by Alcian blue staining (3).

A rim of elastic fibers (3) is present along the length of the duct system, from the nipple (collecting ducts) (fig. 1-9, left) to the extralobular portion of the TDLU complex (fig. 1-9, right), but it is not seen around the acini. It is more abundant in parous women and in the post-menopausal breast (25). It is absent around the ducts in gynecomastia (3).

DEVELOPMENT

In the late stages of embryonic development, breast tissue is visible as an ovoid mass under the epidermis (25). In this early structure, branching channels with evident lumens immersed in a cellular stroma are easily visible.

In the infant breast until 2.5 years after birth, three structures are prominent (1): elongated ducts with bulbous endings; ducts with dichotomous branching; and ducts with dichotomous branching and rudimentary lobules. The latter ducts are composed of 5 to 10 short and blunt-ended acini surrounded by specialized stroma. These rudimentary lobules are reminiscent of the ill-defined glandular proliferation,

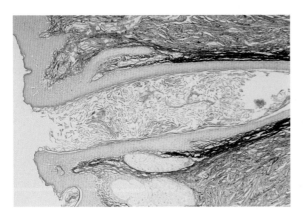
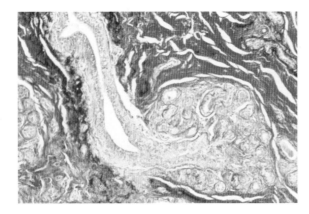

Figure 1-9

COLLECTING DUCT AND TERMINAL DUCT LOBULAR UNIT

A rim of elastic tissue envelops the ductal tree from the squamous-glandular junction (left) to the extralobular portion of the terminal duct lobular unit (TDLU) (right).

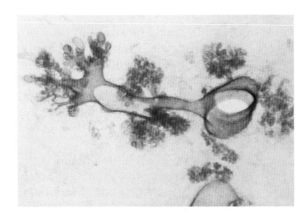
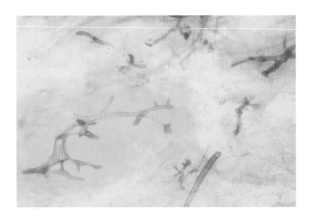

Figure 1-10

POSTMENOPAUSAL BREAST

In the postmenopausal breast, acini have mostly disappeared and the breast glandular tree is composed of ducts and short dilated intralobular ductules.

Figure 1-11

POSTMENOPAUSAL BREAST

In the postmenopausal breast, lobules have disappeared and the remnants of the ducts are surrounded by adipose tissue. (Courtesy of Dr. T. Tot, Falun, Sweden.)

sometimes called blunt duct adenosis, seen in the adult breast.

These structures start to involute at 6 months after birth and only segmental ducts surrounded by dense connective tissue persist. Ducts remain in this fashion until puberty when the first fully formed lobules appear (54).

Involution (So-Called Postmenopausal Breast)

Progressively with age, beginning around menopause, the acini shorten, dilate, and show blunt endings (71). Some acini disappear and eventually the mammary glandular

tree is composed of ducts and short, dilated intralobular ductules (fig. 1-10); the latter may form microcysts. If the tissue around the cyst has the character of the specialized stroma, the cyst is indicative of early involution (3). On the contrary, sclerohyaline stroma is an indication of a permanent status.

Adipose tissue progressively replaces the interlobar and extralobular connective tissue and connective tissue remains confined to periductal areas (fig. 1-11). This is commonly referred to as "postmenopausal" breast. We consider this a "virtual" description, since in most cases, there are

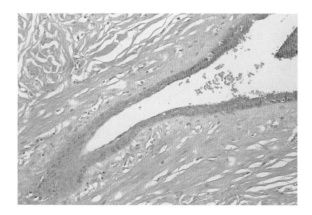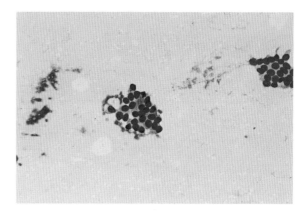

Figure 1-12

SQUAMOUS-GLANDULAR JUNCTION

Left: The transition from the squamous epithelium into the "proper" epithelium is usually smooth.
Right: The secretory cells have round nuclei with inconspicuous nucleoli, are evenly spaced, and show pink and slightly granular cytoplasm.

persistent lobules even at a late age, identical to those seen during reproductive life (71). This is becoming even more frequent since many post-menopausal women are taking hormones. This makes it very difficult to "date" a breast specimen precisely. A direct consequence of this uncertain dating of tissues is that radiologists find it difficult to consider a mammogram "normal."

In a classification of the mammographic features of non-neoplastic breast, Gram et al. (28) described five patterns. Pattern I, which on 3D histologic reconstruction corresponds to the reproductive period of the breast, changes with time into patterns II and III. The latter, when related to 3D reconstructed histology, correspond to the description given above for involuted breast. Mammographic extensive nodular and linear densities, and diffuse fibrosis, regarded as patterns IV and V, respectively, tend to remain unmodified over the years, indicating that the changes described above as involuted breast are not an obligatory pathway. This point will be dealt with in greater detail later in the chapter.

CYTOLOGY OF THE GLANDULAR TREE

Fertile Period

The most external part of the collecting duct is lined by stratified squamous epithelium, which is in continuity with the epidermis via the lactiferous duct orifice. The squamous epithelium ends before entering the lactiferous

sinus. The junction with the glandular epithelium is usually smooth and is here termed the squamous-glandular junction (fig. 1-12, left). The collecting duct in the nonlactating breast is usually sealed by a keratin plug (3,29). Extension of the squamous epithelium into or beyond the lactiferous sinus is an indication of squamous metaplasia (67), most frequently caused by periductal mastitis.

The remainder of the gland is lined predominantly by two cell types surrounded by a basal lamina well delineated by periodic acid–Schiff (PAS) stain, as well as by immunocytochemical stains using collagen IV and laminin antibodies.

Luminal Cells. These vary from cuboidal to columnar in shape and are anchored either to the basal lamina or to myoepithelial cells. The nuclei are located in the middle of the cell and the cytoplasm is abundant. These features are appreciated most closely in fine needle preparations where the round nuclei are evenly spaced by granular and eosinophilic cytoplasm (fig.1-12, right). The cytoplasm contains the typical complement of organelles including electron-dense secretory granules located in the luminal portion of the cell where short microvilli are visible (3). The granules are osmiophilic, stain with uranyl acetate, and can be rendered argyrophilic if the silver solution is overheated.

At the ultrastructural level, the granules stain with ruthenium red (21), indicating an acidic

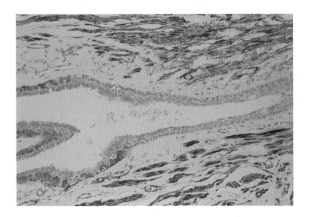

Figure 1-13

MYOEPITHELIAL CELLS

Myoepithelial cells disappear abruptly at the level of the ductal squamous junction.

mucopolysaccharide content. The luminal glycocalix stains with Alcian blue, especially in the secretory phase of the ovulatory cycle, and with EMA. CK19 appears in the breast buds as early as 16 weeks of fetal age and remains for the rest of life confined to the luminal cells (2). CK8, CK15, CK16, and CK18 are also present in the luminal cells (8,53), CK8 and CK18 appear in infant tissue but are not visible in fetuses (2). K-casein positivity is restricted to the first 2 months of the postnatal period (2) while bcl-2 remains positive in the luminal cells but not in the basal myoepithelial cells. Estrogen and progesterone receptors (ER, PR), visualized with monoclonal antibodies, are observed in numerous epithelial cells, mostly in the acini in adult breast, but not in infants and fetuses where these receptors are rare (55). Androgen receptors (AR) are seen in the stroma of fetuses but are absent from the epithelium. The latter receptors disappear in the infant breast. In the adult, they are seen in apocrine cells only (see later in the chapter).

Myoepithelial Cells. These are located between the secretory cells and the basal lamina to which they are anchored. They extend from the collecting ducts to the extreme tip of the acini. In the nipple, they disappear abruptly at the level of the squamous-glandular junction (fig. 1-13). The name of this cell, to use Professor Hamperl's words (30), was adopted to indicate that the cell "belonged to two widely divergent types of tissues," namely, the epithelium and smooth muscle cells. Myoepithelial cells are contractile cells that appear between the 23rd and 24th weeks of fetal life (55). They facilitate the outflow of secretions by increasing pressure on excretory units. Contraction of myoepithelial cells is induced by oxytocin, similar to smooth muscle cells, and indeed they have oxytocin receptors on their surfaces (12). Myoepithelial cells are not readily visible with H&E staining but in fine needle smears their presence around secretory cells is very useful to confirm the benign nature of a given lesion (fig. 1-14, left). The nuclei generally appear thin, elongated, and oriented circumferentially, with the cytoplasm hardly visible when the gland is distended. The nuclei are round and the eosinophilic cytoplasm is prominent when the gland is collapsed or is undergoing atrophy.

Before the immunohistochemical era, phosphotungstic acid-hematoxylin, Masson trichrome (47), and silver impregnation were the methods used, with variable success, to stain myoepithelial cells. In thick sections, however, the dendritic nature of myoepithelial cells enveloping the secretory cells is readily apparent. These methods were followed by ultrastructural studies (58), which consistently showed the presence of microfilaments with dense bodies as well as desmosomes and bundles of tonofilaments (fig. 1-14, right). Enzyme histochemical methods, such as alkaline phosphatase and adenosine triphosphatase, were also used but myoepithelial cells were visualized in their full splendor with the advent of immunohistochemistry. Using monoclonal antibodies against alpha-smooth muscle actin, myoepithelial cells are seen in copious number, being more apparent in the ducts than in the acini . In the gaps between myoepithelial cells, secretory cells are anchored to the basal lamina (58). Several other markers have been used to visualize myoepithelial cells including common acute lymphoblastic leukemia antigen (CALLA), glial fibrillary acidic protein (GFAP), myosin, common actin, vimentin, nerve growth factor receptor, and oxytocin receptors. None of these has achieved widespread routine use for several reasons including the need for a fixative other than formalin or lack of relative specificity for myoepithelial cells.

Smooth muscle actin antibody provided a great improvement in the study of myoepithelial

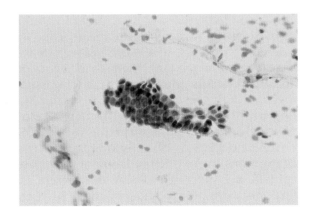 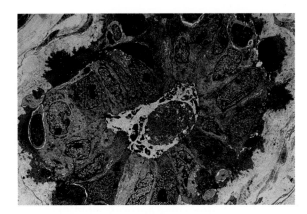

Figure 1-14

MYOEPITHELIAL CELLS

Left: As seen cytologically, the flat myoepithelial layer that envelops secretory, evenly spaced cells, confirms the benign nature of the lesion.

Right: The two layers of "proper" breast epithelium are easily visible at the ultrastructural level. The outer cell layer is formed by myoepithelial cells. (Courtesy of Dr. G. Losa, Locarno, Switzerland.)

cells but it soon was clear that myofibroblasts are also selectively stained since they also contain actin. Calponin, caldesmon, and smooth muscle myosin heavy chain (SMM-HC) were simultaneously studied in the normal breast (24,86). The first two are regulatory proteins of the actin-myosin interaction, while SMM-HC is a structural component of smooth muscle cells. Of these antibodies, the most selective and useful for myoepithelial cells appears to be the one related to myosin, since only rare myofibroblasts are stained (24,86). Myoepithelial cells are heterogeneous cells because caldesmon and myosin stain the periductal myoepithelial cells only, while the periacinar myoepithelial cells are seldom immunoreactive with caldesmon antibodies.

This heterogeneity is also seen when an S-100 protein antibody is used. This protein, also considered a marker for myoepithelial cells, does not stain myoepithelial cells in all cases or in a consistent fashion within the different lobes of the same breast, and unfortunately, intense staining is frequently obtained in luminal cells as well. It appears that the study of S-100 protein content in myoepithelial cells is scientifically interesting, but not practical for diagnostic purposes. The heterogeneity of myoepithelial cells is further evidenced by their constant negativity when S-100 protein antisera are applied to the parotid gland.

CK5, CK14, and CK17 are expressed by myoepithelial cells (8,90); however, they are not exclusive to myoepithelial cells since CK14 is also occasionally seen in secretory cells (90) or is shared with CK5 in basal cells of the epidermis (64) and the prostate gland. Heterogeneity of myoepithelial cells is also revealed by CK17, which is positive in ductal myoepithelial cells but in only 5 percent of acinic myoepithelial cells (90). P63, a p53 homologue, stains the nuclei of myoepithelial cells and is becoming a useful marker because it does not react with secretory cells or myofibroblasts (5). Nevertheless, expression of some markers can change depending on the methodology used (i.e., the variety of antigen retrieval systems).

Stem Cells. Using laser capture microdissection, Lakhani et al. (38) have shown loss of heterozygosity (LOH) in lobules dissected from paraffin-embedded tissues from reduction mammoplasties and implied that normal breast lobules were clonal in nature. The same authors also observed the same LOH in both normal myoepithelial cells and luminal cells, and consequently stated that there is a common stem cell that gives rise to the two cell types.

Despite this evidence, the issue is still far from settled. In spite of numerous accurate ultrastructural studies obtained over 40 years, no ultrastructural evidence for the existence of stem cells has been provided. Stirling and Chandler (75) illustrated basally located lymphocyte-like and macrophage-like cells. The basal clear cell illustrated by Smith et al. (74) is probably a modified myoepithelial cell with hydropic cytoplasmic changes as described by Hamperl (30). If a stem cell had been present, it would not have escaped the notice of these researchers. Sapino et al. (70) obtained two in vitro cell lines (epithelial and myoepithelial) from a single tumor, which, once transplanted into syngenic animals, gave rise to clones of either an epithelial or myoepithelial nature. These authors concluded that the myoepithelial and epithelial cell lines were independent but interactive cell populations. Also, breast epithelial buds in early development are formed by basaloid cells that contain CK19. Myoepithelial cells appear between the 23rd and 24th weeks of fetal life. After this period, the two types of cells (myoepithelial cells and luminal) are clearly recognizable while a common precursor is no longer traceable (2). If the existence of a stem cell is an intellectual necessity, the most suitable candidate is the basaloid cell present in fetal breast buds.

Since no clear-cut evidence of the existence of stem cells in the adult mammary glandular tree is currently available, it seems appropriate to leave the question open. As Sapino et al. (70) suggest, it is possible that mature luminal cells and myoepithelial cells are still capable of transdifferentiation and therefore postulation of the existence of a stem cell is no longer necessary.

Apocrine Cells. Apocrine epithelium was regarded as "a prominent constituent of normal breast" by Haagensen (29). The word apocrine is derived from the ancient Greek "apokrines-thioi," which means "to be secreted." Creighton (1902) first suggested that the pink epithelial cysts were accidental inclusions of sweat glands in the breast tissue, also referred to as "pale cells" (15) and "pink cells" (9). It was Lendrum (41) who first used the term "apocrine metaplasia." The apocrine nature of these cells was also held by Masson (47), who rejected Hamperl's interpretation of the oncocytic nature of these cells and named them "metaplasie hidrosadenoide ou apocrine." An apocrine metaplastic origin was also strongly supported by Azzopardi (3). The noncommittal term of "apocrine change" was adopted by Page and Anderson (61). Nev-

ertheless, the presence of apocrine epithelium in most of the non-neoplastic breast tissue in women over the age of 40 years is a well-established phenomenon (15). The high incidence of apocrine cysts in non-neoplastic breast tissue, together with the clinically apparent correlation with the menstrual cycle, is suggestive of physiologic change rather than true disease (43). This led Eusebi et al. (19) to regard apocrine cells as a normal line of differentiation of the breast epithelium. Apocrine cells are not present in fetal breasts (82) or in patients under 20 years of age (82,87). GCDFP-15, immunohistochemically localized by Viacava et al. (82) to "ordinary" luminal cells of fetal breast, suggests that GCDFP-15–immunoreactive cells are elements programmed to become typical apocrine cells, a phenomenon that is best described as "late" differentiation.

The lobular origin of apocrine cells was proposed by Masson (46). Azzopardi (3) stated that the lobular origin was easily appreciated under the scanning microscope, a view also held by Wellings and Alpers (87). In a 3D study, these authors showed that small apocrine cysts are grouped together, reflecting the expansion of the lobular architecture. Apocrine cells may line as few as one to two acini, but usually all acini in a given lobule show apocrine epithelium (fig. 1-15, left). Ducts are rarely involved by apocrine differentiation.

The apocrine cells appear columnar, cuboidal, or flattened, depending on their location within acini or cysts. With the H&E stain, two distinct types of apocrine cells are recognized. The type A cell shows abundant eosinophilic and granular cytoplasm (20), best visualized at the cytologic level (fig. 1-15, right). A supranuclear vacuole is often observed in which a yellow-brown ceroid-like pigment is present. In columnar cells, a dome-shaped luminal portion containing birefringent granules is easily visible. The nuclei are globoid and generally display one to two prominent nucleoli. The granularity of the cytoplasm reflects electron-dense granules, which vary in size from 303 to 722 nm (20). These granules condense under the luminal pole, which shows short and sparse microvilli.

The type B cell has to be included in the broad category of clear cells in the sense that the cytoplasm is distinctly foamy where minute

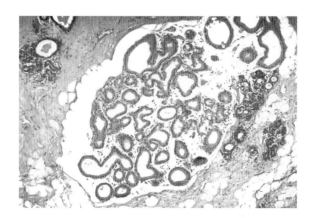
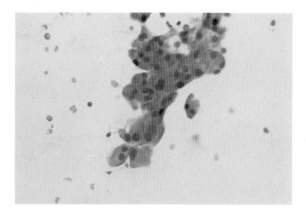

Figure 1-15

APOCRINE CELLS

Left: All acini of this lobule show apocrine differentiation.
Right: The apocrine epithelium cytologically shows ovoid nuclei with nucleoli and abundant pink cytoplasm.

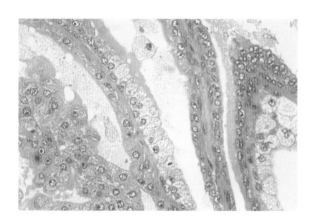
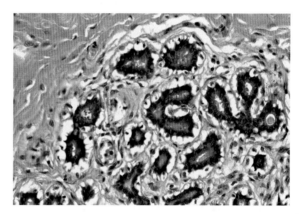

Figure 1-16

APOCRINE CELLS

Left: The apocrine type B cells have microvacuoles in the cytoplasm which correspond to the empty vesicles seen ultrastructurally. They impart a foamy appearance to the cytoplasm.

Right: The foamy appearance contrasts with the empty cytoplasm shown by myoepithelial cells in the postovulatory phase.

vacuoles reminiscent of sebaceous cells are present. These same cells have been designated as sebocrine (77). The microvacuoles correspond at the ultrastructural level to empty vesicles (63) or lipid droplets (77). The empty vesicles are as large as osmiophilic granules (20) and contain GCDFP-15 (49). The type B cell is probably a storage cell. These cells can be distinguished from other clear cells, such as the glycogen-rich myoepithelial cells that are seen during the postovulatory phase (fig. 1-16) (42,85), and show empty cytoplasm because of glycogen extraction during tissue processing.

Histochemically, the supranuclear vacuole of type A apocrine cells contains iron-related substance (3,9). The apical granules are stained by oil red-O, Sudan black, and PAS after diastase digestion, indicating their glycolipid nature (19). These granules are products of secretion and observed in both types of cells. They are visualized ultrastructurally as osmiophilic bodies.

Immunohistochemically, both types of cells are positive for low weight keratins and EMA. Apocrine cells are positive with GCDFP-15 antibody (48). This staining is selective but not confined to the apocrine cells of the breast.

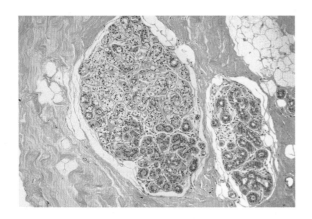

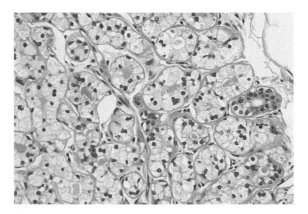

Figure 1-17

CLEAR CELLS

Some of the acini in this lobule have luminal cells with clear empty cytoplasm.

Figure 1-18

CLEAR CELLS

Clear empty cytoplasm does not have the microvacuolar structure of type B apocrine cells.

Positivity has been observed in the apocrine glands of the axilla, anogenital area, and in all apoeccrine glands of the rest of the body as well as in the acini of salivary and bronchial glands (60,83). GCDFP-15 has also been localized in the apocrine epithelium of the breast at the genetic level (14,59). Apocrine cells lack bcl-2 immunostaining as well as S-100 protein, ER, and PR. On the other hand, staining for AR and bax is positive (19,78).

Clear Cells. There are several cells in the breast glandular tree that show clearing of the cytoplasm. This is due to artifactual changes during tissue processing (16). Barwick et al. (6) were "unable to find a single example of clear cell change at the time of frozen section." The intracellular substances that are extracted vary; therefore, the clear cell nature of various cells deserves further characterization.

There are three types of "clear" cells that, although artifactual, deserve recognition. 1) If fixation is delayed, any type of cell can undergo "hydropic" change and hence have empty clear cytoplasm (16). This is easily recognized since cells (luminal and myoepithelial) in the same area show the same changes. 2) Glycogen-rich myoepithelial cells were described by Skorpil (72) in 1943 as "lamproziten" (lampros meaning clear in ancient Greek). These correspond to the clear basal cells described by Smith et al. (74). The cells show clear empty cytoplasm resulting from glycogen extraction, and correspond to the clear cells seen in the postovulatory phase

of the menstrual cycle (fig. 1-16, right) (42,85). 3) Apocrine type B foamy cells are probably the result of GCDFP-15 extraction.

Barwick et al. (6) described a further type of clear cell not well defined as yet. This type of clear cell change can invest part (figs. 1-17, 1-18) or all of the lobule. This cell was also reported by Tavassoli and Yeh (79), who found PAS-positive diastase-resistant granules in the cytoplasm that were mucicarmine and Alcian blue negative. Eusebi et al. (19) found these cells to be occasionally GCDFP-15 positive. The percent of clear cells (1.6 percent [15 cases out of a series of 934]) given by Vina and Wells (84) in non-neoplastic breast tissue is probably high. Usually only one to three lobules are affected per case, although exceptionally, numerous lobules may show clear cell changes.

The Menstrual Cycle

Breast size, density, and nodularity are related to the menstrual cycle (29,51). The water content of the breast shows remarkable variation depending on the phase of the cycle, clearly seen with magnetic resonance imaging (MRI) (51).

As stated by Geschickter (25), there is little agreement on the microscopic changes that accompany the menstrual cycle. This is because the histologic changes of the lobules are remarkably different from area to area within the same breast. It is possible, for instance, to observe in one area lobules showing advanced secretory changes (42) and in other areas lobules showing

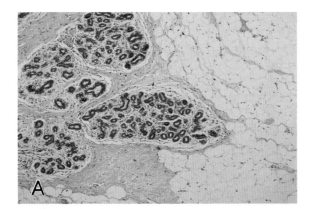

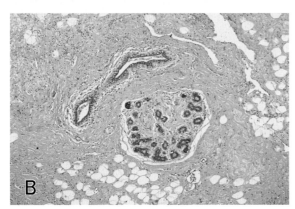

Figure 1-19

BREAST CYCLE

A: The "specialized" lobular stroma is slightly edematous and the acini are numerous.

B: The specialized stroma of this lobule is fibrous, similar to that seen in involuted breast.

C: Clear cell changes of the myoepithelium of the "postovulatory phase." (All figures are images taken from the same large (macro) section from a 45-year-old woman.)

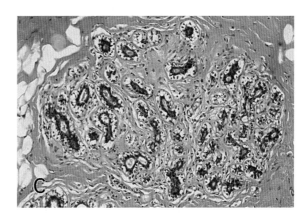

proliferative features (85). This heterogeneity of "menstrual cycle changes" can be best appreciated on macrosections that give an overview of larger samples of breast tissue than that obtained in conventional routine sections (fig. 1-19).

It is possible that the heterogeneity of the hormonal response is due to the fact that breast tissue has a different, and probably longer, reparative/proliferative period than the endometrium. Consequently, the endometrial phase cannot be compared to the breast cycle.

The various changes of the breast cycle have been described in great detail by Vogel et al. (85) and Longacre and Bartow (42). 1) The size of lobules increases from 1.06 mm in greatest diameter in the proliferative phase to 1.82 mm in the late secretory phase; 2) the number of acini per lobule increases as well from a minimum of 8 to a maximum of 200 in the late secretory phase; 3) the lobular specialized stroma is dense after menstruation while it is edematous and strongly alcianophilic in the late progestational phase (fig. 1-19A); 4) lymphocytes are rare in the early phase of the cycle, while they can be as numerous as 350 per lobule in the late

secretory phase. Plasma cells are usually scanty throughout the cycle (3); 5) lumens are closed in the early cycle and open with alcianophilic secretion in the late secretory phase; and 6) the epithelium varies from cuboidal to columnar, with luminal (apical) snouts at the end of the cycle. Myoepithelial vacuoles containing glycogen appear around the late proliferative phase (figs. 1-16, right, 1-19C) and are more conspicuous in the secretory phase.

Pregnancy and Lactational Changes

Enlargement of the breast becomes apparent around the 5th month of pregnancy when there is a tremendous increase in acini. The peak of the proliferative activity is during the first 20 weeks of gestation as proved by the high number of mitotic figures in the acini (76). The lumens of the acini become lined by cuboidal cells and dilate, while the myoepithelial cells become inconspicuous. The specialized stroma of the lobules progressively disappears to become a strand of connective tissue enclosing thin-walled capillary residues. The stroma is progressively compressed by adjacent acini.

Lactation begins 2 to 6 days after delivery. Secretion takes place in the epithelial lining of the acini of the "immense lobules" (25). The luminal secretory cells, which in the resting breast are similar in the whole glandular tree, acquire the secretory features previously described (76). Lumens become filled by secretory material, resulting in distension of the lactiferous ducts. "Virginal" unmodified lobules are seen among those showing pregnancy and lactational changes. The number of these is highly variable and is probably one of the factors associated with individual variability in the quantity of milk produced (25).

On average, it takes 3 to 4 months for the breast to return to the nonlactational status (76), although signs of "recent" pregnancy can be observed even up to 5 years after the end of lactation (7). These signs were described by Battersby and Anderson (7) and consist mainly of irregularity of the shape of the lobules, angulated acini, flattened epithelium, crenulated basal membrane, and, as stressed by Azzopardi (3) and Tavassoli (76), the presence of lymphocytes and plasma cells within the specialized stroma of the lobules.

Occasionally, the acini, which average 400 to 500 per lobule in a lactating breast, undergo exuberant growth. The "focal exaggerated physiologic hyperplasia" causes clinically detectable lumps (73). These can be confused with carcinoma at frozen section, especially when they undergo coagulative necrosis. Cases of infarction of the breast not related to pregnancy, but associated with mitral stenosis or congestive heart failure, have been documented (31). Nevertheless, most of the examples of coagulative necrosis reported in the literature are related to pregnancy and are also seen in hamartomas, fibroadenomas, and tubular adenomas (73).

Focal Lactational Changes and Focal Lactational Hyperplasia

Focal lactational changes are defined as "epithelial changes whose morphology cannot be distinguished from the more diffuse epithelial changes observed during pregnancy or lactation" (35). The only morphologic difference is the lack of prominent secretion within the lumens of distended acini. The condition is not related to lactation since in most cases a prior pregnancy preceded the lesion by several years and in the series reported by Kiaer and Andersen (35) at least three patients had never been pregnant. The reported frequency of such changes varies from 1.7 (67) to 3.0 percent (35) of examined breast specimens. Lactational changes never form tumoral lumps, and isolated foci vary from 1 to 12, according to the size of the specimen (35). Occasionally, only part of a lobule demonstrates the change. The epithelium, which shows PAS-positive, diastase-resistant granules, is immunoreactive with alpha-lactalbumin and S-100 protein antibody (84) as well as lysozyme (66). Focal lactational changes have been seen in postmenopausal women taking tamoxifen for breast cancer as well as in gynecomastia in patients on estrogen therapy for prostatic carcinoma. A variety of other drugs, including phenothiazine, may also cause these changes (62).

Focal lactational hyperplasia is the same phenomenon with micropapillary hyperplasia occasionally associated with nuclear pleomorphism (67). Laminar calcifications can be present in the lumens. Acquaintance with this lesion is necessary as it is often mistaken for in situ carcinoma.

LYMPHATIC NODES AND LYMPHATIC DRAINAGE

Anatomy

Lymphatic drainage in the breast is more complex than in other organs because it is the result of the connection of two systems, the subepithelial plexus of the skin and the lymphatic drainage from the breast parenchyma. It is not clear whether the two lymphatic streams merge or flow separately to specific lymph nodes. In the breast parenchyma, lymphatics lie in the periductal "specialized" stroma (10) and the lymph flows along the ducts to the deep retroareolar plexus (29) and then to the regional lymph nodes. These consist mainly of axillary lymph nodes; up to 97 percent of the lymph from the breast drains into them (77). This is indirectly confirmed by studies on the localization of sentinel lymph nodes which show the tracer at extraaxillary sites in about 3 percent of the cases while in the rest, the tracer is in one to four axillary lymph nodes (69).

Lymphatic drainage to the contralateral breast has not yet been demonstrated. In spite of this, some nonfunctioning lymphatic channels must exist since contralateral metastases occur in routine practice. When the internal mammary trunk is blocked, the direction of lymphatic flow may reverse and tumor emboli from the breast may reach the liver through the rectus muscle lymphatic route (29).

Axillary nodes are anatomically subdivided into apical or subclavicular nodes, which are located medial to the pectoralis muscle; the external mammary nodes, which lie beneath the lateral edge of the pectoralis major; the scapular nodes, which are closely applied to the subcapsular vessels; and the central group, situated in the center of the axilla and containing "the largest and most numerous of the axillary nodes" in Haagensen's words (29). Rotter nodes are one to four nodes located between the pectoralis major and minor muscles (29).

Intramammary lymph nodes are seen in up to 28 percent of cases (18). The internal mammary nodes are very small and measure from 2 to 5 mm in greatest dimension; they are located in the intercostal spaces. They run along the internal mammary lymphatics and are located within 3 cm of the sternal edge (29).

The number of axillary lymph nodes averaged 24 in 195 complete axillary dissections (including level III) (17). The mean was 17 when lymph nodes were reactive or had a maximum of three metastases; 21 was the mean when metastases were present in at least four lymph nodes (22). One patient had 81 axillary nodes.

In clinical practice, axillary lymph nodes are subdivided into three levels (I to III), according to the theoretical path of axillary lymphatic drainage from the breast (77). This subdivision has been challenged by the recent localization of sentinel nodes (i.e., the first nodes to receive lymphatic drainage), which are seen at level II in up to 23 percent of patients (40). Metastases to level III lymph nodes only, without concomitant metastases at levels I and II, are seen in about 2 to 3 percent of cases (52). These findings indicate that our understanding of the anatomy of the lymphatic channels that drain to the axilla is far from complete.

Histology

The axillary nodes, as seen in many other regions of the body, may harbor cells that do not belong strictly to the lymphoid tissue. Nevus cells, similar to those seen in intradermal nevi, were first described by McCarthy et al. (50) in the capsule as well as in the peripheral sinuses, trabeculae, and lymphatic walls and their valves in 6.2 percent of axillary lymph nodes. A much lower incidence (0.33 percent) was reported by Ridolfi et al. (65). Metastatic carcinoma is ruled out by the presence of very regular cells and nevus cells that are negative with antibodies against keratins and positive with S-100 protein antiserum (23). A blue nevus located in the capsule and the trabeculae of an axillary lymph node was first described by Azzopardi et al. (4). This is a rare occurrence documented only in sporadic reports.

Benign epithelial inclusion is a well-established entity in the axillary lymph nodes and is regarded as a distinct histologic pitfall by Holdsworth et al. (32). Normal lobules, apocrine and squamous cysts, papilloma, epithelial hyperplasia, and intraductal papillary carcinoma have been reported at this anatomic site. Fisher et al. (23) concluded that epithelial inclusions are the consequence of an embryonic phenomenon, especially in those cases not preceded by surgery or fine needle aspiration. The use of smooth muscle antibodies, which reveal myoepithelial cells around the epithelial inclusions (23), is very useful in preventing the diagnosis of a metastatic process. Antimyoepithelial cell antibodies are also potentially useful for separating benign epithelial inclusions from "benign" transport of breast epithelium to axillary lymph nodes after a biopsy (13) or needle manipulation (91).

Cytokeratin-positive interstitial reticulum cells were well characterized by Gould et al. (27) with CK8 and CK18 antibodies. These are mostly dendritic cells found in the subcapsular, paracortical, and occasionally, medullary zones. Caution is needed when accepting a metastatic process in a lymph node (and bone marrow) if keratin stains are not coupled and supported by conventional H&E histology. Unfortunately, histology often is bypassed in favor of immunohistochemistry in routine pathology. Some authors have proposed the exclusive use of antikeratin antibody immunohistochemistry to find breast micrometastases in bone marrow (11). This can cause difficulties in interpretation when isolated neoplastic cells have to be distinguished from keratin-positive dendritic cells.

Intramammary Lymph Nodes

Intramammary lymph nodes are routinely found in 0.7 percent of breast samples in a large teaching hospital (33). If mastectomy specimens are systematically sliced into 5-mm–thick sections, the incidence is as high as 28 percent of all the breasts examined (18). Intramammary lymph nodes can be seen in all quadrants and vary from one to nine in different patients; up to three quadrants can be simultaneously involved (18). The size of incidental lymph nodes varies between 3 and 15 mm. They are mainly seen radiologically or macroscopically during tissue processing. Some of these lymph nodes present as palpable masses and are referred for mammography as primary breast tumors (37).

Intramammary lymph nodes can harbor various pathologic processes, such as dermatopathic lymphadenopathy, gold granulomas following chrysotherapy for rheumatoid arthritis, reactive hyperplasia, cat scratch disease (personal case), non-Hodgkin lymphoma, and metastases from breast carcinoma (10 percent of cases) (77). The latter are usually from the same area as the lymph node, indicating that these nodes are located along a lymphatic route. The route needs to be better elucidated since rarely is an intramammary node detected in studies that reveal axillary sentinel lymph nodes. An extraordinary case reported by Lee et al. (40) describes a metastasis to an intramammary lymph node from a carcinoma located in the upper outer quadrant, while the axillary lymph nodes detected with a gamma camera were not involved. When an intramammary lymph node contains a carcinomatous process, primary medullary carcinoma must be excluded before taking into consideration a metastatic process. The presence of the marginal sinus is the only convincing proof of the existence of a lymph node.

DEVELOPMENTAL ABNORMALITIES

Defect in Number or Size

Amastia is the total lack of breast, and atelia is the lack of nipple formation. The two defects appear in combination, but cases are observed of atelia alone and nipples with only amastia. This indicates that the embryologic development of both structures is related, but independent. Amastia is seen when the breast anlage is destroyed in the embryo (77) and is observed (rarely) in families or in diseases with complex genetic defects (67).

Mammary hypoplasia is underdevelopment of the breast and can be unilateral or bilateral. In congenital forms, 90 percent of patients show ipsilateral hypoplasia of the pectoralis muscle (77). Acquired mammary hypoplasia appears in patients who have undergone irradiation of the mammary region in infancy or prepubertal surgical excision of the mammary bud (67).

Excess in Number

Polymastia is a condition in which there are more than two breasts. This is the result of ectopic breast tissue, which can be seen along the milk line, and results from the regression of the milk ridge. Polymastia (with or without atelia) may extend from the axilla to the vulva. The axilla is the most frequent ectopic site in females. Patients may have swelling and premenstrual tenderness at this site.

Several benign mammary processes (including fibroadenoma) as well as malignant conditions (invasive carcinoma) have been reported in *ectopic breast tissue* along the milk line (67,77). Frequently, especially in males, breast tissue is not evident at these ectopic sites, but rather the nipple is (polytelia). An extremely rare condition is the formation of more than one nipple within the same areola (67). Polymastia, more often with atelia, is the result of aberrant breast tissue located outside the milk line (67). Occasional cases of aberrant breast tissue have been described in the shoulder or the dorsum (77,80).

REFERENCES

1. Anbazhagan R, Bartek J, Monaghan P, Gusterson BA. Growth and development of the human infant breast. Am J Anat 1991;192:407-417.
2. Anbazhagan R, Osin PP, Bartkova J, Nathan B, Lane EB, Gusterson BA. The development of epithelial phenotypes in the human fetal and infant breast. J Pathol 1998;184:197-206.
3. Azzopardi JG, Ahmed A, Millis RR. Problems in breast pathology. Major Prob Pathol 1979;11:1-466.
4. Azzopardi JG, Ross CM, Frizzera G. Blue naevi of lymph node capsule. Histopathology 1977;1:451-461.
5. Barbareschi M, Pecciarini L, Cangi MG, et al. p63, a p53 homologue, is a selective nuclear marker of myoepithelial cells of the human breast. Am J Surg Pathol 2001;25:1054-1060.
6. Barwick KW, Kashgarian M, Rosen PP. "Clear-cell" change within duct and lobular epithelium of the human breast. Pathol Annu 1991;17:319-328.
7. Battersby S, Anderson TJ. Histological changes in breast tissue that characterize recent pregnancy. Histopathology 1989;15:415-433.
8. Bocker W, Bier B, Freytag G, et al. An immunohistochemical study of the breast using antibodies to basal and luminal keratins, alpha-smooth muscle actin, vimentin, collagen IV and laminin. Part I: Normal breast and benign proliferative lesions. Virchows Arch A Pathol Anat Histopathol 1992;421:315-322.
9. Bonser GM, Dossett JA, Jull JW. Cystic disease of the human breast. In: Human and experimental breast cancer. London: Pitman Medical Pub. Co. Ltd.; 1961:266-314.
10. Bonser GM, Dossett JA, Jull JW. Duct ectasia in the human breast. In: Human and experimental breast cancer. London: Pitman Medical Pub. Co. Ltd.; 1961:237-265.
11. Braun S, Pantel K, Muller P, et al. Cytokeratin-positive cells in the bone marrow and survival of patients with stage I, II or III breast cancer. N Engl J Med 2000;342:525-533.
12. Bussolati G, Cassoni P, Ghisolfi G, Negro F, Sapino A. Immunolocalization and gene expression of oxytocin receptors in carcinomas and non-neoplastic tissues of the breast. Am J Pathol 1996;148:1895-1903.
13. Carter BA, Jensen RA, Simpson JF, Page DL. Benign transport of breast epithelium into axillary lymph nodes after biopsy. Am J Clin Pathol 2000;113:259-265.
14. Damiani S, Cattani MG, Buonamici L, Eusebi V. Mammary foam cells. Characterization by immunohistochemistry and in situ hybridization. Virchows Arch 1998;432:433-440.
15. Dawson EK. Sweat gland carcinoma of the breast: a morpho-histological study. Edinburgh Med J 1932;39:409-438.
16. Dina R, Eusebi V. Clear cell tumors of the breast. Semin Diagn Pathol 1997;14:175-182.
17. Donegan WL, Spratt JS, eds. Cancer of the breast, 4th ed. Philadelphia: W.B. Saunders; 1995.
18. Egan RL, McSweeney MB. Intramammary lymph nodes. Cancer 1983;51:1838-1842.
19. Eusebi V, Damiani S, Losi L, Millis RR. Apocrine differentiation in breast epithelium. Advances Anat Pathol 1997;4:139-155.
20. Eusebi V, Millis RR, Cattani MG, Bussolati G, Azzopardi JG. Apocrine carcinoma of the breast. Am J Pathol 1986;123:532-541.
21. Eusebi V, Pich A, Macchiorlatti E, Bussolati G. Morpho-functional differentiation in lobular carcinoma of the breast. Histopathology 1977;1:301-314.
22. Fisher B, Slack NH. Number of lymph nodes examined and the prognosis of breast carcinoma. Surg Gynecol Obstet 1970;131:79-88.
23. Fisher CJ, Millis RR. Benign lymph node inclusions mimicking metastatic carcinoma. J Clin Pathol 1994;47:245-247.
24. Foschini MP, Scarpellini F, Gown AM, Eusebi V. Differential expression of myoepithelial markers in salivary, sweat and mammary glands. Int J Surg Pathol 2000;8:29-37.
25. Geschickter CF. Diseases of the breast: diagnosis, pathology, treatment, 2nd ed. Philadelphia: J.B. Lippincott; 1945.
26. Going JJ, Moffat DF. Escaping from flatland: clinical and biological aspects of human mammary duct anatomy in three dimensions. J Pathol 2004;203:538-544.
27. Gould VE, Bloom KJ, Franke WW, Warren WH, Moll R. Increased numbers of cytokeratin-positive interstitial reticulum cells (CIRC) in reactive, inflammatory and neoplastic lymphadenopathies: hyperplasia or induced expression? Virchows Arch 1995;425:617-629.
28. Gram IT, Funkhouser E, Tabar L. The Tabar classification of mammographic parenchymal patterns. Eur J Radiol 1997;24:131-136.
29. Haagensen CD. Diseases of the breast, 3rd ed. Philadelphia: W.B. Saunders; 1986.
30. Hamperl H. The myothelia (myoepithelial cells). Normal state; regressive changes; hypeplasia; tumors. Curr Top Pathol 1970;53:161-220.

31. Hasson J, Pope CH. Mammary infarcts associated with pregnancy presenting as breast tumors. Surgery 1961;49:313-316.

32. Holdsworth PJ, Hopkinson JM, Leveson SH. Benign axillary epithelial lymph node inclusions—a histological pitfall. Histopathology 1988;13:226-228.

33. Jadusingh IH. Intramammary lymph nodes. J Clin Pathol 1992;45:1023-1026.

34. Kanhai RC, Hage JJ, van Diest PJ, Bloemena E, Mulder JW. Short-term and long-term histologic effects of castration and estrogen treatment on breast tissue of 14 male-to-female transsexuals: comparison with two chemically castrated men. Am J Surg Pathol 2000;24:74-80.

35. Kiaer HW, Andersen JA. Focal pregnancy-like changes in the breast. Acta Path Microbiol Scand 1977;85:931-941.

36. Koerner FC, O'Connell JX. Fibroadenoma: morphological observations and a theory of pathogenesis. Pathol Annu 1994;29(Pt. 1):1-19.

37. Kopans DB, Meyer JE, Murphy GF. Benign lymph nodes associated with dermatitis presenting as breast masses. Radiology 1980;137(Pt. 1):15-19.

38. Lakhani SR, Chaggar R, Davies S, et al. Genetic alterations in 'normal' luminal and myoepithelial cells of the breast. J Pathol 1999;189:496-503.

39. Lammie GA, Barnes DM, Millis RR, Gullick WJ. An immunohistochemical study of the presence of c-erbB-2 protein in Paget's disease of the nipple. Histopathology 1989;15:505-514.

40. Lee AH, Ellis IO, Pinder SE, Barbera D, Elston CW. Pathological assessment of sentinel lymph-node biopsies in patients with breast cancer. Virchows Arch 2000;436:97-101.

41. Lendrum AC. On the "pink" epithelium of the cystic breast and the staining of its granules. Pathol Bacteriol 1945;57:267-272.

42. Longacre TA, Bartow SA. A correlative morphologic study of human breast and endometrium in the menstrual cycle. Am J Surg Pathol 1986;10:382-393.

43. Love SM, Gelman RS, Silen W. Sounding board. Fibrocystic "disease" of the breast—a nondisease? N Engl J Med 1982;307:1010-1014.

44. Lundquist K, Kohler S, Rouse RV. Intraepidermal cytokeratin 7 expression is not restricted to Paget cells but is also seen in Toker cells and Merkel cells. Am J Surg Pathol 1999;23:212-219.

45. Marucci G, Betts CM, Golouh R, Peterse JL, Foschini MP, Eusebi V. Toker cells are probably precursors of Paget cell carcinoma: a morphological and ultrastructural description. Virchows Arch 2002;441:117-123.

46. Masson P. Tumeurs-diagnostic histologiques, in diagnostics de laboratoire. In: Ribadeau-Dumas L, Babonneix L, eds. Traitè de Pathologie Médicale et de Thèrapeutique Appliquè. Paris: Maloine et Fils; 1923:277-79.

47. Masson P. Tumeurs humaines. Histologie. diagnostics et techniques. Paris: Librairie Maloine; 1968.

48. Mazoujian G, Pinkus G, Davis S, Haagensen D Jr. Immunoperoxidase localization of a breast gross cystic disease fluid protein. Lab Invest 1982;46:52A-53A.

49. Mazoujian G, Warhol MJ, Haagensen DE. The ultrastructural localization of gross cystic disease fluid protein (GCDFP-15) in breast epithelium. Am J Pathol 1984;116:305-310.

50. McCarthy SW, Palmer AA, Bale PM, Hirst E. Naevus cells in lymph nodes. Pathology 1974;6:351-358.

51. McCarty KS, Nath M. Breast. In: Sternberg SS, ed. Histology for pathologists. Philadelphia: Lippincott-Raven; 1997:71-82.

52. McMasters KM, Giuliano AE, Ross MI, et al. Sentinel lymph-node biopsy for breast cancer—not yet the standard of care. N Engl J Med 1998;339:990-995.

53. Moinfar F, Man Y, Lininger RA, Bodian C, Tavassoli FA. Use of keratin 34betaE12 as an adjunct in the diagnosis of mammary intraepithelial neoplasia-ductal type—benign and malignant intraductal proliferations. Am J Surg Pathol 1999;23:1048-1058.

54. Monaghan P, Perusinghe NP, Cowen P, Gusterson BA. Peripubertal human breast development. Anat Rec 1990;226:501-508.

55. Naccarato AG, Viacava P, Vignati S, et al. Biomorphological events in the development of the human female mammary gland from fetal age to puberty. Virchows Arch 2000;436:431-438.

56. Ohtake T, Abe R, Kimijima I, et al. Intraductal extension of primary invasive breast carcinoma treated by breast-conservative surgery. Computer graphic three-dimensional reconstruction of the mammary duct-lobular system. Cancer 1995;76:32-45.

57. Orr JW, Parish DJ. The nature of the nipple changes in Paget's disease. J Pathol Bacteriol 1962;84:201-206.

58. Ozzello L. Ultrastructure of the human mammary gland. Pathol Annu 1971;6:1-59.

59. Pagani A, Eusebi V, Bussolati G. Detection of PIP-GCDFP-15 gene expression in apocrine epithelium of the breast and salivary glands. Applied Immunohistochemistry: official publication of the Society for Applied Immunohistochemistry 1994;2:29-35.

60. Pagani A, Sapino A, Eusebi V, Bergnolo P, Bussolati G. PIP/GCDFP-15 gene expression and apocrine differentiation in carcinomas of the breast. Virchows Arch 1994;425:459-465.

61. Page DL, Anderson TJ, eds. Diagnostic histopathology of the breast. Edinburgh: Churchill Livingstone; 1987.

62. Pier WJ, Garancis JC, Kuzma JF. Fine structure of tranquilizer-induced changes in rat mammary gland. Am J Pathol 1970;60:119-130.

63. Pier WJ, Garancis JC, Kuzma JF. The ultrastructure of apocrine cells in intracystic papilloma and fibrocystic disease of the breast. Arch Pathol 1970;89:446-452.

64. Purkis PE, Steel JB, Mackenzie IC, Nathrath WB, Leigh IM, Lane EB. Antibody markers of basal cells in complex epithelia. J Cell Sci 1990;97:39-50.

65. Ridolfi RL, Rosen PP, Thaler H. Nevus cell aggregates associated with lymph nodes: estimated frequency and clinical significance. Cancer 1977;39:164-171.

66. Roncaroli F, Lamovec J, Zidar A, Eusebi V. Acinic cell-like carcinoma of the breast. Virchows Arch 1996;429:69-74.

67. Rosen PP. Rosen's breast pathology. Philadelphia: Lippincott-Raven; 1997.

68. Russo J, Gusterson A, Rogers AE, Russo IH, Wellings SR, Van Zwieten MJ. Comparative study of human and rat mammary tumorigenesis. Lab Invest 1990;62:244-278.

69. Sandrucci S, Casalegno PS, Percivale P, Mastrangelo M, Bombardieri E, Bertoglio S. Sentinel lymph node mapping and biopsy for breast cancer: a review of the literature relative to 4791 procedures. Tumori 1999;85:425-434.

70. Sapino A, Papotti M, Sanfilippo B, Gugliotta P, Bussolati G. Tumor types derived from epithelial and myoepithelial cell lines of R3230AC rat mammary carcinoma. Cancer Res 1992;52:1553-1560.

71. Sarnelli R, Orlandi F, Migliori E, Squartini F. Morfologia submicroscopica della mammella: reperti semeiologici, nomenclatura e possibilità di applicazione del metodo. Pathologica 1980;72:139-187.

72. Skorpil F. Uber das vorkommen von sog. hellen zellen (lamproziten) in der milchdruse. Beitr Pathol Anat 1943;108:378-393.

73. Slavin JL, Billson VR, Ostor AG. Nodular breast lesions during pregnancy and lactation. Histopathology 1993;22:481-485.

74. Smith CA, Monaghan P, Neville AM. Basal clear cells of the normal human breast. Virchows Arch A Pathol Anat Histopathol 1984;402:319-329.

75. Stirling JW, Chandler JA. The fine structure of the normal, resting terminal ductal-lobular unit of the female breast. Virchows Arch A Pathol Anat Histopathol 1976;372:205-226.

76. Tavassoli FA. Pathology of the breast. New York: Elsevier Science Pub. Col, Inc.; 1992.

77. Tavassoli FA. Pathology of the breast, 2nd ed. Stamford: Appleton & Lange; 1999.

78. Tavassoli FA, Purcell CA, Bratthauer GL, Man Y. Androgen receptor expression along with loss of bcl-2, ER, and PR expression in benign and malignant apocrine lesions of the breast: implications for therapy. Breast J 1996;2:261-269.

79. Tavassoli FA, Yeh IT. Lactational and clear cell changes of the breast in nonlactating, nonpregnant women. Am J Clin Pathol 1987;87:23-29.

80. Testut L, Jacob O. Trattato di anatomia topografica con applicazioni medico chirurgiche. Torino: Unione Tipografico-Editrice Torinese; 1977.

80a. Toker C. Clear cells of the nipple epidermis. Cancer 1970;25:601-610.

81. Urmacher C. Histology of normal skin. Am J Surg Pathol 1990;14:671-686.

82. Viacava P, Naccarato AG, Bevilacqua G. Apocrine epithelium of the breast: does it result from metaplasia? Virchows Arch 1997;431:205-209.

83. Viacava P, Naccarato AG, Bevilacqua G. Spectrum of GCDFP-15 expression in human fetal and adult normal tissues. Virchows Arch 1998;432:255-260.

84. Vina M, Wells CA. Clear cell metaplasia of the breast: a lesion showing eccrine differentiation. Histopathology 1989;15:85-92.

85. Vogel PM, Georgiade NG, Fetter BF, Vogel S, McCarty KS Jr. The correlation of histologic changes in the human breast with the menstrual cycle. Am J Clin Pathol 1981;104:23-34.

86. Wang NP, Wan BC, Skelly M, Frid MG, Glukhova MA, Gown AM. Antibodies to novel myoepithelium-associated proteins distinguish benign lesions and carcinoma in situ from invasive carcinoma of the breast. Applied Immunohistochem 1997;5:141-151.

87. Wellings SR, Alpers CE. Subgross pathologic features and incidence of radial scars in the breast. Hum Pathol 1984;15:475-479.

88. Wellings SR, Jensen HM. On the origin and progression of ductal carcinoma in the human breast. J Natl Cancer Inst 1973;50:1111-1118.

89. Wellings SR, Wolfe JN. Correlative studies of the histological and radiographic appearance of the breast parenchyma. Radiology 1978;129:299-306.

90. Wetzels RH, Kuijpers HJ, Lane EB, et al. Basal cell-specific and hyperproliferation-related keratins in human breast cancer. Am J Pathol 1991;138:751-763.

91. Youngson BJ, Cranor M, Rosen PP. Epithelial displacement in surgical breast specimens following needling procedures. Am J Surg Pathol 1994;18:896-903.

92. Zeng Z, Melamed J, Symmans PJ, et al. Benign proliferative nipple duct lesions frequently contain CAM 5.2 and anti-cytokeratin 7 immunoreactive cells in the overlying epidermis. Am J Surg Pathol 1999;23:1349-1355.

2 BENIGN LESIONS

FIBROCYSTIC CHANGES

Definition. *Fibrocystic changes* (FCC) of the breast are characterized by a variety of benign mammary alterations: gross and microscopic lobulocentric cysts, apocrine differentiation, and variable stromal fibrosis reflecting exaggerated physiologic phenomena. Close to 40 terms have been used to designate this condition, which is present in a high proportion of surgical and autopsy specimens (18). In 1986, the American Cancer Committee of the College of American Pathologists proposed that FCC is not a disease, but rather an exaggerated physiologic response and that the terminology should be changed to "fibrocystic changes." The Committee also recommended the separation of FCC from the variety of proliferative changes that are associated with an increased risk for the subsequent development of invasive carcinoma (7).

Clinical Features. FCC is seen predominantly in premenopausal women between 20 and 50 years of age; about 75 percent are in their mid 30s or 40s. Many women with FCC are nulliparous, have menstrual abnormalities, and give a history of spontaneous abortions; generally, they have not taken oral contraceptive hormones. While most patients present with multifocal and bilateral disease, FCC may partially or diffusely involve only one breast (23). Premenstrual breast swelling, pain, and tenderness affect 20 percent of women. The cysts of FCC develop from dilatation of the acini and are far from the nipple, in contrast to cysts that develop in duct ectasia and in a subareolar location. Around 20 percent of women complain of axillary tenderness and enlarged lymph nodes.

After menopause, elaboration of estrogen by the ovaries diminishes and FCC involutes. The associated symptomatology disappears within 1 to 2 years of menopause unless the patient is put on estrogen replacement therapy. The peripheral conversion of androstenedione to estrone in adipose tissue serves as a source of estrogen that can sustain FCC in obese women even past the menopause.

The etiology of FCC appears to be an imbalance of estradiol and progesterone levels while elevated estrogen levels alone may induce stromal fibrosis. Women who have taken birth control hormones appear to have a lower risk of developing FCC, possibly due to the progestational component (14). While the cyclic secretions persist, the fibrotic stroma compresses the ductules and causes obstruction, gradual dilatation, and cystic transformation of the ductules. Although a role for methylxanthines in the development of FCC has been suggested by some (11), abstaining from these substances does not seem to affect the course of the alterations (23).

Mammographically, a diffuse density secondary to the extensive stromal fibrosis is characteristic.

Gross Findings. The presence of 1- to 2-mm, clear or blue-domed cysts distributed in fibrofatty tissue is the typical gross appearance of FCC (fig. 2-1); larger cysts (up to 2 cm) also develop. Variable amounts of soft white fibrous tissue replace the normal adipose tissue, and may be several centimeters wide.

Aspiration Cytology. Fine needle aspiration cytology (FNAC) is frequently used for the assessment of cysts, both diagnostically and therapeutically. To qualify as a cyst, more than 1 mL of fluid should be aspirated. Clear fluid indicates low cellularity. The cyst fluid varies from clear to turbid and yellow to brown and bloody. Cytologic assessment of the fluid is performed generally when the aspirated fluid appears blood stained (not considered of traumatic origin), brown, or turbid, and in cases where the cyst does not collapse completely postaspiration or when there remains a residual palpable mass.

Characterized by monolayer sheets of epithelial cells, apocrine cells, foamy histiocytes, naked nuclei, and myoepithelial cells (figs. 2-2, 2-3), aspirates of FCC have generally low

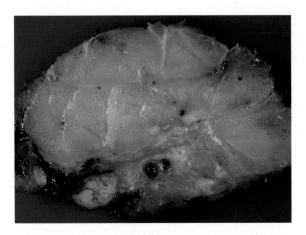

Figure 2-1

FIBROCYSTIC CHANGE

The presence of variably sized cysts (often 1- to 2-mm clear or blue-domed cysts) scattered in a fibroadipose background tissue is typical of fibrocystic changes (FCC).

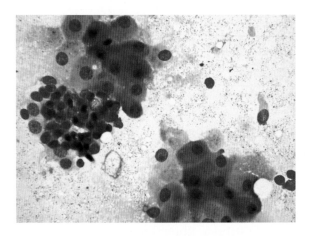

Figure 2-3

FIBROCYSTIC CHANGE

Monolayers of epithelial cells are admixed with myoepithelial cells and clusters of apocrine cells (Diff Quik). (Courtesy of Dr. F. Moinfar, Graz, Austria).

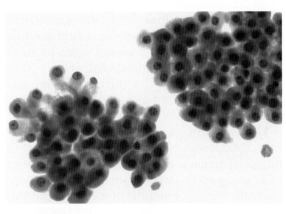

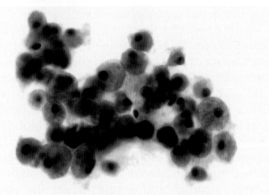

Figure 2-2

FIBROCYSTIC CHANGE

Aspiration cytology shows the clusters of apocrine cells with abundant granular cytoplasm (top) and histiocytes (bottom) that are characteristically present in FCC (Thin Prep; Diff Quik).

to occasionally moderate cellularity and may have fragments of adipose tissue or stroma. The epithelial cells are arranged in cohesive, tight, honeycomb aggregates or in monolayers. The nuclei of the epithelial cells are round to oval, with finely dispersed chromatin and small nucleoli. The apocrine cells have abundant granular cytoplasm, variably sized nuclei, and prominent nucleoli. The cytoplasm stains eosinophilic with the Papanicolaou stain but slate gray-blue with Diff Quik preparations.

Along with the low to moderate cellularity, FCCs feature small clusters of cells with complex configurations, lack or have less than 20 percent cellular dissociation (single epithelial cells), have no or mild nuclear pleomorphism, have myoepithelial cells and/or bipolar naked nuclei, and lack necrosis (16,21). Nonetheless, there are relatively few cytologic features that can separate FCC from proliferative breast disease.

Microscopic Findings. Characteristically, FCC consists of cystically dilated ductules lined by attenuated epithelial and myoepithelial cells; apocrine differentiation of the cyst lining is common (figs. 2-4, 2-5). The type of cyst lining correlates with the composition of the cyst fluid. Many proteins, including gross cystic disease fluid protein (GCDFP)-15, have been isolated from the cyst contents. There is a generalized fibrosclerosis affecting both the intralobular and interlobular stroma. Rupture

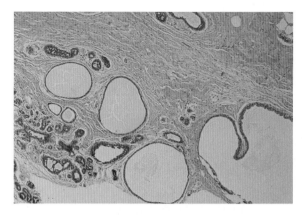

Figure 2-4

FIBROCYSTIC CHANGE

Cysts lined by cells with apocrine differentiation are a common feature of fibrocystic change.

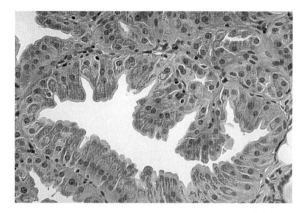

Figure 2-5

FIBROCYSTIC CHANGE

The apocrine cells may develop coarse granularity.

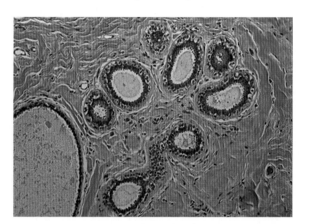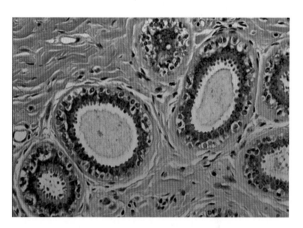

Figure 2-6

BLUNT DUCT ADENOSIS

Left: The ductules are distended in a terminal duct lobular unit (TDLU), with prominence of all components (epithelial, myoepithelial, and stromal cells).

Right: Both the epithelial and myoepithelial cells are prominent.

of the cyst results in an inflammatory infiltrate and eventual stromal fibrosis.

Blunt duct adenosis, in the form of expanded lobules without an increase in the number of acini per lobule, is part of the spectrum of FCC. Blunt duct adenosis is characterized by hypertrophy of the epithelial cells lining distended unit structures (ductules or acini within lobules) that often contain floccular secretory material, with or without microcalcifications (fig. 2-6).

In the absence of epithelial proliferation, FCC does not pose a significant risk for subsequent development of invasive breast carcinoma (7). The 0.89 relative risk for the development of

carcinoma from FCC increases to 1.2 in the presence of a positive family history of breast cancer (6). In the presence of gross cysts, the risk increases from 1.5 in the absence of a family history to 3.0 among women with a positive family history of breast carcinoma (6).

VARIOUS EPITHELIAL ALTERATIONS AND METAPLASIAS

A variety of alterations and metaplastic changes affect the mammary epithelium. The most common among these is *apocrine differentiation.* This most probably represents a variant native cell of the breast that manifests after puberty.

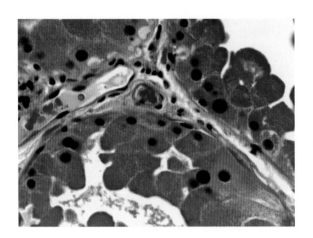

Figure 2-7

ATYPICAL APOCRINE DIFFERENTIATION

There is more than a three-fold increase in nuclear size.

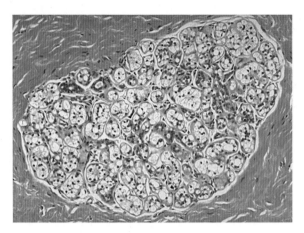

Figure 2-8

CLEAR CELL METAPLASIA

The cells have abundant clear cytoplasm and small eccentric or basal nuclei.

Apocrine Differentiation ("Metaplasia")

Present in 20 to 85 percent of "normal" breasts at autopsy (5,13) and a component of FCC, *apocrine differentiation* (see chapter 1) generally results in a cuboid to columnar configuration, abundant granular eosinophilic cytoplasm, and cytoplasmic protrusions commonly known as "apical snouts." Periodic acid–Schiff (PAS)–positive glycolipid granules are common in the cytoplasm and may form crescents beneath the luminal margin of the cells. Lipofuscin granules and iron pigment are seen less frequently (2,4).

Cystic and hyperplastic apocrine changes have been noted more frequently among breasts harboring cancer (24). It has been suggested that apocrine differentiation may be a precursor to malignant transformation, may reflect a response to the same stimulus that induces carcinoma, or may imply a higher propensity for malignant changes. These hypotheses have not been confirmed.

Apocrine differentiation and hyperplasia are considered atypical (fig. 2-7) when the cells display more than a three-fold nuclear size variation or when the proliferating cells form well-developed epithelial arcades or bridges that cross the lumen (18). Atypia is present in up to 26 percent of adenosis tumors (13) and 70 percent of sclerosing adenosis with apocrine change; atypia in this setting confers a risk of developing cancer of 5.5 times that of control groups for women over 60 years of age (16a).

Apocrine cells in all settings generally fail to express estrogen receptor (ER), progesterone receptor (PR), and bcl-2, while they routinely express androgen receptor (AR) (19). Occasionally, however, they express ER, PR, and AR, implying that ER and PR may have been altered. Microsatellite analysis suggests that a subset of apocrine metaplasias are clonal (15). At the molecular level, apocrine hyperplasias may have some of the same alterations that are present in invasive and in situ apocrine carcinomas (8).

Clear Cell Metaplasia

Clear cell metaplasia is characterized by clearing of the cytoplasm of epithelial cells and may affect a lobule partially or completely (fig. 2-8) (3,20,22); the changes are present in about 1.6 percent of breast biopsies and may also involve areas of adenosis (20). Clear cells may contain PAS-positive granules partly removed by diastase predigestion, but are Alcian blue and mucicarmine negative. This change is termed *hellen Zellen* in the German literature (17).

Immunohistochemically, clear cells are negative for myoepithelial markers (smooth muscle actin, S-100 protein, calponin), but positive for CAM5.2 and E-cadherin. At the ultrastructural level, the cells contain multiple coalescing vacuoles that push the nucleus aside (20). Clear cell change does not appear to be associated with a risk for the subsequent development of clear cell carcinoma.

Lactational Changes in Nonpregnant Women

Lactational changes similar to those occurring in pregnant and lactating women occasionally develop in the lobules of women who are neither pregnant nor lactating; some have never been pregnant (10,20). This change is noted in 3.0 to 3.7 percent of autopsy and surgical specimens (9,20). Microscopically, the changes resemble the Arias-Stella changes in the endometrium (fig. 2-9) (1) or assume a hobnail appearance (20). Lactational changes are believed to reflect either a response to exogenous hormones (e.g., estrogen replacement therapy, tamoxifen) (20,25) or to a variety of nonhormonal drugs (digitalis, dilantin, reserpine) (25).

Squamous Metaplasia

A relatively uncommon form of metaplasia in the breast, the frequency of *squamous metaplasia* has increased substantially with the increasing use of FNAB and core biopsies. Squamous metaplasia is often noted around biopsy sites, areas of infarction, subareolar abscesses, and sometimes in duct ectasia (12).

Mucinous Metaplasia

Mucinous metaplasia is rarely encountered in the breast. When it occurs, it is often noted in a papilloma or an otherwise unaltered lobule (18).

ADENOSIS

Adenosis is a benign proliferation of tubules usually originating in the terminal duct lobular unit. The proliferation may be associated with significant sclerosis, resulting in distortion of the tubules and patterns mimicking invasive carcinoma. Focal or diffuse, it may form a palpable mass.

Adenosis exists in several forms. In its most simple form, adenosis is characterized by an organoid increase in the number of acini within a lobule, most often resulting from hormonal stimulation. When these variably expanded lobules form nodules (up to 2.5 cm), the term *adenosis tumor* is used (fig. 2-10) (37). The tubules are lined by epithelial and myoepithelial cell layers and surrounded by a basement membrane. During gestation, the increase in the number of acini represents physiologic hyperplasia. At least some lesions interpreted as adenosis may reflect incomplete regression of gestational lobular hyperplasia.

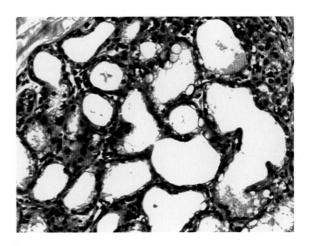

Figure 2-9

LACTATIONAL METAPLASIA

Lactational metaplasia in a postmenopausal woman on antihypertensive medication. Vacuolated secretory transformation is seen in the epithelial cells.

Sclerosing Adenosis

Definition. Among the variants of adenosis, *sclerosing adenosis* (SA) is the most important. Notable for mimicking invasive carcinoma at mammographic (32,36), gross, and microscopic levels, SA is a benign lesion with a lobulated outline that is composed of a compact aggregate of small tubules lined by both epithelial and myoepithelial cells. Most often a microscopic lesion, it may form large, clinically palpable nodules, known as *nodular sclerosing adenosis*.

Clinical Features. SA occurs in a wide age range, but is most frequent in the 3rd and 4th decades. The nodular variant, in particular, may be associated with pain and tenderness. Regression of sclerosing adenosis has been noted among postmenopausal women. The presence of fine, punctate or granular and sometimes clustered microcalcifications (48) on mammography is common, leading to frequent core biopsies (fig. 2-11).

Gross Findings. SA results from a proliferation of numerous tubules parallel to the mammary duct system (44). These tubules grow either into the ducts, remain periductal, or grow both in an intraductal and periductal fashion. About 2 percent of SA lesions grow into perineural spaces (fig. 2-12D) (47). In rare cases, extension into the walls of veins and, exceptionally, arteries has been reported (2).

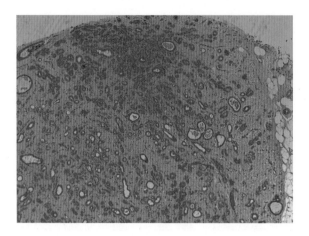
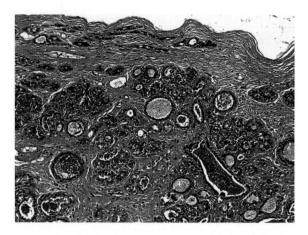

Figure 2-10

ADENOSIS TUMOR

Left: Nodular aggregation of adjacent areas of adenosis can result in clinically palpable nodules.
Right: Compression of surrounding ducts and lobules is often noted at the periphery.

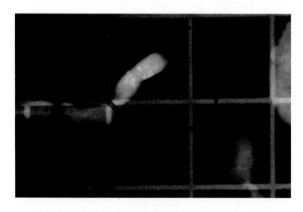

Figure 2-11

SCLEROSING ADENOSIS

Specimen mammography shows coarse microcalcifications in a needle core biopsy.

Microscopic Findings. SA is characterized by a compact aggregation of ductules that are variably compressed and distorted by the background collagen (fig. 2-12). The tubules are lined by both epithelial and myoepithelial cells. The myoepithelial cells are frequently prominent and sometimes hyperplastic. They often assume a spindle cell configuration. SA is the most common lesion with myoepithelial proliferation in a periductal fashion. Occasionally, the myoepithelial cells become myoid and dominant, with minimal epithelial elements left behind; these nodular proliferations are often referred to as *myoid hamartomas* (75a). SA may

be more cellular at its center, or vice versa, with sclerosis dominating at the periphery. As the lesion ages, the sclerosis and myoepithelial cell prominence become more notable. The two cell layers are best appreciated in the peripheral tubules. Microcalcification is noted in 50 percent of cases (fig. 2-13). When florid with diffuse involvement of the breast, various stages of the lesion (cellular to sclerotic) are evident in different areas of the biopsy.

The epithelial cells in SA may undergo a variety of metaplastic and proliferative changes. Apocrine differentiation is the most common alteration; when the entire nodule of SA is replaced by apocrine cells, the term *apocrine adenosis* has been used (fig. 2-14) (16a). Atypia may develop in the apocrine cells (26). A variety of ductal and lobular intraepithelial neoplasias may involve SA (fig. 2-15) (31,38–40). This may be mistaken for invasive carcinoma, particularly in a core biopsy of the lesion. Careful assessment for the identification of a myoepithelial cell layer resolves the problem; sometimes it is necessary to use an immunostain (29) to unmask the myoepithelial cells or the basement membrane surrounding the neoplastic cells.

Differential Diagnosis. The differential diagnosis of SA includes mainly tubular carcinoma and microglandular adenosis (MA). At low magnification, the lobulated distribution of the tubules in SA is in sharp contrast to the haphazard arrangement of the tubules in

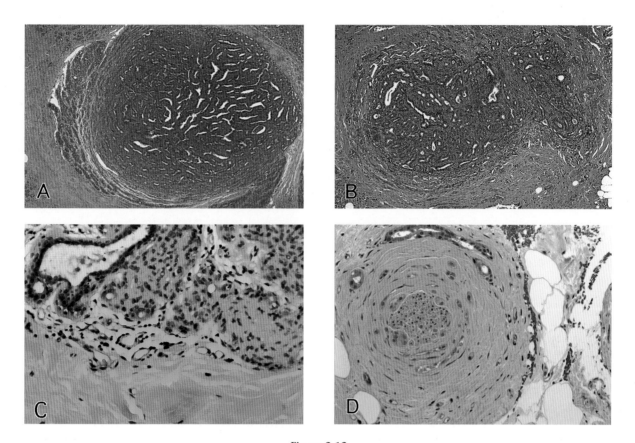

Figure 2-12

SCLEROSING ADENOSIS

A,B: Sclerosing adenosis is characterized by a compact, lobulated aggregate of tubules. Those at the periphery are compressed and streaming.

C: The myoepithelial cells may constitute the dominant proliferating cells. They may proliferate in a periductal fashion, expanding the myoepithelial cell layers around the tubules.

D: Perineural invasion is seen in 2 percent of lesions. The tubules retain the myoepithelial cell layer, distinguishing them from invasive carcinoma.

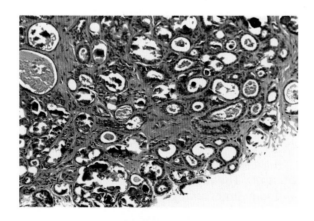

Figure 2-13

SCLEROSING ADENOSIS

Microcalcification is a common feature of sclerosing adenosis.

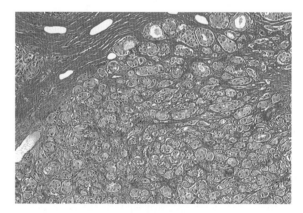

Figure 2-14

APOCRINE ADENOSIS

There is diffuse apocrine metaplasia involving sclerosing adenosis.

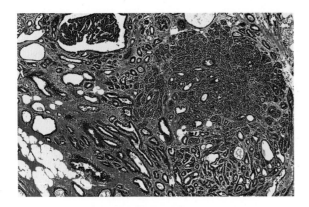

Figure 2-15

LOBULAR INTRAEPITHELIAL NEOPLASIA (LIN) INVOLVING SCLEROSING ADENOSIS

In this setting, LIN may be misdiagnosed as invasive carcinoma.

Table 2-1

MORPHOLOGIC FEATURES OF SCLEROSING ADENOSIS (SA) AND MICROGLANDULAR ADENOSIS (MGA)

Features	SA	MGA
Configuration	Lobulated	Irregular
Lumens	Compressed	Open, containing colloid-like secretory material
Myoepithelial cells	Present	Absent
Basement membrane	Present	Present, multi-layered

tubular carcinoma and the zonal distribution in MA. The tubules of SA are compressed, while those of MA and tubular carcinoma are open. MA tubules contain colloid-like secretory material, while those of tubular carcinoma are generally empty. Particularly when the sample does not include the entire lesion outline (e.g., core biopsy), it is necessary to assess other features at higher magnification. The tubules of SA are lined by two layers, luminal epithelial cells and outer myoepithelial cells, while the tubules of both tubular carcinoma and MA are lined by a single layer of epithelial cells. The tubules of SA are compressed by the surrounding collagen, resulting in a streaming effect. The tubules of tubular carcinoma are separated by abundant reactive fibroblastic stroma, while those of MA are separated by abundant collagen or fibroadipose tissue. The tubules of SA are invested by basement membrane that can be enhanced with a PAS stain; those of tubular carcinoma are devoid of basement membrane, while those of MA are surrounded by a multilayered basement membrane, although the multilayering is not easy to appreciate on light microscopy (Table 2-1).

Prognosis. When present in pure form, SA is associated with a relative risk of 1.7 for the subsequent development of infiltrating carcinoma (33); this risk appears to be unaffected by a positive family history of breast carcinoma (28). A relative risk of 5.5 has been noted for SA with atypical apocrine cells (*atypical apocrine adenosis*) (43). A proportion of apocrine adenosis

has been found to be monoclonal and may be a precancerous lesion (8,15).

Tubular Adenosis

While the tubules in *tubular adenosis* are lined by two cell layers, similar to those of SA, they proliferate as branching tubules (fig. 2-16) that extend into the adipose tissue without forming the lobulated, clustered arrangement typical of SA. They also lack the collagenous stroma of SA (35).

The differential diagnosis includes tubular adenomyoepithelioma, which is characterized by a compact proliferation of tubules and multilayered myoepithelial proliferation in at least some of the tubules, in contrast to the branching dispersed tubules with only a single layer of myoepithelial cells surrounding the epithelial cell layer in tubular adenosis.

Secretory Adenosis

Secretory adenosis is adenosis in its most simple form. It is composed of generally lobulated aggregates of tubules lined by two cell layers, but with intraluminal secretory material (fig. 2-17) (18). The importance of recognizing this lesion is to prevent its misinterpretation as microglandular adenosis.

Adenomyoepithelial Adenosis

Adenomyoepithelial adenosis is a rare variant of adenosis. The myoepithelial cells are prominent and sometimes arranged in two to three layers.

Microglandular Adenosis

A rare lesion, *microglandular adenosis* (MA) is characterized by a proliferation of small, round tubules with open lumens in a background of

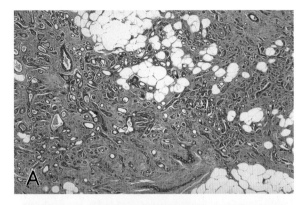

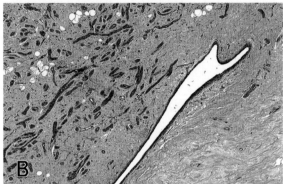

Figure 2-16

TUBULAR ADENOSIS

A, B: A branching tubular pattern and lack of a lobulated, compact distribution distinguish tubular adenosis from sclerosing adenosis.

C: Both epithelial and myoepithelial cells line the tubules that have small to obliterated lumens.

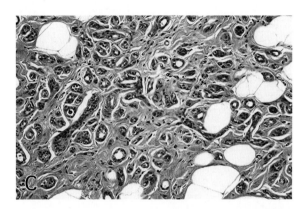

dense collagenous stroma (fig. 2-18) (27,42,46). At least focally, the tubules contain colloid-like secretory material. The tubules are lined by a single layer of cuboidal (fig. 2-19A), often clear cells with a truncated luminal margin; the cell cytoplasm may be eosinophilic and, rarely, displays a coarsely granular change reminiscent of apocrine/acinic differentiation (fig. 2-19B). Atypia is uncommon (fig. 2-19C) but when present, is often noted in cases that also harbor a carcinoma. Myoepithelial cells are absent (30,46). The basement membrane is thick, but may be unrecognizable as it often blends with the surrounding dense collagenous stroma. Electron microscopy reveals the presence of a multilayered basement membrane (46).

Importantly, the epithelial cells of MA are uniformly positive for S-100 protein (fig. 2-20) in addition to a variety of cytokeratin epithelial markers (33a,45). Myoepithelial markers (actin, calponin, p63) confirm the absence of myoepithelial cells.

A variety of types of carcinoma may arise in MA (fig. 2-21). The carcinomas may be of the more common intraepithelial and invasive ductal types or they may assume patterns of spe-

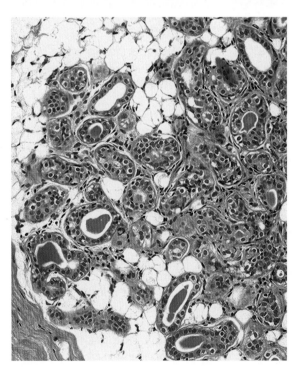

Figure 2-17

SECRETORY ADENOSIS

The tubules contain eosinophilic secretory material.

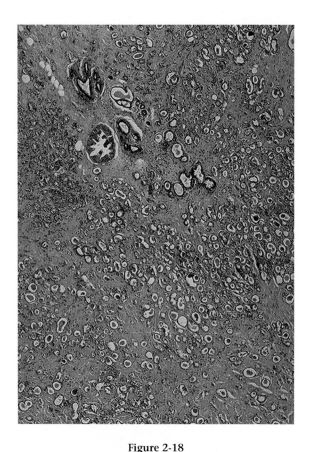

Figure 2-18

MICROGLANDULAR ADENOSIS

A proliferation of rounded tubules with open lumens in a background of dense collagenous stroma.

cial type carcinomas. The majority of carcinomas arising in MA retain immunoreactivity for S-100 protein regardless of their subtype (34,41,45,46); these carcinomas are generally ER and PR negative (33a,41,46). They are also negative for HER2, in the author's experience, qualifying as a triple negative. Rare carcinomas coexisting, but not arising in MA may not be triple negative, however. About one third of MAs harbor an invasive carcinoma. MA with epithelial atypia or pure noninvasive carcinoma is rare; it has been suggested that once atypias develop, progression to an invasive carcinoma occurs rapidly due to the absence of the myoepithelial cell layer, an important barrier to invasion (34,46).

When consideration is given to conservative therapy for carcinomas arising in MA, it is prudent to excise completely the surrounding MA, which often shows atypia, to preclude recurrence from progression of residual MA (41).

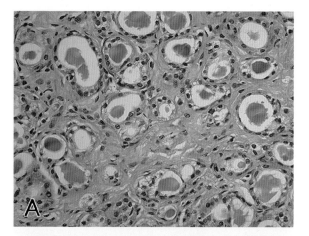

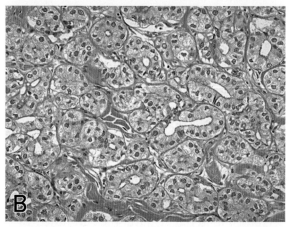

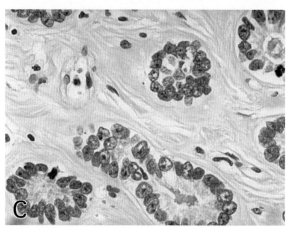

Figure 2-19

MICROGLANDULAR ADENOSIS

A: The tubules are lined by a single layer of epithelial cells; the lumens contain colloid-like material.

B: The epithelial cells rarely undergo granular apocrine-like/acinic metaplasia.

C: Atypical microglandular adenosis consists of epithelial atypia with occasional mitotic figures and often loss of the colloid-like intraluminal secretory material.

ADENOMAS

Tubular Adenoma

Tubular adenoma is a benign lesion composed of a nodular, compact proliferation of small round tubules lined by epithelial and myoepitheial cell layers. Accounting for 0.13 to 1.7 percent of benign breast lesions (56,71), tubular adenomas occur mainly in young women. Although rare prior to menarche and after the menopause (56,64,65), cases have been reported even in elderly women, including an 84-year-old woman (67a). Mammographically, they resemble a fibroadenoma.

Grossly, tubular adenoma is firm and well circumscribed, with a uniform, yellow cut surface. Microscopically, there is a compact proliferation of round to ovoid tubules with open or obliterated lumens lined by epithelial and myoepithelial cells and invested by a circumferential basement membrane (fig. 2-22). The epithelial cells have vesicular nuclei; the myoepithelial cells are less conspicuous. The sparse intervening stroma is vascular and may contain a mild lymphocytic infiltrate. The lumens may contain proteinaceous material, but are often empty. Rarely, elongated profiles of tubules with early branching are evident. Mitotic activity is generally low, but may be abundant if the lesion is removed during the early stages of pregnancy. The lesion may be combined with fibroadenoma

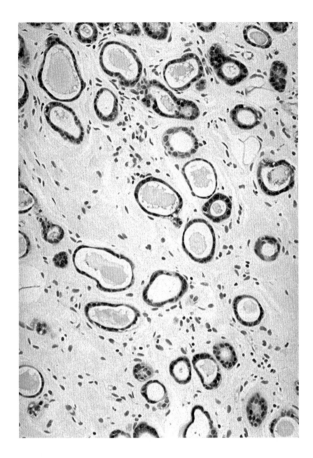

Figure 2-20

MICROGLANDULAR ADENOSIS

The cells lining the tubules are uniformly immunoreactive with S-100 protein.

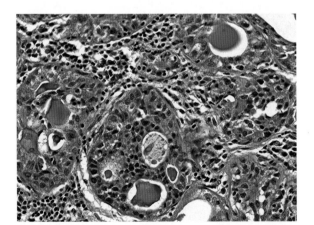
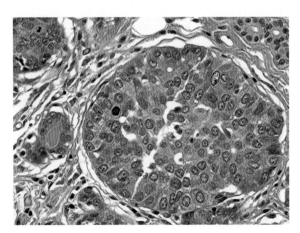

Figure 2-21

MICROGLANDULAR ADENOSIS WITH DUCTAL CARCINOMA IN SITU (DCIS)/DUCTAL INTRAEPITHELIAL NEOPLASIA (DIN)

Left: There is epithelial bridging by uniform atypical cells qualifying as DCIS, grade 1/DIN1.
Right: The tubules, filled and distended by neoplastic cells, coalesce to form larger nodules.

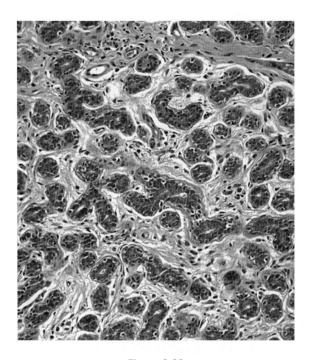

Figure 2-22

TUBULAR ADENOMA

The tubules are lined by epithelial and myoepithelial cells and separated by scant intervening stroma.

(56,71); such a lesion is appropriately designated as *combined tubular and fibroadenoma*.

Lactating Adenoma

Lactating adenoma is the secretory, lactating counterpart of tubular adenoma and is detected during pregnancy and lactation (57,65). The epithelial cells show extensive secretory/lactational activity, with distension of the tubules by variable amounts of secretory material (fig. 2-23). These lesions may sometimes result from coalescence of adjacent gestational hyperplastic lobules.

Apocrine Adenoma

So-called *apocrine adenomas* (52,61,67) most probably represent nodular sclerosing adenosis with apocrine differentiation (see section on sclerosing adenosis).

Pleomorphic Adenoma

Definition. *Pleomorphic adenoma* is a neoplasm characterized by an admixture of abundant myoepithelial cells and ductal type epithelial cells, along with myxoid and cartilaginous tissue.

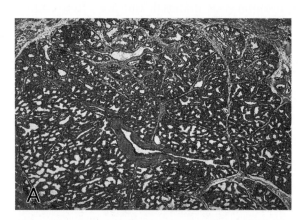

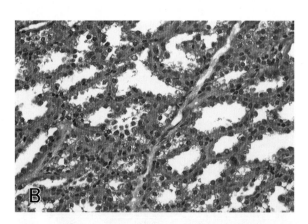

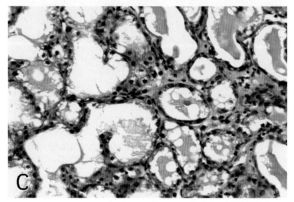

Figure 2-23

LACTATING ADENOMA

A: A compact aggregate of tubules is variably distended by secretory material.

B: Some tubules lack secretory material.

C: Others contain abundant secretory material and are lined by cells resembling the Arias-Stella reaction of the endometrium.

Clinical Features. Although common in the salivary glands, pleomorphic adenoma is rare in the mammary glands. All but 4 of the nearly 70 reported cases have occurred in women (50, 51,53–55,61–63,66,68–70,72). The patients range in age from 19 to 85 years; with a median age in the early 60s. Most patients present with a solitary, palpable, mobile mass that is frequently located in the subareolar region. The duration of symptoms varies from a few weeks to 30 years. Mammographically, the lesions simulate, and are often mistaken for, a carcinoma (68,72).

Gross Findings. The tumor is generally well delineated and firm to hard, with a gritty consistency. The size ranges from 0.6 to 17.0 cm, with a median of 1.7 to 2.0 cm.

Microscopic Findings. Abundant sheaths of spindled or rounded myoepithelial cells proliferate around a few epithelial-lined spaces; myxochondroid and cartilaginous areas, with or without osseous foci, are typically present (fig. 2-24). Core biopsies may be misinterpreted as metaplastic carcinoma. Satellite nodules are common around the main tumor mass. The myoepithelial component is positive with myoepithelial cell markers (smooth muscle actin, muscle-specific actin, calponin, CK34betaE12, p63, vimentin, S-100 protein, and cytokeratin [AE1/AE3/LP34]). Rarely, atypia develops in the form of atypical myoepithelial cells, focally increased mitotic activity, or focally infiltrating margins.

Treatment and Prognosis. Most pleomorphic adenomas behave in a benign fashion, with only a few recurrences reported. Treatment is directed at complete excision; follow-up of lesions with atypical features is recommended.

Pleomorphic adenoma probably represents the benign counterpart of the mixed epithelial and mesenchymal variant of metaplastic carcinoma.

SCLEROSING PAPILLOMA ("DUCTAL ADENOMA")

Sclerosing papilloma is characterized by a compact proliferation of tubules lined by epithelial and myoepithelial cells, sometimes in or around a sclerotic region (49,59). The lesion either protrudes as a polyp into a duct that displays a thick hyalinized wall or it forms a solid mass occluding the duct lumen (fig. 2-25); the latter is also referred to as "*ductal adenoma*." Sclerosing papil-

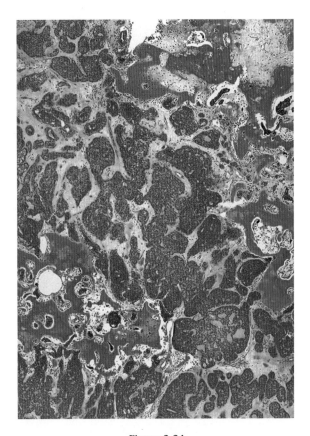

Figure 2-24

PLEOMORPHIC ADENOMA

Sheets of spindled myoepithelial cells proliferate around epithelial-lined spaces and chondroosseous aggregates.

loma occurs most often in women over 40 years of age and presents as a mass or sometimes as nipple discharge. Mammographically, it appears as a density that may mimic a carcinoma.

When there is extensive sclerosis, sclerosing papilloma may mimic a hyalinized fibroadenoma. Additional sections of the lesion often show a few more typical papillary projections or residual lumens at the side or tip of the solid area. Apocrine differentiation and pseudoinvasive areas are common; the latter are easily mistaken for invasive carcinoma, particularly on core biopsies. This benign lesion is not associated with increased risk for the subsequent development of carcinoma and does not recur if adequately excised.

HAMARTOMA

Hamartoma is a nodule composed of a variable aggregation of mature cells and tissues that occur

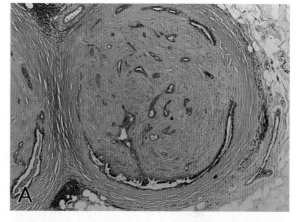

Figure 2-25

SCLEROSING PAPILLOMA/DUCTAL ADENOMA

A: Ducts sometimes appear occluded by a nodular proliferation of often distorted tubules in a fibrosclerotic background. This feature is generally noted in a sclerosing papilloma that is cut in a plane of section that does not show the entire duct lumen and may mimic a fibroadenoma.

B,C: The lesion may appear as a polypoid intraductal nodule formed of a compact proliferation of tubular structures and lined by epithelial and myoepithelial cells.

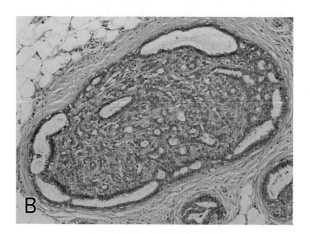

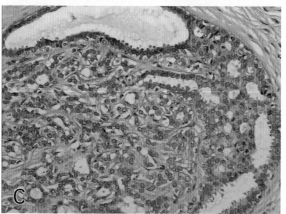

normally in the breast, but is generally devoid of normal mammary structural organization or any of the patterns associated with recognized entities found in the breast.

Described in 1968 by Hogeman and Ostberg (78), hamartoma presents either as a palpable, most often solitary, mass or a discrete mammographically detected lesion in women predominantly in the 5th and 6th decades of life, but over a wide range including young women (77a). Occasionally the mass is tender. The development of hamartomas appears to be independent of hormonal stimulation during pregnancy or lactation. Mammographically, the lesion is a well-delineated electron-dense mass with a rim of radiolucency and generally lacks microcalcifications. While hamartomas usually arise within the breast proper, rare examples have been described in accessory breast tissue in the axilla (76a).

The tumor is round to ovoid, with an average size of 3 cm, but it may exceed 10 cm and weigh over 1 kg (79–81). Hamartomas are softer than

fibroadenomas and are gray-white to yellow on cut surface. An intracystic papillary variant occurs, but is rare (82).

The microscopic appearance depends on the proportion of fibroadipose and glandular elements in the lesion. The lesion consists of a partially to completely encapsulated nodule of sequestered normal to minimally altered mammary tissue (fig. 2-26, left); adipose tissue comprises between 5 and 90 percent of the lesion (74,83). Fibrocystic changes, sclerosing adenosis, and pseudoangiomatous stromal changes may occur (76,77,83). Ductal carcinoma in situ (DCIS)/ductal intraepithelial neoplasia (DIN) 1-3 arising in a hamartoma has been reported (83), as well as rare examples of invasive carcinoma (73). The so-called *myoid hamartoma* (fig. 2-26, right) composed of ducts, lobules, fat, and fibrous and abundant smooth muscle stroma, is believed to reflect nodular sclerosing adenosis with hyperplasia of myoid myoepithelial cells by some and an adenomyoepithelioma by others.

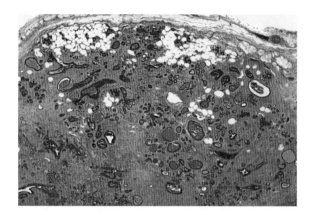
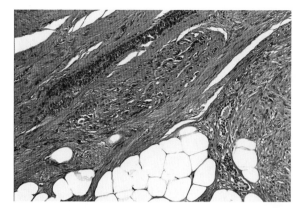

Figure 2-26

HAMARTOMA

Left: An encapsulated nodule of normal to minimally altered mammary tissue lacks the features of any distinct entity.

Right: "Myoid hamartoma" reflects myoid myoepithelial hyperplasia in sclerosing adenosis and is considered an adenomyoepithelioma by others.

Hamartomas are benign, but "recurrences" have been noted in 8 percent of patients (75). These most probably reflect multifocal disease rather than a true recurrence. Because of the encapsulated nature of the nodules, they are easily enucleated.

RADIAL SCAR

Definition. Closely mimicking an invasive carcinoma on imaging, gross inspection, and low-power microscopy, *radial scar* is characterized by ducts and ductules often containing a variety of proliferative epithelial lesions radiating from a central scar region that contains distorted entrapped tubules.

Clinical Features. The term radial scar is a translation of the German "Strahlige Narben" proposed for this lesion by Hamperl in 1975 (92), although the lesion had been described much earlier with a variety of terms. It has been suggested that radial scar starts as a reaction to injury and forms areas of fibrosis and elastosis as it heals (100). Manfrin et al. (95a) have suggested that pure radial scar progresses in some cases to radial scar with atypical epithelial proliferation and ultimately to low-grade carcinoma.

A common lesion found as an incidental microscopic finding in many breast biopsies, the true incidence of radial scar is not known. A frequency of less than 2 percent to over 25 percent has been reported in association with benign lesions or carcinomas (85,86,91,92); in one study,

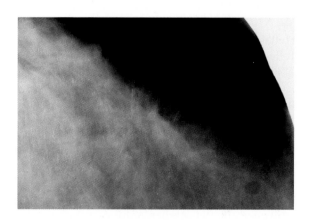

Figure 2-27

RADIAL SCAR

The mammographic appearance of this spiculated lesion simulates an invasive carcinoma.

radial scar was present in 28 percent of women with breast cancer, and was multicentric in 67 percent and bilateral in 43 percent (96). Radial scars are very common even in association with benign breast lesions and their frequency may increase further as a result of needle aspirations and biopsies that result in scar formation.

Mammographically, radial scars appear as stellate lesions simulating invasive carcinoma (fig. 2-27) (88). Microcalcifications are uncommon in radial scar and, when present, suggest superimposed proliferative changes (98).

Gross Findings. The larger lesions are grossly detectable as an irregular, firm area exhibiting a

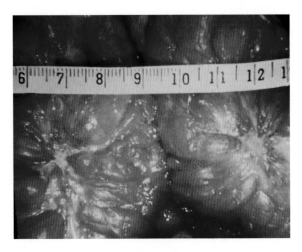

Figure 2-28

RADIAL SCAR

The stellate appearance of radial scar is indistinguishable from an invasive carcinoma.

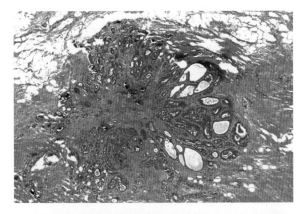

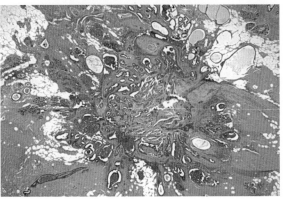

Figure 2-29

RADIAL SCAR

Top, Bottom: Ducts are often radially arranged around a central scar with entrapped tubules. Various patterns of epithelial proliferation may be present in the ducts (bottom).

stellate configuration. Occasional yellow streaks reflect elastosis. This appearance is indistinguishable from an invasive carcinoma (fig. 2-28) (90).

Microscopic Findings. Radial scar displays a mixture of benign changes often inclusive of some form of adenosis. At low magnification, a stellate configuration is typical, with a central area of hyalinization that contains distorted ducts and areas of elastosis (fig. 2-29). Entrapped, distorted ductules in the central scar raise further concern for an invasive carcinoma (fig. 2-30); however, the persistence of myoepithelial cells around the distorted ductules rules out an invasive process. The ducts and ductules at the periphery of the lesion may be dilated, sclerotic, or contain various patterns of epithelial hyperplasia. Intraductal hyperplasia (low-risk DIN) is frequently seen in the peripheral ducts. Other types of intraepithelial neoplasia are rare, but among these, lobular intraepithelial neoplasia (atypical lobular hyperplasia and lobular carcinoma in situ) is the most common (84). Involvement of radial scar by apocrine differentiation makes interpretation of the lesion on cytology preparations difficult (95); the presence of atypia in the metaplastic apocrine cells further aggravates the difficulty whether involving a radial scar or areas of adenosis (97a).

It is appropriate to refer to a radial scar that contains abundant epithelial proliferation in its peripheral ducts, often inclusive of an sclerosing

papilloma, as a *complex sclerosing lesion*, implying that such a lesion is basically a giant radial scar with more abundant epithelial proliferation. Others prefer the designation of *infiltrative epitheliosis* for these complex proliferations. The term infiltrative epitheliosis is more appropriate for lesions that, in addition to the features described, show infiltrative cell clusters emanating from ducts that contain the epithelial proliferation and extend into the periductal stroma, not into the scar region (see Infiltrative Epitheliosis below).

Distinguishing radial scars from invasive carcinomas relies on the recognition of the typical architecture of radial scar as well as the presence of a myoepithelial cell layer and circumferential basement membrane around the tubules of radial scar. Immunohistochemical confirmation may be necessary (see chapter 9). In core biopsies

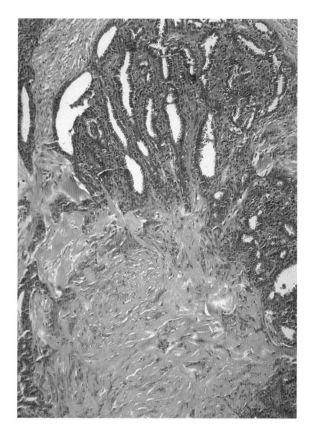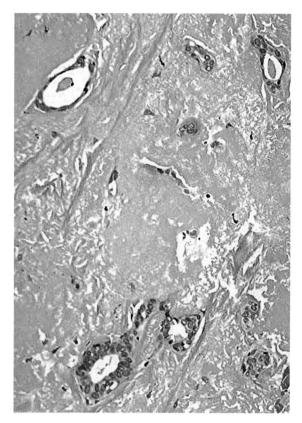

Figure 2-30

RADIAL SCAR

Left: The distorted, entrapped tubules in the scar mimic an invasive carcinoma.
Right: The presence of myoepithelial cells around the tubules confirms their benign nature.

containing sclerotic lesions, it is prudent to exercise caution in diagnosing an invasive carcinoma. Utilization of immunostains in this setting is particularly helpful, but radial scar can be reliably diagnosed on biopsies that show the lesion in its entirety. For large, mammographically detected radial scars, excision is prudent.

Prognosis. It has been suggested that radial scars are preneoplastic and may reflect an early stage of tubular carcinoma (94), or are a marker of increased risk for the subsequent development of invasive carcinoma, particularly the larger lesions that exceed 6 mm and those that occur in women over 50 years of age (93,99). It appears, however, that any increased risk is attributable to the presence of epithelial proliferations within the lesion. It is doubtful that radial scar without significant epithelial proliferation poses a risk for the subsequent development of invasive carcinoma.

INFILTRATIVE EPITHELIOSIS

Infiltrative epitheliosis is a lesion described by Azzopardi (87) and often included within the spectrum of radial scar. The lesion is characterized by a central area of florid intraductal hyperplasia/low-risk DIN surrounded by admixed elastotic tissue and desmoplastic stroma (fig. 2-31). Emanating from and spindling off the duct with epithelial proliferation, strands of polygonal to spindled cells intermingle with elastosis and a desmoplastic stroma. These cells occasionally develop squamous differentiation, a feature corroborated by positivity for CK5/6. Myoepithelial cells are seen as an attenuated rim at the edge of the epithelial strand. Infiltrative epitheliosis is associated with florid intraductal hyperplasia/low-risk DIN in contrast to radial scar, which may have no epithelial proliferation. In addition, as depicted in Table 2-2, the central

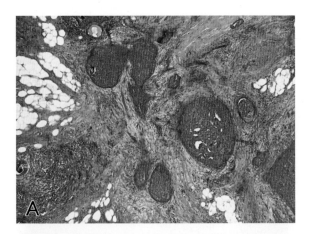

Figure 2-31

INFILTRATIVE EPITHELIOSIS

A: The ducts surrounding the central scar show intraductal hyperplasia (IDH)/low-risk DIN.

B: Small clusters and strands of epithelial and squamoid myoepithelial cells emanate from the periphery of the ducts and into the scar.

C: Both epithelial and myoepithelial cells are present in these clusters and strands.

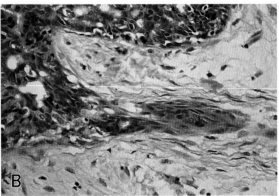

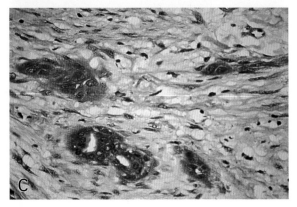

Table 2-2

MORPHOLOGIC FEATURES OF RADIAL SCAR (RS) AND INFILTRATING EPITHELIOSIS (IE)

Features	RS	IE
Sclerotic tissue	yes	little
Elastosis	yes	yes
Desmoplastic stroma	No	yes
Obliterated ducts	yes	no
CD34	yes	little
Tubules	yes	uncommon
Strands/threads	no	yes
CK5/6[a]	No	yes

[a]CK = cytokeratin, in epithelial cells.

core of radial scar differs in many respects from infiltrative epitheliosis.

Infiltrating epitheliosis is also found in the setting of complex sclerosing papilloma and may be seen adjacent to a variety of ducts with florid epithelial prolferation. Since the tubules

of SA also show perineural invasion, it should be noted that "invasion" does not necessarily imply malignancy. Five examples of this lesion have been reported as metaplastic carcinoma (89), although no evidence of malignant behavior was provided.

Complex sclerosing lesions with infiltrating epitheliosis may have a different biologic implication and should be separated from radial scar.

DUCT ECTASIA

Duct ectasia is characterized by dilatation of ducts associated with variable degrees of periductal inflammatory reaction and progressive fibrosis. It usually affects the major ducts and may be bilateral. While the term duct ectasia, proposed by Haagensen (105), is the most widely used designation for this lesion, Azzopardi (101) considers *periductal mastitis* a more appropriate designation. Dixon (103a), however, considers periductal mastitis and duct ectasia two different conditions with different etiologies.

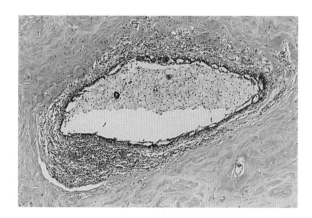 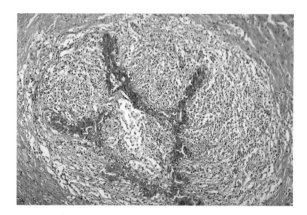

Figure 2-32

DUCT ECTASIA

Left: The duct is distended and surrounded by an inflammatory infiltrate.
Right: In obliterative duct ectasia, the histiocytic infiltrate surrounds and/or fills the duct, obliterating the duct lumen.

Women with duct ectasia range in age from 33 to 79 years, with a mean age of 54 years (105). Patients present with serous, bloody, or pus-like nipple discharge. Nipple retraction, pain, fistula formation, and subareolar abscess are the presenting features in some patients. Sometimes, it presents as a palpable worm-like mass beneath the areola (9). A blue cystic dilatation may be evident at the time of exploration of the ducts. Upon rupture of the dilated ducts, the secretory content escapes into the surrounding stroma, inciting an inflammatory response. Recurrent episodes are heralded by acute pain, tenderness, and edema of the overlying skin; the acute phase generally subsides within 7 to 10 days. With disease progression, the acute inflammation is replaced by progressive fibrosis.

Clinically, duct ectasia may be confused with invasive carcinoma. In 23 to 40 percent of women, duct ectasia remains asymptomatic (101,104).

The pathogenesis and etiology of duct ectasia are unknown. Some believe the inflammation is the original insult to the ducts (103), while others consider the inflammation a reaction to leakage of irritant duct contents (104). The squamous metaplasia that obstructs portions of the duct may result in duct ectasia and formation of fistula tracts (106).

Mammographically, duct ectasia shows a variety of appearances ranging from tubular shadows to focal or extensive calcifications. Spiculated and nodular masses may be present in the obliterative stage (107,108).

The distended ducts are surrounded by an inflammatory infiltrate and may be empty or contain abundant secretory material in the initial stages (fig. 2-32). Foamy histiocytes migrate into the duct lumen, dislodging, lifting, and folding the epithelial layer in patches; the epithelial layer may eventually desquamate. With progression of the disease, the acute inflammatory cells are replaced by a lymphoplasmacytic infiltrate. Eventually, fibrosis develops and may obliterate the duct lumen. When plasma cells dominate and diffusely involve the surrounding stroma, the term *plasma cell mastitis* has been used (109,117).

MASTITIS

Mastitis may have an infectious etiology, reflect a localized manifestation of a systemic disease, or be idiopathic. In some of its various manifestations, it may mimic carcinoma (109).

Acute Mastitis and Abscess

Acute mastitis is seen mainly in the lactating breast, often secondary to a crack in the nipple, and is often localized. Progression to an abscess may result in the formation of a thick wall, with redness and edema of the overlying skin, simulating an inflammatory carcinoma.

Abscesses develop in the breast during lactation as a result of obstruction of the lactiferous ducts. Often sterile in the early phase, the nipple discharge may contain streptococcus, *Staphylococcus aureus* (the most common pathogen), or coagulase-negative *Staphylococcus* (143).

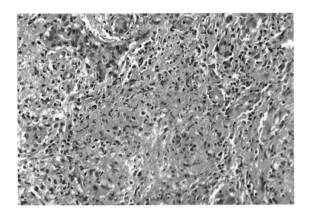

Figure 2-33

GRANULOMATOUS MASTITIS

Noncaseating granulomas are present adjacent to ducts and lobules.

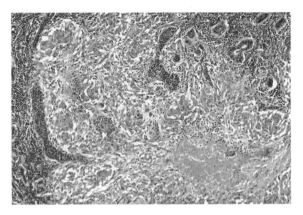

Figure 2-34

TUBERCULOUS MASTITIS

Granulomas with central necrosis disrupt ducts and lobules. (Fig. 15-27 from Tavassoli F. Pathology of the breast, 2nd ed. Stamford, CT: Appleton & Lange/McGraw Hill, 1999:795.)

Subareolar abscesses that are a result of obstruction caused by squamous metaplasia occur in nonlactating women. These abscesses may evolve into sinus tracts and fistulas (121,124). Excision of the abscess and the affected duct and sinus tract is necessary.

Idiopathic Granulomatous Mastitis

Idiopathic granulomatous mastitis (IGM) is diagnosed after the exclusion of specific infections, sarcoidosis, trauma, or foreign material as a cause of the inflammation. The average age of the patient with IGM is 30 years and most women develop the disease within 3 years of pregnancy (119,120). Hyperprolactinemia, associated with a pituitary adenoma or drug induced, has been reported in rare patients (120). Patients present with a palpable mass, and about 25 percent have associated pain or bilateral disease. Rarely, IGM results in nipple inversion and sinus tract formation, mimicking inflammatory carcinoma.

With an average size of 3 cm, there is usually plenty of material for a variety of special studies and cultures. The microscopic hallmark of the lesion is the presence of lobulocentric granulomas distorting the lobules; in advanced disease, the granulomas extend to the surrounding stroma and adjacent duct (fig. 2-33). Giant cells, plasma cells, lymphocytes, neutrophils, and eosinophils, may be present.

The presence of mycobacteria, corynebacteria, and other microorganisms should be ruled out with special stains and microbial cultures (aerobic and anaerobic) (126b,132,141,142). The possibility of sarcoidosis should be excluded by appropriate clinical tests. Chest X ray and measurement of serum angiotensin converting enzyme (ACE) and lysozyme (134) may be necessary.

Tuberculous Mastitis

In most Western countries, mammary tuberculosis is rare and accounts for a fraction of 0.1 percent of treated breast diseases. The majority of cases occur in women in the 3rd and 4th decades of life (110,111,122). Patients present with either a mass or an abscess; the masses are often mistaken for carcinoma (138).

Microscopically, granulomas with caseation necrosis (fig. 2-34) disrupt ducts and lobules (110,111). Acid-fast bacilli are identified in only a small proportion of cases (122). The isolation of *Mycobacterium tuberculosis* is required for the diagnosis of tuberculous mastitis, particularly when acid-fast bacilli are not detected (142) and there is no clinical evidence of pulmonary or extrapulmonary tuberculosis.

Lymphocytic Mastitis

Lymphocytic mastitis is a generally lobulocentric lymphocytic infiltrate associated with a poorly defined area of stromal fibrosis. The stroma contains myofibroblasts, histiocytes, and occasionally, epithelioid cells. Referred to by a variety of designations, including *diabetic mastopathy* (125,126) and *fibrous mastopathy* (130),

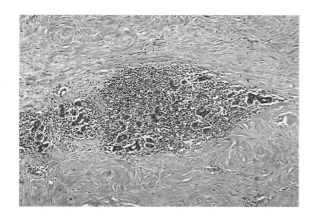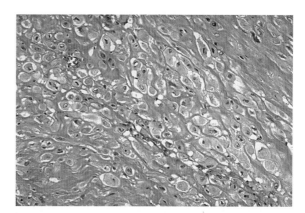

Figure 2-35

LYMPHOCYTIC MASTITIS

Left: A prominent and often lobulocentric lymphocytic infiltrate is typical.
Right: Large epithelioid cells in the stroma are often mistaken for an infiltrating carcinoma.

lymphocytic mastitis is a clinically palpable, usually painless and poorly defined mass that occurs in women 24 to 72 years of age; it may be noted in association with DCIS/DIN (117) and it may also affect the male breast (113,126,127).

Microscopically, a lymphocytic infiltrate is noted in the lobules, and may involve ducts and vascular channels (fig. 2-35, left). The infiltrate consists of a polyclonal B-cell population (125–127,144) and may be quite intense, forming follicular centers in some cases. B-cell lymphoepithelial changes occasionally occur. The lobules may also display sclerosis and involutional type changes. Plasma cells may be admixed with the lymphocytic infiltrate. In some cases, large epithelioid cells are noted in the stroma, either singly or in clusters (fig. 2-35, right); these cells simulate an invasive carcinoma. The epithelioid cells fail to show immunoreactivity with epithelial markers, but contain actin-positive intracytoplasmic fibrils (113).

The microscopic changes are nonspecific for the most part, but an association with thyroiditis, arthropathy, and diabetes mellitus has raised the possibility of autoimmune disease (113,127,139). The patients with the most florid lymphocytic mastitis in one study subsequently developed Hashimoto thyroiditis (127). Among those women whose human leukocyte antigen (HLA) status was determined, some were positive for HLA-DR3, -DR4 (associated with type 1 diabetes mellitus), and -DR5 (associated with Hashimoto thyroiditis), either singly or in combination (127,139). Lymphocytic mastitis may coexist with a variety of breast carcinomas (116) and lymphomas (112,135), but does not appear to be associated with an increased risk for lymphoma (144).

Fungal, Parasitic, and Other Infections

It is uncommon to encounter mycotic and parasitic infections of the breast. Among these, actinomycosis (*Actinomyces bovis*) may develop through the nipple, leading to formation of a sinus tract or a mass simulating carcinoma (126a, 141); histoplasmosis (*Histoplasma capsulatum*) presents as a solitary mass consisting of necrotizing granulomas, often in young women of reproductive age (134,137); blastomycosis (*Blastomyces dermatididis*) may present as a periareolar abscess containing the organism (137); and cryptococcosis may be mistaken for mucinous carcinoma (141).

Among parasitic infections, mammary filariasis (*Filaria bancroftii*) occurs during the chronic phase of the infection in endemic areas (115,129). The breast involvement is in the form of one or more nodules that may be fixed to the overlying skin. Associated microfilarial lymphadenitis contributes to a clinical picture mimicking carcinoma. The firm gray-white nodules occasionally contain grossly visible white worms. An adult worm surrounded by a granulomatous inflammation is the typical microscopic picture.

Dirofilaria tenuis (common hosts are cats and dogs) and *D. repens* (main host is raccoon)

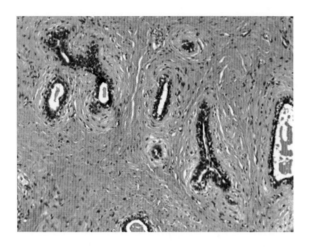

Figure 2-36

JUVENILE HYPERTROPHY

Normal ducts and lobules proliferate in a dense, fibrocollagenous stroma.

infections also occur in the breast (114,123). A few examples of cat-scratch disease have presented in the breast as granulomatous lesions within intramammary or axillary lymph nodes (128); the necrotic center of the granulomas contains filamentous, branching, gram-negative, Warthin-Starry–positive bacilli.

MISCELLANEOUS LESIONS

Sarcoidosis

Among the reported cases of mammary *sarcoidosis*, few have both clinical and histologic documentation (118,136). On the rare occasions when the breast is involved, there is generally clinical evidence of the disease elsewhere. An association with silicone implants and paraffinomas has been noted (131,145); this association is probably coincidental.

The clinical presentation of sarcoidosis is in the form of either solitary, multiple, or bilateral mammary nodules. Microscopically, typically noncaseating granulomas with multinucleated giant cells are dispersed in the lobules and interlobular stroma; asteroid bodies are occasionally present in the giant cells.

In the absence of clinical evidence of sarcoidosis, and absence of serum lysozyme (133) and angiotensin-converting enzyme (140), other granulomatous lesions should be considered and systematically excluded. Occasionally,

noncaseating granulomas occur in association with duct ectasia.

Juvenile Hypertrophy

Juvenile hypertrophy is the excessive enlargement of one or both breasts by the proliferation of normal ductal/lobular and stromal elements during adolescence. The proliferation may assume a gynecomastoid pattern.

Most often seen in young girls between 11 and 14 years of age, the onset of the hypertrophy often coincides with the first menstruation and continues for up to 6 months (146–153). Rarely, the proliferation continues for longer, requiring one or more reduction mammoplasties (146).

There is often no distinct gross lesion evident, but simply very firm mammary tissue with a paucity of adipose tissue elements. Microscopically, there is proliferation of ducts and lobules, similar to normal structures in a distinctly more fibrocollagenous background (fig. 2-36). Sometimes, proliferating ducts are surrounded by dense concentric stromal proliferations similar to the pattern of gynecomastia. Prominent pseudoangiomatous stromal hyperplasia (PASH) is present in some cases. While both the stroma and the duct system are involved in the proliferation, the stromal/epithelial relationship characteristic of fibroadenoma is not evident. In some cases, particularly those associated with PASH, the epithelial cells in the hypertrophic area are conspicuously larger than those in the surrounding normal breast tissue (152).

An increased sensitivity of mammary tissue to normal hormonal surges (particularly estrogens) during puberty may be the major cause of the hypertrophy (151). Tamoxifen may be a useful adjunct in the management of this lesion, particularly for stabilizing the results of reduction mammoplasty (146).

Collagenous and Mucinous Spheruloses

Collagenous and *mucinous spheruloses* are two types of benign intraductal proliferation of epithelial and myoepithelial cells and are comparable to low-risk DIN (intraductal hyperplasia). The myoepithelial cells surround spaces filled by 20- to 100-µm spherules of collagen or mucoid material (fig. 2-37) (154,161). The collagenous spherules are composed of basement membrane-like material; the mucinous type may contain

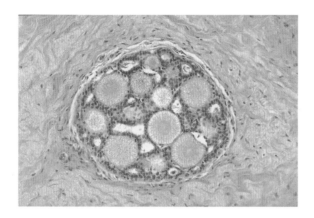

Figure 2-37

COLLAGENOUS SPHERULOSIS

Characterized by a cribriform architecture mimicking DCIS/DIN1, the spaces are filled by collagenous material and surrounded by myoepithelial cells.

mucicarmine-positive secretory material. Mucinous spherulosis sometimes appears as a thin membrane retracting from the space-lining cells. Both types of spherules may be present simultaneously and may show foci of calcification.

Spherulosis of either type is generally an incidental finding in 1 to 2 percent of breast biopsies, but appears to be preferentially located at the periphery of large complex papillary and sclerosing lesions. Occasionally, intraepithelial neoplasia (lobular and ductal in situ carcinoma) extends into the ducts harboring collagenous spherulosis (162).

Microcalcifications/Liesegang Rings/Inclusions/Foreign Bodies

Microcalcifications in the breast are an important contributor to early detection of carcinoma by mammography. Approximately 40 to 50 percent of mammary carcinomas have mammographically detectable microcalcifications (160), and at least half of these are intraepithelial lesions (155). Microcalcifications are not exclusive to carcinomas, however, as nearly 50 percent of sclerosing adenosis cases also have microcalcifications (see figs. 2-11, 2-13); these are widely scattered, more uniform in size, and smoother than those of carcinoma. Hyalinized fibroadenomas also often show coarse, chunky calcifications (fig. 2-38); microcalcifications in benign ductules may be quite prominent as well (fig. 2-38C). Calcifications associated with carcinoma have been

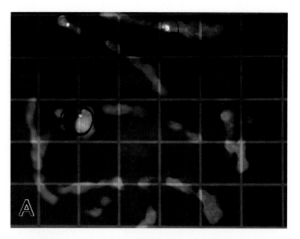

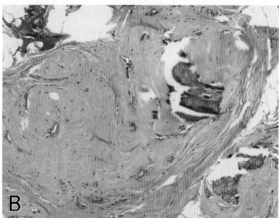

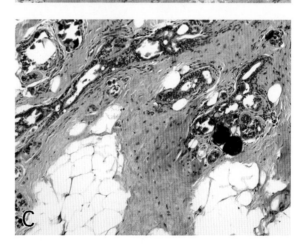

Figure 2-38

MICROCALCIFICATIONS IN HYALINIZED FIBROADENOMATOUS NODULES

A: The calcifications appear coarse and chunky.

B: Microscopically, these are large fragments of calcium phosphate in a hyalinized nodule.

C: Microcalcifications in benign ductules, in contrast, are small and either within the duct lumens or in the surrounding stroma.

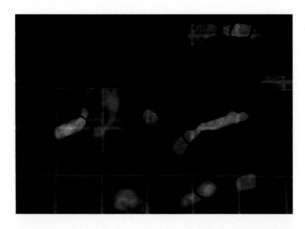
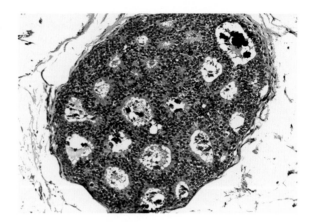

Figure 2-39

MICROCALCIFICATIONS IN DUCTAL CARCINOMA IN SITU

These microcalcifications appear as fine, irregularly shaped granules on specimen radiograms (left) and as small granules of calcium phosphate within the secondary lumens (right). There is significant variation in the appearance of the microcalcifications both on mammographic and histologic evaluation.

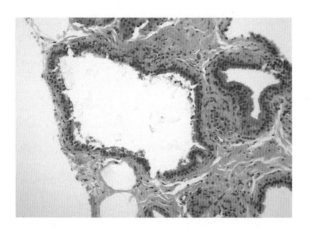
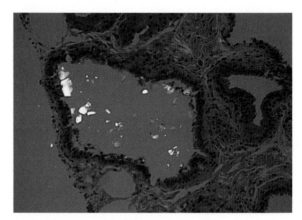

Figure 2-40

CALCIUM OXALATE CRYSTALS

Left: Calcium oxalate crystals have geometric shapes, are colorless, and can be overlooked easily; they are most often found in apocrine-lined dilated ducts or cysts.

Right: Assessment with polarized light shows birefringent material.

described as being irregular and fine rather than coarse in appearance (fig. 2-39) (156).

The calcifications also vary in their chemical composition. The laminated psammoma body type calcification represents calcium phosphate in the form of hydroxyapatite and occurs most often in noninvasive carcinomas (158). The calcification associated with necrosis is also often composed of calcium phosphate. Calcium oxalate, mainly in the form of weddelite, is another mammographically detectible microcalcification that appears as amorphous, poorly stained, cloud-shaped intraluminal birefringent bodies (157); calcium oxalate is generally associated with benign lesions (fig. 2-40) (168).

Intraluminal crystalloids appear most often in areas of atypical intraductal hyperplasia and low-grade DCIS/DIN1. They vary in size, shape, and number (fig. 2-41) (163). They lack periodicity on ultrastructural analysis, are not birefringent, have no mineral content, but contain sulfur (163). These crystals probably represent an unusual condensation of proteinaceous material.

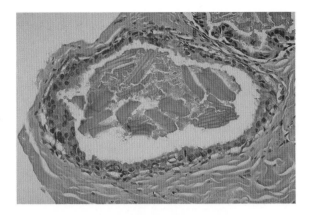

Figure 2-41

INTRALUMINAL CRYSTALLOIDS

Often present as multiple crystalloids of variable size and shape, the intraluminal crystalloids are not birefringent and are present in ducts that show apocrine differentiation or may have a variety of DIN patterns.

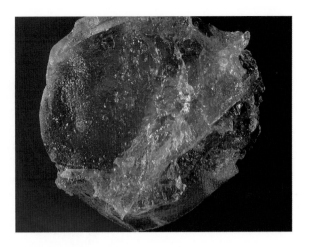

Figure 2-42

RUPTURED SILICONE IMPLANT

The implant was removed because of rupture and leakage of silicone.

An unusual combination of calcium with iron (hemosiderin), silicone, and sulfur forms laminated inclusions known as *Liesegang rings* which are often mistaken for parasites (166,167). These clearly lack the internal organs of parasites and are often observed in areas of fat necrosis in the breast.

Intranuclear helioid bodies are inclusions that can be seen in a variety of DIN lesions (166). With the hematoxylin and eosin (H&E) stain, they appear as rounded, eosinophilic bodies within the nucleus. At the ultrastructural level, these are single, membrane-bound, rounded structures containing a laminated or homogeneously electron-dense core with a corona of radiating filaments resembling the sun's rays (Greek helios, meaning sun). They probably reflect intranuclear sequestration of cytoplasmic secretory material.

The major foreign body of concern in the breast is the *silicone* used in augmentation mammoplasty. While several decades ago one occasionally encountered paraffinomas, these are rare and basically nonexistent today (159). Silicone implants consist of the elastomere dispersion that forms the outer shell and the compliant gel within the shell; these can rupture (fig. 2-42). It is the leakage of the gel that can lead to the development of a variety of complications and a granulomatous reaction characterized by rounded spaces of highly variable

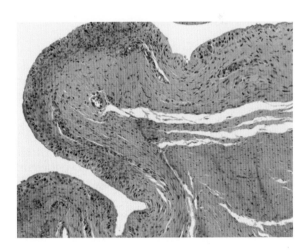

Figure 2-43

SYNOVIAL METAPLASIA

Synovial-like metaplasia covers the fibrous capsule around an implant.

size with numerous clusters of small vacuoles surrounded by giant cells (165). The complications associated with silicone breast implants occur earlier among patients undergoing reconstruction than in patients with cosmetic augmentation (164). Angulated polyurethane crystals and synovial-like metaplasia (fig. 2-43) are rarely found in the fibrous capsule around the implant (165). Axillary and intramammary lymph nodes that drain the breast may show *silicone lymphadenitis* (fig. 2-44).

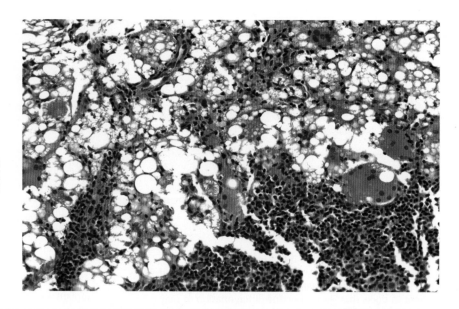

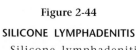

Figure 2-44

SILICONE LYMPHADENITIS

Silicone lymphadenitis with numerous vacuolated histiocytes disrupting the nodal architecture.

REFERENCES

Fibrocystic Changes and Metaplasias

1. Arias-Stella J. A topographic study of uterine epithelial atypia associated with chorionic tissue; demonstration of alteration in the endocervix. Cancer 1959;12:782-790.
2. Azzopardi JG. Problems in breast pathology. Philadelphia: Saunders; 1979:57-72.
3. Barwick KW, Kashgarian M, Rosen PP. "Clear-cell" change within duct and lobular epithelium of the human breast. Pathol Annu 1982;17(Pt. 1):319-328.
4. Bonser GM, Dossett JA, Jull JW. Human and experimental breast cancer. London: Pitman; 1961.
5. Cowan DF, Bherbert TA. Involution of the breast in women aged 50 to 104 years: a histopathologic study of 102 cases. Surg Pathol 1989;2:323-333.
6. Dupont WD, Page DL. Risk factors for breast cancer in women with proliferative disease. N Engl J Med 1985;312:146-151.
7. Is "fibrocystic disease" of the breast precancerous? Arch Pathol Lab Med 1986;110:171-173.
8. Jones C, Damiani S, Wells D, Chaggar R, Lakhani SR, Eusebi V. Molecular cytogenetic comparison of apocrine hyperplasia and apocrine carcinoma of the breast. Am J Pathol 2001;158:207-214.
9. Kiaer HW, Andersen JA. Focal pregnancy-like changes in the breast. Acta Pathol Microbiol Scand [A] 1977;85:931-941.
10. Mills SE, Fechner RE. Focal pregnancy-like change of the breast. Diagn Gynecol Obstet 1980;2:67-70.
11. Minton JP, Foecking MK, Webster DJ, Matthews RH. Response of fibrocystic disease to caffeine withdrawal and correlation of cyclic nucleotides with breast disease. Am J Obstet Gynecol 1979;135:157-158.
12. Ng WK, Kong JH. Significance of squamous cells in fine needle aspiration cytology of the breast. A review of cases in a seven-year period. Acta Cytol 2003;47:27-35.
13. Nielsen M, Thomsen JL, Primdahl S, Dyreborg U, Andersen JA. Breast cancer and atypia among middle-aged women: a study of 110 medicolegal autopsies. Br J Cancer 1987;56:814-819.
14. Pastides H, Kelsey JL, LiVolsi VA, Holford TR, Fischer DB, Goldenberg IS. Oral contraceptive use and fibrocystic breast disease with special reference to its histopathology. J Natl Cancer Inst 1983;71:5-9.
15. Selim AG, Ryan A, El-Ayat G, Wells CA. Loss of heterozygosity and allelic imbalance in apocrine metaplasia of the breast: microdissection microsatellite analysis. J Pathol 2002;196:287-291.
16. Sidawy MK, Tabbara SO, Bryan JA, Poprocky LA, Frost AR. The spectrum of cytologic features in nonproliferative breast lesions. Cancer 2001;93:140-145.
16a. Simpson JF, Page DL, Dupont WD. Apocrine adenosis. A mimic of mammary carcinoma. Surg Pathol 1990;3:289-299.
17. Skorpil F. Uber das Vorkommen von sog. hellen Zellen (Lamprocyten) in der Milchdruse. Beitr Pathol Anat 1943;108:378-393.
18. Tavassoli FA. Pathology of the breast, 2nd ed. Stamford, CT: Appleton & Lange/McGraw Hill; 1999:115-204.

19. Tavassoli FA, Purcell CA, Bratthauer GL et al. Androgen receptor expression along with loss of bcl-2, ER and PR expression in benign and malignant apocrine lesions of the breast. Implications for therapy. Breast J 1996;4:261-269.
20. Tavassoli FA, Yeh IT. Lactational and clear cell changes of the breast in nonlactating, nonpregnant women. Am J Clin Pathol 1987;87:23-29.
21. The uniform approach to breast fine-needle aspiration biopsy. National Cancer Institute Fine-Needle Aspiration of Breast Workshop Subcommittees. Diagn Cytopathol 1997;16:295-311.
22. Vina M, Wells CA. Clear cell metaplasia of the breast: a lesion showing eccrine differentiation. Histopathology 1989;15:85-92.
23. Vorherr H. Fibrocystic breast disease: pathophysiology, pathomorphology, clinical picture and management. Am J Obstet Gynecol 1986;154:161-179.
24. Wellings SR, Alpers CE. Apocrine cystic metaplasia: subgross pathology and prevalence in cancer-associated versus random autopsy breasts. Hum Pathol 1987;18:381-386.
25. Wellings SR, Jensen HM, Marcum RG. An atlas of subgross pathology of the human breast with special reference to possible precancerous lesions. J Natl Cancer Inst 1975;55:231-273.

Adenosis

26. Carter DJ, Rosen PP. Atypical apocrine metaplasia in sclerosing lesions of the breast: a study of 51 patients. Mod Pathol 1991;4:1-5.
27. Clement PB, Azzopardi JG. Microglandular adenosis of the breast—a lesion simulating tubular carcinoma. Histopathology 1983;7:169-180.
28. Eusebi V, Azzopardi JG. Vascular infiltration in benign breast disease. J Pathol 1976;118:9-16.
29. Eusebi V, Collina G, Bussolati G. Carcinoma in situ in sclerosing adenosis of the breast: an immunohistochemical study. Semin Diagn Pathol 1989;6:146-152.
30. Eusebi V, Foschini MP, Betts CM, et al. Microglandular adenosis, apocrine adenosis, and tubular carcinoma of the breast. An immunohistochemical comparison. Am J Surg Pathol 1993;17:99-109.
31. Fechner RE. Lobular carcinoma in situ in sclerosing adenosis. A potential source of confusion with invasive carcinoma. Am J Surg Pathol 1981;5:233-239.
32. Gunhan-Bilgen I, Memis A, Ustun EE, Ozdemir N, Erhan Y. Sclerosing adenosis: mammographic and ultrasonographic findings with clinical and histopathological correlation. Eur J Radiol 2002;44:232-238.
33. Jensen RA, Page DL, Dupont DW, Rogers LW. Invasive breast cancer risk in women with sclerosing adenosis. Cancer 1989;64:1977-1983.
33a. Khalifeh IM, Albarracin C, Diaz LK, et al. Clinical, histopathologic and immunohistochemical features of microglandular adenosis and transition into in situ and invasive carcinoma. Am J Surg Pathol 2008;32:544-552.
34. Koenig C, Dadmanesh F, Bratthauer GL, Tavassoli FA. Carcinoma arising in microglandular adenosis: an immunohistochemical analysis of 20 intraepithelial and invasive neoplasms. Int J Surg Pathol 2000;8:303-315.
35. Lee KC, Chan JK, Gwi E. Tubular adenosis of the breast. A distinctive benign lesion mimicking invasive carcinoma. Am J Surg Pathol 1996;20:46-54.
36. MacErlean DP, Nathan BE. Calcification in sclerosing adenosis simulating malignant breast calcification. Br J Radiol 1972;45:944-945.
37. Nielsen BB. Adenosis tumour of the breast—a clinicopathological investigation of 27 cases. Histopathology 1987;11:1259-1275.
38. Oberman HA, Markey BA. Noninvasive carcinoma of the breast presenting in adenosis. Mod Pathol 1991;4:31-45.
39. Popper HH, Gallagher JV, Ralph G, Lenard PD, Tavassoli FA. Breast carcinoma arising in microglandular adenosis: a tumor expressing S-100 immunoreactivity. Report of five cases. Breast J 1996;2:154-9.
40. Rasbridge SA, Millis RR. Carcinoma in situ involving sclerosing adenosis: a mimic of invasive breast carcinoma. Histopathology 1995;27:269-273.
41. Resetkova E, Flanders DJ, Rosen PP. Ten-year follow-up of mammary carcinoma arising in microglandular adenosis treated with breast conservation. Arch Pathol Lab Med 2003;127:77-80.
42. Rosen PP. Microglandular adenosis: a benign lesion simulating invasive mammary carcinoma. Am J Surg Pathol 1983;7:137-144.
43. Seidman JD, Ashton M, Lefkowitz M. Atypical apocrine adenosis of the breast: a clinicopathologic study of 37 patients with 8.7-year follow-up. Cancer 1996;77:2529-2537.
44. Tanaka Y, Oota K. A stereomicroscopic study of the mastopathic human breast. 1. Three-dimensional structures of abnormal duct evolution and their histologic entity. Virchows Arch A Pathol Anat Histopathol 1970;349:195-214.
45. Tavassoli FA, Bratthauer GL. Immunohistochemical profile and differential diagnosis of microglandular adenosis. Mod Pathol 1993;6:318-322.
46. Tavassoli FA, Norris HJ. Microglandular adenosis of the breast. A clinicopathologic study of 11 cases with ultrastructural observations. Am J Surg Pathol 1983;7:731-784.
47. Taylor HB, Norris HJ. Epithelial invasion of nerves in benign diseases of the breast. Cancer 1967;20:2245-2249.
48. Tse GM, Tan PH, Pang AL, Tang AP, Cheung HS. Calcification in breast lesions: pathologists' perspective. J Clin Pathol 2008;61:145-151.

Adenomas

49. Azzopardi JG, Salm R. Ductal adenoma of the breast: a lesion which can mimic carcinoma. J Pathol 1984;144:15-23.
50. Ballance WA, Ro JY, el Naggar AK, Grignon DJ, Ayala AG, Romsdahl MG. Pleomorphic adenoma (benign mixed tumor) of the breast. An immunohistochemical, flow cytometric, and ultrastructural study and review of the literature. Am J Clin Pathol 1990;93:795-801.
51. Chen KT. Pleomorphic adenoma of the breast. Am J Clin Pathol 1990;93:792-794.
52. Costa A. [A little known variant of pure adenoma of the breast: pure apocrine cell adenoma (with a classification of breast adenomas)]. Arch De Vecchi Anat Patol 1974;60:393-401. [Italian.]
53. Cuadros CL, Ryan SS, Miller RE. Benign mixed tumor (pleomorphic adenoma) of the breast: ultrastructural study and review of the literature. J Surg Oncol 1987;36:58-63.
54. Diaz NM, McDivitt RW, Wick MR. Pleomorphic adenoma of the breast: a clinicopathologic and immunohistochemical study of 10 cases. Hum Pathol 1991;22:1206-1214.
55. Fiks T. Pleomorphic adenoma (benign "mixed" tumor) of the human female breast. Case report. Pol J Pathol 1999;50:297-299.
56. Hertel BF, Zaloudek C, Kempson RL. Breast adenomas. Cancer 1976;37:2891-2905.
57. James K, Bridger J, Anthony PP. Breast tumour of pregnancy ('lactating' adenoma). J Pathol 1988;156:37-44.
58. Kanter MH, Sedeghi M. Pleomorphic adenoma of the breast: cytology of fine-needle aspiration and its differential diagnosis. Diagn Cytopathol 1993;9:555-558.
59. Lammie GA, Millis RR. Ductal adenoma of the breast—a review of fifteen cases. Hum Pathol 1989;20:903-908.
60. Lecene PP. Les tumeurs mixtes du sein. Rev Chir (Paris) 1906;33:434-449.
61. Lui M, Dahlstrom JE, Bell S, James DT. Apocrine adenoma of the breast: diagnosis on large core needle biopsy. Pathology 2001;33:149-152.
62. Moran CA, Suster S, Carter D. Benign mixed tumors (pleomorphic adenomas) of the breast. Am J Surg Pathol 1990;14:913-921.
63. Narita T, Matsuda K. Pleomorphic adenoma of the breast: case report and review of the literature. Pathol Int 1995;45:543-548.
64. Nishimori H, Sasaki M, Hirata K, et al. Tubular adenoma of the breast in a 73-year-old woman. Breast Cancer 2000;7:169-172.
65. O'Hara MF, Page DL. Adenomas of the breast and ectopic breast under lactational influences. Hum Pathol 1985;16:707-712.
66. Parham DM, Evans A. Pleomorphic adenoma of the breast; a potential for the misdiagnosis of malignancy on fine needle aspiration (FNA). Cytopathology 1998;9:343-348.
67. Rosen PP, Oberman HA. Tumors of the mammary gland. Atlas of Tumor Pathology, 3rd Series, Fascicle 7. Washington DC: Armed Forces Institute of Pathology; 1993.
67a. Rovera F, Ferrari A, Carcano G, et al. Tubular adenoma of the breast in an 84-year-old woman: report of a case simulating breast cancer. Breast J 2006;12:257-259.
68. Sheth MT, Hathway D, Petrelli M. Pleomorphic adenoma ("mixed" tumor) of human female breast mimicking carcinoma clinico-radiologically. Cancer 1978;41:659-665.
68a. Shum J, Obeid J, Smith P, Allevato P, Liebman S, Shum DT. Pleomorphic adenoma of the breast. Breast J 2007;13:94-102.
69. Simha MR, Doctor VM, Udwadia TE. Mixed tumor of salivary gland type of the male breast. Indian J Cancer 1992;29:14-17.
70. Soreide JA, Anda O, Eriksen L, Holter J, Kjellevold KH. Pleomorphic adenoma of the human breast with local recurrence. Cancer 1988;61:997-1001.
71. Tavassoli FA. Pathology of the breast. New York: Elsevier; 1992:157-168.
72. Willen R, Uvelius B, Cameron R. Pleomorphic adenoma in the breast of a human female. Aspiration biopsy findings and receptor determinations. Case report. Acta Chir Scand 1986;152:709-713.

Hamartoma

73. Anani PA, Hessler C. Breast hamartoma with invasive ductal carcinoma. Report of two cases and review of the literature. Pathol Res Pract 1996;192:1187-1194.
74. Charpin C, Mathoulin MP, Andrac L, et al. Reappraisal of breast hamartomas. A morphological study of 41 cases. Pathol Res Pract 1994;190:362-371.
75. Daya D, Trus T, D'Souza TJ, Minuk T, Yemen B. Hamartoma of the breast, an underrecognized breast lesion. A clinicopathologic and radiographic study of 25 cases. Am J Clin Pathol 1995;103:685-689.
75a. Filho OG, Gordan AN, Mello Rde A, Neto CS, Heinke T. Myoid hamartomas of the breast: report of 3 cases and review of the literature. Int J Surg Pathol 2004;12:151-153.
76. Fischer CJ, Hanby AM, Robinson L, Millis RR. Mammary hamartoma—a review of 35 cases. Histopathology 1992;20:99-106.
76a. Hattori H. Mammary hamartoma of the axillary subcutis. Breast J 2006;12:181-182.
77. Helvie MA, Adler DD, Rebner M, Oberman HA. Breast hamartoma: variable mammographic appearance. Radiology 1989;170:417-421.

77a. Hernanz F, Vega A, Palcios A, Fleitas MG. Giant hamartoma of the breast treated by the mammoplasty approach. ANZ J Surg 2008;78:216-217.

78. Hogeman KE, Ostberg G. Three cases of postlactational breast tumour of a peculiar type. Acta Pathol Microbiol Scand 1968;73:169-176.

79. Jones MW, Norris HJ, Wargotz ES. Hamartomas of the breast. Surg Gynecol Obstet 1991;173:54-56.

80. Ljungqvist U, Anderson I, Hildell J, Linell F. Mammary hamartoma: a benign breast lesion. Acta Chir Scand 1979;145:227-230.

81. Oberman HA. Hamartomas and hamartoma variants of the breast. Semin Diagn Pathol 1989;173:135-145.

82. Tavassoli FA. Pathology of the breast, 2nd ed. Stamford, CT: Appleton & Lange/McGraw Hill; 1999:168-171.

83. Tse GM, Law BK, Ma TK, et al. Hamartoma of the breast: a clinicopathological review. J Clin Pathol 2002;55:951-954.

Radial Scar/Infiltrating Epitheliosis

84. Alvarado-Cabrero I, Tavassoli FA. Neoplastic and malignant lesions involving or arising in a radial scar: a clinicopathologic analysis of 17 cases. Breast J 2000;6:96-102.

85. Andersen JA, Gram JB. Radial scar in the female breast. A long-term follow-up study of 32 cases. Cancer 1984;53:2557-2560.

86. Anderson TJ, Battersby S. Radial scars and complex sclerosing lesions. Histopathology 1994;24:296-297.

87. Azzopardi JG. Problems in breast pathology. Philadelphia: WB Saunders; 1979.

88. Ciatto S, Morrone D, Catarzi S, et al. Radial scars of the breast: review of 38 consecutive mammographic diagnoses. Radiology 1993;187:757-760.

89. Denley H, Pinder SE, Tan PH, et al. Metaplastic carcinoma of the breast arising within complex sclerosing lesions: a report of five cases. Histopathology 2000;36:203-209.

90. Eusebi V, Grassigli A, Grosso F. [Breast sclero-elastotic focal lesions simulating infiltrating carcinoma.] Pathologica 1976;68:507-518. [Italian.]

91. Fisher ER, Palekar AS, Kotwal N, Lipana N. A nonencapsulated sclerosing lesion of the breast. Am J Clin Pathol 1979;71:240-246.

92. Hamperl H. Strahlige Narben und obliterierende Mastopathie. Beitrage zur pathologischen Histologie der Mamma XI. Virchows Arch A Pathol Anat Histopathol 1975;369:55-68.

93. Jacobs TW, Byrne C, Colditz G, Connoly JL, Schnitt SJ. Radial scars in benign breast-biopsy specimens and the risk of breast cancer. N Engl J Med 1999;340:430-436.

94. Linnel F, Ljungberg O, Andersson I. Breast carcinoma: aspects of early stages, progression and related problems. Acta Pathol Microbiol Scand Suppl 1980;272:1-233.

95. Makunura CN, Curling OM, Yeomans P, Perry N, Wells CA. Apocrine adenosis within a radial scar. A case of false positive breast cytodiagnosis. Cytopathology 1994;5:123-128.

95a. Manfrin E, Remo A, Falsipollo F, Reghellin D, Bonetti F. Risk of neoplastic transformation in asymptomatic radial scar. Analysis of 117 cases. Breast Cancer Res Treat 2008;107:371-377.

96. Nielsen M, Christensen L, Andersen J. Radial scars in women with breast cancer. Cancer 1987;59:1019-1025.

97. Nielsen M, Jensen J, Andersen JA. An autopsy study of radial scars in the female breast. Histopathology 1985;9:287-295.

97a. Perez-Campos A, Perez F, Tejerina E, Sanchez-Yuste R, Jimenez-Heffernan JA. Fine needle aspiration cytology of atypical apocrine adenosis of the breast. Cytopathology 2007 [Epub ahead of print.]

98. Orel SG, Evers K, Yeh IT, Troupin RH. Radial scar with microcalcifications: radiologic pathologic correlation. Radiology 1992;183:479-484.

99. Sloane JP, Mayers MM. Carcinoma and atypical hyperplasia in radial scars and complex sclerosing lesions: importance of lesion size and patient age. Histopathology 1993;23:225-231.

100. Wellings SR, Alpers CE. Subgross pathologic features and incidence of radial scars in the breast. Hum Pathol 1984;15:475-479.

Duct Ectasia

101. Azzopardi JG. Problems in breast pathology. Philadelphia: WB Saunders; 1979:72-87.

102. Bloodgood JC. The clinical picture of dilated ducts beneath the nipple frequently to be palpated as a doughy worm-like mass—the varicocele tumor of the breast. Surg Gynecol Obstet 1923;36:486-495.

103. Davies JD. Inflammatory damage to ducts in mammary dysplasia. A cause of duct obliteration. J Pathol 1975;117:47-54.

103a. Dixon JM, Ravisekar O, Chetty U, Anderson TJ. Periductal mastitis and duct ectasia: different conditions with different etiologies. Br J Surg 1996;83:820-822.

104. Frantz VK, Pickren JW, Melcher GW, Auchincloss H Jr. Incidence of chronic cystic disease in so-called "normal breasts". A study based on 225 postmortem examinations. Cancer 1951;4:762-783.

105. Haagensen CD. Mammary duct ectasia—a disease that may simulate carcinoma. Cancer 1951;4:749-761.

106. Habif DV, Perzin KH, Lipton R, Lattes R. Subareolar abscess associated with squamous metaplasia of lactiferous ducts. Am J Surg 1970;119: 523-526.

106a. Hari S, Kumar J, Chumber S. Bilateral severe mammary duct ectasia. Acta Radiologica 2007;48:398-400.

107. Webb AJ. Mammary duct ectasia—periductal mastitis complex. Br J Surg 1995;82:1300-1302.

108. Young GB. Mammography in carcinoma of the breast. J R Coll Surg Edinb 1968;13:12-33.

Mastitis

109. Adair FE. Plasma cell mastitis—a lesion simulating mammary carcinoma. A clinical and pathologic study with a report of 10 cases. Arch Surg 1933;26:735-749.

110. Alagaratnam TT, Ong GB. Tuberculous of the breast. Br J Surg 1980;67:1225-1226.

111. Al Soub H, Chacko K. Tuberculous mastitis: a rare disease. Br J Clin Pract 1996;50:50-51.

112. Aozasa K, Ohsawa M, Saeki K, Horiuchi K, Kawano K, Taguchi T. Malignant lymphoma of the breast—immunologic type and association with lymphocytic mastopathy. Am J Clin Pathol 1992;97:699-704.

113. Ashton MA, Lefkowitz M, Tavassoli FA. Epithelioid stromal cells in lymphoctyic mastitis—a source of confusion with invasive carcinoma. Mod Pathol 1994;7:49-54.

114. Bennett IC, Furnival CM, Searle J. Dirofilariasis in Australia: unusual cause of a breast lump. Aust N Z J Surg 1989;59:671-673.

115. Chen Yuehan, Xie Qun. Filarial granuloma of the female breast: a histopathological study of 131 cases. Am J Trop Med Hyg 1981;30:1206-1210.

116. Chetty R, Butler AE. Lymphocytic mastopathy associated with infiltrating lobular breast carcinoma. J Clin Pathol 1993;46:376-377.

117. Coyne JD, Baildam AD, Asbury D. Lymphocytic mastopathy associated with ductal carcinoma in situ of the breast. Histopathology 1995;26:579-580.

118. Fitzgibbons PL, Smiley DF, Kern WH. Sarcoidosis presenting initially as breast mass: report of two cases. Hum Pathol 1985;16:851-852.

119. Fletcher A, Magrath IM, Riddel RH, Talbot IC. Granulomatous mastitis: a report of seven cases. J Clin Pathol 1982;35:941-945.

120. Going JJ, Anderson TJ, Wilkinson S, Chetty U. Granulomatous lobular mastitis. J Clin Pathol 1987;40:535-540.

121. Golinger RC, O'Neal BJ. Mastitis and mammary duct disease. Arch Surg 1982;117:1027-1029.

122. Gottschalk FA, Decker GA, Schmaman A. Tuberculosis of the breast. S Afr J Surg 1976;14:19-22.

123. Gutierrez Y, Paul GM. Breast nodule produced by Dirofilaria tenius. Am J Surg Pathol 1984;8:463-465.

124. Habif DV, Perzin KH, Lipton R, Lattes R. Subareolar abscess associated with squamous metaplasia of lactiferous ducts. Am J Surg 1970;119:523-526.

125. Hunfeld KP, Bassler R. Lymphocytic mastitis and fibrosis of the breast in long-standing insulin-dependent diabetics. A histopatholgic study on diabetic mastopathy and report of ten cases. Gen Diagn Pathol 1997;143:49-58.

126. Hunfeld KP, Bassler R, Kronsbein H. "Diabetic mastopathy" in the male breast—a special type of gynecomastia. A comparative study of lymphocytic mastitis and gynecomastia. Pathol Res Pract 1997;193:197-205.

126a. Jain BK, Sehgal VN, Jagdish S, Ratnakar C, Smile SR. Primary actinomycosis of the breast: a clinical review and a case report. J Dermatol 1994;21:497-500.

126b. Kieffer P, Dukic R, Hueber M, et al. [A young woman with granulomatous mastitis: a corynebacteria may be involved in the pathogenesis of this disease.] Rev Med Interne 2006;27:550-554. [French]

127. Lammie GA, Bobrow LG, Staunton MD, Levison DA, Page G, Millis RR. Sclerosing lymphocytic lobulitis of the breast—evidence for an autoimmune pathogenesis. Histopathology 1991;19:13-20.

128. Lefkowitz M, Wear DJ. Cat-scratch disease masquerading as a solitary tumor of the breast. Arch Pathol Lab Med 1989;113:473-475.

129. Miller MJ, Moore S. Nodular breast lesion caused by Bancroft's filariasis. Can Med Assoc J 1965;93:711-714.

130. Minkowitz S, Hedayati H, Hiller S, Gardner B. Fibrous mastopathy. A clinical histopathologic study. Cancer 1973;32:913-916.

131. Montagnac R, Collet E, Schillinger F, Chapelon C. [Sarcoidosis secondary to bilateral breast paraffinoma.] Presse Med 1993;22:1707. [French.]

132. Osborne BM. Granulomatous mastitis caused by histoplasma and mimicking inflammatory breast carcinoma. Hum Pathol 1989;20:47-52.

133. Pascual RS, Gee JB, Finch SC. Usefulness of serum lysozyme in the diagnosis and evaluation of sarcoidosis. N Engl J Med 1973;289:1074-1076.

134. Pemberton M. A case of actinomycosis of the breast. Br J Surg 1955;42;29:353.

135. Rooney N, Snead D, Goodman S, Webb AJ. Primary breast lymphoma with skin involvement arising in lymphocytic lobulitis. Histopathology 1994;24:81-84.

136. Ross MJ, Merino MJ. Sarcoidosis of the breast. Hum Pathol 1985;16:185-187.

137. Salfelder K, Schwarz J. Mycotic "pseudotumors" of the breast. Report of four cases. Arch Surg 1975;110:751-754.

138. Shinde SR, Chandawarkar RY, Deshmukh SP. Tuberculosis of the breast masquerading as carcinoma: a study of 100 patients. World J Surg 1995;19:379-381.

138a. Shousha S. Diabetic mastopathy: strong CD10+ immunoreactivity of the atypical stromal cells. Histopathology 2008;52:648-649.

139. Soler NG, Khardori R. Fibrous disease of the breast, thyroiditis, and cheiroarthropathy in type I diabetes mellitus. Lancet 1984;1:193-195.

140. Studdy PR, Lapwork R, Bird R. Angiotensin-converting enzyme and its clinical significance—a review. J Clin Pathol 1983;36:938-947.

141. Symmers WS. Deep-seated fungal infections currently seen in the histopatholgic service of a medical school laboratory in Britain. Am J Clin Pathol 1966;46:514-537.

143. Thomsen AC, Espersen T, Maigard S. Course and treatment of milk stasis, noninfectious inflammation of the breast, and infectious mastitis in nursing women. Am J Obstet Gynecol 1984;149:492-495.

142. Tuberculosis of the breast. Br Med J (Clin Res Ed) 1984;289:48-49.

144. Valdez R, Thorson J, Finn WG, Schnitzer B, Kleer CG. Lymphocytic mastitis and diabetic mastopathy: a molecular, immunophenotypic, and clinicopathologic evaluation of 11 cases. Mod Pathol 2003;16:223-228.

145. Yoshida T, Tanaka M, Okamoto K, Hirai S. Neurosarcoidosis following augmentation mammoplasty with silicone. Neurol Res 1996;18:319-320.

Juvenile Hypertrophy

146. Baker SB, Burkey BA, Thornton P, LaRossa D. Juvenile gigantomastia: presentation of four cases and review of the literature. Ann Plast Surg 2001;46:517-525.

147. Farrow JH, Ashikari H. Breast lesions in young girls. Surg Clin North Am 1969;49:261-269.

148. Geschikter CF. Diseases of the breast; diagnosis, pathology, treatment, 2nd ed. Philadelphia: JB Lippincott; 1945:97-132.

149. Griffith JR. Virginal breast hypertrophy. J Adolesc Health Care 1989;10:423-432.

150. Oberman HA. Breast lesions in the adolescent female. Pathol Ann 1979;14(Pt. 1):175-201.

151. Sagot P, Mainguene C, Barriere P, Lopes P. Virginal breast hypertrophy at puberty: a case report. Eur J Obstet Gynecol Reprod Biol 1990;34:289-292.

152. Tavassoli FA. Pathology of the breast, 2nd ed. Stamford, CT: Appleton & Lange/McGraw Hill; 1999:171-177.

153. Uribe Barreto A. Juvenile mammary hypertrophy. Plast Reconstr Surg 1991;87:583-584.

Spherulosis, Microcalcifications, Inclusions, and Foreign Bodies

154. Clement PB, Young RH, Azzopardi JG. Collagenous spherulosis of the breast. Am J Surg Pathol 1987;11:411-417.

155. Fandos-Morera A, Prats-Esteve M, Tura-Soteras JM, Traveria-Cros A. Breast tumors: composition of microcalcifications. Radiology 1988;169:325-327.

156. Galkin BM, Feig SA, Frasca P, et al. Photomicrographs of breast calcifications: correlation with histopathologic diagnosis. Radiographics 1983;3:450-417.

157. Gonzalez JE, Caldwell RG, Valaitis J. Calcium oxalate crystals in the breast. Pathology and significance. Am J Surg Pathol 1991;15:586-591.

158. Holland R, Hendriks JH. Microcalcifications associated with ductal carcinoma in situ: mammographic-pathologic correlation. Semin Diagn Pathol 1994;11:181-192.

159. Merckx L, Lamote J, Sacre R. Bilateral ulcerating paraffinoma of the breast in a man. Breast Dis 1993;6:41-44.

160. Millis RR, Davis R, Stacey AJ. The detection and significance of calcifications in the breast: a radiological and pathological study. Br J Radiol 1976;49:12-26.

161. Mooney EE, Kayani N, Tavassoli FA. Spherulosis of the breast. A spectrum of mucinous and collagenous lesions. Arch Pathol Lab Med 1999;123:626-630.

162. Pesutic-Pisac V, Bezic J, Tomic S. Collagenous spherulosis of the breast in association with in situ carcinoma. Pathologica 2002;94:317-319.

163. Ro JY, Ngadiman S, Sahin A, et al. Intraluminal crystalloids in breast carcinoma. Immunohistochemical, ultrastructural, and energy-dispersive x-ray element analysis in four cases. Arch Pathol Lab Med 1997;121:593-598.

164. Siggelkow W, Klosterhalfen B, Klinge C, et al. Analysis of local complications following explantation of silicone breast implants. Breast 2004;13:122-128.

165. Tavassoli FA Pathology of the breast, 2nd ed. Stamford, CT: Appleton & Lange/McGraw Hill; 1999:187-193.

166. Tavassoli FA, Majeste RM, Snyder RC. Intranuclear helioid inclusions in mammary intraductal hyperplasias. Ultrastruct Pathol 1991;15:267-279.

167. Tuur SM, Nelson AM, Gibson DW, et al. Liesegang rings in tissue. How to distinguish Liesegang rings from giant kidney worm, Dioctophyma renale. Am J Surg Pathol 1987;11:598-605.

168. Winston JS, Yeh IT, Evers K, Friedman AK. Calcium oxalate is associated with benign breast tissue. Can we avoid biopsy? Am J Clin Pathol 1993;100:488-492.

3 LOBULAR INTRAEPITHELIAL NEOPLASIA

Lobular intraepithelial neoplasia (LIN) is a solid, often occlusive proliferation of generally small and loosely cohesive cells. LIN refers to the entire spectrum of atypical epithelial proliferations (inclusive of *atypical lobular hyperplasia* [ALH] and *lobular carcinoma in situ* [LCIS]) originating in and confined predominantly to the terminal duct lobular unit (TDLU), with or without pagetoid extension to the terminal ducts. An important defining characteristic of LIN cells is the absence of immunoreactivity for E-cadherin and a polarized positive reaction with high molecular weight cytokeratin (CK) 34betaE12 (CK903).

In 1941, Foote and Stewart (27) used the term lobular carcinoma in situ for a distinctive proliferation affecting the TDLU. The uniform proliferating cells grew in a solid, occlusive fashion, with or without distension of the affected acini; the cells were loosely cohesive and the lesion was frequently multicentric, but inconspicuous on macroscopic evaluation of tissue samples. The same lesion had been described before, but without a specific designation (19). Subsequently, these lesions were divided into ALH and LCIS based variably and predominantly on involvement of more than one TDLU, distension of more than half of the acini within a TDLU by neoplastic lobular cells, or persistence of lumens.

Two series published in 1978 (33,58) concluded that the qualitative and quantitative features generally used to subdivide the lobular changes into LCIS and ALH are not of prognostic significance. Some of the main features evaluated by these studies included persistence of central lumen, distension of acini, involvement of one or more lobules, presence of macroacini, variation in cell type, loss of cell cohesion, and presence of an admixture of small and large cells. Despite the findings, one group continued to separate the changes into ALH and LCIS, while the other recommended the term *lobular neoplasia*. More recently, the latter term has been modified to lobular intraepithelial neoplasia (LIN) to distinguish it from invasive lobular neoplasms (10–12). The term LIN will be used throughout this chapter.

LIN is almost always an incidental finding. It generally does not form a palpable mass, is not associated with specific mammographic findings, is bilateral in a high proportion of cases, and may progress to invasive carcinoma (33,39,52,58,66–69). With follow-up of about 30 years, up to a third of women with LIN develop an invasive carcinoma in either breast and of either ductal or lobular type (56–59).

CLINICAL FEATURES

LIN ranges in frequency from less than 0.3 to 3.8 percent of breast "carcinomas" (33,38,68). Recent epidemiologic studies have noted an increase in the frequency of LIN (39). Over a period of 20 years (1978–1998), the overall incidence of LIN increased four-fold, from 0.90/100,000 person-years in 1978–80 to 2.83/100,000 person-years in 1987–89, and then increased modestly up to 1996–98 when the incidence rate was 3.19/100,000 person-years (38). The incidence rates increased continuously over the study period for women 50 to 59 years of age, who had the highest incidence of 11.47/100,000 person-years and an absolute increase in incidence of 9.48/100,000 person-years over the study period; obesity and hormone replacement therapy may have a role in this change. Although patients range in age from 15 (1) to over 90 years of age (67), LIN occurs most frequently in premenopausal women. The frequency of bilaterality ranges from 30 percent to as high as 67 percent (32,35,69) among women treated by bilateral mastectomy.

An increase in the risk for subsequent invasive carcinoma has been noted by Haagensen et al. (33,34) in patients with LIN who have a family history of breast carcinoma and gross cystic disease. The ratio of observed-to-expected subsequent carcinomas rose from 7.2 for all women with LIN but without such a history to 11.8 for

Table 3-1

GRADING OF LOBULAR INTRAEPITHELIAL NEOPLASIA (LIN) BASED ON EXTENT OF LOBULAR INVOLVEMENT[a,b]

LIN1	There is partial or complete replacement of the normal epithelial cells of the acini within one or more lobules by a proliferation of generally uniform cells with poorly defined margins which may fill, but do not distend, the acinar lumens (in comparison to adjacent uninvolved acini).
LIN2	There is more abundant proliferation of similar cells than in LIN1, which fill and actually distend some or all acini, but the acinar outlines remain distinct and separate from one another with persistence of intervening lobular stroma; residual lumens may persist in some acini.
LIN3	There is proliferation of cells similar to those of LIN1 or LIN2, but there is a massive degree of acinar distension to the point that the acini appear almost confluent; the interacinar stroma is barely evident. When there is necrosis or the proliferating cells are completely of the pleomorphic or signet ring cell type, significant acinar distension is not required.

[a]Adapted from reference 67.
[b]The myoepithelial cells may remain in their usual location or may be dislodged in any of these variants. In a small number of LIN3 lesions, the myoepithelial cell layer is hardly visible on hematoxylin and eosin (H&E)-stained slides. Immunostain for actin shows widening of the intermyoepithelial cell gaps.

those who had a positive family history and gross cystic disease. Rosen et al. (58,59) found that 5 of 12 (42 percent) women with LIN and a family history of breast carcinoma subsequently developed invasive carcinoma, compared with 22 of 62 (36 percent) women with LIN but without a positive family history; the differences between a positive and negative family history were not significant. Interestingly, Page et al. (49) concluded that family history did not further affect the risk among women with LCIS, but it did double the risk for those with ALH (21,46,47).

Mammographic abnormalities were absent in one series (45), but were noted in 52 percent (68) and 56 percent (8) of women in other series. The mammographic findings are not localized or specific to the LIN (51). LIN is sometimes detected incidentally when a biopsy is performed for microcalcifications that turn out to be localized in benign disease (65). It is possible, however, to mammographically detect LIN that is characterized by calcification often in association with central necrosis (22a,61).

PATHOLOGIC FEATURES

Gross and Microscopic Findings

LIN does not generally produce a grossly visible lesion. Microscopically, LIN lesions (ALH and LCIS) are located within the TDLU. Pagetoid involvement of the terminal ducts is present in 65 to 75 percent of patients (3–5,31,32).

LIN assumes a variety of appearances depending on the degree of acinar distension, the proportion of acini involved within a lobule, and the cytologic features. Typically uniform, the cells are often small, loosely cohesive, with rather indistinct cell margins and sparse cytoplasm. Deviations from this "classic appearance" are common. The cells may occasionally develop significant nuclear pleomorphism and/or abundant granular, eosinophilic cytoplasm with apocrine differentiation (67). Often, at least some of the proliferating cells contain intracytoplasmic lumens, and less commonly, even a signet ring cell appearance is seen. The nuclei of LIN cells are generally round and uniform. The native epithelial cells in the TDLU are either completely replaced or simply displaced and lifted by the neoplastic cells. The myoepithelial cells may remain in their original basal location or they may be dislodged (14,15). The basement membrane is generally intact. The neoplastic cells may extend to adjacent terminal ducts in a pagetoid fashion. This pagetoid pattern may be the only change evident in some biopsy specimens (4,24,46).

Based mainly on the extent of proliferation (Table 3-1) in a majority of cases and on the cytologic features in a small proportion of the lesions, Tavassoli (12,67) subdivided over 750 LIN cases sent to the Armed Forces Institute of Pathology (AFIP) into three grades (LIN1 to LIN3) to determine whether this division would correlate with any clinical features of the lesion. To qualify as LIN1, the normal epithelial cells of the acini have to be partially or completely replaced or displaced within one or more lobules by typical neoplastic lobular cells, which

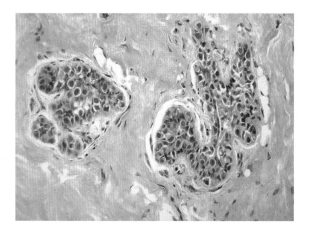

Figure 3-1

LOBULAR INTRAEPITHELIAL NEOPLASIA

In a postmenopausal woman, a few neoplastic lobular cells proliferate in atrophic lobules (lobular intraepithelial neoplasia grade 1 [LIN1]).

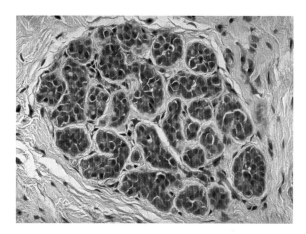

Figure 3-2

LOBULAR INTRAEPITHELIAL NEOPLASIA

The native epithelial cells are mostly replaced by neoplastic lobular cells, but there is no distension or even filling of the acini (LIN1).

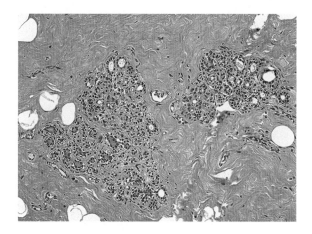

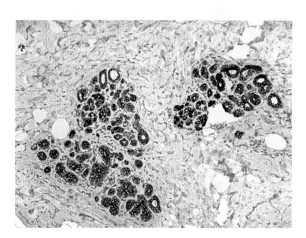

Figure 3-3

LOBULAR INTRAEPITHELIAL NEOPLASIA

Left: Little abnormality is seen in the adjacent lobules, except for a few neoplastic lobular cells (LIN1).

Right: Double staining with E-cadherin (brown) and CK34betaE12 (magenta) unmasks the few neoplastic lobular cells (CK34betaE12 positive) within these otherwise normal-appearing lobules (LIN1).

may fill the lumens, but without any evidence of acinar distension (figs. 3-1–3-3). LIN2 displays more abundant proliferation of LIN cells, which fill and distend some or all acini, but the acinar outlines remain distinct, often with persistence of intervening lobular stroma (figs. 3-4, 3-5); residual lumens may persist in some acini. Pagetoid extension into adjacent ducts is a common feature (fig. 3-6). To warrant a designation of LIN3, there is either necrosis, an occlusive epithelial proliferation that maximally distends the acini to near confluence (macroacini), a population of nearly 100 percent signet ring cell proliferation, or proliferating cells that show significant pleomorphism and bizarre nuclei (pleomorphic lobular carcinoma in situ of other authors); maximal acinar distension is not required for the latter two variants (figs. 3-7–3-10).

Among consultation cases reviewed at AFIP (12), LIN2 comprised about 80 percent of all LIN cases, while LIN1 and LIN3 each represented about 10 percent (Table 3-2). In actual general practice

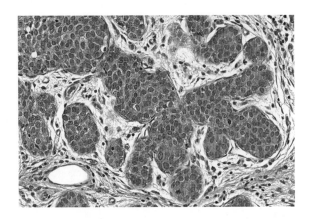
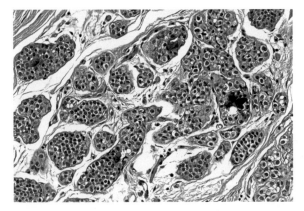

Figure 3-4

LOBULAR INTRAEPITHELIAL NEOPLASIA

Left: A proliferation of uniform neoplastic lobular cells distends the acini, but not to the point of confluence (LIN2).
Right: Rarely, microcalcifications may develop in LIN.

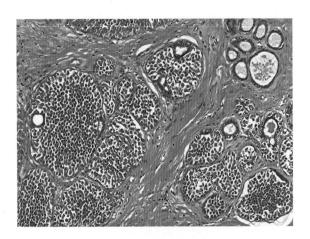

Figure 3-5

LOBULAR INTRAEPITHELIAL NEOPLASIA

The acini are distended and residual lumens are apparent in some.

of pathology, LIN2 probably represents over 90 percent of the cases. Correlating with the ALH/LCIS subdivision, LIN1 always falls into the ALH category, while LIN3 always falls in the LCIS category; due to the variability of the criteria used, LIN2 may qualify as either ALH or LCIS.

The National Surgical Adjuvant Breast Project (NSABP) confirmed that the three-tier grading system effectively separates those lesions with a limited likelihood of progression (LIN1) from those with a greater chance of recurrence or subsequent progression within 5 to 12 years after diagnosis (Table 3-3) (26). Fisher et al. (26,26a) used the

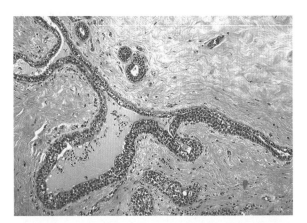
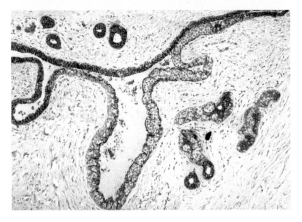

Figure 3-6

LOBULAR INTRAEPITHELIAL NEOPLASIA

Top: Pagetoid extension into adjacent ducts.
Bottom: The neoplastic lobular cells are E-cadherin negative beneath luminal epithelial cells that are E-cadherin positive.

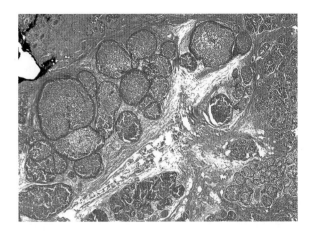
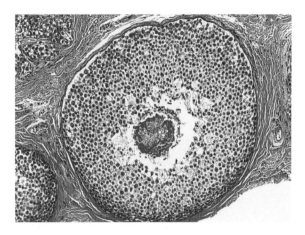

Figure 3-7

LOBULAR INTRAEPITHELIAL NEOPLASIA, GRADE 3

Left: There is massive distension of acini compared to adjacent normal acini (LIN3).
Right: Necrosis is apparent in some distended acini, mimicking ductal intraepithelial neoplasia (DIN). This is LIN, necrotic type.

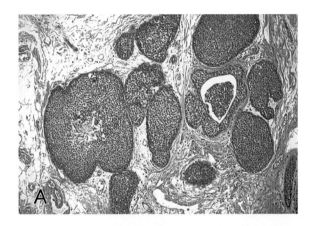

Figure 3-8

LOBULAR INTRAEPITHELIAL NEOPLASIA: NECROTIC TYPE, GRADE 3

A: Necrosis is most evident in one of the distended acini.

B: E-cadherin is negative in the neoplastic cells; the residual native epithelial cells lining the only visible lumen are E-cadherin positive.

C: A massively distended acinus shows loosely cohesive cells. Intracytoplasmic lumens are seen in some.

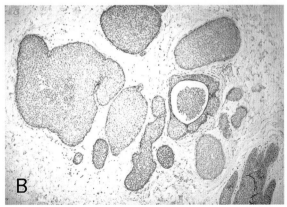
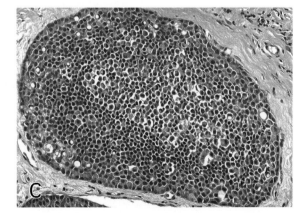

three-tier grading system proposed by Tavassoli, but retained the designation of LCIS.

As the grade of LIN increases, the likelihood that the associated invasive carcinoma will be lobular in nature increases from 11 percent for LIN1 to 47 percent for LIN2 and ultimately to 86 percent for LIN3 (Table 3-2) (12). Basically, LIN3 identifies those lesions mainly committed to

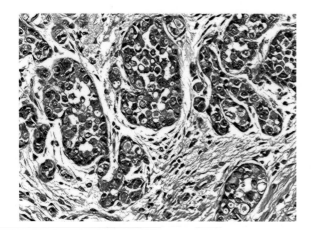

Figure 3-9

**LOBULAR INTRAEPITHELIAL
NEOPLASIA: PLEOMORPHIC TYPE**

The acini are not massively distended, but there is nuclear atypia. The intracytoplasmic lumens and targetoid secretions are prominent.

progression into an invasive lobular carcinoma. For practical purposes, it is advocated that LIN be used for all lesions; when appropriate, the designation of LIN should be qualified as necrotic type, pleomorphic type, macroacinar type (which may present as a mass lesion), or signet ring cell type to draw attention to the variants that need further attention (Table 3-4).

While some have continued to separate LIN into ALH and LCIS, requiring involvement of at least 50 percent of the acini within one lobule for a diagnosis of LCIS (48,49), the management of the lesion has evolved to the point that most patients are followed regardless of whether the diagnosis is ALH or LCIS. Management will continue to evolve since it appears that the necrotic (9a), pleomorphic, signet ring cell, and macroacinar types of LIN may benefit from a different management approach.

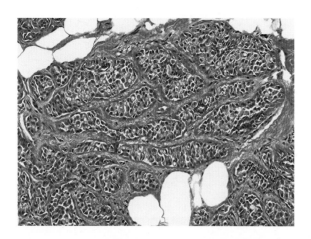

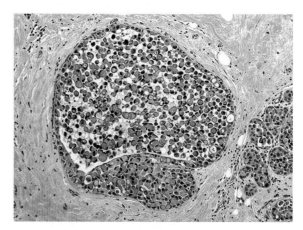

Figure 3-10

LOBULAR INTRAEPITHELIAL NEOPLASIA: SIGNET RING CELL TYPE

Left: The neoplastic cells are of signet ring cell type without much acinar distension (LIN3).
Right: Another example with significant distension of the involved acini by loosely cohesive signet ring cells.

Table 3-2				
RELATIONSHIP OF GRADE OF LOBULAR INTRAEPITHELIAL NEOPLASIA (LIN) TO TYPE OF ASSOCIATED INVASIVE CARCINOMA[a]				
Grade of LIN	Number (%)	Total Inv Ca[b]	Inv DCa	Inv LCa
LIN1	65 (8%)	9 (14%)	8 (89%)	1 (11%)
LIN2	618 (80%)	110 (18%)	58 (53%)	52 (47%)
LIN3	92 (12%)	21 (23%)	3 (14%)	18 (86%)

[a]Modified from Tables 1 and 2 from Bratthauer GL, Tavassoli FA. Lobular intraepithelial neoplasia. Previously unexplored aspects assessed in 775 cases and their clinical implications. Virchows Arch 2002;440:137.
[b]Inv Ca = invasive carcinoma; DCa = ductal carcinoma; LCa = lobular carcinoma.

Cytologic Findings

On fine needle aspiration cytology (FNAC) (60,71), the presence of loosely cohesive cell clusters composed of uniform cells with frequent eccentric nuclei, minimal nuclear atypia, and occasional intracytoplasmic lumens is suggestive of LIN (fig. 3-11). Invasive lobular carcinomas may be more cellular and have a higher proportion of noncohesive (dissociated) single cells (60). It is almost impossible to distinguish between an intraepithelial and invasive lobular carcinoma based on aspiration cytology, however. In most cases, a biopsy is obtained to determine whether the lobular lesion is invasive or intraepithelial. The limitations of FNAC should be kept in mind; a negative FNAC does not exclude the possibility of LIN.

Ultrastructural Findings

At the ultrastructural level, LIN cells frequently display intracytoplasmic lumens with microvilli containing secretory droplets (45), and often a prominent Golgi apparatus. The myoepithelial cells and basement membrane generally persist (14,15,43).

Hormone Receptors and Tumor Markers

LINs are positive for estrogen receptors (ERs) in up to 90 percent of cases and for progesterone receptors (PRs) in a slightly lower proportion (13,26,29). They are negative for c-erbB-2 (26, 52,53) and E-cadherin (2,35).

Table 3-3

RELATIONSHIP OF GRADE OF LOBULAR INTRAEPITHELIAL NEOPLASIA (LIN) TO RECURRENCE[a]

Grade	No. of Patients	% of Patients	No. of IBTR[b]	Avg. An. Rate/100 Patient Yrs.
1	63	34.6	0	0
2	81	44.5	3	0.84
3	38	20.9	4	2.36

[a]Modified from Table 4 from Fisher ER, Constantino J, Fisher B, et al. Pathologic findings from the National Surgical Adjuvant Breast Project (NSABP) protocol B-17. Five year observations concerning lobular carcinoma in situ. Cancer 1996;78:1412.

[b]IBTR = ipsilateral breast tumor recurrence; Avg. An. = average annual.

Table 3-4

PRACTICAL CLASSIFICATION OF LOBULAR INTRAEPITHELIAL NEOPLASIA (LIN)

LIN1 and 2 are combined and designated simply as:	LIN
Lesions within LIN3 category are specified:	LIN, necrotic type
	LIN, pleomorphic type
	LIN, signet ring cell
	LIN, macroacinar type

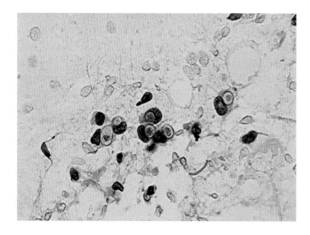
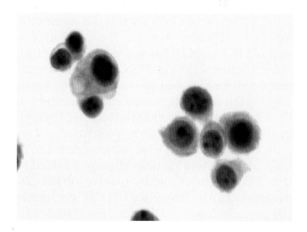

Figure 3-11

LOBULAR INTRAEPITHELIAL NEOPLASIA: ASPIRATION CYTOLOGY

Left: There are small clusters of neoplastic cells with intracytoplasmic lumens. It is impossible to determine whether the lesion is intraepithelial or invasive.

Right: Another case with loosely cohesive cells and a rare, somewhat inconspicuous, intracytoplasmic lumen. (Courtesy of Dr. G. Rasty, Toronto, Canada.)

One example of LCIS evaluated by Nesland et al. (44) displayed a positive reaction for carcinoembryonic antigen (CEA), prekeratin, and casein, but failed to react with lactalbumin. Casein has been found in the cytoplasm of 5 examples of LCIS and 21 infiltrating lobular carcinomas (22). In addition, alpha-lactalbumin has been identified in both infiltrating and in situ lobular carcinomas.

Ploidy and Molecular Findings

LIN is predominantly diploid (50). The rare pleomorphic variant is often aneuploid (7a), but these lesions have not been studied in detail.

Application of molecular techniques, including assessment of loss of heterozygosity (LOH) in lobular lesions, may unravel some of the early events in the development of LIN (36,42) and its progression to more advanced lesions. LOH on chromosome 16q, the site of the E-cadherin gene, has been detected in 30 percent of cases (36). Interestingly, loss of chromosomal material from 16p, 16q, 17p, and 22q, and gain of material in 6q were detected in almost equal frequency among both ALH and LCIS lesions by comparative genomic hybridization; this finding confirms that both ALH and LCIS are neoplastic in nature.

Perrone et al. (50a) assessed the expression of cyclooxygenase 2 (Cox-2) in the three grades of LIN and found predominantly membranous and some cytoplasmic immunoreactions in 16/17 (94 percent) of LIN1, 22/25 (88 percent) of LIN2, and 2/9 (22 percent) of LIN3. There was a statistically significant difference between the Cox-2 expression of LIN1 and LIN3 as well as LIN2 and LIN3, but not between LIN1 and LIN2. The authors suggest a role for Cox-2 in the early developmental stages of this neoplastic process and exploration of Cox-2 inhibitors as a potential targeted therapy in the management of these patients.

In another study, LOH at chromosome 11q13 (INT2, PYGM) was identified in about a third of the ALH/LCIS cases, and in invasive lobular carcinoma (42). The frequency of LOH was higher (50 percent) among LCIS cases associated with invasive carcinoma (42). The genetic relationship between synchronous LCIS and infiltrating lobular carcinoma suggests clonality in a majority of paired specimens studied by array comparative genomic hybridization, and supports a progression pathway from the former

to the latter (63). Using microarray comparative genomic hybridization (array CGH), loss of 16q21-23.1 was identified in both "ALH" and "LCIS" (38a). The majority of alterations identified occurred in both "ALH" and "LCIS" further confirming a genomic signature common to both and providing additional support for combining the two under the term LIN.

Lesions Associated with LIN

LIN occurs simultaneously with high-grade ductal intraepithelial neoplasia (DIN) or invasive carcinomas in 12 to 16 percent of cases (31,32,55). The association of LIN with flat DIN1 (flat epithelial atypia), however, is reportedly as high as 88 percent (37a). Patients in whom LIN occurs alone are generally younger than those having LIN associated with other forms of intraepithelial or invasive breast carcinoma (31,32). About 86 percent of the carcinomas that are present simultaneously with LIN3 are lobular in type in contrast to 47 percent of those associated with LIN2 and 11 percent of those associated with LIN1 (12).

Among 775 patients with LIN, 22 percent of the 65 with LIN1, 33 percent of the 618 with LIN2, and 41 percent of the 92 with LIN3 had either in situ or invasive carcinoma (12). Benign intraductal proliferations were present in 78 percent of the LIN1 cases, 67 percent of the LIN2 cases, and 59 percent of LIN3 cases. With more extensive sampling of breast biopsy specimens and emphasis on specifying the various pathologic findings in the current practice of surgical pathology, it is not surprising that we are observing an increase in the frequency of LIN associated with various intraductal proliferations.

DIFFERENTIAL DIAGNOSIS

Since both ductal and lobular neoplasia originate in the TDLU (73), distinction of LIN from solid ductal intraepithelial neoplasias can be difficult and a source of confusion (23). Features that help identify the relatively solid variants of DIN include formation of multiple, albeit minuscule, secondary lumens; rosette-like arrangements of the nuclei; distinctive cell margins; and immunoreactivity with E-cadherin. Among these features, a distinctive cell margin is the least reliable since some lobular lesions have distinctive cell margins. Features in favor of LIN include

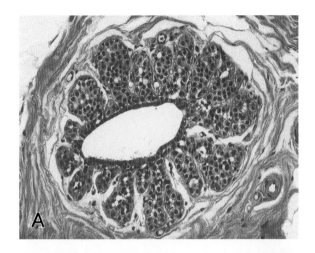

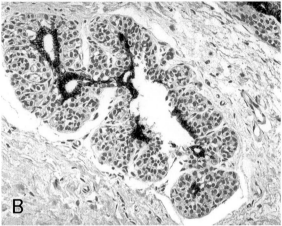

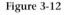

Figure 3-12

LOBULAR INTRAEPITHELIAL NEOPLASIA

A: The neoplastic cells are barely evident. (Fig. 8-13C from Tavassoli F. Pathology of the breast, 2nd ed. Stamford, CT: Appleton & Lange/McGraw Hill; 1999:388.)
B: The neoplastic cells are unmasked by the E-cadherin-negative immunoreaction; residual native epithelial cells are positive.
C: The cells are CK34betaE12 positive.

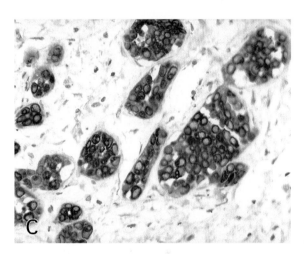

loosely cohesive cells, the presence of intracytoplasmic lumens (7) or secretory globules (6), and mucin positivity. Gad and Azzopardi (27a) found that the mucosubstance in the LIN cells is Alcian blue positive and periodic acid–Schiff (PAS) positive after diastase digestion.

The necrotic variant of LIN (with or without microcalcifications) is particularly prone to misdiagnosis as a ductal process. Since the presence of necrosis and microcalcification is generally associated with advanced ductal neoplasias, the presence of intracytoplasmic lumens in loosely cohesive cells and a negative immunoreaction with E-cadherin help identify the necrotic variant of LIN. Microcalcification may occur in all grades of LIN, but its frequency appears to increase with increasing grade.

Despite the variety of helpful features mentioned earlier, it is impossible to distinguish some lobular lesions from a ductal process on the basis of hematoxylin and eosin (H&E) morphology

alone. In these cases, the immunoprofile of the lesion should be assessed. As noted earlier, LIN is E-cadherin negative, but high molecular weight CK34betaE12 positive (fig. 3-12). DIN, on the other hand, is E-cadherin positive (100 percent), but CK34betaE12 negative (90 percent) when atypias develop (41). The usefulness of this immunoprofile in separating ductal and lobular lesions has been noted in several studies (10,11,35). It is important to use both markers, as there are lesions that may be negative or positive for both markers; these are lesions that we designate as mammary intraepithelial neoplasia (MIN) with morphologic and immunohistochemical hybrid (either negative hybrid or positive hybrid) features (Table 3-5) (see also chapter 4.)

Involvement of a variety of other lesions by LIN can be a source of diagnostic problems. When confined to sclerosing adenosis (25), LIN may be confused with an invasive carcinoma. Evaluation of the lesion at low magnification is

Table 3-5

IMMUNOEXPRESSION OF E-CADHERIN AND CK34BETAE12 IN LOBULAR INTRAEPITHELIAL NEOPLASIA (LIN)[a]

	E-K+[b]	E+K-	E+K+	E-K-
Classic LIN1-3 (n = 40)	40	0	0	0
Classic DIN1c-DIN3[c] (n = 20)	0	20	0	0
MIN by H&E[d] (n = 50)	17	6	16	11
Ultimate LIN	17			
Ultimate DIN		6		
Positive hybrid MIN			16	
Negative hybrid MIN				11

[a]Adapted from reference 11.

[b]E-K+ = negative for E-cadherin, positive for CK-34BetaE12.

[c]DIN = ductal intraepithelial neoplasia.

[d]MIN by H&E = mammary intraepithelial neoplasia assessed by hematoxylin and eosin [H&E] stain.

crucial to its recognition. Maintenance of a lobulated outline at low magnification is the first clue that the lesion is not invasive carcinoma. If doubts persist concerning the possibility of invasion, immunostains for calponin or p63 (or any other marker of myoepithelial cells) can be used to unmask the myoepithelial cell layer around the ductules of sclerosing adenosis filled by neoplastic lobular cells.

Involvement of collagenous or mucinous spherulosis by LIN (fig. 3-13) may be confused with cribriform ductal carcinoma in situ (62). The distinctive spherules and the orientation of myoepithelial cells around the spherules help resolve the problem.

Prominent and/or hyperplastic myoepithelial cells with clear or vacuolated cytoplasm that assume a pagetoid appearance can be confused with LIN. Nearly every ductule or acinus with prominent/hyperplastic myoepithelial cells retains its original lumen, however; tangential cutting through the myoepithelial cell region may mask the persistent acinus lumen. Often, comparison with adjacent normal myoepithelial cells helps resolve the problem. Sometimes, the only way to exclude this possibility is to immunostain the myoepithelial cells with any of its markers (calponin, actin, p63, CD10, and others).

Involvement of radial scars and fibroadenomas by LIN is discussed in chapters 2 and 12, respectively.

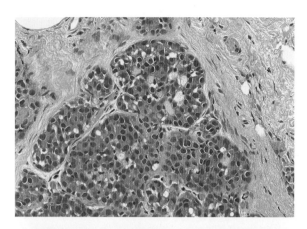

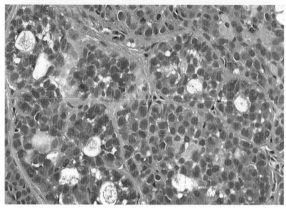

Figure 3-13

LOBULAR INTRAEPITHELIAL NEOPLASIA

Top: Mucinous spherulosis involved by LIN.

Bottom: The neoplastic cells contain intracytoplasmic mucin (mucicarmine stain).

PROGNOSTIC/PREDICTIVE FEATURES

The results of numerous studies containing over 1,100 patients have shown that among women with either LCIS or LN (as designated in these studies) and treated by biopsy alone, about 15 percent eventually develop invasive carcinoma (within 15 to 20 years); 8.7 percent of the subsequent carcinomas are in the ipsilateral breast, while 6.7 percent are in the contralateral breast (67). Over half (55 percent) of the subsequent invasive carcinomas are ductal in type and the rest (45 percent) are lobular. The relative risk (RR) of developing carcinoma increased substantially from 4.9 after one biopsy with LIN to 16.1 after a second biopsy also showed LIN (9). Using the three-tier grading system for LIN and with a follow-up of 12 years, the NSABP found that patients with LIN2 and LIN3 have an increased risk for the subsequent development of invasive carcinoma, whereas those with LIN1 had minimal, if any, increased risk (26,26a).

TREATMENT

In the past, a diagnosis of LIN led almost invariably to mastectomy. Following significant debate over the value of mastectomy and alternative therapeutic approaches for these lesions (16,18,20,30,31,34,37,69,70,72), and evolution of our understanding of these lesions, both ALH and LCIS came to be regarded as risk factors and nonobligate precursors for the subsequent development of invasive carcinoma. Studies have shown that invasive carcinoma may develop in either breast in at most 30 percent of women with long-term (30+ years) follow-up, and it may be of either ductal or lobular type (44,48,49,57,58). Patients with LIN require lifelong follow-up, with or without tamoxifen therapy. Reexcision should be considered only in those rare cases (less than 5 percent of all LIN cases encountered in general practice) that would qualify as the necrotic, pleomorphic, signet ring cell, or macroacinar variants of LIN and mainly when the lesion is at or close to the inked resection margin or when these variants are detected in core biopsies.

It is important to note that patients have a highly variable perception of the risk for the subsequent development of invasive carcinoma after a diagnosis of "LCIS" (28). It is the surgeons and the oncologists who provide the majority of the counseling; most patients will adhere to suggested follow-up recommendations (28). For this reason, it is best to avoid the alarming and emotionally charged term of carcinoma and use the designation of LIN.

Radiation therapy is not generally used in the management of LIN. A single recent study has found radiation therapy reduces the frequency of subsequent invasive cancer (17a). While giving radiation therapy to all women with LIN is unnecessary, it is not unreasonable to explore the efficacy of alternative and preferably targeted therapies for patients with the necrotic, pleomorphic, macroacinar, and signet ring cell variants of LIN.

In core biopsies, LIN is generally an incidental finding associated with a variety of lesions that present with microcalcifications or mass densities. Correlation with mammographic findings is crucial for all core biopsies. When the main lesion (the source of mammographic detection) does not require reexcision, follow-up is appropriate for most incidentally detected LIN lesions. LIN cases that are the source of mammographically detected lesions either produce a mass (macroacinar) or are necrotic with or without microcalcifications. While there is not sufficient data available on these rare subtypes, these variants should be reexcised if detected on a core biopsy given the high frequency (66 percent) of association with invasive carcinoma in the necrotic and macroacinar variants (22a). These lesions are rarely encountered in pure form; this may be a reflection of more rapidly progressive cell populations that have only a brief intraepithelial phase.

Of patients with a diagnosis of LIN on core biopsy, 21 percent also have ductal intraepithelial or invasive neoplasms (64). Of those LIN tumors immediately reexcised or excised after follow-up of up to 3 years, 24 percent show invasive carcinoma (17). After excluding the necrotic and pleomorphic variants, Middleton et al. (40) recommended excisional biopsy for LIN (ALH/LCIS) only when associated with a mass lesion. Without addressing specific subtypes, others have concluded that follow-up is sufficient for patients with pure LIN on core biopsy (54,64a). Clearly, there are diverse opinions on this issue and a consensus viewpoint is lacking.

In order to clarify the indications for surgical excision, Bowman et al. (9a) analyzed the findings in 19 studies that had evaluated the incidence of high-risk lesions associated with LIN diagnosed on core needle biopsy in a total of 504 patients. Based on the literature review, the authors concluded that even though some cases of LIN are associated with higher-risk lesions on subsequent surgical excision, the findings do not support routine excision for all patients.

It appears that some institutions routinely reexcise all LINs detected on core needle biopsies, some routinely do not reexcise such lesions, and still others manage the lesions case by case. Regardless of the routine institutional policy, reexcision would be prudent, in our opinion, for all cases of LIN3 (necrotic, pleomorphic, pure signet ring cell, and the often mass-forming macroacinar variants) until additional data based on larger numbers of cases becomes available.

REFERENCES

1. Ackerman BL, Otis C, Steuber K. Lobular carcinoma in situ in a 15-year-old girl: a case report and review of the literature. Plast Reconstr Surg 1993;94:714-718.
2. Acs G, Lawton TJ, Rebbeck TR, LiVolvsi VA, Zhang PJ. Differential expression of E-cadherin in lobular and ductal neoplasms of the breast and its biologic and diagnostic implications. Am J Clin Pathol 2001;115:85-98.
3. Anderson JA. Lobular carcinoma in situ. A histologic study of 52 cases. Acta Pathol Microbiol Scand [A] 1974;82:735-741.
4. Andersen JA. Lobular carcinoma in situ of the breast with duct involvement. Frequency and possible influence on prognosis. Acta Pathol Microbiol Scand [A] 1974;82:655-662.
5. Anderson JA. Multicentric and bilateral appearance of lobular carcinoma in situ of the breast. Acta Pathol Microbiol Scand [A] 1974;82:730-734.
6. Andersen JA, Vendelboe ML. Cytoplasmic mucous globules in lobular carcinoma in situ. Diagnosis and prognosis. Am J Surg Pathol 1981;5:251-255.
7. Battifora H. Intracytoplasmic lumina in breast carcinoma. A helpful histopathologic feature. Arch Pathol 1975;99:614-617.
7a. Bentz JS, Yassa N, Clayton F. Pleomorphic lobular carcinoma of the breast: clinicopathologic features of 12 cases. Mod Pathol 1998;18:814-822.
8. Beute BJ, Kalisher L, Hutter RV. Lobular carcinoma in situ of the breast: clinical, pathologic, and mammographic features. AJR Am J Roentgenol 1991;157:257-265.
9. Bodian CA, Perzin KH, Lattes R. Lobular neoplasia. Long-term risk of breast cancer and relation to other factors. Cancer 1996;78:1024-1034.
9a. Bowman K, Munoz A, Mahui DM, Breslin TM. Lobular neoplasia diagnosed at core biopsy does not mandate surgical excision. J Surg Res 2007;142:275-280.
10. Bratthauer GL, Miettinen M, Tavassoli FA. Cytokeratin immunoreactivity in lobular intraepithelial neoplasia. J Histochem Cytochem 2003;51:1527-1531
11. Bratthauer GL, Moinfar F, Stamatakos MD, et al. Combined E-cadherin and high molecular weight cytokeratin immunoprofile differentiates lobular, ductal and hybrid mammary intraepithelial neoplasias. Hum Pathol 2003;33:620-627.
12. Bratthauer GL, Tavassoli FA. Lobular intraepithelial neoplasia. Previously unexplored aspects assessed in 775 cases and their clinical implications. Virchows Arch 2002;440:134-138.
13. Bur ME, Zimarowski MJ, Schnitt SJ, Baker S, Lew R. Estrogen receptor immunohistochemistry in carcinoma in situ of the breast. Cancer 1992;69:1174-1181.
14. Bussolati G. Actin-rich (myoepithelial) cells in lobular carcinoma in situ of the breast. Virchows Arch B Cell Pathol Incl Mol Pathol 1980;32:165-176.
15. Bussolati G, Botto Micca F, Eusebi V, Betts CM. Myoepithelial cells in lobular carcinoma in situ of the breast: a parallel immunocytochemical and ultrastructural study. Ultrastruct Pathol 1981;2:219-230.
16. Carson W, Sanchez-Forgach E, Stomper P, Penetrante R, Tsangaris TN, Edge SB. Lobular carcinoma in situ without surgery as an appropriate therapy. Ann Surg Oncol 1994;1:141-146.
17. Crisi GM, Mandavilli S, Cronin E, Ricci A Jr. Invasive mammary carcinoma after immediate and short-term follow-up for lobular neoplasia on core biopsy. Am J Surg Pathol 2003;27:325-333.
17a. Cutuli B, de Lafontan B, Quentin P, Mery E. Breast-conserving surgery and radiotherapy: a possible treatment for lobular carcinoma in situ? Eur J Cancer 2005;41:380-385.
18. Dall'Olmo CA, Ponka JL, Horn RC Jr, Riu R. Lobular carcinoma of the breast in situ. Are we too radical in its treatment? Arch Surg 1975;110:537-542.
19. Dawson EK. Carcinoma in the mammary lobule and its origin. Edinb Med J 1933;40:57-82.
20. Donegan WL, Perez-Mesa CM. Lobular carcinoma—an indication for elective biopsy of the second breast. Ann Surg 1972;176:178-187.
21. Dupont WD, Page DL. Risk factors for breast cancer in women with proliferative breast disease. N Engl J Med 1985;312:146-151.
22. Eusebi V, Pich A, Macchiorlatti E, Bussolati G. Morpho-functional differentiation in lobular carcinoma of the breast. Histopathology 1977;1:307-314.
22a. Fadare O, Dadmanesh F, Alvarado-Cabrero I, et al. Lobular intraepithelial neoplasia (lobular carcinoma in situ) with comedo-type necrosis. A clinico-pahtologic study of 18 cases. Am J Surg Pathol 2006;30:1445-1453.
23. Fechner RE. Ductal carcinoma involving the lobule of the breast. A source of confusion with lobular carcinoma in situ. Cancer 1971;28:274-281.
24. Fechner RE. Epithelial alterations in the extralobular ducts of breasts with lobular carcinoma. Arch Pathol 1972;93:164-171.

25. Fechner RE. Lobular carcinoma in situ in sclerosing adenosis. A potential source of confusion with invasive carcinoma. Am J Surg Pathol 1981;5:233-239.

26. Fisher ER, Costantino J, Fisher B, et al. Pathologic findings from the National Surgical Adjuvant Breast Project (NSABP) protocol B-17. Five-year observations concerning lobular carcinoma in situ. Cancer 1996;78:1403–1416.

26a. Fisher ER, Land SR, Fisher B, Mamounas E, Gilarski L, Wolmark N. Pathologic findings from the National Surgical Adjuvant Breast and Bowel Project: twelve-year observations concerning lobular carcinoma in situ. Cancer 2004;100:238-244.

27. Foote FW, Stewart FW. Lobular carcinoma in situ: a rare form of mammary cancer. Am J Pathol 1941;17:491-495.

27a. Gad A, Azzopardi JG. Lobular carcinoma of the breast: a special variant of mucin-secreting carcinoma. J Clin Pathol 1975;28:711-716.

28. Garreau JR, Nelson J, Look R, et al. Risk counseling and management in patients with lobular carcinoma in situ. Am J Surg 2005;189:610-615.

29. Giri DD, Dundas SA, Nottingham JF, Underwood JC. Oestrogen receptors in benign epithelial lesions and intraduct carcinomas of the breast: an immunohistochemical study. Histopathology 1989;15:575-584.

30. Gump FE. Lobular carcinoma in situ. Pathology and treatment. Surg Clin North Am 1990;70:873-883.

31. Haagensen CD. Diseases of the breast, 3rd ed. Philadelphia: WB Saunders; 1986:192-249.

32. Haagensen CD, Lane N, Lattes R. Neoplastic proliferation of the epithelium of the mammary lobules: adenosis, lobular neoplasia, and small cell carcinoma. Surg Clin North Am 1972;52:497-524.

33. Haagensen CD, Lane N, Lattes R, Bodian C. Lobular neoplasia (so-called lobular carcinoma in situ) of the breast. Cancer 1978;42:737-769.

34. Hutter RV. The management of patients with lobular carcinoma in situ of the breast. Cancer 1984;53:798-802.

35. Jacobs TW, Pliss N, Kouria G, Schnitt SJ. Carcinoma in situ of the breast with indeterminate features: role of E-cadherin staining in categorization. Am J Surg Pathol 2001;25:229-236.

36. Lakhani SR, Collins N, Sloane JP, Stratton MR. Loss of heterozygosity in lobular carcinoma in situ of the breast. Clin Mol Pathol 1995;48:M74-M78.

37. Lattes R. Lobular neoplasia (lobular carcinoma in situ) of the breast—a histological entity of controversial clinical significance. Pathol Res Pract 1980;166:415-429.

37a. Leibl S, Regitnig P, Moinfar F. Flat epithelial atypia (DIN1a atypical columnar change): an underdiagnosed entity very frequently co-existing with lobular neoplasia. Histopathology 2007;50:859-865.

38. Li CI, Anderson BO, Daling JR, Moe RE. Changing incidence of lobular carcinoma in situ of the breast. Breast Cancer Res Treat 2002;75:259-268.

38a. Mastracci TL, Shadeo A, Colby SM, et al. Genomic alterations in lobular neoplasia: a microarray comparative genomic hybridization signature for early neoplastic proliferation in the breast. Genes Chromosomes Cancer 2006;45:1007-1017.

39. McDivitt RW, Hutter RV, Foote FW Jr, Stewart FW. In situ lobular carcinoma. A prospective follow-up study indicating cumulative patient risks. JAMA 1967;201:82-86.

40. Middleton LP, Grant S, Stephens T, Stelling CB, Sneige N, Sahin AA. Lobular carcinoma in situ diagnosed by core needle biopsy: when should it be excised? Mod Pathol 2003;16:120-129.

41. Moinfar F, Man YG, Lininger RA, Bodian C, Tavassoli FA. Use of keratin 35betaE12 as an adjunct in the diagnosis of mammary intraepithelial neoplasia-ductal type—benign and malignant intraductal proliferations. Am J Surg Pathol 1999;23:1048-1058.

42. Nayar R, Zhuang Z, Merino MJ, Silverberg SG. Loss of heterozygosity on chromosome 11q13 in lobular lesions of the breast using tissue microdissection and polymerase chain reaction. Hum Pathol 1997;28:277-282.

43. Nesland JM, Holm R, Johannessen JV. Ultrastructural and immunohistochemical features of lobular carcinoma of the breast. J Pathol 1985;145:39-52.

44. Ottesen GL, Graversen HP, Blichert-Toft M, Zedeler K, Andersen JA. Lobular carcinoma in situ of the female breast. Short-term results of a prospective nationwide study. The Danish Breast Cancer Cooperative Group. Am J Surg Pathol 1993;17:14-21.

45. Ozzello L. Ultrastructure of intra-epithelial carcinomas of the breast. Cancer 1971;28:1508-1515.

46. Page DL, Dupont WD. Anatomic markers of human premalignancy and risk of breast cancer. Cancer 1990;66:1326-1335.

47. Page DL, Dupont WD, Rogers LW. Ductal involvement by cells of atypical lobular hyperplasia in the breast: a long term follow-up study of the cancer risk. Hum Pathol 1988;19:201-207.

48. Page DL, Dupont WD, Rogers LW, Rados MS. Atypical hyperplastic lesions of the female breast. A long-term follow-up study. Cancer 1985;55:2698-2708.

49. Page DL, Kidd TE Jr, Dupont WD, Simpson JF, Rogers LW. Lobular neoplasia of the breast: higher risk for subsequent invasive cancer predicted by more extensive disease. Hum Pathol 1991;22:1232-1239.

50. Pallis L, Skoog L, Falkmer U, et al. The DNA profile of breast cancer in situ. Eur J Surg Oncol 1992;18:108-111.

50a. Perrone G, Zagami M, Santini D, et al. COX-2 expression in lobular in situ neoplasia of the breast: correlation with histopathological grading system according to the Tavassoli classification. Histopathology 2007;51:33-39.

51. Pope TL Jr, Fechner RE, Wilhelm MC, Wanebo HJ, de Paredes ES. Lobular carcinoma in situ of the breast: mammographic features. Radiology 1988;168:3-66.

52. Porter PL, Garcia R, Moe R, Corwin DJ, Gown AM. C-erbB-2 oncogene protein in in-situ and invasive lobular neoplasia. Cancer 1991;68:331-334.

53. Ramachandra S, Machin L, Ashley S, Monaghan P, Gusterson BA. Immunohistochemical distribution of c-erbB-2 in in situ breast carcinoma—a detailed morphologic analysis. J Pathol 1990;161:7-14.

54. Renshaw AA, Cartagena N, Derhagopian RP, Gould EW. Lobular neoplasia in breast core needle biopsy specimens is not associated with an increased risk of ductal carcinoma in situ or invasive carcinoma. Am J Clin Pathol 2002;117:797-799.

55. Rosen PP. Coexistent lobular carcinoma in situ and intraductal carcinoma in a single lobular-duct unit. Am J Surg Pathol 1980;4:241-246.

56. Rosen PP. Lobular carcinoma in situ: recent clinicopathologic studies at Memorial Hospital. Pathol Res Pract 1980;166:430-455.

57. Rosen PP, Braun DW Jr, Lyngholm B, Urban JA, Kinne DW. Lobular carcinoma in situ of the breast. Preliminary results of treatment by ipsilateral mastectomy and contralateral breast biopsy. Cancer 1981;47:813-819.

58. Rosen PP, Kosloff C, Lieberman PH, Adair F, Braun DW Jr. Lobular carcinoma in situ of the breast. Detailed analysis of 99 patients with average follow-up of 24 years. Am J Surg Pathol 1978;2:225-251.

59. Rosen PP, Senie RT, Farr GH, Schottenfeld D, Ashikari R. Epidemiology of breast carcinoma: age, menstrual status, and exogenous hormone usage in patients with lobular carcinoma in situ. Surgery 1979;85:219-224.

60. Salhany KE, Page DL. Fine-needle aspiration of mammary lobular carcinoma in situ and atypical lobular hyperplasia. Am J Clin Pathol 1989;92:22-26.

61. Sapino A, Frigerio A, Peterse JL, Arisio R, Coluccia C, Bussolati G. Mammographically detected in situ lobular carcinomas of the breast. Virchows Arch 2000;436:421-430.

62. Sgroi D, Koerner FC. Involvement of collagenous spherulosis by lobular carcinoma in situ. Potential confusion with cribriform ductal carcinoma in situ. Am J Surg Pathol 1995;19:1366-1370.

63. Shelley Hwang E, Nyante SJ, Yi Chen Y, et al. Clonality of lobular carcinoma in situ and synchronous invasive lobular carcinoma. Cancer 2004;100:2562-2572.

64. Shin SJ, Rosen PP. Excisional biopsy should be performed if lobular carcinoma in situ is seen on needle core biopsy. Arch Pathol Lab Med 2002;126:697-701.

64a. Sohn VY, Arthurs ZM, Kim FS, Brown TA. Lobular neoplasia: is surgical excision warranted. Am Surg 2008;74:172-177.

65. Sonnenfeld MR, Frenna TH, Weidner N, Meyer JE. Lobular carcinoma in situ: mammographic-pathologic correlation of results of needle-directed biopsy. Radiology 1991;181:363-367.

66. Sunshine JA, Moseley HS, Fletcher WS, Krippaehne WW. Breast carcinoma in situ. A retrospective review of 112 cases with a minimum 10 year follow-up. Am J Surg 1985;150:44-51.

67. Tavassoli FA. Pathology of the breast, 2nd ed. Stamford, CT: Appleton & Lange; 1999:373-400.

68. Tulusan AH, Egger H, Ober KG. Lobular carcinoma in situ and its relation to invasive breast cancer. In: Zander J, Baltzer J, eds. Early breast cancer. Histopathology, diagnosis, and treatment. New York: Springer-Verlag; 1985:48-51.

69. Urban JA. Bilaterality of cancer of the breast. Biopsy of the opposite breast. Cancer 1967;20:1867-1870.

70. Urban JA. Biopsy of the "normal" breast in treating breast cancer. Surg Clin North Am 1969;49:291-301.

71. Ustun M, Berner A, Davidson B, Risberg B. Fine-needle aspiration cytology of lobular carcinoma in situ. Diagn Cytopathol 2002;27:22-26.

72. Walt AJ, Simon M, Swanson GM. The continuing dilemma of lobular carcinoma in situ. Arch Surg 1992;127:904-909.

73. Wellings SR, Jensen HM, Marcum RG. An atlas of subgross pathology of the human breast with special reference to possible precancerous lesions. J Natl Cancer Inst 1975;55:231-273.

4 DUCTAL INTRAEPITHELIAL NEOPLASIA

Ductal intraepithelial neoplasia (DIN) refers to a group of cytologically and architecturally diverse proliferations confined to the duct system, generally multifocal, and associated with an increased risk for the subsequent development of invasive carcinoma. The magnitude of this risk increases with the increasing grade of the lesion.

Segmentally distributed, most DIN lesions originate in the terminal duct lobular unit (TDLU) (118). A substantially smaller proportion originates in larger and lactiferous ducts; the latter may be associated with Paget's disease through epidermotropic extension to the squamous epithelium of the nipple.

CLASSIFICATION

In the conventional classification, the variety of intraductal epithelial proliferations has been considered as either benign or malignant and divided into three categories: *intraductal hyperplasia* (IDH), *atypical intraductal hyperplasia* (AIDH), and *ductal carcinoma in situ* (DCIS). While several subtypes of DCIS (comedo, cribriform, micropapillary, spindle cell, apocrine, clear cell, and others) are recognized, for a long time the diagnosis of DCIS was either not further qualified or simply subdivided into one of these subtypes.

Gradually, the impact of nuclear grade (82) or nuclear grade and necrosis (55) resulted into a classification system for DCIS with four subtypes: comedo, cribriform with necrosis, comedo with anaplasia, and micropapillary (55). As a further refinement of the grading system, several approaches have been proposed for a three-tier grading system for DCIS (Table 4-1); the number of features used to determine the various grades ranges from a minimum of only two features (necrosis and nuclear atypia) (106,107) to a maximum of 17 features (48). A more rapid rate of recurrence and progression has been noted for higher-grade lesions following conservative therapy. Microcalcification, a common finding in DCIS and a major basis for its mammographic detection, is not a helpful feature in either the morphologic diagnosis or grading of DCIS. The European Commission's Working Group on Breast Pathology found that the most robust histologic features for separating the various grades were high- and low-grade nuclei and necrosis, provided that the latter did not require recognition of a comedo growth pattern (101).

Because of the variety of grading systems and failure to agree on any one as optimal, a consensus conference proposed that regardless of which grading system is used, a number of features should be noted in reporting on DCIS to facilitate communication and understanding of various aspects (20). These features include type, size, overall grade, nuclear grade, and presence or absence of necrosis and microcalcification, along with the proximity to various margins (Table 4-2).

An increased risk for the subsequent development of invasive carcinoma has been determined for the varieties of intraductal proliferative lesions. The magnitude of this risk varies with the severity of the lesion and increases with progression from ordinary hyperplasia (low risk) to high-grade intraductal carcinoma (high risk). Initially, even cases of florid ordinary IDH were designated as AIDH (74); as such, AIDH was not found to be associated with a further increased risk for the subsequent development of invasive carcinoma. Subsequently, IDH was separated from AIDH based on morphologic features, while most AIDH lesions were separated from low-grade DCIS based mainly on the quantity of the proliferation (75,100).

The DIN classification (105a,106) considers all these intraductal proliferations as risk factors, albeit of different magnitude, for the subsequent development of invasive carcinoma. It was Rosai (87) who first suggested applying the concept of intraepithelial neoplasia to mammary intraductal proliferations. With the accumulation of supportive evidence at the immunohistochemical and molecular levels, the intraepithelial neoplasia concept was expanded into a working

67

Table 4-1

SUMMARY OF THE BASIC FEATURES OF VARIOUS THREE-TIERED CLASSIFICATION SYSTEMS FOR DUCTAL CARCINOMA IN SITU (DCIS)

Classification	Low	Grade Intermediate	High
Ottesen et al. 1992 (73) (growth pattern, size, circumscription, stromal fibrosis)	*Microfocal.* DCIS localized to one or more lobules or ducts and measuring 5 mm or less in diameter	*Diffuse.* An ill-defined DCIS at macroscopic and microscopic level exceeding 5 mm with segmental-like distribution; minimal to moderate periductal fibrosis is present	*Tumor Forming.* Compact aggregate of DCIS exceeding 5 mm grossly and with abundant confluent periductal stromal fibrosis
Tavassoli 1992 (107) (nuclear grade, necrosis)	*Low Grade.* Cribriform, solid, and micropapillary patterns; uniform population of cells lacking necrosis or nuclear pleomorphism	*Intermediate Grade.* DCIS lacking cellular atypia and forming solid, cribriform, or micropapillary patterns with either moderate atypia, central necrosis, or minimal amounts of both; many special types of DCIS also fall in this category due to moderate nuclear atypia	*High Grade.* DCIS showing severe cytologic atypia with or without necrosis; includes all comedo carcinomas and signet ring cell variants of intraductal carcinoma and many intraductal apocrine carcinomas
European Pathologists Working Group 1994 (48) (differentiation, nuclear grade, polarization)	*Well Differentiated.* Evenly spaced, markedly polarized, nuclei of uniform size and regular contour with uniformly dispersed fine chromatin, inconspicuous nucleoli, and rare mitotic figures; necrosis absent or minimal; laminated and rarely amorphous calcifications may be present	*Intermediately Differentiated.* Mildly or moderately pleomorphic nuclei with some polarization, and variation in size, contour, and distribution; fine to coarse nuclear chromatin and small nucleoli; occasional mitotic figures; variable central or individual cell necrosis; calcifications amorphous or laminated	*Poorly Differentiated.* Highly pleomorphic, poorly polarized nuclei with irregular contour and distribution, coarse clumped chromatin and prominent nucleoli; mitotic figures common; centeral and individual cell necrosis often present; amorphous calcification common
Van Nuys 1995 (84, 96) (nuclear grade and size, necrosis)	*Nonhigh Grade without Necrosis.* The proliferating cells have low- or intermediate-grade nuclei; there is no comedo necrosis	*Nonhigh Grade with Necrosis.* Low-grade nuclei (1-1.5 red blood cells in diameter) with inconspicuous nucleoli and diffuse chromatin or intermediate-grade nuclei (1-2 red blood cells) with occasional nucleoli, coarse chromatin, and comedo type necrosis; individual necrotic cells not accepted	*High Grade.* High-grade nuclei (> 2 red blood cells in diameter) with $\geq$ 1 nucleoli; comedo necrosis is surrounded by either large pleomorphic cells or cribriform and micropapillary patterns; necrosis may be absent

Table 4-2

PATHOLOGIC FEATURES OF DIN 1-3/DCIS THAT SHOULD BE INCLUDED IN THE SURGICAL PATHOLOGY REPORT SINCE THEY VARIABLY IMPACT MANAGEMENT/OUTCOME

Type of lesion: cribriform, micropapillary, solid, apocrine (apocrine lesions are estrogen receptor [ER] and progesterone receptor [PR] negative, but androgen receptor [AR] positive; important for hormonal therapies)

Size/extent/distribution of disease (small, localized lesions are better)

Necrosis (present or absent)

Nuclear grade (1, 2, 3)

Overall grade of lesion and proportion of highest grade when more than one grade is present (higher-grade lesions recur faster and more frequently)

Marginal status (positive or specify distance to the nearest lesion)

ER and PR status

Table 4-3

TRANSLATIONAL TABLE FOR CONVERSION OF THE TRADITIONAL CLASSIFICATION TO THE DUCTAL INTRAEPITHELIAL NEOPLASIA (DIN) CLASSIFICATION

Traditional	DIN	Reexcision, if in core or at margin
Intraductal hyperplasia[a]	DIN, low risk	No
Flat epithelial atypia	flat DIN1	No[b]
Atypical intraductal hyperplasia	DIN1, quantify (≤2mm)	Yes
Ductal carcinoma in situ, grade 1 (low grade)	DIN1, quantify (>2mm)	Yes
Ductal carcinoma in situ, grade 2 (intermediate grade)	DIN2, quantify	Yes
Ductal carcinoma in situ, grade 3 (high grade)	DIN3, quantify	Yes

[a]Recent molecular studies confirm earlier studies that a proportion of intraductal hyperplasia lesions are clonal and share molecular alterations with the more advanced lesions, supporting a neoplastic nature (50,61).

[b]When extensive with rare micropapillae (minimal AIDH), reexcision may be prudent; some prefer to reexcise when flat epithelial atypia is extensive regardless of the presence or absence of micropapillae. Sufficient data on the management of flat DIN1 do not exist.

Table 4-4

EXTENT OF LOSS OF HETEROZYGOSITY (LOH) IN VARIOUS GRADES OF DUCTAL INTRAEPITHELIAL NEOPLASIA (DIN)[a]

Grade of DIN	LOH at Any One Locus	Overall LOH at Multiple Loci (No. of Loci)	Total Number of Cases Evaluated
IDH = DIN, low risk (-CA)[b]	1-12%	37% (15)	163
IDH = DIN, low risk (+CA)	0-20%	40% (15)	48
DIN1, flat (-CA) (flat epithelial atypia)	0-50%	78% (8)	9
DIN1, flat (+CA) (flat epithelial atypia)	25-57%	77% (8)	13
ADH = DIN1, ≤2mm (-CA)	0-15%	42% (15)	26
ADH = DIN1, ≤2mm (+CA)	0-38%	44% (15)	25
Noncomedo DCIS (-CA) (DIN1, >2mm and DIN2)	2-35%	70% (15)	67
Noncomedo DCIS (+CA)c (DIN1, >2mm and DIN2)	0-75%	93% (15)	14
Comedo DCIS (-CA) (DIN2 and DIN3)	0-39%	79% (15)	42
Comedo DCIS (+CA) (DIN2 and DIN3)	0-44%	79% (15)	14

[a]Adapted from reference 69 (assessed all lesions, but DIN1, flat type = flat epithelial atypia) and reference 66 (assessed DIN1, flat type = flat epithelia atypia only).

[b]IDH = intraductal hyperplasia; -CA = without an associated invasive carcinoma; +CA = associated with invasive carcinoma.

classification for both ductal (DIN) and lobular (lobular intraepithelial neoplasia [LIN]) lesions (106,107). A translational table providing the equivalents in the traditional systems for various grades of DIN enables one to convert easily from one system to the other (Table 4-3).

The DIN classification system considers all of these intraductal proliferations as neoplasms since none serves a physiologic purpose, none is known to be reversible, and all share some molecular features of invasive carcinoma. It is emphasized that a neoplasm may be either benign or malignant. As such, IDH/low-risk DIN has a benign course, while grade 3 DCIS/DIN3 is more likely to follow an aggressive course, particularly if incompletely excised. The only unequivocal hyperplastic process in the breast is gestational hyperplasia, a reversible process that is induced by the hormonal alterations of pregnancy and subsides once the hormonal stimulation has ceased.

As molecular data accumulate, it appears that the term hyperplasia has been used inappropriately in the conventional system for "atypical" and most probably also for "ordinary" hyperplasias. Some investigators require molecular alterations similar to those of clearcut in situ and invasive carcinoma or clonality to designate a proliferation as neoplastic. The presence of molecular alterations or clonality in a significant number of ordinary intraductal hyperplasias studied by comparative genomic hybridization (CGH) further supports the inclusion of IDH among neoplasias (3,44,50).

It has been argued that too few of the ordinary hyperplasias show evidence of clonal expansion or loss of heterozygosity (LOH) to qualify as a neoplastic process. As shown in Table 4-4, however, nearly the same proportion of IDH and AIDH lesions show LOH at loci altered in DCIS and invasive carcinomas. Using high-resolution chromosome 3p allelotyping, 7 of 25 (28 percent) IDH lesions studied had LOH of at least one 3p locus compared to 87 percent of invasive carcinomas and 92 percent of DCIS cases (61). Interestingly, nearly 20 percent of even unequivocal low- or high-grade DCIS lesions fail to show LOH for the loci assessed (69). Therefore, if molecular alterations were a requirement or justification for considering a process neoplastic, even some of the DCIS lesions would not qualify as neoplastic. It is quite possible that the low-risk IDH lesions have distinctive alterations such as expression of high molecular weight cytokeratin (CK) 5 (9) and lead to distinctive types of invasive carcinoma, albeit rarely and slowly; clearly, we have not yet identified these molecular alterations in their entirety. Expression of CK5 mRNA, as validated by immunoreactivity with monoclonal antibodies to CK5/6, has been associated with poor clinical outcome, and positivity for CK17 and CK5 is also believed to identify a group of breast carcinomas with poor clinical outcome (113). Therefore, it is likely that IDH progresses to its own distinctive type of invasive carcinoma, albeit on rare occasions. There are probably a multitude of additional molecular changes even in AIDH and DCIS that have not been detected or identified by current methodologies.

Early attempts at classification of a small number of ductal carcinomas in situ by gene expression profiling have shown upregulation of bcl-2 (an antiapoptotic protein) in low-grade lesions, and upregulation of HER2 in 43 percent of high-grade DCIS lesions. Ultimate subdivision of DCIS into two groups (low grade and high grade) was proposed after supervised classification. The four groups of DCIS (well, well-intermediately, intermediately-poorly, and poorly differentiated) were rearranged into two groups by combining the first two into a well-differentiated group and the last two into a poorly differentiated DCIS (45a).

The DIN classification system combines AIDH and low-grade DCIS based on its consideration of AIDH as a smaller version or a more limited quantity of low-grade DCIS. By providing the size of the DIN1 lesion, this approach allows for variation in management based on lesion size, since smaller lesions often do not have the same clinical implications as larger ones. It avoids the use of different terms merely because of differences in lesion size. By analogy, it is well accepted that a small, 3.0-mm invasive breast carcinoma does not behave and is not managed the same way as a larger, 2.8-cm invasive carcinoma. Nonetheless, both are designated as invasive carcinomas.

The suggestion that the separation of AIDH from low-grade DCIS is justified since carcinomas that develop post-AIDH may occur in either breast while those following low-grade DCIS occur in the same breast (74,75,88) is questionable. If this claim were true, then there should be a higher incidence of contralateral breast carcinomas among low-grade DCIS cases at institutions where a single space completely involved by either cribriform or micropapillary patterns is sufficient for a diagnosis of low-grade DCIS, contrary to the requirement of two spaces by Page et al. (76). Over a period of 23 years, three publications have appeared on this topic based on a group of 28 women with a median follow-up of 31 years (74,75,88). They note that the invasive carcinomas that occur following low-grade DCIS treated by biopsy alone develop in the same breast and in the same quadrant from which the original DCIS specimen was taken. Eleven of the 28 women (39.3 percent) developed subsequent invasive carcinoma, 5 of whom died of metastatic disease. Seven of these were diagnosed within 10 years of the DCIS biopsy, 1 was diagnosed within 12 years, and the remaining 3 developed infiltrating carcinomas over 23 to 42 years (88). The authors conclude that these results indicate a striking dividing point biologically and histopathologically between low-grade DCIS and the cytologically similar but smaller lesions of AIDH (88).

We believe, however, upon careful review of reference 75 in which the macroscopic and microscopic features of these cases are described in detail, that a significant proportion of patients who died within 10 years probably had residual disease after resection and/or higher-grade DCIS. The outcome of these inadequately sampled 28 cases of allegedly "low-grade DCIS," with clearly undetermined margins, undocumented extent, and even poorly documented in situ status, appears worse than the 22 percent frequency of

Table 4-5

ADVANTAGES OF THE DUCTAL INTRAEPITHELIAL NEOPLASIA (DIN) CLASSIFICATION

1. It diminishes the impact of having two drastically different designations of cancer and noncancer applied to the same lesion by different observers.

2. It incorporates the flat epithelial atypias that have been proven to have molecular alterations similar to those of cells in low-grade ductal carcinoma in situ (DCIS) and tubular carcinoma in the classification system as flat DIN1, while the high-grade polymorphous flat lesions are categorized as DIN3.

3. It allows for management approaches based on the size/extent of distribution of either the low- or higher-grade lesions.

4. It diminishes the anxiety and emotional stress associated with a diagnosis of cancer for the patient and her family, while allowing for an individualized approach to managing the disease.

5. It eliminates the term cancer and the likelihood of mastectomy—a possibility that persists due to geographic variations in practice standards even for small low-grade DCIS lesions.

6. It applies the unifying concept of intraepithelial neoplasia as it is already used in many other organs including cervix, vagina, vulva, prostate, pancreas, and colorectum.

7. Modifications can be made easily as we learn more about distinctive subgroups within the system.

8. DIN obviates upstaging up to 63% of core biopsy diagnoses from atypical intraductal hyperplasia (AIDH) to grade 1 DCIS on subsequent excisional biopsies.

subsequent invasive carcinoma observed among a group of 130 women without prior breast carcinomas and with varied types of DCIS lesions definitely inclusive of high-grade DCIS following local excision alone who had at least 3 years of follow-up (5). Thus, we believe that it is far more likely that the studies reported in references 74, 75, and 88 reflect the natural history of a wide variety of intraductal carcinomas including some low-grade DCIS; therefore, these studies do not provide any support for separating AIDH from low-grade DCIS.

A simpler explanation for any differences in the frequency of subsequent progression between AIDH and low-grade DCIS would be that a minuscule lesion, once totally removed, results in near equalization of the risk for the subsequent development of carcinoma in the two breasts of that individual patient. A more extensive process is less likely to be completely excised, leading to the development of recurrences at the same site due to residual disease.

The 28 patients in these three studies (74,75,88) probably already had more advanced disease that was missed due to highly inadequate sampling of the specimen. This speculation is supported by a recent study of epithelial atypia in biopsies performed for microcalcifications (23b); in this study, where thorough sampling was a crucial step, 31 percent of the cases with epithelial atypia had concomitant carcinoma (DCIS/DIN1, microinvasive and invasive carcinoma).

The DIN classification does not necessarily imply a continuous progression from one grade to the next, but rather a progression in level of risk for the subsequent development of invasive carcinoma. A proportion of these intraepithelial neoplasias, the precise quantity of which has not been established, may progress from a lower grade to higher grades, however. The finding of various stages in the same biopsy and the identification of shared molecular features among some of the higher- and lower-grade lesions (Table 4-4) (54,69) support this. While any of these lesions has the potential to progress to an invasive carcinoma and may serve as a marker or precursor of such, none necessarily represents an obligate precursor of invasive carcinoma within the current life expectancy of most women, with the probable exception of grade 3 DCIS/DIN3.

Based on routine morphologic assessment, the most readily visible evidence for progression or continuity is noted within the DIN1 category, in which cases of flat epithelial atypia/flat DIN1 advance to AIDH and low-grade DCIS/DIN1 through development of epithelial tufts and bridges. Further advancement to grade 2 DCIS/DIN2 is noted through the development of either focal intraluminal necrosis or focal moderate nuclear pleomorphism. Most low-grade intraepithelial lesions remain low grade on recurrence and develop into a low-grade invasive carcinoma when they invade, while the high-grade intraepithelial lesions develop into intermediate or high-grade invasive carcinomas (7,65,103). Recurrent DCIS lesions may and do acquire additional molecular changes (58,115), but this is not always readily reflected in the phenotype of the lesion. The frequency of invasive carcinoma (ductal or lobular) increases from 2 percent in association with IDH/low-risk DIN to 37 percent for grades 2 and 3 DCIS/DIN2 and 3 (13).

From a psychological standpoint, it has been shown that women who are diagnosed as having DCIS suffer the same level of anxiety and depression as those with a diagnosis of invasive breast carcinoma (86). The DIN classification has eliminated the emotionally charged term "carcinoma" from the designation, potentially preventing such distress; the advantages of using the term DIN are listed in Table 4-5.

There is clearly significant confusion as to the nature of DCIS. In a review of the complexities and challenges of ductal carcinoma in situ, Leonard and Swain (58a) state "Although DCIS is a benign disease, women with DCIS have an increased propensity to develop invasive disease..." One wonders why we should call a benign disease cancer? Similarly, a recent textbook that beautifully illustrates DCIS is entitled "Preneoplasia of the Breast," implying that DCIS is not even neoplastic (8a). One might argue that the entire normal breast is in a potentially "preneoplastic" state!

Whichever terminology (traditional or DIN) is used, it is suggested that the alternative system be provided as well until familiarity with the DIN system obviates the need of any other terminology, in the same manner that transition from the older terminology to the currently accepted designations of cervical, vulvar, vaginal, and prostatic intraepithelial neoplasia has taken place. In her practice, the author of this chapter gives preference to DIN and puts the traditional system in parentheses. As the first step in the application of the new DIN terminology, however, in this book, the conventional classification is noted first followed by a slash and the DIN equivalent. The simultaneous use will facilitate and expedite the ultimate switch to the DIN system. With modification of the "in situ carcinoma" terminology to "intraepithelial neoplasia," the TNM classification also should be modified to Tin rather than Tis (113a).

ROUTE OF LESION PROGRESSION

DIN progresses within the duct system from its origin in a TDLU, toward the nipple, and into adjacent branches of a given segment of the duct system (70–72). The rare lesions that develop within the lactiferous ducts may progress toward the nipple, resulting in Paget's disease, or to the adjacent branches of the reference duct. Progression beyond the duct system and into the surrounding stroma may occur at any point along the intraductal route in DCIS/DIN1-3. This important feature should be utilized in the surgical excision of the lesion (70–72).

EPIDEMIOLOGY AND PREDISPOSING (RISK) FACTORS

Proliferative changes are present in nearly 60 percent of breast biopsies. The reported frequency of atypical proliferations ranges from 1.7 to 19.0 percent of breast biopsies (10,26, 27,53,57,76,77). DCIS/DIN1-3 of the breast has been reported in 12.6 percent (6) to 14.0 percent (68) of forensic autopsies. The precise frequency of atypia is difficult to determine, however, and the range reflects variations in criteria or in application of the same criteria. In general, the factors that are associated with an increased risk for the development of invasive breast carcinoma are also associated with an increased risk for the development of various grades of DIN (51,57,89).

A substantial increase in the prevalence of DCIS/DIN1-3 lesions has been noted with the introduction of widespread screening mammography. The average annual increase in the incidence rate of DCIS in the decade of 1973 to 1982 was 3.9 percent compared to 17.5 percent annually in the decade between 1983 to 1992, increasing from 2.4/100,000 women in 1973 to 15.8/100,000 in 1992 for women of all races, an overall increase of 557 percent (31). In the United States, the proportion of breast carcinomas diagnosed as DCIS increased from 2.8 percent in 1973 to 14.4 percent in 1995 (32). Nearly 60 percent of mammographically detected lesions are noncomedo type and this percentage is increasing. Among women 40 to 84 years of age, approximately 20 percent of breast cancers detected by mammographic screening are DCIS: approximately, 1 in every 1,300 screening mammographic examinations leads to a diagnosis of DCIS/DIN1-3 (30).

Absolute Risk

Between 2.6 percent (53,110) and 10.0 percent (9,25) of women with intraepithelial proliferative breast lesions develop an invasive carcinoma. Among those with IDH/low-risk DIN, 2.6 percent develop subsequent invasive carcinoma within an average interval of 14.3 years (110). Following a breast biopsy diagnosis of AIDH/DIN1 ($\leq$2 mm), 3.7 percent to 22.0 percent of the women develop an invasive carcinoma within 8.3 years (9,27,54,110). On the other hand, AIDH/DIN1 is also present in 2.2 percent (80) to 10.5 percent (59) of controls who do not develop subsequent carcinoma. Among women with all types of DCIS/DIN1-3 treated with lumpectomy alone, the incidence of ipsilateral invasive breast cancer is 13.4 percent (37). Despite this elevated risk, most women with DCIS/DIN1-3 do not develop an invasive carcinoma within the first 10 to 15 years after diagnosis (30,32).

Relative Risk

Women with IDH/low-risk DIN have a low risk (relative risk [RR], 1.6 to 1.9) for the subsequent development of invasive carcinoma (8,63,74). The highest relative risk reported for flat epithelial atypia/flat DIN1 has been 1.1 (33). Using the same criteria, drastically different RR figures, ranging from a low of 2.4 to a high of 13.0 (15,25, 59,62,63,76,80), have been reported for AIDH/ DIN1 ($\leq$2 mm); the RR of 2.4 is closer to the RR of 1.9 associated with IDH/low-risk DIN (63), while the RR of 13 is even higher than the RR of 8 to 11 suggested for DCIS/DIN1-3 (26,27).

The Cancer Committee of the College of American Pathologists (39) has assigned IDH/ low-risk DIN a slightly increased RR value (1.5 to 2.0) for the subsequent development of invasive carcinoma. AIDH/DIN1 ($\leq$2 mm) was assigned to a moderately increased risk (4.0 to 5.0) category. A meta-analysis of 15 reports containing 182,980 women found an overall odds ratio (OR) of 3.67 (95 percent confidence interval [CI] = 3.16–4.26) for AIDH/DIN1 ($\leq$2 mm) (60).

CLINICAL FEATURES

The age range of women with DIN is wide and spans 8 decades postadolescence. DIN is extremely rare prior to puberty; when it occurs in infants and children, it is generally a reflection of exogenous or abnormal endogenous hormonal stimulation. The mean age of patients with DCIS/DIN1-3 lesions is between 50 and 59 years. Although most often unilateral, about 22 percent of women with DCIS in one breast develop either in situ or invasive carcinoma in the contralateral breast (116). Prior to the introduction of screening mammography, 50 to 65 percent of women presented with a palpable mass (2,119). While presentation with a palpable mass continues to occur, the proportion of lesions that present as a mass has decreased in countries where screening mammography is widely utilized. An increasing number of these lesions is detected mammographically. Approximately 1 in every 1,300 screening mammography examinations leads to a diagnosis of DCIS/DIN1-3 (30). Patients who present with nipple discharge appear to have more aggressive lesions, possibly indicating a more advanced/extensive process, i.e., extension of the lesion from its origin in the TDLU to the major and lactiferous ducts.

MAMMOGRAPHIC DETECTION

Among mammographically detected nonpalpable lesions, 25 to 30 percent are DCIS/DIN1-3 (18,47,83). Of carcinomas detected on the initial screening mammography, about 20 percent (range, 8 to 43 percent) are DCIS/DIN1-3 (30,95). The presence of microcalcifications is the major basis of mammographic detection (72 to 98 percent) for DCIS/DIN1-3 lesions (24,49,104). Approximately 15 percent of DCIS/DIN1-3 lesions are incidental findings in biopsies performed for other unrelated and usually palpable lesions (18,81,95).

The mammographic calcifications in DCIS/ DIN1-3 form linear casts, clustered granularities with either a "crushed stone" or a powdery appearance, or a combination of the two. The clustered or dispersed arrangement may outline the distribution of one or more branching involved ducts (fig. 4-1) (104). The linear, branching casts are more frequently encountered among the comedo variant of grade 3 DCIS/DIN3, whereas clustered granularity, occasionally with a "snakeskin" pattern corresponding to cribriform architecture, is more common among the lower-grade non-necrotic DCIS/DIN1 lesions (34). About 17 percent of the lesions lack histologic evidence of microcalcifications (43); a significant proportion of these are non-necrotic, low-grade DCIS/DIN1. Because microcalcifications

Figure 4-1

DUCTAL CARCINOMA IN SITU (DCIS)/ DUCTAL INTRAEPITHELIAL NEOPLASIA (DIN)

Mammographically, microcalcifications in the form of linear, branching casts (A) are more commonly observed in the comedo variant of grade 3 DCIS/DIN3. Clustered granularity, which on rare occasion forms a "snakeskin" appearance (B,C), is more common in low-grade DCIS/ DIN1. (4-1B courtesy of Dr. Enzo Lattanzio, Bari, Italy.)

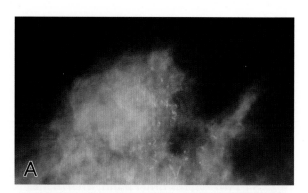

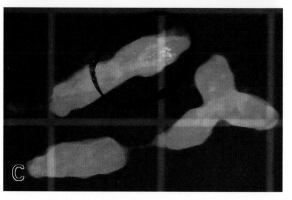

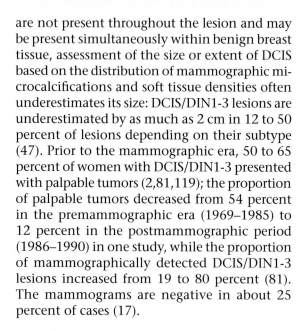

are not present throughout the lesion and may be present simultaneously within benign breast tissue, assessment of the size or extent of DCIS based on the distribution of mammographic microcalcifications and soft tissue densities often underestimates its size: DCIS/DIN1-3 lesions are underestimated by as much as 2 cm in 12 to 50 percent of lesions depending on their subtype (47). Prior to the mammographic era, 50 to 65 percent of women with DCIS/DIN1-3 presented with palpable tumors (2,81,119); the proportion of palpable tumors decreased from 54 percent in the premammographic era (1969–1985) to 12 percent in the postmammographic period (1986–1990) in one study, while the proportion of mammographically detected DCIS/DIN1-3 lesions increased from 19 to 80 percent (81). The mammograms are negative in about 25 percent of cases (17).

FINE NEEDLE ASPIRATION CYTOLOGY OF PROLIFERATIVE BREAST DISEASE WITH AND WITHOUT ATYPIA

While separation of low-risk lesions (non-proliferative breast disease and proliferative breast disease without atypia) from high-risk lesions is possible, further separation into more distinctive groups is associated with difficulty and lack of interobserver agreement (94). There are a number of features that allow a distinction of proliferative breast disease without atypia (PBD) from proliferative breast disease with atypia (PBDA)/DCIS. Compared with PBD, PBDA/DCIS smears are more likely to be cellular, and have single cells, necrosis, nuclear overlap, cytoplasmic vacuoles, large nuclei, macronucleoli, pleomorphism, and hyperchromasia. PBD is more likely to form monolayers and complex cell groups, and display swirling and cohesion, with myoepithelial cells present both in the epithelial sheets and the background (41). A recent study by Sauer et al. (90) noted that it is even possible to specify the subtype of DCIS if the samples are carefully assessed for nuclear size; monolayer sheets; solid, cribriform, micropapillary, and papillary aggregates; comedo type necrosis; microcalcifications; myoepithelial cells; and dyscohesion. The patterns identified in the smears correlate with the histologic pattern. Monolayer sheets are interpreted as the equivalent of a flat growth pattern in 49 percent of histologic specimens from nonhigh-grade DCIS and 16 percent of high-grade DCIS lesions.

Table 4-6
INTRADUCTAL HYPERPLASIA/LOW-RISK DUCTAL INTRAEPITHELIAL NEOPLASIA (DIN)

Architectural Features
  Irregular fenestrations
  Peripheral fenestrations
  Stretched or twisted epithelial bridges
  Streaming
  Uneven distribution of nuclei and overlapped nuclei

Cellular Features[a]
  Multiple cell types
  Variation in appearance of epithelial cells
  Indistinct cell margins and deviation from a round
    contour
  Variation in the appearance of nuclei

[a]One of the most important indicators of low-risk DIN is the presence of an admixture of two or more cell types (epithelial, myoepithelial, and metaplastic apocrine cells) in the proliferation.

Table 4-7
ATYPICAL INTRADUCTAL HYPERPLASIA, NONAPOCRINE TYPE/DUCTAL INTRAEPITHELIAL NEOPLASIA (DIN), (≤2 MM)

Architectural Features
  Arcade, cribriform, and/or micropapillary pattern
    involving anywhere from part of a single duct to
    multiple ducts or ductules (measurement of lesion
    size is required).
  High molecular weight cytokeratin (CK34betaE12) is
    extremely useful in unmasking atypical cells in both
    DIN1, flat type and DIN1 lesions with intraluminal
    projections.

Cellular Features
  Monotonous, uniform rounded cell population
  Subtle increase in nuclear-cytoplasmic ratio
  Equidistant or highly organized nuclear distribution
  Round nuclei
  Hyperchromasia may or may not be present

PATHOLOGIC FEATURES

Gross Findings

Most DIN lesions, particularly those detected mammographically, are not evident on macroscopic inspection of the specimen. A small proportion of grade 3 DCIS/DIN3 lesions are extensive enough and contain such an abundance of intraluminal necrosis that they are detectable as multiple areas of round, pale comedonecrosis or a firm, gritty mass.

Microscopic Findings

The criteria for the diagnosis of several of the more difficult grades of intraductal proliferation are illustrated in Tables 4-6 and 4-7 (110). Proper assessment of the lesions requires evaluation of both architectural features at low magnification and cytologic features at higher magnification. Grading of DIN relies on the assessment of cytologic features, and to a lesser extent, the presence or absence of intraluminal necrosis. The myoepithelial cell layer generally persists, but may become very attenuated with increased size of intermyoepithelial cell gaps (patchy loss of myoepithelial cells). The surrounding basement membrane is also generally retained. A myxoid periductal stromal change may develop around the ducts in the higher-grade lesions, particularly grade 3 DCIS/DIN3; this may be associated with significant lymphoplasmacytic infiltration. Both the myxoid change and the pronounced

lymphoplasmacytic infiltrate contribute to the size of the mass when the lesions are palpable. A range of DIN lesions is often present in a given biopsy.

IDH/Low-Risk DIN. Architecturally, this lesion is characterized by irregularly shaped, variably sized and often peripherally distributed fenestrations, with streaming of the central bolus of cells (figs. 4-2–4-5). Epithelial bridges are thin and stretched; nuclei are unevenly distributed. Cytologically, the lesion is composed of cells with indistinct cell margins, variation in the tinctorial features of the cytoplasm, and characteristic variation in shape and size of the nuclei (Table 4-6). An admixture of epithelial, myoepithelial, and metaplastic apocrine cells may occur (fig. 4-4). The presence or absence of either microcalcifications or necrosis does not impact on the diagnosis; the latter is a frequent cause of misdiagnosis as grade 2 DCIS/DIN2. IDH/low-risk DIN shows a diffuse or mosaic pattern of immunoreactivity with high molecular weight cytokeratin (CK) 34betaE12 (fig. 4-2C) and CK5/6. The myoepithelial cell layer persists (fig. 4-5).

Flat Epithelial Atypia/Flat DIN1. Flat epithelial atypia is characterized by replacement of the native epithelial cells by either one layer of atypical cells, often with apical snouts, or proliferation of a monotonous atypical cell population in the form of stratification of uniform cells with round, ovoid, or spindled nuclei, generally of

Figure 4-2

INTRADUCTAL HYPERPLASIA (IDH)/LOW-RISK DIN

A: Solid and fenestrated areas are seen.

B: The secondary spaces are variable in size and shape. The nuclei are irregularly distributed and bland.

C: Immunostain for CK34betaE12 is positive in most cells.

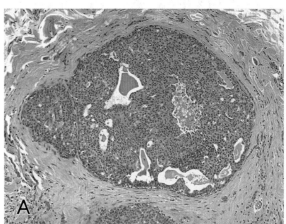

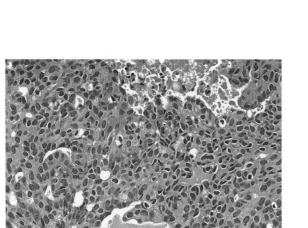

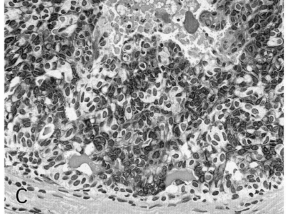

three to five cell layers with occasional mounding (fig. 4-6). The atypical cells are similar to those of AIDH and low-grade DCIS/DIN1. The ducts involved are often variably distended and may contain secretory or floccular material and/ or lamellar microcalcifications (fig. 4-7). The myoepithelial cell layer, although invariably present, is generally not prominent.

This pattern has also been referred to as "clinging carcinoma" (4). It was designated in 1992, in the American literature, as flat epithelial atypia because of the replacement of the native epithelial cell layer by atypical cells without intraluminal projections or bridging (107). Subsequently, this lesion was included among variants of columnar alterations with prominent apical snouts (40). A wide variety of mammary epithelial cells are columnar in their native state, however, with or without apical snouts; making the designation of "columnar alterations" imprecise. It is the presence of cytologic atypia comparable to that of low-grade DCIS/DIN1 that is the relevant

feature of flat epithelial atypias; mitotic figures are rarely observed (fig. 4-8).

More recently, the spectrum of columnar cell alterations has been subdivided into four or six categories to accommodate the fact that atypia is present in some of these lesions, with preference given to the WHO proposed designation of flat epithelial atypia by one group (91). A word of caution to readers of such articles: inclusion of examples of atypical IDH characterized by arcades and micropapillae among flat epithelial atypia would render any findings attributed to the lesion irrelevant. We believe that subdivision of flat epithelial atypia/flat DIN into various categories is unnecessary and likely to cause more confusion than help with the diagnosis of this lesion. The pathologist should focus on recognizing this flat pattern of atypia regardless of the setting in which it is found; furthermore, as soon as a single epithelial micropapilla or arcade develops, the lesion is no longer flat epithelial atypia/flat DIN1, but rather, minimal AIDH/DIN1 (≤2 mm).

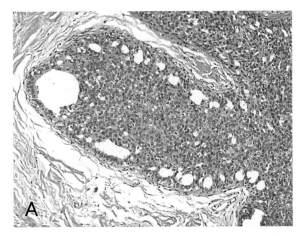

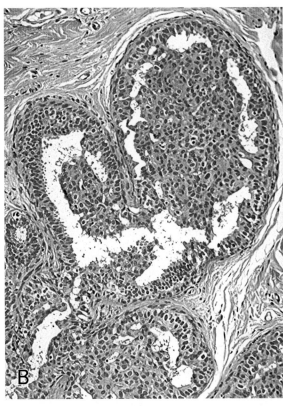

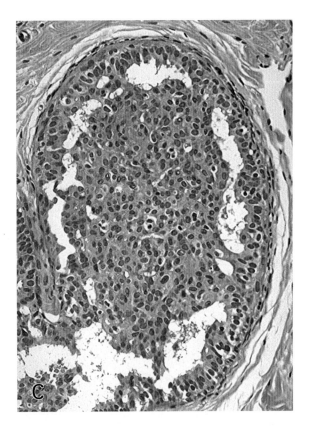

Figure 4-3

IDH/LOW-RISK DIN

A: Numerous irregularly shaped secondary spaces are peripherally distributed.

B: A solid bolus of central epithelial proliferation is surrounded by a residual lumen at the periphery.

C: The nuclei of the proliferating cells are banal and irregularly distributed, overlapping in some areas.

The atypical cells fail to immunoreact with CK34betaE12 or CK5/6, but are generally positive for ER. Flat epithelial atypia/flat DIN1 is detected increasingly in core biopsies—approximately 8.5 percent of 736 core needle biopsies in a recent study (62a). Whether or not reexcision should be performed when this is the only lesion and the cause of mammographic detection (often due to microcalcifications) is not well established. In this situation, evaluation of deeper levels is advised to exclude the presence of a more advanced process.

Periodic follow-up for 3 years (mammography at 6-month intervals) is advised for early detection of any carcinomas (62a). In a study of 2,628 excisional biopsies with various forms of DIN, lobular intraepithelial neoplasia (LIN) was associated with flat epithelial atypia/ flat DIN1 in 26 percent of cases (13). Interestingly, flat epithelial atypia/flat DIN1 is often multifocal, similar to the multifocality of LIN, and it also shares some of the molecular alterations noted in LIN (66).

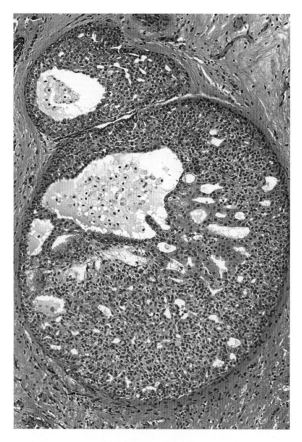

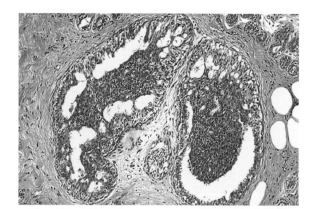

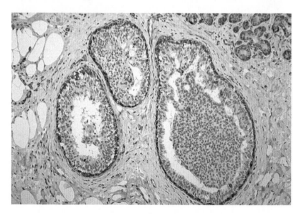

Figure 4-5

IDH/LOW-RISK DIN

Top: The characteristic pattern of ordinary IDH is evident.

Bottom: Retention of the myoepithelial cell layer is evident with an immunostain for smooth muscle actin.

Figure 4-4

IDH/LOW-RISK DIN

This lesion shows an admixture of metaplastic apocrine cells and proliferating epithelial cells.

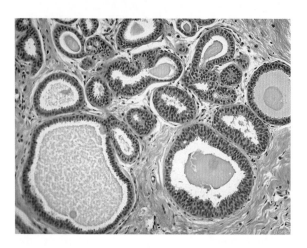

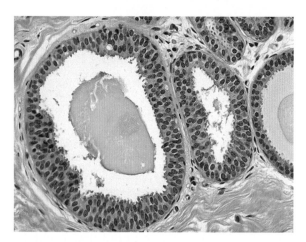

Figure 4-6

FLAT EPITHELIAL ATYPIA/FLAT DIN1

Left: Some of the spaces in a terminal duct lobular unit are distended.

Right: The native epithelial cell layer is replaced by a flat proliferation of stratified columnar cells.

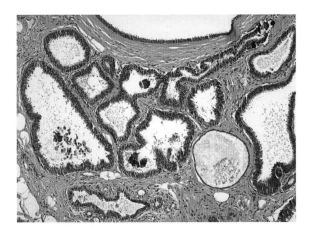
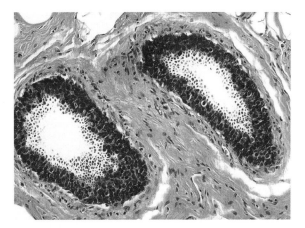

Figure 4-7

FLAT EPITHELIAL ATYPIA/FLAT DIN1

Left: Some of the distended ductules contain microcalcifications.
Right: The ductules are lined by two to three layers of mildly atypical cells.

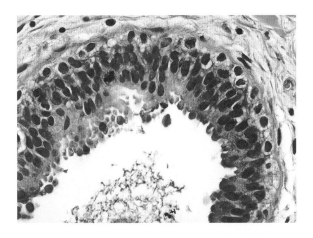
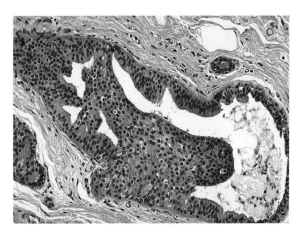

Figure 4-8

FLAT EPITHELIAL ATYPIA/FLAT DIN1
Occasional mitotic figures are present.

Figure 4-9

ATYPICAL INTRADUCTAL HYPERPLASIA (AIDH)/DIN1

The ductal spaces are partially involved by a proliferation of uniform cells overlying flat epithelial atypia.

At the molecular level, flat epithelial atypia/flat DIN1 has shown LOH at the same loci as seen for in situ and invasive ductal carcinoma, even when it is present as the only lesion in a biopsy. The most common alterations are at chromosomes 11q21-23 (50 percent), 16q23.1-24.2 (45 percent), and 3p14.2 (41 percent) (66). These alterations suggest that flat epithelial atypia/flat DIN1 reflects the earliest morphologically recognizable neoplastic alteration in the breast. These molecular alterations, first noted in an Armed Forces Institute of Pathology (AFIP) study in 2000 (66), have been confirmed in a subsequent study (98).

AIDH and Grade 1 DCIS/DIN1. The most distinctive feature of this lesion is the proliferation of evenly distributed, monomorphic cells, with generally ovoid to rounded nuclei, which protrude into, bridge across, or fill the duct lumens. These cells are similar to those seen in flat epithelial atypia/flat DIN1. The cells grow in micropapillae, tufts, fronds, arcades, Roman bridges, and solid and cribriform patterns (figs. 4-9–4-12). Lesion size is assessed by measurement of duct cross sections completely involved by one of these patterns; lesions of partially

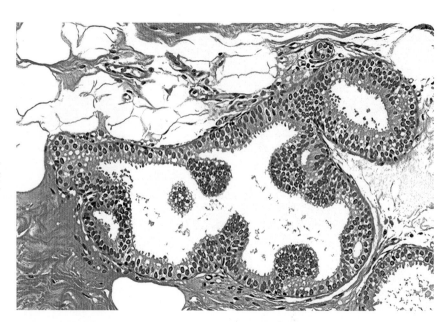

Figure 4-10

AIDH/DIN1

The ductal spaces are partially involved by a proliferation of uniform cells in a micropapillary pattern.

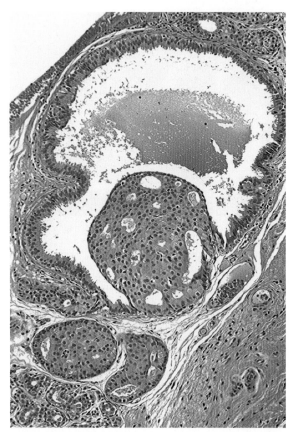

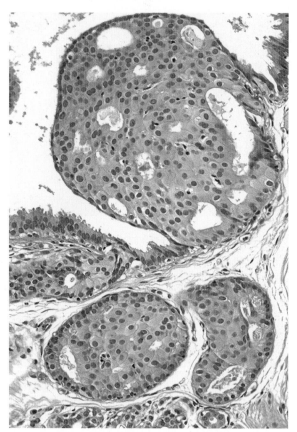

Figure 4-11

AIDH/DIN1, ≤2 MM

Left: Partial involvement of a distended ductal space by a proliferation of uniform cells.

Right: Higher magnification shows cells with relatively uniform rounded nuclei polarized around secondary lumens. One minuscule adjacent duct in cross section is completely involved by a similar proliferation.

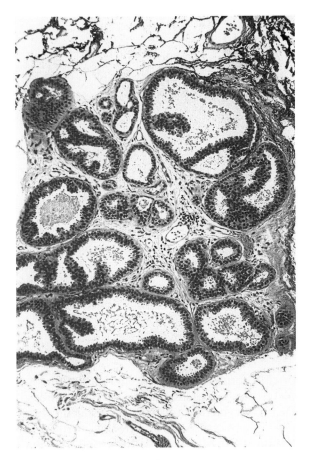

Figure 4-12

AIDH/DIN1, ≤2 MM

Partial involvement of ducts by a few micropapillae or epithelial bridges in a background of flat epithelial atypia.

involved ducts are placed in the AIDH/DIN1 (≤2 mm) category and are not measured.

In the traditional system, lesions are designated as AIDH when: characteristic cells are admixed with the pattern and/or cells of ordinary hyperplasia; there is partial duct involvement by classic cribriform/arcade morphology; characteristic cytology and architecture completely involve either only one duct cross section (size not specified) or involve one or more duct cross sections that measure ≤2 mm in aggregate (Table 4-7).

In the DIN system, all these lesions as well as those that would qualify as low-grade DCIS in the conventional system (figs. 4-13–4-15) are combined under the designation of DIN1, and their size is specified; management is based on the quantity/size of the lesion. The completely

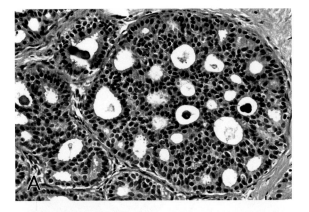

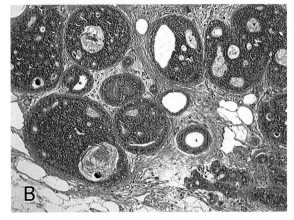

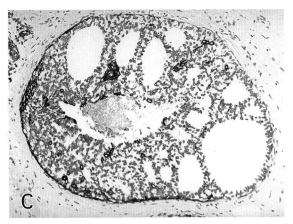

Figure 4-13

AIDH AND GRADE 1 DCIS/DIN1, CRIBRIFORM TYPE

A: This single duct is completely involved by the cribriform pattern, which measured 1.2 mm in maximum extent and qualifies as AIDH in the conventional system.

B: A cribriform proliferation of uniform, low nuclear grade cells is the most common phenotype of grade 1 DCIS. This lesion involved multiple adjacent ducts and measured 5 mm.

C: Immunostain for CK34betaE12 shows an absence of reactivity in the neoplastic cells, while the myoepithelial cell layer and a few residual native epithelial cells stain intensely.

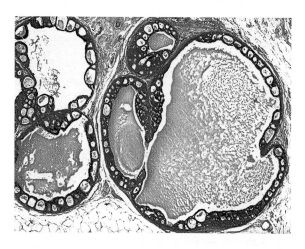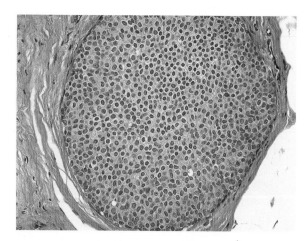

Figure 4-14

GRADE 1 DCIS/DIN1, CRIBRIFORM TYPE, >2 MM

Left: Several adjacent and distended ducts seen in cross section show complete involvement by arcades of uniform, rounded proliferating cells. When either one duct or the aggregate measures over 2 mm in maximum cross-sectional diameter, it qualifies as low-grade DCIS in the conventional classification; when the entire aggregate measures less than that, it qualifies as AIDH.

Right: A solid pattern of proliferation of uniform cells is seen.

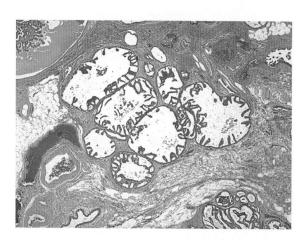

Figure 4-15

DCIS/DIN1, MICROPAPILLARY TYPE, >2 MM

Micropapillae protrude into the lumens of many ducts. The micropapillae lack fibrovascular cores, are rigid, and show early arcade formation.

involved duct cross sections are measured and the size provided in all cases. When duct cross sections are only partially involved, it is so specified and the conventional term of AIDH is put in parenthesis; partial involvement of duct cross sections may be focal or extensive (over 20 duct cross sections involved) and is so specified. When longitudinal segments of the duct are involved by typical micropapillae, arcades, or cribriform patterns, whether partial or complete, the size is measured and the designation of DCIS is placed next to DIN1. Microcalcifications may be absent, focal, or extensive within the lumen of involved ducts; their presence does not impact on diagnosis. By current grading convention, the presence of necrosis in any of these DIN1 settings propels the lesion into the DIN2 category. The micropapillary grade 1 DCIS/DIN1 lesion (fig. 4-15) appears to be associated with a more extensive distribution in multiple quadrants of the breast compared to other variants (93). Some grade 1 DCIS/DIN1 lesions grow in a solid fashion. The extent (distribution in multiple blocks or one block if limited to a single block) of DCIS/DIN1-3 lesions should be provided in all cases.

Significant interobserver variability in the cytologic classification of proliferative breast disease has been documented (94). In general, fine needle aspiration cytology is most accurate when experienced breast cytopathologists are available and when immediate evaluation of sample adequacy is assessed by the cytopathologist in order to perform additional aspirations if needed. Aspiration cytology of grade 1 DCIS/DIN1 is characterized by cords and clusters of loosely cohesive, uniform cells without myoepithelial cells (fig. 4-16); these features are quite

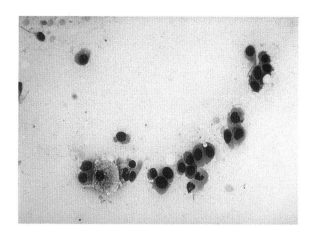
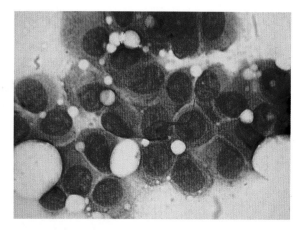

Figure 4-16

DCIS/DIN1, CRIBRIFORM TYPE: ASPIRATION CYTOLOGY

Left: A case interpreted as proliferative disease with atypia shows monotonous atypical cells in small aggregates of three to four cells as well as individual cells. It is not possible to distinguish invasive and intraepithelial lesions on the basis of aspirates (Diff Quik stain). (Courtesy of Dr. G. Rasty, Toronto, Canada.)

Right: Another case shows a monotonous population of cells with low-grade nuclei forming a monolayer cellular aggregate (Papanicolaou stain). (Courtesy of Dr. F. Moinfar, Graz, Austria.)

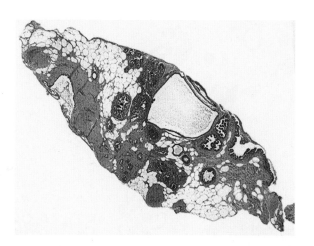
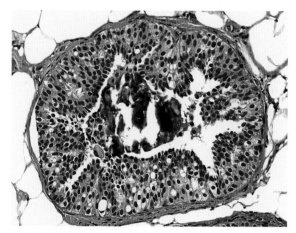

Figure 4-17

GRADE 1 DCIS/DIN 1, >2 MM

Left: A core biopsy specimen shows several ducts with epithelial proliferation.
Right: Higher magnification of one of the ducts shows microcalcification and grade 1 DCIS/DIN1 >2 mm.

similar to those for AIDH/DIN1 ($\leq$2 mm). In one study of nine AIDH lesions assessed by cytologic and architectural features, two were diagnosed as carcinoma and seven were inconclusive (102); the presence of overlapping features between AIDH/DIN1 ($\leq$2 mm) and grade 1 DCIS/DIN1 (>2 mm) makes separation of these lesions difficult. Cytology preparations cannot distinguish intraepithelial from invasive carcinomas with certainty either (see Appendix).

Identification of DIN1 (whether AIDH or DCIS) on a core biopsy (fig. 4-17) requires reexcision for exclusion of a more advanced process. When AIDH is present in the core biopsy, invasive carcinoma and DCIS have been reported in up to 52 percent of the reexcision specimens (46,120). The reexcision shows low-grade DCIS in up to 63 percent of the 52 percent that is upgraded (10,120); this is one more reason to use the designation of DIN1 with quantity specified.

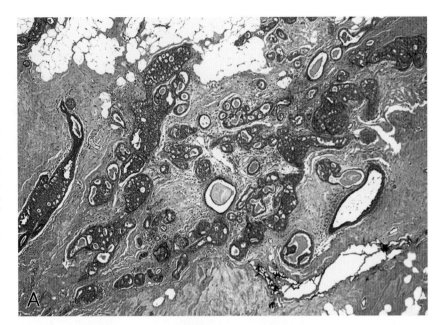

Figure 4-18

DCIS/DIN1, CRIBRIFORM TYPE, >2 MM

A: The lesion stained with hematoxylin and eosin (H&E).

B: A significantly reduced to completely negative immuno-reaction with CK34betaE12 is a common finding; the residual native epithelial cells show intense positivity.

C: Positive immunoreaction for E-cadherin.

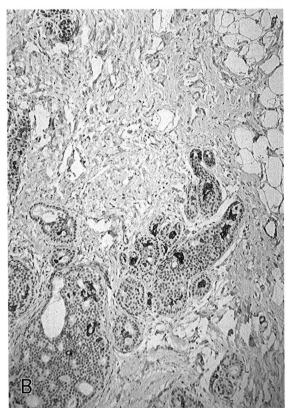

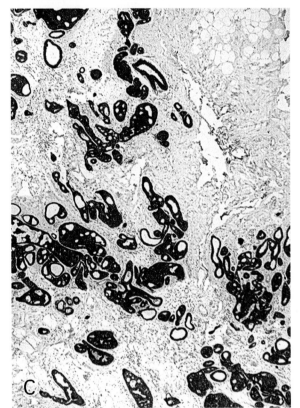

There would be no change in the diagnosis but only the quantity of DIN1.

The vast majority (about 90 percent) of DIN1 lesions are negative with CK34betaE12 and CK5/6, and positive with E-cadherin (fig. 4-18).

Grade 2 DCIS/DIN2. In either classification system, this lesion is generally composed of cells cytologically similar to those of AIDH and low-grade DCIS, but some ducts contain intraluminal necrosis (figs. 4-19, 4-20). Alternatively, the cells

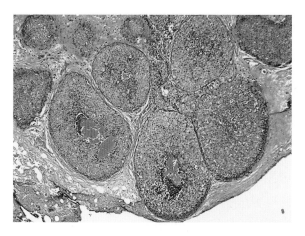
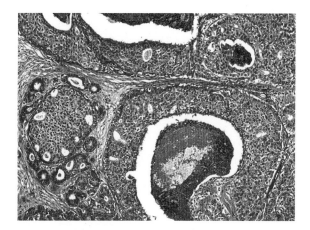

Figure 4-19

GRADE 2 DCIS/DIN2

DIN2 is usually characterized by a cribriform proliferation of uniform, low nuclear grade cells with intraluminal necrosis.

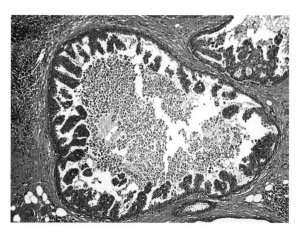
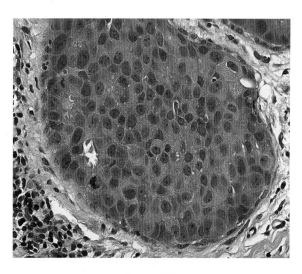

Figure 4-21

GRADE 2 DCIS/DIN2

The moderate nuclear pleomorphism qualifies this lesion as DIN2.

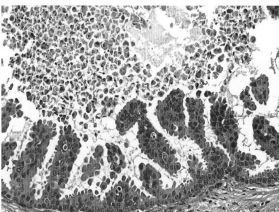

Figure 4-20

GRADE 2 DCIS/DIN2

The architecture and cytology are those of micropapillary DIN1, but the presence of intraluminal necrosis qualifies the lesion as DIN2.

may display moderate variation in nuclear size and shape, with or without intraluminal necrosis (fig. 4-21), or even have a flat architecture (fig. 4-22). The distribution of microcalcifications is similar to that of DIN1.

Grade 3 DCIS/DIN3. This is most frequently characterized by a solid proliferation of highly atypical, anaplastic cells, with or without intraluminal necrosis (figs. 4-23–4-25); the former is designated as the comedo type. Occasionally, only a single layer of pleomorphic

85

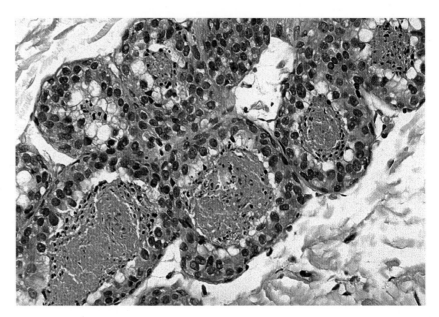

Figure 4-22

GRADE 2 DCIS/DIN2, FLAT TYPE

There is mild cytologic atypia with necrosis in every duct lumen, but only a single layer of mildly atypical cells.

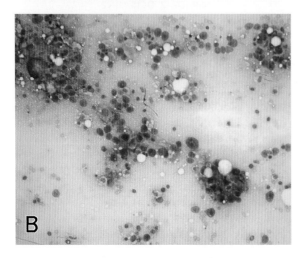

Figure 4-23

GRADE 3 DCIS/DIN3

A: The lesion displays significant cytologic atypia but no intraluminal necrosis.

B,C: Fine needle aspiration shows numerous highly atypical epithelial cells in clusters and as isolated cells.

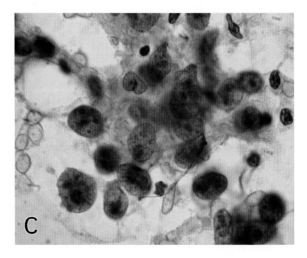

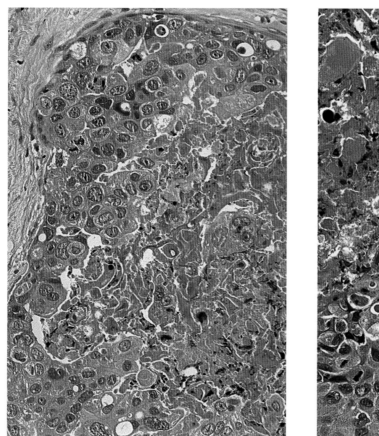
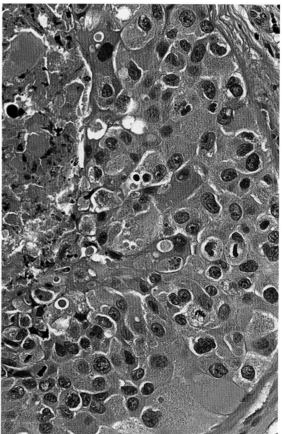

Figure 4-24

COMEDO DCIS/DIN3, COMEDO TYPE

The presence of high-grade nuclei with necrosis is the hallmark of this variant.

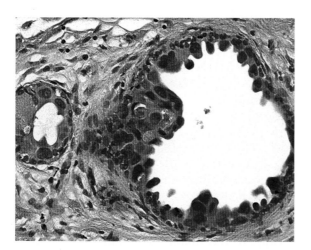
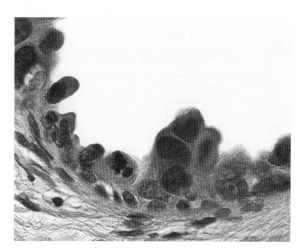

Figure 4-25

GRADE 3 DCIS/DIN3

Highly atypical, anaplastic cells replace the single layer of native epithelial cells with rare tufting.

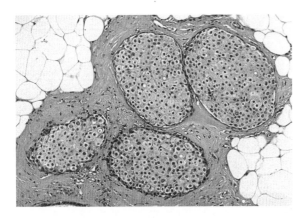
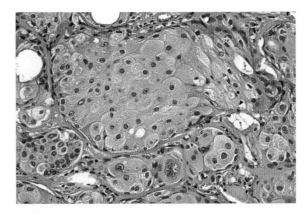

Figure 4-26

GRADE 2 APOCRINE DCIS/DIN2, APOCRINE TYPE

Left: There is a solid proliferation of apocrine cells with moderate nuclear pleomorphism within several ducts.

Right: Higher magnification shows the prominent nucleoli and abundant cytoplasm; the ductules in an area of adenosis are variably involved and distended by the neoplastic apocrine cells. (Fig. 6-46D from Tavassoli FA. Pathology of the breast, 2nd ed. Stamford, CT: Appleton & Lange/McGraw Hill; 1999:282.)

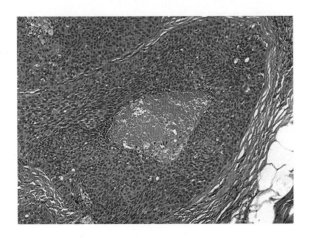

Figure 4-27

SPINDLE CELL DCIS/DIN2, SPINDLE CELL TYPE

The proliferating cells show spindled nuclei and minimal intraluminal necrosis. This variant is generally positive for neuroendocrine granules. (Fig. 6-54A from Tavassoli FA. Pathology of the breast, 2nd ed. Stamford, CT: Appleton & Lange/McGraw Hill; 1999:292.)

cells replaces the native epithelial cell layer; this is the high-grade counterpart of flat DIN1. Mitotic figures may or may not be abundant. Microcalcifications may or may not be present and do not impact on diagnosis.

Histologic Variants of DCIS/DIN1-3. A minority of DCIS/DIN1-3 lesions is composed of apocrine (109,111), spindle cell (35,105), signet ring, neuroendocrine (112), squamous (46a), or clear cells (figs. 4-26–4-29). The clear and spindle

cell DIN lesions are sometimes admixed and continuous with typical grade 1 DCIS/DIN1, but often the nuclei are moderately atypical, qualifying the lesions as grade 2 DCIS/DIN2. High nuclear grade, spindle or clear cell DIN is extremely rare. Spindle cell DCIS/DIN1-2 may be confused with IDH/low-risk DIN; positivity with neuroendocrine markers and negative immunoreactivity with high molecular weight CK34betaE12 point to a diagnosis of spindle cell DCIS/DIN1-2.

The apocrine DCIS lesions are generally grade 3 and of comedo type, with significant cytologic atypia and necrosis. A small proportion displays minor to moderate nuclear atypia, with or without necrosis, qualifying as grade 1 or 2 DCIS/DIN1-2. Prominent enlarged nucleoli are characteristic of the apocrine cells and their presence does not have any impact on the grade of the lesion. The 2-mm quantitative rule (based on assessment of completely involved duct cross sections) has been used to distinguish between low-grade apocrine DCIS and atypical apocrine hyperplasia (82) in the conventional classification. Irregularities in nuclear outline and variation in nuclear size are used for nuclear grading. If grading were based purely on nuclear features, a smaller proportion of clear cell and apocrine lesions would qualify as grade 1 DCIS/DIN1. Grading based mainly on nuclear grade and complemented by necrosis can be used to grade these DCIS variants as well, unless future studies provide evidence to the contrary.

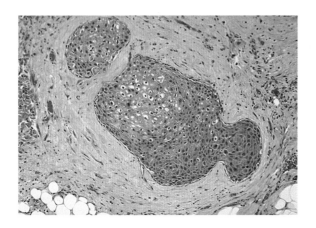
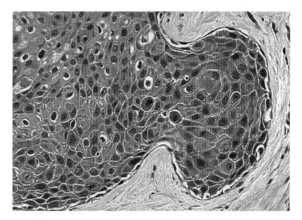

Figure 4-28

GRADE 2 SQUAMOUS DCIS/DIN2, SQUAMOUS TYPE

Top: The proliferating cells show squamous differentiation and grow in a solid fashion.
Bottom: Mitotic figures are noted occasionally.

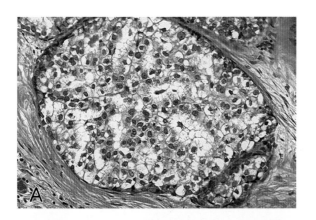
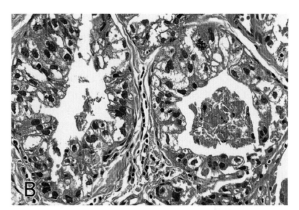

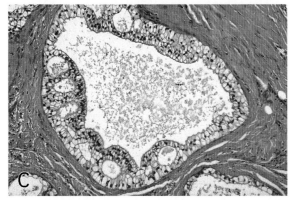

Figure 4-29

DCIS/DIN2-3, CLEAR CELL TYPE

This uncommon cytologic variant often displays intermediate-grade nuclei (A), may have high-grade nuclei with necrosis (B), or a cribriform pattern with low to intermediate-grade nuclei (C).

The proliferation of apocrine cells in solid and cribriform patterns generally implies AIDH or grade 1 DCIS/DIN1, even when there is nuclear uniformity. For solid patterns in small caliber ductules, the possibility of tangential cutting should be excluded.

Among these variants, the apocrine type is generally negative for estrogen and progesterone receptors, but positive for androgen receptors regardless of grade (111). At the molecular level, however, the cells do have the mRNA for estrogen receptor even though they lack the protein expression (11).

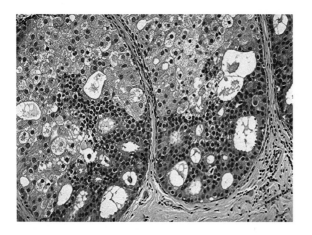 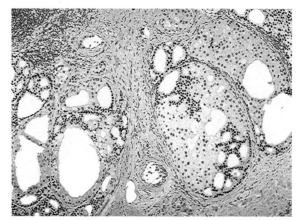

Figure 4-30

HETEROGENEITY OF DCIS/DIN

Left: Several adjacent ducts show a combination of typical cribriform and solid apocrine cell proliferation.
Right: Immunostain for estrogen receptor is positive in the cribriform, but not the apocrine, areas.

Heterogeneity of DCIS/DIN1-3

It is common to find a mixture of various grades of DIN as well as various cytologic variants of DIN/DCIS within the same biopsy or even within the same ductal space (fig. 4-30). The variation reflects biologic heterogeneity (1) that could benefit from and might require different therapeutic approaches. When more than one grade of DCIS is present, the proportion of the highest grade should be noted since recurrences may be derived from any of the components (58). It is also important to note the presence of different cytologic variants (apocrine, clear cell, squamous, spindle cell), whether present in pure form or admixed with other forms.

PROCESSING THE EXCISIONAL BIOPSY/LUMPECTOMY

There is no standardized approach for processing excisional biopsies for lesions that are not grossly visible (see Appendix). For practical purposes, we recommend processing the entire sample when the size of the sample is about 5 x 5 x 5 cm. The sample should be inked (color coded if orientation has been provided by the surgeon), serially sliced at 2- to 3-mm intervals from lateral to medial or perpendicular to the long axis of the specimen if there is no sample orientation, and submitted in sequence in appropriately coded blocks. For larger samples, sections should be taken preferentially from the nonadipose, fibrous parenchyma and submitted sequentially as for smaller samples. Having more than 30 to 40 slides per case may detract from the level of concentration required for assessing these samples, given the increasing number of such samples and the increasing number of features that need to be evaluated in every slide. The optimal approach would be assessment of whole mounts (see Appendix).

SIZE/EXTENT/DISTRIBUTION OF DIN

The extent or size of IDH/low-risk DIN does not impact on outcome or therapy, whereas the size and/or extent of DCIS, low- to high-grade/DIN1-3 does influence the management of the lesion. Assessment of size is difficult and there are many unresolved problems. Correlation of the mammogram, specimen radiograph, and histologic findings is important (34), but the ultimate decision in many cases is based on the histologic features. The mammographically determined size, based on microcalcifications, underestimates the pathologically determined size in 23 percent of DCIS lesions (21). When the entire biopsy sample has been sequentially processed, small localized lesions can be measured directly on one microscopic slide. When larger lesions are present in multiple consecutive tissue blocks (e.g., in three consecutive blocks of 2.5-mm thickness), the number of involved blocks is multiplied by the thickness of the tissue block

Table 4-8

IMMUNOHISTOCHEMICAL EXPRESSION OF VARIOUS MARKERS IN DUCTAL INTRAEPITHELIAL NEOPLASIA (DIN)

p53: Expression of p53 is noted mainly in ductal carcinoma in situ (DCIS), grade 3/DIN3 and may be associated with an increased risk for subsequent invasive carcinoma (29,108).

c-erbB2: Expression of c-erbB2 is associated mainly with higher-grade DCIS/DIN2-3, particularly the comedo subtype (34).

bcl-2: Expression of bcl-2 is diminished with increasing grade (85,108).

Estrogen Receptor (ER): Expression of ER diminishes in higher grades of DCIS/DIN (31,42). Apocrine DIN of all grades generally lacks expression of ER (42,108).

Progesterone Receptor (PR): Expression of PR diminishes in higher grades of DCIS/DIN (31). Apocrine DIN of all grades generally lacks expression of PR (108).

Cytokeratin 34betaE12 (CK1, 5, 10, 14): Expression of this marker diminishes significantly or is completely absent in 87% of atypical intraductal hyperplasia (AIDH)/DIN1 ($\leq$ 2mm) and 92% of grade 1 DCIS/DIN1 (> 2mm) lesions (9,67).

E-Cadherin: Expression of this adhesion molecule is characteristic of all variants of DIN, but it may be slightly diminished in some high-grade DIN lesions (12,45)

to obtain the extent of the disease. When there is involvement of ducts at opposing poles on a tissue block, with normal intervening breast tissue, either the extent of lesion distribution is assessed or individual foci are measured and the distance between them noted. If the entire sample has not been processed, the size/extent of lesions could be conveyed by providing the proportion of slides containing the lesion; the size/extent of the lesion appears to influence the chance of recurrence (52).

An alternative approach is to measure the extent of involved ducts/ductules in the most extensively involved slide of the sample. Using whole mounts would facilitate assessment of the lesion size/extent regardless of which approach is preferred.

Substantial differences exist in how low-grade DCIS/DIN1 lesions are measured. Of 230 pathologists who responded to a questionnaire, 43.5 percent included ducts partially involved by cribriform or micropapillary patterns around areas of grade 1 DCIS/DIN1 in the measurement, while others measured only completely involved ducts for size assessment (42a). Our preference is to include partially involved ducts, in this setting, when assessing the size/extent of grade 1 DCIS/DIN1.

MARKERS AND SPECIAL STUDIES

There are no markers or special studies that consistently, accurately, or independently separate the various grades of DIN (IDH, AIDH, and DCIS). Immunohistochemical expression of a variety of markers and hormone receptors is summarized in Table 4-8.

Proliferation Rate. In vivo labeling with bromodeoxyuridine (BrdU) found no significant difference in the proliferating cell fraction between IDH and AIDH, but it was significantly increased in DCIS (16). The thymidine labeling index is significantly lower for cribriform DCIS (median, 1.3 percent) compared to the comedo variant (median, 4.4 percent) (64). With the Ki-67 antibody, the highest proliferating index of 21.9 (median) is noted for comedo type DCIS/DIN3, while the median for low-grade DCIS/DIN1 is 5.6 (99).

DNA Ploidy. Aneuploidy has been found in 7 percent of IDH lesions, 13 to 36 percent of AIDH lesions, and 30 to 72 percent of low- to high-grade DCIS/DIN1-3 (14,22,32).

DIFFERENTIAL DIAGNOSIS

The solid variant of low-grade DCIS/DIN1 is often misinterpreted as LIN. Immunohistochemistry for E-cadherin and CK34betaE12 is helpful in separating the two: grade 1 DCIS/DIN1 is E-cadherin positive in nearly 100 percent of cases and CK34betaE12 negative in 92 percent of cases (12,67), whereas LIN is E-cadherin negative (12,45,114), but CK34betaE12 positive in nearly all cases (13).

IDH/low-risk DIN with necrosis, although rare, is often mistaken for DCIS. IDH has bland cytology and generally displays a mosaic pattern of positivity with CK34betaE12 and CK5/6; it is also positive for E-cadherin.

REPRODUCIBILITY OF DIAGNOSIS

Many studies have assessed reproducibility in diagnosing the range of DIN lesions, especially AIDH and low-grade DCIS (9,19,78,79,87,91). The results have ranged from a lack of a unanimous diagnosis on any case by expert breast pathologists (87) to a poor kappa value of agreement of 0.33 for atypical hyperplasias (79). It has been concluded that there are sufficient problems with reproducibility of the criteria to suggest caution in making precise risk estimates for specific features of borderline conditions, particularly at the individual level (8). In studies that have had the benefit of using a single set of criteria and intensive training in its application, either at multiple centers or within the same department (the latter following many years of working as a team and reflecting ideal circumstances for improved reproducibility), disagreement in diagnosis occurred in 33 percent (92) to 37 percent (78) of cases, respectively. Consistency in diagnosis and classification of the range of intraepithelial proliferations does not change significantly when interpretation is confined to specific images versus the assessment of the entire tissue section on a slide (100). Kappa statistics for diagnosing low-risk DIN/IDH; AIDH/DIN1 ($\leq$2 mm); and low-grade DCIS/DIN1 (>2 mm), DIN3/DCIS were 0.54, 0.35, and 0.78 for tissue sections and 0.47, 0.29, and 0.78 for images (100), respectively, reflecting inconsistencies secondary to differences in morphologic interpretations.

There are no such reproducibility studies available for the DIN system. It should be noted, however, that a major advantage of the DIN system is the reduction of the impact of different terms (DCIS versus AIDH) used for the same lesion by different observers. It is easier to accept that a 1.5-mm DIN1 lesion diagnosed on a core biopsy becomes a 6-mm DIN1 lesion rather than an AIDH lesion diagnosed on core biopsy being upgraded to DCIS on a reexcision biopsy. Since one of the major problem areas in reproducibility is diagnosing AIDH versus DCIS, the use of the DIN classification, which combines the two under one designation (DIN1), improves reproducibility.

It is important to emphasize that significant interobserver variability persists in the interpretation of the same morphologic changes by different pathologists, with significant impact on ultimate patient management and cancer statistics (42a).

RECURRENCE

Features of Recurrent DCIS/DIN1-3

Recurrences generally have the same morphology as the original lesion. When there is cytologic heterogeneity or more than one grade in the original lesion, any one of these subtypes or grades may be reflected in the recurrence, however.

At the molecular level, recurrences have alterations similar to the original lesion but may gain additional ones when patients have not received radiation or hormonal therapy for their DCIS (58,115). Given the heterogeneity of these lesions, it is important to analyze multiple foci from both the primary and the recurrent lesions to ascertain adequate representation for molecular analysis. It is also important not to mix cells from morphologically heterogeneous areas in a sample for molecular studies. Whether the recurrence developed following radiation and/or hormonal therapy should also be specified; these interventions may have eradicated one component of the initial DCIS/DIN1-3 while another progressed, and the therapies themselves may induce alterations at the molecular level.

By comparative genomic hybridization (CGH), the most common findings in the paired specimen (primary and recurrent DCIS) are gains involving chromosome 17q and losses involving chromosomes 8p and 17p (115). In one case, the recurrent lesions had the same LOH as that found in an area of AIDH/DIN1 $\leq$2 mm within the original biopsy rather than the LOH profile of the original DCIS/DIN1-3 (58). These findings support focusing on total eradication of the primary DIN1 lesion (whether AIDH or grade 1 DCIS) by requiring clear margins and/or postoperative radiation therapy for the larger lesions.

Factors Influencing Recurrence and Prognosis of DCIS/DIN1-3

The most important factor influencing the possibility of recurrence is the persistence of neoplastic cells postexcision. The significance of margins is mainly to ascertain complete excision. The amount of disease-free margin of breast tissue for optimal prognosis is not established, although some require a 1-cm margin. When disease is at or close to the margin, the amount or linear extent of disease at the margin correlates with outcome: those with disease of 1 cm or greater at the margin have higher likelihood of residual disease in the reexcision specimen (23). In both univariate and multivariate analysis, age over 50 years and negative margins are associated with a lower risk of local failure among 1,003 women with mammographically detected lesions treated with breast conserving surgery followed by irradiation (102a). The presence of immunohistochemically detected occult micrometastasis in axillary lymph nodes, identified in 13 percent of 102 women with a minimum of 10 years of follow-up, appears to have no impact on the outcome (56). The clinical and pathologic factors that influence recurrence and prognosis are listed in Table 4-9.

Behavior

Interestingly, despite the more limited surgical excisions in recent years, mortality from DCIS has declined. While 3.4 percent of women with a diagnosis of DCIS diagnosed between 1978 and 1983 (premammographic era) died of breast cancer at 10 years even though a majority of these women were treated by mastectomy, only 1.9 percent of women diagnosed with DCIS between 1984 and 1989 died of breast cancer at 10 years despite the increasing trend toward lumpectomy (30). Based on the 10-year follow-up period available for these women, it was concluded that "DCIS per se is not a life-threatening disease." The limited data available from several autopsy studies suggest that DCIS is common among women who die of causes unrelated to breast cancer. The median prevalence of DCIS in autopsy studies is 8.9 percent (range, 0 to 14.7 percent); possibly not all of these would have been mammographically detectable (117). The deaths that do occur following a diagnosis of mammographically detected DCIS are probably related to an undetected invasive carcinoma present at the time of the initial diagnosis of DCIS, progression of residual incompletely excised DCIS to invasive carcinoma, or development of a de novo invasive carcinoma elsewhere

Table 4-9
CLINICAL FACTORS THAT INFLUENCE MANAGEMENT, RECURRENCE, AND PROGNOSIS IN DUCTAL CARCINOMA IN SITU (DCIS)/DUCTAL INTRAEPITHELIAL NEOPLASIA (DIN)1-3
Lesion size within a quadrant (smaller, asymptomatic ones are better)
Lesion extension beyond a single quadrant (generally results in mastectomy, particularly for grade 2 and 3 lesions)
Status of lumpectomy margins and extent of positivity, when positive
Visibility on imaging procedures (image definition facilitates proper excision)
Radiation therapy (reduces chances of recurrence)

in the breast (32). When DCIS/DIN1-3 is diagnosed in a core biopsy, invasive carcinoma is found in the surgical specimen in 26.2 percent of cases (63a).

TREATMENT

Complete excision of grades 1-3 DCIS/DIN1-3 should eliminate the chance of recurrence or progression. In practice, however, it is difficult to ascertain complete excision of all neoplastic cells. Optimal management no longer requires mastectomy for unifocal or localized small lesions. A variety of factors influence the ultimate choice of therapy (97), with mastectomy used for the larger and multicentric tumors with positive margins.

Radiation therapy and tamoxifen have significantly reduced the recurrence rate (36–38). A follow-up of 1,003 women with mammographically detected DCIS treated by conservative surgery and irradiation noted an overall survival of 89 percent at 15 years (median follow-up, 8.5 years), cause-specific survival of 98 percent at 15 years, and freedom from distant metastases of 97 percent at 15 years; these findings support a treatment regimen of irradiation following breast-conserving surgery for mammographically detected lesions (102a). Patients whose lesions involve more than one quadrant would probably benefit from mastectomy since complete excision of extensive disease is more difficult to accomplish by conservative surgery. Optimal management is still evolving as data are accumulating from a variety of prospective studies.

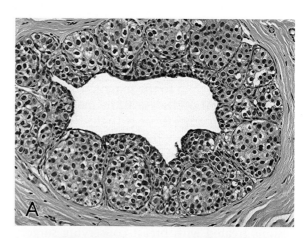

Figure 4-31

MAMMARY INTRAEPITHELIAL NEOPLASIA, POSITIVE HYBRID

The solid architecture suggests a lobular intraepithelial neoplasm (A). Immunoreaction for CK34betaE12 is positive (B), but so is the immunoreaction for E-cadherin (C).

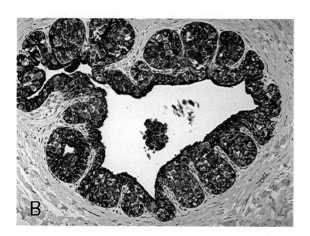

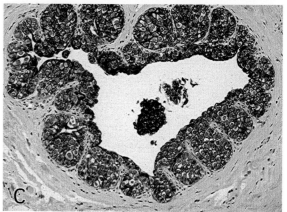

The clinical relevance of axillary node metastases, which are found in 1 to 2 percent of women with DCIS, has been debated. Such nodal involvement is often due to a missed area of invasive carcinoma. Whether patients with DCIS/DIN1-3 should routinely have sentinel node biopsies has not been established; sentinel node assessment is often included in the workup of extensive DCIS/DIN1-3. Follow-up immunohistochemical assessment of initially negative nodes (by hematoxylin and eosin [H&E] staining), using anticytokeratin antibodies, has shown a frequency of "metastases" of 6 percent in 219 women in one study (28), and 13 percent in 102 women in another study (55); the latter study found only micrometastases. The immunodetected metastases had no impact on outcome or survival in either study regardless of the type or extent of the disease.

The contralateral breast should be included in the follow-up regimen since contralateral breast carcinoma was recorded in 44 of 350 patients with DCIS (17). In another study, 5.6 percent of 799 patients with DCIS developed a second event (either DIN/DCIS or invasive carcinoma); 63 percent of the second events were in the contralateral breast. The incidence of further metachronous carcinoma in the other breast was 10 times higher than expected in normal breast in that study.

MAMMARY INTRAEPITHELIAL NEOPLASIA

A small proportion of intraepithelial neoplasias cannot be separated into either ductal or lobular type on the basis of pure H&E morphology (fig. 4-31). Using immunostains for E-cadherin and CK34betaE12, some of these qualify as ductal (E-cadherin positive, CK34betaE12 negative), some as lobular (E-cadherin negative, CK34betaE12 positive), while others, referred to as mammary intraepithelial neoplasia (MIN), are either negative for both markers (negative hybrid) or positive for both (positive hybrid) (see Table 3-5) (12). This important group requires further evaluation as it may reflect a neoplasm of mammary stem cells (particularly the negative hybrids) or immediate poststem cells with plasticity and potential to evolve into either a ductal or lobular intraepithelial or invasive neoplasm. For management purposes, morphologically hybrid "MIN" lesions are interpreted and graded according to their immunoprofile. Since

E-cadherin positively is currently considered a feature of ductal lesions, hybrid positive lesions are generally managed as ductal proliferations, whereas E-cadherin-negative lesions are managed as lobular intraepithelial neoplasia.

REFERENCES

1. Albonico G, Querzoli P, Ferretti S, Rinaldi R, Nenci I. Biological heterogeneity of breast carcinoma in situ. Ann N Y Acad Sci 1996;784:458-461.

2. Ashikari R, Hajdu SI, Robbins GF. Intraductal carcinoma of the breast (1960-1969). Cancer 1971;28:1182-1187.

3. Aubele MM, Cummings MC, Mattis AE, et al. Accumulation of chromosomal imbalances from intraductal proliferative lesions to adjacent in situ and invasive ductal breast cancer. Diagn Mol Pathol 2000;9:14-19.

4. Azzopardi JG. Problems in breast pathology, vol 11. In: Bennington JL, ed. Major problems in pathology. Philadelphia: WB Saunders; 1979:193-203.

5. Bellamy CO, McDonald C, Salter DM, Chetty U, Anderson TJ. Noninvasive ductal carcinoma of the breast: the relevance of histologic categorization. Hum Pathol 1993;24:16-23.

6. Bhathal PS, Brown RW, Lesueur GC, Russell IS. Frequency of benign and malignant breast lesions in 207 consecutive autopsies in Australian women. Br J Cancer 1985;51:271-278.

7. Bijker N, Peterse JL, Duchateau L, et al. Histological type and marker expression of the primary tumor compared with its local recurrence after breast-conserving therapy for ductal carcinoma in situ. Br J Cancer 2001;84:539-544.

8. Bodian CA, Perzin KH, Lattes R, Hoffman P, Abernathy TG. Prognostic significance of benign proliferative breast disease. Cancer 1993;71:3896-3907.

8a. Boecker W. Preneoplasia of the breast: a new conceptual approach to proliferative breast disease. Munich: Elsevier Saunders; 2006.

9. Boecker W, Buerger H, Schmitz K, et al. Ductal epithelial proliferations of the breast: a biological continuum? Comparative genomic hybridization and high-molecular-weight cytokeratin expression patterns. J Pathol 2001;195:415-421.

10. Bonnett M, Wallis T, Rossmann M, et al. Histopathologic analysis of atypical lesions in image-guided core breast biopsies. Mod Pathol 2003;16:154-160.

11. Bratthauer GL, Lininger RA, Man YG, Tavassoli FA. Androgen and estrogen receptor mRNA status in apocrine carcinomas. Diagn Mol Pathol 2002;11:113-118.

12. Bratthauer GL, Moinfar F, Stamatkos MD, et al. Combined E-cadherin and high molecular weight cytokeratin immunoprofile differentiates lobular, ductal, and hybrid mammary intraepithelial neoplasia. Hum Pathol 2002;33:620-627.

13. Bratthauer GL, Tavassoli FA. Assessment of lesions coexisting with various grades of ductal intraepithelial neoplasia of the breast. Virchows Arch 2004;444:340-344.

14. Carpenter R, Gibbs N, Matthews J, Cooke T. Importance of cellular DNA content in premalignant breast disease and pre-invasive carcinoma of the female breast. Br J Surg 1987;74:905-906.

15. Carter CL, Corle DK, Micozzi MS, Schatzkin A, Taylor PR. A prospective study of the development of breast cancer in 16,692 women with benign breast disease. Am J Epidemiol 1988;128:467-477.

16. Christov K , Chew KL, Ljung BM, et al. Cell proliferation in hyperplastic and in situ carcinoma lesions of the breast estimated by in vivo labeling with bromodeoxyuridine. J Cell Biochem Suppl 1994;19:165-172.

17. Ciatto S, Bonardi R, Cataliotti L, Cardona G. Intraductal breast carcinoma. Review of a multicenter series of 350 cases. Coordinating Center and Writing Committee of FONCAM (National Task Force for Breast Cancer), Italy. Tumori 1990;76:552-554.

18. Ciatto S, Cataliotti L, Distante V. Nonpalpable lesions detected with mammography: review of 512 consecutive cases. Radiology 1987;165:99-102.

19. Clayton F, Bodian CA, Banogon P, et al. Reproducibility of diagnosis in noninvasive breast disease. Lab Invest 1992;66:12A.

20. Consensus Conference on the classification of ductal carcinoma in situ. The Consensus Conference Committee. Cancer 1997;80:1798-1802.

21. Coombs JH, Hubbard E, Hudson K, et al. Ductal carcinoma in situ of the breast: correlation of pathologic and mammographic features with extent of disease. Am Surg 1997;63:1079-1083.

22. Crissman JD, Visscher DW, Kubus J. Image cytophotometric DNA analysis of atypical hyperplasia and intraductal carcinoma of the breast. Arch Pathol Lab Med 1990;114:1249-1253.

23. Darvishian F, Hajdu SI, DeRisi DC. Significance of linear extent of breast carcinoma at surgical margins. Ann Surg Pathol 2003;10:48-51.

23a. Dawood S, Broglio K, Gonzalez-Angulo AM, et al. Development of new cancers in patients with DCIS: the M.D. Anderson experience. Ann Surg Oncol 1008;15:244-249.

23b. de Mascarel I, MacGrogan G, Mathoulin-Pelissier S, et al. Epithelial atypia in biopsies performed for microcalcifications. Practical considerations about 2,833 serially sectioned surgical biopsies with a long follow-up. Virchows Arch 2007;451:1-10.

24. Dershaw DD, Abramson A, Kinne DW. Ductal carcinoma in situ: mammographic findings and clinical implications. Radiology 1989;170:411-415.

25. Dupont WD, Page DL. Breast cancer risk associated with proliferative disease, age at first birth, and family history of breast cancer. Am J Epidemiol 1987;1225;769-779.

26. Dupont WD, Page DL. Risk factors for breast cancer in women with proliferative disease. N Engl J Med 1985;312:146-151.

27. Dupont WD, Parl FF, Hartmann WH, et al. Breast cancer risk associated with proliferative breast disease and atypical hyperplasia. Cancer 1993;71:1258-1265.

28. El-Tamer M, Chun J, Gill M, et al. Incidence and clinical significance of lymph node metastasis detected by cytokeratin immunohistochemical staining in ductal carcinoma in situ. Ann Surg Oncol 2005;12:254-259.

29. Eriksson ET, Schimmelpenning H, Aspenblad U, Zetterberg A, Auer GU. Immunohistochemical expression of the mutant p53 protein and nuclear DNA content during the transition from benign to malignant breast disease. Hum Pathol 1994;25:1228-1233.

30. Ernster VL, Ballard-Barbash R, Barlow WE, et al. Detection of ductal carcinoma in situ in women undergoing screening mammography. J Natl Cancer Inst 2002;94:1546-1554.

31. Ernster VL, Barclay J, Kerlikowski K, Grady D, Henderson C. Incidence of and treatment for ductal carcinoma in situ of the breast. JAMA 1996;275:913-918.

32. Ernster VL, Barclay J, Kerlikowski K, Wilkie H, Ballard-Barbash R. Mortality among women with ductal carcinoma in situ of the breast in the population-based surveillance, epidemiology and end results program. Arch Intern Med 2000;160:953-958.

33. Eusebi V, Feudale E, Foschini MP, et al. Long-term follow-up of in situ carcinoma of the breast. Semin Diagn Pathol 1994;11:223-235.

34. Evans AJ, Pinder S, Wilson R, et al. Ductal carcinoma in situ of the breast: correlation between mammographic and pathologic findings. AJR Am J Roentgenol 1994;162:1307-1311.

35. Farshid G, Moinfar F, Meredith DJ, Peiterse S, Tavassoli FA. Spindle cell ductal carcinoma in situ. An unusual variant of ductal intra-epithelial neoplasia that simulates ductal hyperplasia or a myoepithelial proliferation. Virchows Arch 2001;439:70-77.

36. Fisher B, Dignam J, Wolmark N, et al. Lumpectomy and radiation therapy for the treatment of intraductal breast cancer: findings from the National Surgical Adjuvant Breast and Bowel Project B-17. J Clin Oncol 1998;16:441-452.

37. Fisher B, Dignam J, Wolmark N, et al. Tamoxifen in treatment of intraductal breast cancer: National Surgical Adjuvant Breast and Bowel Project B-24 randomised controlled trial. Lancet 1999;353:1993-2000.

38. Fisher ER, Costantino J, Fisher B, Palekar AS, Redmond C, Mamounas E. Pathologic findings from the National Surgical Adjuvant Breast Project (NSABP) Protocol B-17. Intraductal carcinoma (ductal carcinoma in situ). The National Surgical Adjuvant Breast and Bowel Project Collaborating Investigators. Cancer 1995;75:1310-1319.

39. Fitzgibbons PL, Henson DE, Hutter RV. Benign breast changes and the risk for subsequent breast cancer: an update of the 1985 consensus statement. Cancer Committee of the College of American Pathologists. Arch Pathol Lab Med 1998;122:1053-1055.

40. Fraser JL, Raza S, Chorny K, Connolly JL, Schnitt SJ. Columnar alteration with prominent apical snouts and secretions: a spectrum of changes frequently present in breast biopsies performed for microcalcifications. Am J Surg Pathol 1998;22:1521-1527.

41. Frost AR, Tabbara SO, Poprocky LA, Weiss H, Sidawy MK. Cytologic features of proliferative breast disease: a study designed to minimize sampling error. Cancer 2000;90:33-40.

42. Giri DD, Dundas SA, Nottingham JF, Underwood JC. Oestrogen receptors in benign epithelial lesions and intraduct carcinomas of the breast: an immunohistochemical study. Histopathology 1989;15:575-584.

42a. Ghofrani M, Tapia B, Tavassoli FA. Discrepancies in the diagnosis of intraductal proliferative lesions of the breast and its management implications: results of a multinational survey. Virchows Arch 2006;449:609-616.

43. Goldstein NS, Kestin L, Vicini F. Intraductal carcinoma of the breast: pathologic features associated with local recurrence in patients treated by breast-conserving therapy. Am J Surg Pathol 2000;24:1058-1067.

44. Gong G, DeVries S, Chew KL, Cha I, Ljung BM, Waldman FM. Genetic changes in paired atypical and usual ductal hyperplasia of the breast by comparative genomic hybridization. Clin Cancer Res 2002;7:2410-2414.

45. Gupta SK, Douglas-Jones AG, Jasani B, Morgan JM, Pignatelli M, Mansel RE. E-cadherin (E-Cad) expression in duct carcinoma in situ (DCIS) of the breast. Virchows Arch 1997;430:23-28.

45a. Hannemann J, Velds A, Halfwerk JB, Kreike B, Peterse JL, van de Vijver MJ. Classification of ductal carcinoma in situ by gene expression profiling. Breast Ca Res 2007;8:R61.

46. Harvey JM, Sterrett GF, Frost FA. Atypical ductal hyperplasia and atypia of uncertain significance in core biopsies from mammographically detected lesions: correlation with excision diagnosis. Pathology 2002;34:410-416.

46a. Hayes MM, Peterse JL, Yavuz E, Vischer GH, Eusebi V. Squamous cell carcinoma in situ of the breast: a light microscopic and immunohistochemical study of a previously undescribed lesion. Am J Surg Pathol 2007;31:1414-1419.

47. Holland R, Hendriks JH, Vebeek AL, Mravunac M, Schuurmans Stekhoven JH. Extent, distribution, and mammographic/histological correlations of breast ductal carcinoma in situ. Lancet 1990;335:519-522.

48. Holland R, Peterse JL, Millis RR, et al. Ductal carcinoma in situ: a proposal for a new classification. Sem Diagn Pathol 1994;11:167-180.

49. Ikeda DM, Andersson I. Ductal carcinoma in situ: atypical mammographic appearances. Radiology 1989;172:661-666.

50. Jones C, Merret S, Thomas VA, Barker TH, Lakhani SR. Comparative genomic hybridization analysis of bilateral hyperplasia of usual type of the breast. J Pathol 2003;1992:152-156.

51. Kerlikowske K, Barclay J, Grady D, Sickles EA, Ernster V. Comparison of risk factors for ductal carcinoma in situ and invasive breast cancer. J Natl Cancer Inst 1997;89:76-82.

52. Kestin LL, Goldstein NS, Lacerna MD, et al. Factors associated with local recurrence of mammographically detected ductal carcinoma in situ in patients given breast-conserving therapy. Cancer 2000;88:596-607.

53. Kodlin D, Winger EE, Morgenstern NL, Chen U. Chronic mastopathy and breast cancer. A follow-up study. Cancer 1977;39:2603-2607.

54. Krieger N, Hiatt RA. Risk of breast cancer after benign breast diseases. Variation by histologic type, degree of atypia, age at biopsy, and length of follow-up. Am J Epidemiol 1992;135:619-631.

55. Lagios MD. Ductal carcinoma in situ. Pathology and treatment. Surg Clin N Am 1990;70:853-871.

56. Lara JF, Young SM, Velilla RE, Santoro EJ, Templeton SF. The relevance of occult axillary micrometastasis in ductal carcinoma in situ: a clinicopathologic study with long term follow-up. Cancer 2003;98:2105-2113.

57. La Vecchia C, Parazzini F, Franceschi S, Decarli A. Risk factors for benign breast disease and their relation with breast cancer risk. Pooled information from epidemiologic studies. Tumori 1985;71:167-178.

58. Lininger RA, Fujii H, Man YG, Gabrielson E, Tavassoli FA. Comparison of loss of heterozygosity in primary and recurrent ductal carcinoma in situ of the breast. Mod Pathol 1998;11:1151-1159.

58a. Leonard GD, Swain SM. Ductal carcinoma in situ, complexities and challenges. J Natl Cancer Inst 2004;96:906-920.

59. London SJ, Connolly JL, Schnitt SJ, Colditz GA. A prospective study of benign breast disease and the risk of breast cancer. JAMA 1992;267:941-944.

60. Ma L, Boyd NF. Atypical hyperplasia and breast cancer risk: a critique. Cancer Causes Control 1992;3:517-525.

61. Maitra A, Wistuba II, Washington C, et al. High-resolution chromosome 3p allelotyping of breast carcinomas and precursor lesions demonstrates frequent loss of heterozygosity and a discontinuous pattern of allele loss. Am J Pathol 2001;159:119-130.

62. Marshall LM, Hunter DJ, Connolly JL, et al. Risk of breast cancer associated with atypical hyperplasia of lobular or ductal types. Cancer Epidemiol Biomarkers Prev 1997;6:297-301.

62a. Martel M, Barron-Rodriguez P, Tolgay Ocal I, Dotto J, Tavassoli FA. Flat DIN1 (flat epithelial atypia) on core needle biopsy: 63 cases identified retrospectively among 1,751 core biopsies performed over an 8-year period (1992-1999). Virchows Arch 2007;451:883-891.

63. McDivitt RW, Stevens JA, Lee NC, Wingo PA, Rubin GL, Gersell D. Histologic types of benign breast disease and the risk for breast cancer. The Cancer and Steroid Hormone Study Group. Cancer 1992;69:1408-1414.

63a. Meijnen P, Oldenberg HS, Loo CE, Nieweg OE, Peterse JL, Rutgers EJ. Risk of invasion and axillary node metastasis in ductal carcinoma in situ diagnosed by core-needle biopsy. Br J Surg 2007;94:952-956.

64. Meyer JS. Cell kinetics of histologic variants of in situ breast carcinoma. Breast Cancer Res Treat 1986;7:171-180.

65. Millis RR, Barnes DM, Lampejo OT, Egan MK, Smith P. Tumour grade does not change between primary and recurrent mammary carcinoma. Eur J Cancer 1998;34:548-553.

66. Moinfar F, Man YG, Bratthauer GL, Ratschek M, Tavassoli FA. Genetic abnormalities in mammary ductal intraepithelial neoplasia-flat type ("clinging carcinoma in situ"): a simulator of normal mammary epithelium. Cancer 2000;88:2072-2081.

67. Moinfar F, Man YG, Lininger RA, Bodian C, Tavassoli FA. Use of keratin 35betaE12 as an adjunct in the diagnosis of mammary intraepithelial neoplasia-ductal type—benign and malignant intraductal proliferations. Am J Surg Pathol 1999;23:1048-1058.

68. Nielsen M, Thomsen JL, Primdahl S, Dyreborg U, Andersen JA. Breast cancer and atypia among young and middle-aged women: a study of 110 medicolegal autopsies. Br J Cancer 1987;56:814-819.

69. O'Connell P, Pekkel V, Fuqua SA, Osborne CK, Clark GM, Allred DC. Analysis of loss of heterozygosity in 399 premalignant breast lesions at 15 genetic loci. J Natl Cancer Inst 1998;90:697-703.

70. Ohtake T, Abe R, Kimijima I, et al. Intraductal extension of primary invasive breast carcinoma treated by breast-conserving surgery. Computer graphic three-dimensional reconstruction of the mammary duct-lobular systems. Cancer 1995;76:32-45.

71. Ohuchi N. Breast-conserving surgery for invasive cancer: a principle based on segmental anatomy. Tohoku J Exp Med 1999;188:103-118.

72. Ohuchi N, Furuta A, Mori S. Management of ductal carcinoma in situ with nipple discharge. Intraductal spreading of carcinoma is an unfavorable pathologic factor for breast-conserving surgery. Cancer 1994;74:1294-1302.

73. Ottesen GL, Graversen HP, Blichert-Toft M, Zedeler K, Andersen JA. Ductal carcinoma in situ of the female breast. Short-term results of a prospective nationwide study. The Danish Breast Cancer Cooperative Group. Am J Surg Pathol 1992;16:1183-1196.

74. Page DL, Dupont WD, Rogers LW, Jensen RA, Schuyler PA. Continued local recurrence of carcinoma 15-25 years after a diagnosis of low grade ductal carcinoma in situ of the breast treated only by biopsy. Cancer 1995;76:1197-1200.

75. Page DL, Dupont WD, Rogers LW, Landenberger M. Intraductal carcinoma of the breast: follow-up after biopsy only. Cancer 1982;49:751-758.

76. Page DL, Dupont WD, Rogers LW, Rados MS. Atypical hyperplastic lesions of the female breast. A long term follow-up study. Cancer 1985;55:2698-2708.

77. Page DL, Vander Zwaag R, Rogers LW, Williams LT, Walker WE, Hartmann WH. Relation between component parts of fibrocystic disease complex and breast cancer. J Natl Cancer Inst 1978;61:1055-1063.

78. Palazzo JP, Hyslop T. Hyperplastic ductal and lobular lesions and carcinoma in situ of the breast: reproducibility of current diagnostic criteria among community- and academic-based pathologists. Breast J 1998;4:230-237.

79. Palli D, Galli M, Bianchi S, et al. Reproducibility of histological diagnosis of breast lesions: results of a panel in Italy. Eur J Cancer 1996;32A:603-607.

80. Palli D, Rosselli del Turco M, Simoncini R, Bianchi S. Benign breast disease and breast cancer: a case-control study in a cohort in Italy. Int J Cancer 1991;47:703-706.

81. Pandya S, Mackarem G, Lee AK, McLellan R, Heatley GJ, Hughes KS. Ductal carcinoma in situ: the impact of screening on clinical presentation and pathologic features. Breast J 1998;4:146-151.

82. Patchefsky AS, Schwartz GF, Finkelstein SD, et al. Heterogeneity of intraductal carcinoma of the breast. Cancer 1989;63:731-741.

83. Patchefsky AS, Shaber GS, Schwartz GF, Feig SA, Nerlinger RE. The pathology of breast cancer detected by mass population screening. Cancer 1977;40:1659-1670.

84. Poller DN, Silverstein MJ, Galea M, et al. Ideas in pathology. Ductal carcinoma in situ of the breast: a proposal for a new simplified histological classification association between cellular proliferation and c-erb-B-2 protein expression. Mod Pathol 1994;7:257-262.

85. Quinn CM, Ostrowski JL, Harkins L, Rice AJ, Loney DP. Loss of bcl-2 expression in ductal carcinoma in situ of the breast relates to poor histological differentiation and to expression of p53 and c-erbB-2 proteins. Histopathology 1998;33:531-536.

86. Rakovitch E, Franssen E, Kim J, et al. A comparison of risk perception and psychological morbidity in women with ductal carcinoma in situ and early invasive breast cancer. Breast Cancer Res Treat 2003;77:285-293.

87. Rosai J. Borderline epithelial lesions of the breast. Am J Surg Pathol 1991;15:209-221.

88. Sanders ME, Schuyler PA, Dupont WD, Page DL. The natural history of low-grade ductal carcinoma in situ of the breast in women treated by biopsy only revealed over 30 years of long-term follow-up. Cancer 2005;103:2481-2484.

89. Sartwell PE, Arthes FG, Tonascia JA. Benign and malignant breast tumours: epidemiological similarities. Int J Epidemiol 1978;7:217-221.

90. Sauer T, Lomo J, Garred O, Naess O. Cytologic features of ductal carcinoma in situ in fine-needle aspiration of the breast mirror the histopathologic growth pattern heterogeneity and grading. Cancer 2005;105:21-27.

91. Schnitt SJ. The diagnosis and management of pre-invasive breast disease: flat epithelial atypia—classification, pathologic features and clinical significance. Breast Cancer Res 2003;5:263-268.

92. Schnitt SJ, Connolly J, Tavassoli FA, et al. Interobserver reproducibility in the diagnosis of ductal proliferative breast lesions using standardized criteria. Am J Surg Pathol 1992;16:1133-1143.

93. Schwartz GF, Patchefsky AS, Finkelstein SD, et al. Nonpalpable in situ ductal carcinoma of the breast. Predictors of multicentricity and microinvasion and implications for treatment. Arch Surg 1989;124:29-32.

94. Sidawy MK, Stoler MH, Frale WJ, et al. Interobserver variability in the classification of proliferative breast lesions by fine needle aspiration: results of the Papanicolaou Society of Cytopathology Study. Diagn Cytopathol 1998;18:150-165.

95. Sigfusson BF, Andersson I, Aspergren K, Janzon L, Linell F, Ljungberg O. Clustered breast calcifications. Acta Radiol Diagn (Stockh)1983;24:273-281.

96. Silverstein MJ, Poller DN, Waisman JR, et al. Prognostic classification of breast ductal carcinoma in situ. Lancet 1995;345:1154-1157.

97. Silverstein MJ, Waisman JR, Gamagami P, et al. Intraductal carcinoma of the breast (208 cases). Clinical factors influencing treatment choice. Cancer 1990;66:102-108.

98. Simpson PT, Gale T, Reis-Filho JS, et al. Columnar cell lesions of the breast: the missing link in breast cancer progression? A morphological and molecular analysis. Am J Surg Pathol 2005;29:734-746.

99. Siziopikou KP, Schnitt SJ. MIB-1 proliferation index in ductal carcinoma in situ of the breast: relationship to the expression of apoptosis-regulating protein bcl-2 and p53. Breast J 2000;6:400-406.

100. Sloane JP, Amendoeira I, Apostolikas N, et al. Causes of inconsistency in diagnosing and classifying intraductal proliferations of the breast. European Commission Working Group on Breast Screening Pathology. Eur J Cancer 2000;36:1769-1772.

101. Sloane JP, Amendoeira I, Apostolikas N, et al. Consistency achieved by 23 European pathologists in categorizing ductal carcinoma in situ of the breast using five classifications. European Commission Working Group on Breast Screening Pathology. Hum Pathol 1998;29:1056-1062.

102. Sneige N, Staerkel GA. Fine needle aspiration cytology of ductal hyperplasia with and without atypia and ductal carcinoma in situ. Hum Pathol 1994;25:485-492.

102a. Solin LJ, Fourquet A, Vicini FA, et al. Long-term outcome after breast-conservation treatment with radiation for mammographically detected ductal carcinoma in situ of the breast. Cancer 2005;103:1137-1146.

103. Stanta G, Bonin S, Losi L, Eusebi V. Molecular characterization of intraductal breast carcinomas. Virchows Arch 1998;432:107-111.

104. Stomper PC, Connolly JL, Meyer JE, Harris JR. Clinically occult ductal carcinoma in situ detected with mammography: analysis of 100 cases with radiologic-pathologic correlation. Radiology 1989;172:235-241.

105. Tan PH, Lui GG, Chiang G, Yap WM, Poh WT, Bay BH. Ductal carcinoma in situ with spindle cells: a potential diagnostic pitfall in the evaluation of breast lesions. Histopathology 2004;45:343-351.

105a. Tavassoli FA. Breast pathology: rationale for adopting the ductal intraepithelial neoplasia (DIN) classification. Nat Clin Pract Oncol 2005;2:116-117.

106. Tavassoli FA. Ductal intraepithelial neoplasia of the breast. Virchows Arch 2001;438:221-227.

107. Tavassoli FA. Pathology of the breast. New York: Elsevier; 1992:238-239.

108. Tavassoli FA, Man Y. Morphofunctional features of intraductal hyperplasia, atypical intraductal hyperplasia, and various grades of intraductal carcinoma. Breast J 1995;1:155-162.

109. Tavassoli FA, Norris HJ. Intraductal apocrine carcinoma: a clinicopathologic study of 37 cases. Mod Pathol 1994;7:813-818.

110. Tavassoli FA, Norris HJ. A comparison of the results of long-term follow-up for atypical intraductal hyperplasia and intraductal hyperplasia of the breast. Cancer 1990;65:518-529.

111. Tavassoli FA, Purcell CL, Bratthauer GL, Man YG. Androgen receptor expression along with loss of bcl-2, ER, and PR expression in benign and malignant apocrine lesions of the breast: implications for therapy. Breast 1996;2:261-79.

112. Tsang WY, Chan JK. Endocrine ductal carcinoma in situ (E-DCIS) of the breast: a form of low grade DCIS with distinctive clinicopathologic and biologic characteristics. Am J Surg Pathol 1996;20:921-943.

113. van de Rijn M, Perou CM, Tibshirani R, et al. Expression of cytokeratins 17 and 5 identifies a group of breast carcinomas with poor clinical outcome. Am J Pathol 2002;161:1991-1996.

113a. Veronesi U, Viale G, Rotmensz N, Goldhirsch A. Rethinking TNM: breast cancer TNM classification for treatment decision-making and research. Breast 2006;15:3-8.

114. Vos CB, Cleton-Janson AM, Berx G, et al. E-cadherin inactivation in lobular carcinoma in situ of the breast: an early event in tumorigenesis. Br J Cancer 1977;76:1131-1133.

115. Waldman FM, DeVries S, Chew KL, Moore DH 2nd, Kerlikowske K, Ljung BM. Chromosomal alterations in ductal carcinoma in situ and their in situ recurrences. J Natl Cancer Inst 2000;92:313-320.

116. Ward BA, McKhann CF, Ravikumar TS. Ten-year follow-up of breast carcinoma in situ in Connecticut. Arch Surg 1992;127:1392-1395.

117. Welch HG, Black WC. Using autopsy series to estimate the disease "reservoir" for ductal carcinoma in situ of the breast: how much more breast cancer can we find? Ann Intern Med 1997;127:1023-1028.

118. Wellings SR, Jensen HM, Marcum RG. An atlas of subgross pathology of the human breast with special reference to possible precancerous lesions. J Natl Cancer Inst 1975;55:231-273.

119. Westbrook KC, Gallager HS. Intraductal carcinoma of the breast. A comparative study. Am J Surg 1975;130:667-670.

120. Yeh IT, Dimitrov D, Otto P, Miller AR, Kahlenberg MS, Cruz A. Pathologic review of atypical hyperplasia identified by image-guided breast needle core biopsy. Correlation with excision specimen. Arch Pathol Lab Med 2003;127:49-54.

5 PAPILLARY LESIONS OF THE BREAST

Whether benign or malignant, a papillary lesion should have papillary processes supported by a fibrovascular stalk. The fibrovascular stalk may be inconspicuous, due to an abundant epithelial proliferation, particularly in some carcinomas, or it may be quite prominent and sclerotic in some benign papillary lesions.

Papillary lesions of the breast occur in patients with a wide age range, including children and adolescent females. Papillomas, the most common papillary lesion, account for less than 10 percent of benign mammary lesions (2). Papillary carcinomas are rare prior to the age 30 years.

Papillary lesions of the breast assume a variety of appearances and presentations (Table 5-1). They may be solitary, visible to the naked eye, and centrally located beneath the nipple or they may be multiple, microscopic, and located in the smaller peripheral ducts. The latter originate in the terminal duct lobular unit (TDLU). A papillary lesion may be benign or malignant regardless of its size or location. Included among the benign lesions are solitary papilloma, papillomatosis, and sclerosing papilloma. Malignant lesions include papillary carcinomas. Whether benign or malignant, a solitary (or multiple), large, centrally located papillary lesion may be associated with nipple discharge. The most important, and actually the only, feature that invariably indicates a malignant process is the complete or nearly complete (in 90 percent or more of the papillary processes) absence of the myoepithelial cell layer. This rule holds regardless of the size, number, or location of the papillary lesion. The presence of a myoepithelial cell layer does not exclude a diagnosis of papillary carcinoma, however.

Radiologically, papillary carcinomas, when solitary, most often manifest as round, lobulated lesions but may have an ill-defined appearance. When there is irregularity in an otherwise well-circumscribed outline, the possibility of invasion is raised (14). Mammographically, it may be difficult to distinguish a papillary carcinoma with an invasive component from one without invasion (31).

VARIANTS OF PAPILLARY LESIONS

Papilloma

Papillomas may be central or peripheral in location; the former are generally solitary, while the latter are multifocal involving TDLUs.

Central Papilloma. These are centrally located solitary lesions. They are associated with nipple discharge in 64 to 88 percent of the cases (38). Mammographically, cental papilloma presents as a retroareolar circumscribed mass or a dilated duct; microcalcifications are rare (38). Grossly, the lesion is a sharply circumscribed papillary projection protruding into a dilated cystic duct containing serous or serosanguineous fluid (fig. 5-1) or a solid mass without a discernable duct lumen. Central papillomas may become quite large, but generally do not exceed 2.5 cm.

Microscopically, the arborescent proliferation is characterized by a central fibrovascular stalk covered by a myoepithelial cell layer and an overlying luminal layer of epithelial cells (fig. 5-2).

Table 5-1

CLASSIFICATION OF PAPILLARY LESIONS OF THE BREAST

I. **Benign**
   Papilloma: central, solitary
   Papillomatosis: peripheral, multiple, arises in TDLU[a]

II. **Atypical Papillary Lesions**
   Atypical papilloma: central, solitary or complex
   Atypical papillomatosis: peripheral, multiple

III. **Malignant**
   Noninvasive papillary carcinoma (intraductal papillary carcinoma): central, solitary, palpable or peripheral, multiple, nonpalpable (malignant counterpart of papillomatosis)
   Invasive papillary carcinoma: either central or peripheral, generally the former, with areas of regular infiltrating duct carcinoma or invasive micropapillary carcinoma

[a]TDLU = terminal duct lobular units.

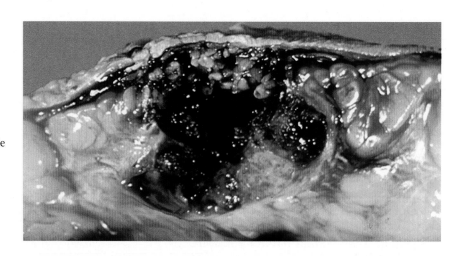

Figure 5-1

PAPILLOMA

Papillary excrescences protrude into a cystically dilated duct.

The epithelial (fig. 5-3) or the myoepithelial (fig. 5-4) cell layer may become hyperplastic, the latter generally in a more focal distribution. The epithelial cells often undergo apocrine metaplasia (fig. 5-5) and less frequently, squamous, mucinous, and sebaceous metaplasia; squamous metaplasia is seen most often around areas of infarction and needle instrumentation (fig. 5-6) (7,8,17,27,29). Sclerosis (*sclerosing papilloma*) or infarction may occur; the infarction is usually hemorrhagic (fig. 5-7) and secondary to torsion of one or more papillary processes.

When various degrees of sclerosis, hyalinization, distortion, and the pseudoinvasive patterns that are easily mistaken for carcinoma are present, the lesion qualifies as sclerosing papilloma (fig. 5-8). None of the 30 patients with sclerosing papillomas reported by Fenoglio and Lattes (5) developed recurrences after a median follow-up of 6 years.

Some papillomas appear as a relatively solid proliferation of tubules occluding the lumen of the involved duct in some planes of section. The term *intraductal adenoma* has been used for this presentation. Generally, the papillary nature of the process becomes apparent when additional levels or sections are assessed.

Peripheral Papilloma. Patients with peripheral papilloma are about the same age or slightly younger than those with solitary central papilloma. When multiple and located in the terminal ducts and TDLUs, the term *papillomatosis* is appropriate. Papillomatosis is invisible to the naked eye. Microscopically, papillomatosis involves multiple TDLUs (figs. 5-9, 5-10), but may extend into the larger ducts (22).

Peripheral papillomas are generally occult clinically and mammographically unless extensive; when extensive, they may present as a palpable mass. Microcalcifications are rare and are mammographically occult as well (3). The basic microscopic appearance is similar to that of solitary central papilloma.

The association of multiple papillomas, whether located in TDLUs (papillomatosis) or in larger ducts, with atypical ductal hyperplasia (ADH)/ductal intraepithelial neoplasia grade 1 (DIN1), lobular intraepithelial neoplasia (LIN), malignant lesions, and bilaterality suggests that they may represent a marker of increased breast cancer risk (1,17,21,22,24).

Atypical papillomatosis is rare. It usually consists of stratified spindle luminal cells overlying fibrovascular stalks with partial loss of the myoepithelial cell layer.

Atypical Papilloma. Atypical papilloma is characterized by areas of stratification of epithelial cells with loss of the myoepithelial cell layer or by areas of solid, cribriform, or micropapillary proliferation of uniform atypical cells confined to less than one third of the lesion, with or without the loss of the underlying myoepithelial cell layer. Areas composed of cribriform, solid, or micropapillary proliferations of monotonous cells may occupy less than 90 percent of an otherwise benign papilloma, complex papilloma, or sclerosing papilloma. The term atypical papilloma is used when the DCIS1/DIN1 component involves less than 30 percent of the lesion (fig. 5-11); the term DCIS arising in a papilloma may be used for lesions with 30 to less than 90 percent involvement by DCIS1/DIN1 (14).

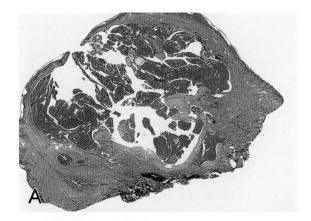

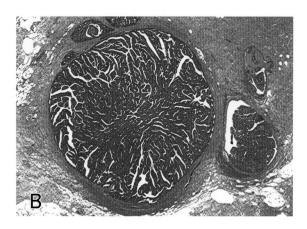

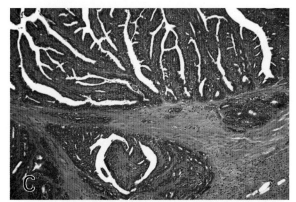

Figure 5-2

PAPILLOMA

A: A subareolar papilloma has characteristic branching papillary processes.

B: A complex papilloma extends into the adjacent branches of the duct.

C: Branching papillae show delicate fibrovascular cores.

D: The papillary processes are lined by luminal epithelial cells overlying myoepithelial cells.

E: Immunostain for actin decorates the myoepithelial cells.

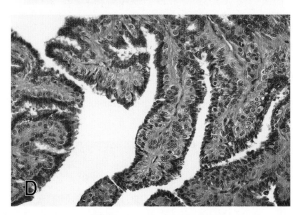

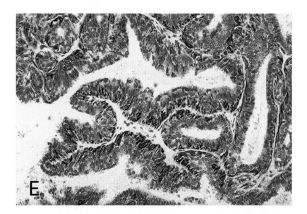

Clinical Significance of Papillomas and Atypical Papillomas

Atypical papillomas are associated with a slightly increased risk for the subsequent development of invasive carcinoma (23). In most cases, the atypia is localized in a lesion confined to a duct that is completely excised. Atypical papillomas may be associated with various grades of DIN in the surrounding mammary tissue; the presence of these proliferations has a significant impact on the outcome for the patient.

A study of 119 centrally located papillary lesions with areas of atypia (cribriform or micropapillary proliferation similar to low-grade DCIS/ DIN1) noted a progression rate of 7.5 percent (5 subsequent invasive and 4 noninvasive ductal carcinomas) whether the atypia comprised 5 percent or 60 percent of the papillary lesion (14). When the criterion of up to 90 percent was used, there were no cases that actually had 70 percent or more involvement by an atypical epithelial proliferation. Progression was observed

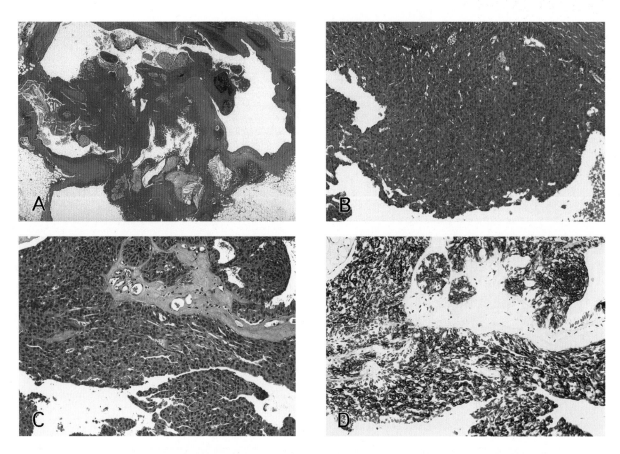

Figure 5-3

PAPILLOMA

A: Papilloma with diffuse epithelial hyperplasia.

B: The epithelial proliferation has the architecture of intraductal hyperplasia (IDH)/low-risk ductal intraepithelial neoplasia (DIN).

C: The proliferating cells have bland cytologic features.

D: The proliferating cells show immunoreactivity for CK34betaE12, reflecting a low-risk proliferating cell population comparable to IDH.

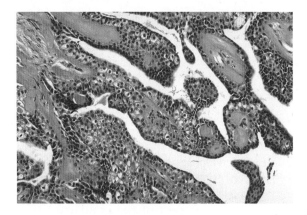

Figure 5-4

PAPILLOMA

Focal prominence and hyperplasia of myoepithelial cells in a papilloma.

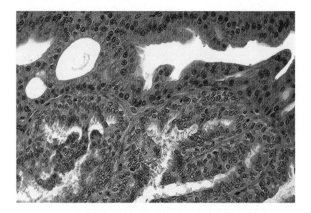

Figure 5-5

PAPILLOMA

Apocrine metaplasia is a common feature.

mainly in cases with IDH/low-risk DIN, AIDH/DIN1 ($\leq$2 mm), or LIN in the surrounding breast tissue (13). In the absence of an atypical proliferation in the surrounding mammary tissue, the risk associated with these papillary lesions does not seem to be substantially different from that of papillomas in general (14). Therefore, papillary lesions with any amount of atypia up to 90 percent can be designated as atypical papilloma or papilloma with DIN1, avoiding the term carcinoma arising in a papilloma.

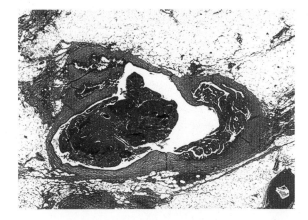

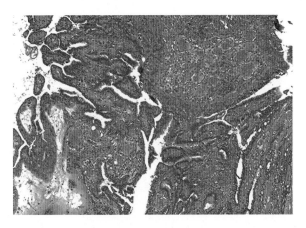

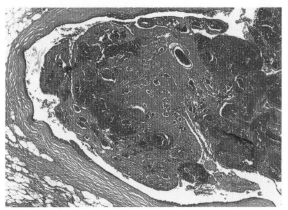

Figure 5-6

PAPILLOMA

Squamous metaplasia in the needle tract following aspiration.

Figure 5-7

INFARCTED PAPILLOMA

Top: On the right, residual viable papillae are evident.
Bottom: Hemorrhagic infarction is often due to torsion of a papillary process.

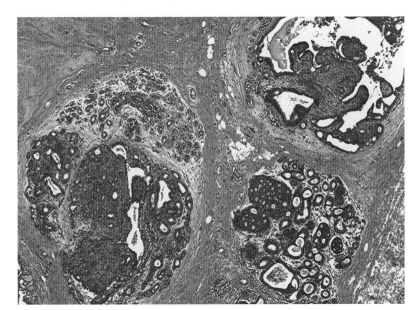

Figure 5-8

PERIPHERAL PAPILLOMA

Several adjacent terminal duct lobular units (TDLUs) show small peripheral papillomas (papillomatosis) and atypical intraductal hyperplasia (AIDH)/DIN1 (<2 mm).

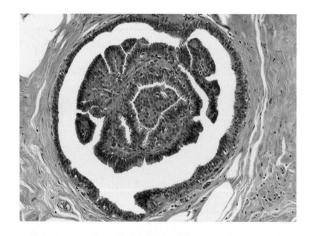

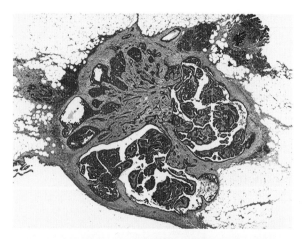

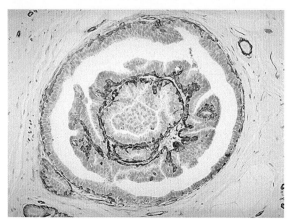

Figure 5-9

PERIPHERAL PAPILLOMA

Top: The TDLU is unfolded by a small peripheral papilloma.

Bottom: Immunostain for actin shows the myoepithelial cell layer beneath the epithelial cells.

Papillary Carcinoma

Papillary carcinomas are either noninvasive (intraductal) or invasive. The former are central or peripheral in type. When papillary carcinomas invade, they generally assume the pattern of an infiltrating duct carcinoma. A rare invasive micropapillary pattern occurs either in pure form or admixed with other patterns.

Mammographically, distinguishing a papillary carcinoma with an invasive component from one without invasion can be difficult (31). The chance of recurrence of a solitary intraductal papillary carcinoma after lumpectomy is increased when it displays high-grade cytologic features or when there is AIDH or DCIS/DIN1 in the adjacent breast tissue (2).

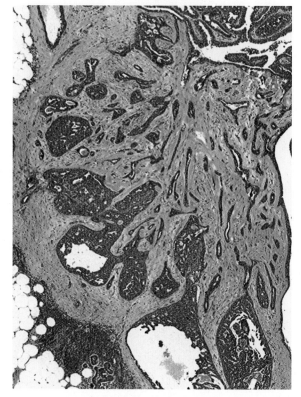

Figure 5-10

SCLEROSING PAPILLOMA

Top: Sclerotic changes are seen in about a third of the lesion.

Bottom: Distorted, elongated tubules are trapped in the sclerotic region.

Papillary intraductal carcinomas (PICs) are solitary and centrally located or multiple and peripheral in distribution. Since all PICs cause some cystic distension of the duct in which they are growing, they may all be considered as

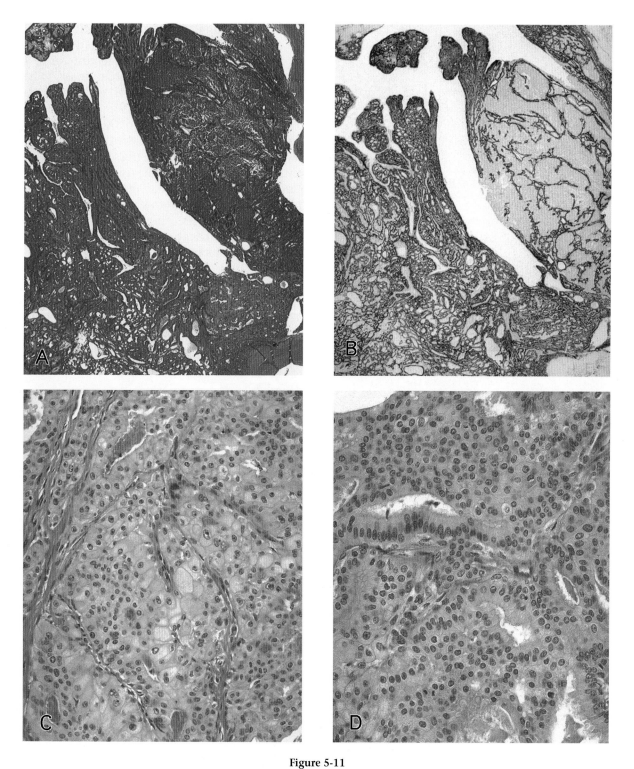

Figure 5-11

ATYPICAL PAPILLOMA

A: There is a relatively solid expansion of one papilla.
B: Immunostain for actin unmasks the areas of atypical epithelial proliferation.
C: A relatively solid proliferation of apocrine cells is in the expanded epithelial region.
D: Mitotic figures are rare.

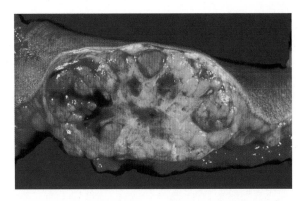

Figure 5-12

PAPILLARY INTRADUCTAL CARCINOMA

Papillary intraductal carcinoma may have a solid cut surface and assume massive proportions.

"intracystic" papillary carcinomas; both intracystic and intraductal papillary designations refer to noninvasive lesions. They account for less than 2 percent of mammary carcinomas (2,17). Patients range in age from 34 to 92 years, with an average age of 65 years (2,9).

Papillary carcinomas cannot be distinguished from benign papillomas on the basis of presentation or gross appearance (fig. 5-12). A majority of papillary carcinomas, usually intraductal carcinomas with a papillary growth pattern, are noninvasive and, therefore, associated with an excellent prognosis. They may form papillae supported by delicate fibrovascular cores with the absence of a myoepithelial cell layer (fig. 5-13). They may also form cribriform to relatively

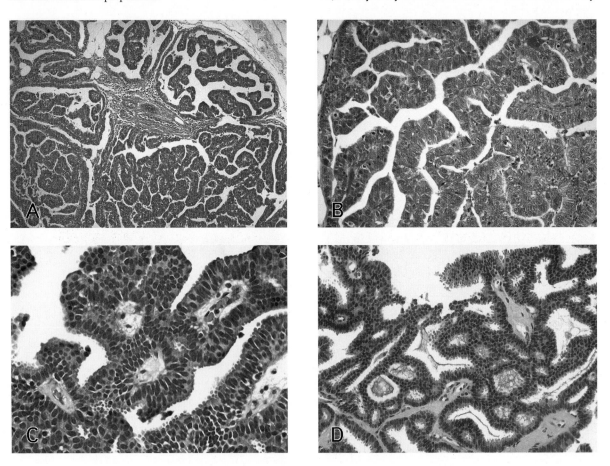

Figure 5-13

PAPILLARY INTRADUCTAL CARCINOMA

A: Delicate fibrovascular cores support the arborescent architecture.

B: The papillary processes are devoid of myoepithelial cells, and the cells are more atypical than those of typical papillary intraductal carcinoma.

C: There are stratified spindled cells and an absence of myoepithelial cells.

D: A cribriform proliferation of uniformly atypical cells overlies the fibrovascular cores.

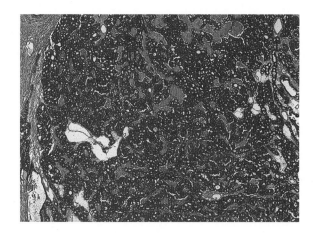
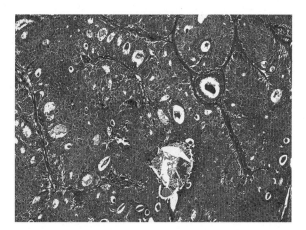

Figure 5-14

PAPILLARY INTRADUCTAL CARCINOMA

Left: A relatively solid, cribriform papillary intraductal carcinoma.
Right: Another compact solid variant of papillary carcinoma shows a fenestrated pattern.

solid patterns of epithelial proliferation generally comparable to DIN1 overlying a sometimes completely retained myoepithelial cell layer (figs. 5-14, 5-15). While complete absence of the myoepithelial cell layer or even its absence in 90 percent of the papillary processes qualifies the papillary proliferation as carcinoma, the presence of this cell layer does not exclude the diagnosis of papillary carcinoma.

Well-delineated, encapsulated, or intracystic papillary carcinomas lack a myoepithelial cell layer not only in the intraluminal papillary processes, but often also in the distended duct walls (3a,7a,16a). A basement membrane or sometimes a thickened multilayered basement membrane/fibrous capsule surrounds some of these intraductal papillary carcinomas. Importantly, despite the absence of a myoepithelial cell layer, management of these lesions as a noninvasive process is favored (3a,7a).

Microscopic papillary carcinoma confined to one or more TDLUs is generally referred to as *intraductal carcinoma, papillary type*. This pattern is often admixed with other patterns of non-necrotic intraductal carcinoma (DIN1). The so-called *micropapillary intraductal carcinoma* is composed of epithelial tufts lacking fibrovascular support and does not qualify as a true papillary lesion since the presence of fibrovascular support is required for a papillary lesion by definition.

The epithelial cells in PIC assume a variety of phenotypes ranging from uniform small

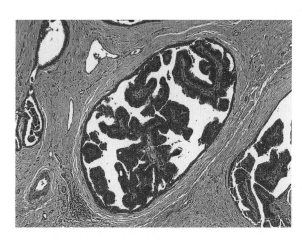

Figure 5-15

INTRADUCTAL PAPILLARY CARCINOMA, PERIPHERAL TYPE

This variant originates in the TDLU.

rounded or spindle cells to apocrine or columnar cells with subnuclear vacuoles resembling secretory phase endometrial epithelium (4a). Rarely, significant cytologic atypia and pleomorphism develop as well.

Distinction of papillomas from PIC can be problematic, particularly when tissue preparation and/or staining is suboptimal. Immunostains for myoepithelial cells are helpful in distinguishing subtypes of papillary lesions (3b). Absence of the myoepithelial cell layer can be confirmed using any of the myoepithelial cell markers (p63,

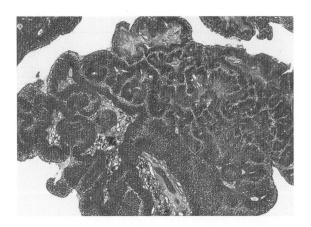 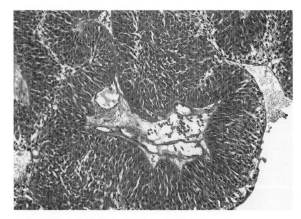

Figure 5-16

PAPILLARY TRANSITIONAL CELL CARCINOMA

Left: The papillae have a compact arrangement.

Right: The fibrovascular stalk supports a proliferation of transitional cells, resembling grade 1 or 2 papillary transitional cell carcinoma.

CD10, calponin). Myoepithelial cells do not uniformly express every myoepithelial marker, probably due to the variable functional state of the cells. In cases with abundant and solid epithelial proliferation, CK903 and CK5/6 are useful. Benign, low-risk epithelial proliferations are positive with these markers, while atypical and malignant cells are negative in nearly 90 percent of cases. Uniform and diffuse positivity for estrogen receptor (ER) is also a feature of low-grade PICs; it should be noted, however, that the rare apocrine PIC and the rare highly anaplastic PIC generally do not express ER.

It has been suggested that CD44 may help distinguish benign papilloma from papillary carcinoma. Normal breast epithelial cells and intraductal papillomas express CD44 in more than 70 percent of the epithelial cells, whereas papillary carcinomas express CD44 in less than 10 percent (30). More experience with this marker is needed before its routine application.

Some solid variants of PIC are characterized by neuroendocrine differentiation and are associated with mucin production and occasionally mucinous carcinoma (12). Lesions composed of cells resembling the tall cell variant of papillary thyroid carcinoma also rarely occur in the breast, forming a solid and papillary architecture; this morphology appears to have no clinical significance (4).

A rare variant, *papillary carcinoma with transitional cell differentiation,* has also been described

(16). This variant generally presents as a solitary, nodular papillary lesion. Microscopically, it shows a solid proliferation of numerous layers of epithelial cells overlying a fibrovascular core, with flattening of the superficial cells (fig. 5-16). The behavior of the small number of reported cases parallels that of PIC, not otherwise specified (NOS).

When a PIC invades or metastasizes, it generally assumes the pattern of an infiltrating duct carcinoma (fig. 5-17). We do not consider a papillary lesion as an invasive carcinoma simply due to the absence of the myoepithelial cell layer in the duct wall. *Invasive ductal carcinomas associated with PIC* account for less than 2 percent of invasive breast carcinomas. A disproportionate number occur in non-Caucasian women. Enlarged axillary nodes are common, due to reactive changes (6). Metastases to lymph nodes rarely, if ever, retain the classic papillary configuration if the invasive component is of typical ductal type. Early invasion may occur around the duct in which the intraepithelial component is proliferating. Both papillomas and intraductal papillary carcinomas may entrap epithelium within the sclerotic, hyalinized duct wall. Entrapment of the epithelial component into a sclerotic duct wall should not be confused with true invasion, however (fig. 5-18). Needle aspiration and core biopsies of papillomas can dislodge tumor cells into the surrounding stroma, mimicking invasive carcinoma. The presence of hemorrhage and reactive changes around such

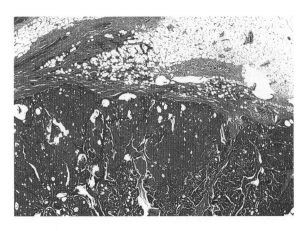
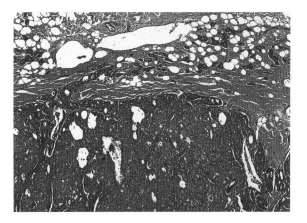

Figure 5-17

INVASIVE PAPILLARY INTRADUCTAL CARCINOMA

Left: A solid papillary intraductal carcinoma with early stromal invasion extends into the adipose tissue.
Right: The invasive component assumes the pattern of an infiltrating duct carcinoma.

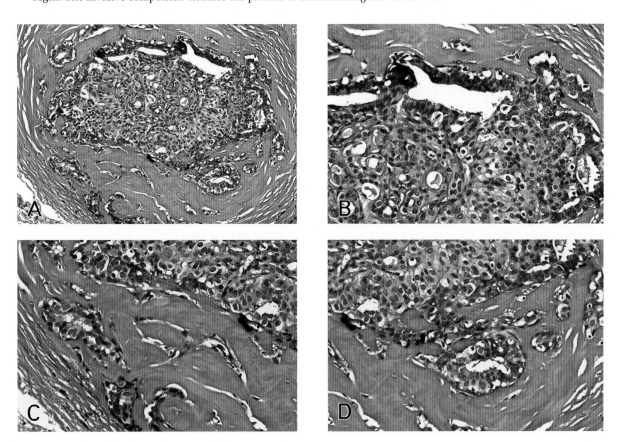

Figure 5-18

PSEUDOINVASION INTO FIBROUS DUCT WALL

A: There are irregular extensions of the epithelial elements into the thick fibrous duct wall.

B,C: The angulated shape of the entrapped epithelial elements may raise concern for invasion, but persistence of the myoepithelial cell layer around them is useful in their recognition as pseudoinvasion.

D: The myoepithelial cell layer is more attenuated here and not quite as readily apparent, but the rounded configuration is helpful.

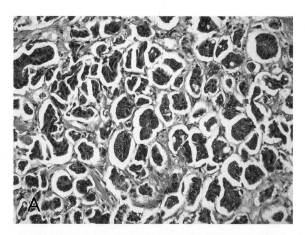

Figure 5-19

INVASIVE MICROPAPILLARY CARCINOMA

A,B: Micropapillae float in stromal spaces. The tumor cells often show grade 1 to 2 nuclear atypia.

C: The in situ (intraepithelial) carcinoma associated with this case was DCIS1/DIN1, micropapillary type.

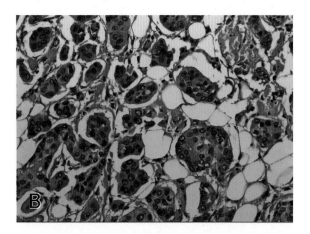

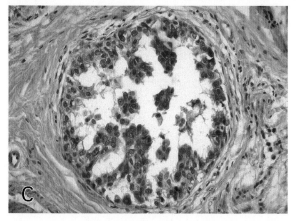

cells favors dislodgement. When there is any doubt about the possibility of entrapment or dislodgement, it is prudent not to call the lesion invasive since early invasion of less than 1 to 2 mm is probably unlikely to change the prognosis significantly. Immunostains for actin or any other marker of myoepithelial cells may help identify the myoepithelial cells that surround suspicious clusters; most dislodged clusters lack a myoepithelial cell layer as well, however.

Patients with PIC in the absence of either concomitant DCIS/DIN1-3 or invasive carcinoma in the surrounding breast tissue have a very favorable prognosis. Lymph node metastases or disease-related deaths have not been reported.

Invasive Micropapillary Carcinoma

In 1993, the term *invasive micropapillary carcinoma* was coined for an unusual variant of invasive carcinoma that retains the papillary or micropapillary configuration in the areas of invasion (33). Invasive carcinomas with a dominant or pure micropapillary pattern account for less than 2 percent of all invasive carcinomas (11,18,25); focal micropapillary change is present in 3 to 6 percent of the common types of invasive carcinoma (18,25).

The small invasive papillae of micropapillary carcinoma appear to float in empty stromal spaces or within vascular channels (fig. 5-19); peritumoral vascular invasion may occur in up to 60 percent of cases. The associated noninvasive component is generally DIN1 (ADH or low-grade DCIS of the micropapillary or cribriform type). When a noninvasive component is absent, the possibility of metastatic ovarian carcinoma (serous papillary) should be considered and excluded. Micropapillary carcinoma occurs either in pure form or admixed with regular infiltrating duct carcinoma. Metastases and recurrences retain the micropapillary configuration.

The micropapillary growth pattern has no independent significance for survival on multivariate analyses (18,25). There is a higher frequency of lymph node metastases and lymphovascular space involvement in this subtype, resulting in a worse overall prognosis. Several reports have elaborated the characteristics of this lesion. One group suggested that these tumors have a high incidence of axillary node metastases and early recurrence rate (35). A report on 14 cases of micropapillary carcinoma from the National Institutes of Health (NIH) also suggested that this is an aggressive tumor with an unfavorable prognosis (15). In another study of 21 invasive micropapillary carcinomas, patients had survival rates similar to those of patients with other breast cancers and equivalent numbers of lymph node metastases (18). A larger series of 80 invasive micropapillary carcinomas included a substantial number of tumors combined with other types of invasive carcinoma (37); axillary lymph node involvement was noted in 72 to 77 percent of patients at presentation.

MOLECULAR ALTERATIONS ASSOCIATED WITH PAPILLARY LESIONS

Clonal analysis of solitary intraductal papilloma has shown that it is monoclonal in origin, suggesting that the lesion originates from a common precursor cell capable of differentiating into epithelial and myoepithelial cells (20). The few studies that have compared the molecular profiles of papilloma and papillary carcinoma indicate chromosome 16 as the most frequently altered, with changes in 16q noted in 52 to 67 percent of lesions. Two studies noted that over 40 percent (3c) and 60 to 63 percent (10) of benign papillomas and papillary lesions harboring carcinoma have loss of heterozygosity (LOH) on chromosome 16p13. Chromosome 16p may contain a tumor-suppressing gene that is mutated in papillary lesions (10). Numerical and structural alterations at chromosomes 16q and 1q, with fusion of chromosomes 16 and 1 [der(1;16)], have been described in low-grade papillary carcinomas by fluorescence in situ hybridization (36). LOH on chromosome 16q was detected in 67 percent of 12 intracystic papillary adenocarcinomas but none of 11 papillomas (36a). In one study, 4 of 5 invasive micropapillary carcinomas had LOH on locus 17p13.1 (p53) (15). Abnormalities of chromosome 8 have been detected in invasive micropapillary carcinoma by comparative genomic hybridization (34). Papillary lesions are highly

Table 5-2

CYTOLOGIC FINDINGS IN MAMMARY PAPILLARY LESIONS ON FINE NEEDLE ASPIRATION BIOPSY[a]

Cytologic Findings	Papilloma	Intracystic Papillary Carcinoma
Cellularity	1-3+ Hypocellular in marked cystic and sclerotic change	3+
Architecture	LCBS[b] and 3D clusters FVC (72%)	LCBS and 3D clusters Rare FVC
Columnar cells	Present (70%)	Present
Single cells	Present (75%) 2-3+ (38%)	2-3+
Atypia	Present in 7% (2+)	3+
Background	Cystic/bloody (72%)	Cystic/bloody

[a]Adapted from reference 32.
[b]LCBS = large complex branching sheets; FVC = fibrovascular cores.

complex and the current molecular studies have barely touched on many of the possible variations that occur in this group of lesions.

ASPIRATION CYTOLOGY, CORE BIOPSY, AND FROZEN SECTION EVALUATION OF PAPILLARY LESIONS

Aspiration cytology of papillary lesions should be interpreted with caution. Many aspirates displaying "papillary" clusters of cells are nonpapillary on excisional biopsies. Fibrocystic changes and fibroadenomas are among those simulating a papilloma on cytology preparations. Simsir et al. (32) suggest that despite overlapping features, it is possible to separate papillary lesions into benign or atypical categories based on the features enumerated in Table 5-2.

Fine needle aspiration cytology of micropapillary carcinoma is characterized by a "dual" pattern formed by round or angulated, three-dimensional, cohesive clusters of neoplastic cells with a pseudopapillary configuration and two-dimensional, dyscohesive aggregates and single cells with high-grade nuclei and intact cytoplasm (26). A micropapillary pattern of mucinous carcinoma is characterized by micropapillary cell clusters lacking fibrovascular cores in a mucoid background (19).

Core biopsies of a papillary lesion should be interpreted cautiously because of the heterogeneity within a papillary lesion and the possible presence of simultaneous benign and morphologically malignant areas. Even if the sampled tissue cores show only benign papillary fragments, the possibility that the remainder of the lesion may have atypical or in situ carcinoma/DIN1-3 within it cannot be excluded (1b). On the other hand, if a small sample is morphologically identical to a papillary carcinoma, the lesion may prove to be an atypical papilloma if the changes are limited to the small portion of the papillary structures that were sampled by the core. The presence of atypia in the core biopsy (1a,28) and patient age of 65 or older are important risk factors for the presence of malignancy in the subsequent excisional biopsy (1a). Some small peripheral (located in TDLUs) papillomas are completely excised by the core biopsy, however, and can be accurately interpreted by this procedure. The pathologic findings should be correlated with the clinical and mammographic findings.

Requests for frozen section evaluation of breast carcinomas are rare and should be abandoned; this is particularly crucial for papillary lesions. Freezing diminishes the tinctorial differences between the epithelial and myoepithelial cells, making recognition of the latter difficult. In this setting, a definitive diagnosis of the papillary lesion should be deferred to permanent sections.

MANAGEMENT OF PAPILLARY LESIONS

Because different areas of a papillary lesion may have variable morphologic appearances, complete excision is prudent if a papillary lesion is detected on needle core biopsy. Solitary intraductal/intracystic papillary carcinomas should be excised with a rim of uninvolved mammary tissue to assess the alterations in the surrounding breast tissue. The likelihood of recurrence increases when either AIDH or DCIS/DIN1-3 is present in the surrounding ducts. Multifocal, peripheral intraductal papillary carcinoma should be approached and managed as DCIS/DIN1-3, whether diagnosed on a core or an excisional biopsy.

The management of patients with papillomatosis diagnosed on core biopsies requires a cautious approach and consideration of family history and mammographic findings. If the lesion is an incidental finding, localized in its distribution to one or two TDLUs and small enough to have been removed by the biopsy, no more than follow-up is required. If there is widespread calcification, however, management depends on the degree of clinical suspicion for malignancy; definitive guidelines for this issue are difficult to establish. About 20 percent of in situ ductal carcinomas/DIN1-3 have papillomatosis in the surrounding area, somewhat complicating the recommendation for the management of papillomatosis based entirely on a core biopsy.

REFERENCES

1. Ali-Fehmi R, Carolin K, Wallis T, Visscher DW. Clinicopathologic analysis of breast lesions associated with multiple papillomas. Hum Pathol 2003;34:234-239.
1a. Arora N, Hill V, Hoda SA, Rosenblatt R, Pigalarga R, Tousimis EA. Clinicopathologic features of papillary lesions on core needle biopsy of the breast predictive of malignancy. Am J Surg 2007;194:444-449.
1b. Ashkenazi I, Ferrer K, Sekosan M, et al. Papillary lesions of the breast discovered on percutaneous large core and vacuum-assisted biopsies: reliability of clinical and pathological parameters in identifying benign lesions. Am J Surg 2007;194:183-188.
2. Carter D, Orr SL, Merino MI. Intracystic papillary carcinoma of the breast. After mastectomy, radiation therapy or excisional biopsy alone. Cancer 1983;52:14-19.
3. Cardenosa G, Eklund GW. Benign papillary neoplasms of the breast: mammographic findings. Radiology 1991;181:751-755.
3a. Collins LC, Carlo VP, Hwang H, Barry TS, Gown AM, Schnitt SJ. Intracystic papillary carcinomas of the breast: a reevaluation using a panel of myoepithelial cell markers. Am J Surg Pathol 2006;30:1002-1007.

3b. de Moraes Schenka NG, Schenka AA, de Souza Queiroz L, de Almeida Matsura M, Vassallo J, Alvarenga M. Use of p63 and CD10 in the differential diagnosis of papillary neoplasms of the breast. Breast J 2008;14:68-75.

3c. DiCristofano, Mrad K, Zavaglia K, et al. Papillary lesions of the breast: a molecular progression? Breast Cancer Res Treat 2005;90:71-76.

4. Eusebi V, Damiani S, Ellis IO, Azzopardi JG, Rosai J. Breast tumor resembling the tall cell variant of papillary thyroid carcinoma: report of 5 cases. Am J Surg Pathol 2003;27;1114-1118.

4a. Fadare O, Rose TA, Tavassoli FA. Papillary intraductal carcinoma with extensive secretory endometrium-like subnuclear vacuolization. Breast J 2005;11:470-471.

5. Fenoglio C, Lattes R. Sclerosing papillary proliferations in the female breast. A benign lesion often mistaken for carcinoma. Cancer 1974;33:691-700.

6. Fisher ER, Palekar AS, Redmond C, Barton B, Fisher B. Pathologic findings from the National Surgical Adjuvant Breast Project (protocol no. 4). VI. Invasive papillary cancer. Am J Clin Pathol 1980;73:313-322.

7. Flint A, Oberman HA. Infarction and squamous metaplasia of intraductal papilloma: a benign breast lesion that may simulate carcinoma. Hum Pathol 1984;15:764-767.

7a. Hill CB, Yeh IT. Myoepithelial cell staining patterns of papillary breast lesions: from intraductal papillomas to invasive papillary carcinomas. Am J Clin Pathol 2005;123:36-44.

8. Jiao YF, Nakamura S, Oikawa T, Sugai T, Uesugi N. Sebaceous gland metaplasia in intraductal papilloma of the breast. Virchows Arch 2001;438:505-508.

9. Lefkowitz M, Lefkowitz W, Wargotz ES. Intraductal (intracystic) papillary carcinoma of the breast and its variants: a clinicopathologic study of 77 cases. Hum Pathol 1994;25:802-809.

10. Lininger RA, Park WS, Man YG, et al. LOH at 16p13 is a novel chromosomal alteration detected in benign and malignant microdissected papillary neoplasms of the breast. Hum Pathol 1998;29:1113-1118.

11. Luna More S, Casquero S, Perez-Mellado A, Ruis F, Weill B, Gornemann I. Importance of estrogen receptors for the behavior of invasive micropapillary carcinoma of the breast. Review of 68 cases with follow-up of 54. Pathol Res Pract 2000;196:35-39.

12. Maluf HM, Koerner FC. Solid papillary carcinoma of the breast. A form of intraductal carcinoma with endocrine differentiation associated frequently with mucinous carcinoma. Am J Surg Pathol 1995;19:1237-1244.

13. MacGrogan G, Tavassoli FA. Central atypical papillomas of the breast: a clinicopathological study of 119 cases. Virchows Arch 2003;443:609-617.

14. McCullough GL, Evans AJ, Yeoman L, et al. Radiologic features of papillary carcinoma of breast. Clin Radiol 1997;52:865-868.

15. Middleton LP, Tressera F, Sobel ME, et al. Infiltrating micropapillary carcinoma of the breast. Mod Pathol 1999;12:499-504.

16. Mooney EE, Tavassoli FA. Papillary transitional cell carcinoma of the breast: a report of five cases with distinction from eccrine acrospiroma. Mod Pathol 1999;12:287-294.

16a. Moritani S, Ichihara S, Kushima R, et al. Myoepithelial cells in solid variant of intraductal papillary carcinoma of the breast: a potential diagnostic pitfall and a proposal of an immunohistochemical panel in the differential diagnosis with intraductal papilloma with usual ductal hyperplasia. Virchows Arch 2007;450:539-547.

17. Murad T, Contesso G, Mouriesse H. Papillary tumors of large lactiferous ducts. Cancer 1981;48:122-133.

18. Nassar H, Wallis T, Andea A, Dey J, Adsay V, Visscher D. Clinicopathologic analysis of invasive micropapillary differentiation in breast carcinoma. Mod Pathol 2001;14:836-841.

19. Ng WK. Fine-needle aspiration cytology findings of an uncommon micropapillary variant of pure mucinous carcinoma of the breast: review of patients over an 8-year period. Cancer 2002;96:280-288.

20. Noguchi S, Motomura K, Inaji H, Imaoka S, Koyama H. Clonal analysis of solitary intraductal papilloma of the breast by means of polymerase chain reaction. Am J Pathol 1994;144:1320-1325.

21. Ohuchi N, Abe R, Kasai M. Possible cancerous change of intraductal papillomas of the breast. A 3-D reconstruction study of 25 cases. Cancer 1984;54:605-611.

22. Ohuchi N, Abe R, Takahashi T, Tezuka F. Origin and extension of intraductal papillomas of the breast: a three-dimensional reconstruction study. Breast Cancer Res Treat 1984;4:117-128.

23. Page DL, Salhany KE, Jensen RA, Dupont WD. Subsequent breast carcinoma risk after biopsy with atypia in a breast papilloma. Cancer 1996;78:258-266.

24. Papotti M, Guggliotta P, Ghiringhello B, Bussolati G. Association of breast carcinoma and multiple intraductal papillomas: an histological and immunohistochemical investigation. Histopathology 1984;8:963-975.

25. Paterakos M, Watkin WG, Edgerton SM, Moore DH 2nd, Thor AD. Invasive micropapillary carcinoma of the breast: a prognostic study. Hum Pathol 1999;30:1459-1463.

26. Pettinato G, Pambuccian SE, Di Prisco B, Manivel JC. Fine needle aspiration cytology of invasive micropapillary (pseudopapillary) carcinoma of the breast. Report of 11 cases with clinicopathologic findings. Acta Cytol 2002;46:1088-1094

27. Raju U, Vertes D. Breast papillomas with atypical ductal hyperplasia: a clinicopathologic study. Hum Pathol 1996;27:1231-1238.

28. Rosen EL, Bentley RC, Baker JA, Soo MS. Imaging-guided core needle biopsy of papillary lesions of the breast. AJR Am J Roentgenol 2002;179:1185-1192.

29. Rosen PP. Arthur Purdy Stout and papilloma of the breast. Comments on the occasion of his 100th birthday. Am J Surg Pathol 1986;10(Suppl 1):100-107.

30. Saddik M, Lai R. CD44s as a surrogate marker for distinguishing intraductal papilloma from papillary carcinoma of the breast. J Clin Pathol 1999;52:862-864.

31. Schneider JA. Invasive papillary carcinoma: a mammographic and sonographic appearance. Radiology 1989;171:377-379.

32. Simsir A, Waisman J, Thorner K, Cangiarella J. Mammary lesions diagnosed as "papillary" by aspiration biopsy. 70 cases with follow-up. Cancer 2003;99:156-165.

33. Siriaunkgul S, Tavassoli FA. Invasive micropapillary carcinoma of the breast. Mod Pathol 1993;6:660-662.

34. Thor AD, Eng C, Devries S, et al. Invasive micropapillary carcinoma of the breast is associated with chromosome 8 abnormalities detected by comparative genomic hybridization. Hum Pathol 2002;33:628-631.

35. Tresserra F, Grases PJ, Fabregas R, Fernandez-Cid A, Dexeus S. Invasive micropapillary carcinoma. Distinct features of a poorly recognized variant of breast carcinoma. Eur J Gynaecol Oncol 1999;20:205-208.

36. Tsuda H, Takarabe T, Sasumu N, Inazawa J, Okada S, Hirohashi S. Detection of numerical and structural alterations and fusion of chromosomes 16 and 1 in low grade papillary breast carcinoma by fluorescence in situ hybridization. Am J Pathol 1997;151:1027-1034.

36a. Tsuda H, Uei Y, Fukutomi T, Hiroshi S. Different incidence of loss of heterozygosity on chromosome 16q between intraductal papilloma and intracystic papillary carcinoma of the breast. Jpn J Cancer Res 1994;85:992-996.

37. Walsh MM, Bleiweiss IJ. Invasive micropapillary carcinoma of the breast: eighty cases of an under-recognized entity. Hum Pathol 2001;32:583-589.

38. Woods ER, Helvie MA, Ikeda DM, Mandell SH, Chapel KL, Adler DD. Solitary breast papilloma: comparison of mammographic galactographic and pathologic findings. Am J Roentgenol 1992;159:487-491.

6 MICROINVASIVE CARCINOMA

Microinvasive carcinoma is characterized by the extension of a few cancer cells beyond the basement membrane of the in situ component and into the adjacent stroma. If there is any uncertainty concerning the presence of invasion, the lesion should be interpreted as noninvasive.

Microinvasive carcinomas are rare and occur mostly in association with ductal carcinoma in situ (DCIS)/ductal intraepithelial neoplasia grade 2-3 (DIN2-3), papillary intraductal carcinoma, and lobular intraepithelial neoplasia (LIN) (12,21). Even in pure consultation practices where the largest number of microinvasive carcinomas are sent for second opinion, microinvasive carcinomas account for significantly less than 1 percent of breast carcinomas (18).

CLINICAL FEATURES

The clinical presentation of microinvasive carcinoma is the same as that of the associated DCIS/DIN and LIN. DCIS/DIN1-3 is most frequently mammographically detected and less commonly associated with nipple discharge or a palpable mass. LIN is generally an incidental finding and has no specific clinical presentation.

PATHOLOGIC FINDINGS

The definition, and hence, the histopathologic criteria for a diagnosis of microinvasive carcinoma, remain contentious. The few points everyone agrees on include: 1) the areas of microinvasion are composed of irregular clusters, small aggregates, or single tumor cells devoid of a myoepithelial cell layer and basement membrane; 2) microinvasion occurs in association with not only all grades of DCIS/DIN1-3 (figs. 6-1–6-3), but also with LIN (fig. 6-4) (11,21) as well as papillary DCIS; and 3) microinvasion is most often present when there is a significant periductal/perilobular lymphocytic infiltrate or an altered periductal desmoplastic stroma, features often present in cases of comedo DCIS/DIN3 (18,23). When there is doubt about the presence of invasion and particularly if uncertainty persists even after rebiopsy and immunostaining for the detection of myoepithelial cells, the case should be diagnosed as noninvasive.

A variety of markers are helpful in unmasking myoepithelial cells (24). These include smooth muscle actin, CD10, calponin, p63 (nuclear), cytokeratin (CK) 14, and smooth muscle myosin-heavy chain (SMM-HC). SMM-HC shows the least cross reactivity with stromal myofibroblasts, which may mimic a myoepithelial cell layer when apposed to the invasive cells.

Some studies on microinvasive carcinoma have provided no maximum size (16,22) or criteria (8) for diagnosis. Some have described subtypes, separating those purely composed of single cells from those that also contain cell clusters and/or tubules of nongradable tumor, without providing information about maximum size, extent, or number of microinvasive foci (3). Others have defined the microinvasive component as a percentage of the surface of the histologic sections (17). More precise definitions accept an unlimited number of clearly separate foci of infiltration into the stroma with none exceeding 1 mm in diameter (1), one or two foci of microinvasion with none exceeding 1 mm (19), a single focus not exceeding 2 mm, or three foci, none exceeding 1 mm in maximum diameter (18).

To qualify as invasive, some require extension of the individual cells or clusters of tumor cells beyond the specialized lobular stroma (4,5). The definitive presence of vascular channels both within the specialized lobular stroma and immediately surrounding the basement membrane that invests the ductules makes this requirement untenable since vascular invasion can occur even within the lobular stroma. Others have required loss of continuity of invasive cells from the intraductal/intraepithelial component. Tumor cells are not known to leap or jump or disassociate from the remaining intraepithelial component in order to invade the stroma, however. Furthermore, the unequivocal influence of the plane of section on the detection of continuity between

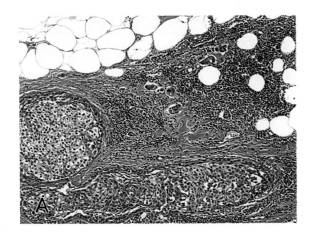

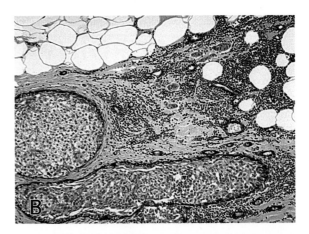

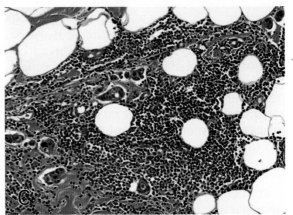

Figure 6-1

MICROINVASIVE CARCINOMA

A: A few small clusters of invasive carcinoma are associated with low-grade ductal carcinoma in situ (DCIS)/ductal intraepithelial neoplasia (DIN1).

B: The immunostain for actin contrasts the myoepithelial-bound DIN and the loose clusters of invasive tumor cells.

C: Higher magnification of the invasive cell clusters.

D: Immunostain for actin shows a lack of myoepithelial cells around the invasive cells; the vascular channels are positive.

E: Microinvasive carcinoma associated with atypical intraductal hyperplasia (AIDH)/DIN1 (<2 mm).

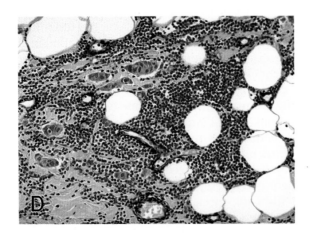

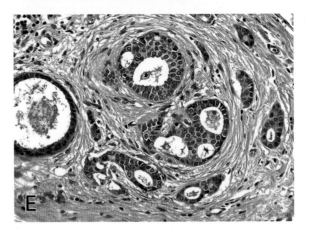

the in situ and invasive components renders this requirement invalid.

DIFFERENTIAL DIAGNOSIS

The most important entity in the differential diagnosis is the artifactual displacement of cells from an in situ process into the surrounding stroma secondary to tissue manipulation (fig. 6-5) or needle punctures (25). Suboptimal slides, a tangential cut through the edge of acini, and the presence of branching points and crush or cautery artifact, particularly in areas with a lymphocytic infiltrate, are other sources of diagnostic problems. Recuts and immunostains are helpful in resolving these problems in a majority of cases. Double immunolabeling with cytokeratin and smooth muscle actin is particularly helpful for assessing microinvasion and early

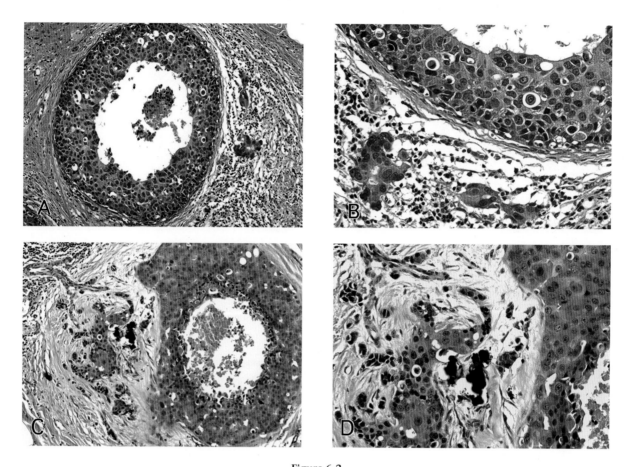

Figure 6-2

MICROINVASIVE CARCINOMA

A: Grade 3 DCIS/DIN3 with microinvasion.
B: The invasive tumor cells are in a lymphoplasmacytic background; there was no history of prior needle core biopsy.
C: Grade 3 DCIS/DIN3 with microinvasion microcalcification is evident in the microinvasive focus.
D: Higher magnification shows a vessel stretching toward the invasive focus.

stromal invasion (13). A diagnosis of noninvasive carcinoma is the prudent approach when doubts persist despite additional studies.

PROGNOSIS AND PREDICTIVE FACTORS

Given the lack of a standardized definition for the lesions in published studies, the clinical significance of "microinvasion" remains controversial. There are not many studies on microinvasive carcinomas or even invasive carcinomas that are 5 mm or smaller in size. The design of many available studies is such that they do not answer some crucial questions (e.g., Is the presence of rare axillary lymph node metastases due to sampling limitations that may have missed a larger focus of invasive carcinoma in the mammary tissue?).

For management purposes, it is important to determine the largest size of an invasive carcinoma that may be safely managed without axillary lymph node dissection, particularly when the associated in situ carcinoma is small and limited in extent. The size of an invasive mammary carcinoma with no risk of distant metastases has not been established; given the size of the breast and the routine sampling limitations, we may never have a definitive definition of such a lesion. At this time, there is no study that provides a basis for considering innumerable foci of invasion less than 1 mm as microinvasive, although this is the recommended definition of microinvasive carcinoma by the American Joint Commission on Cancer (AJCC) (1). This is not an evidence based recommendation. Multifocal disruption of the

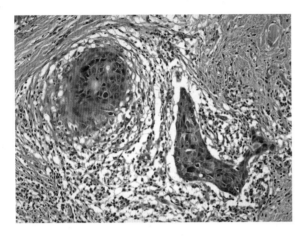
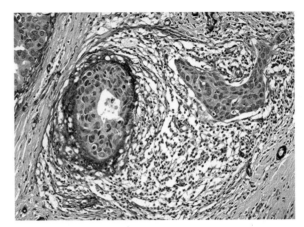

Figure 6-3

MICROINVASIVE CARCINOMA

Left: An angulated cluster of invasive cells is next to a duct with few but highly atypical cells and a significant periductal lymphoplasmacytic reaction.

Right: The immunostain for actin shows the absence of myoepithelial cells around the invasive cell cluster.

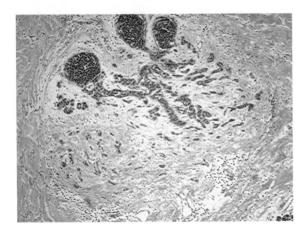
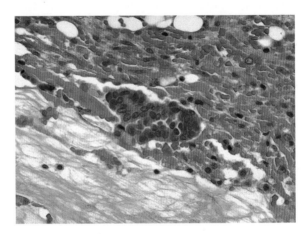

Figure 6-4

MICROINVASIVE CARCINOMA ASSOCIATED WITH LOBULAR INTRAEPITHELIAL NEOPLASIA

The invasive carcinoma is within and outside the stroma of the terminal duct lobular unit (TDLU).

Figure 6-5

PSEUDOINVASION BY DISLODGED CELLS

These cytologically benign tumor cells within the hemorrhagic needle tract were artifactually dislodged during needle aspiration and do not represent microinvasion.

boundaries of an in situ carcinoma and the volume of invasive tumor cells may be crucial factors implying a generalized instability. It is, therefore, conceivable that patients with such lesions may have a worse prognosis compared to those with in situ lesions and a single or multiple, but a finite and small, number of invasive foci.

A few studies that have found no evidence of axillary lymph node metastases associated with a finite number of invasive foci 1 mm or less in maximum dimension or a single invasive focus of 2 mm or less (18,19,21). Using the AJCC definition of microinvasion, axillary node metastases have been identified in up to 10 percent of mainly sentinel nodes (10,15,20,26). Others have described axillary node metastases in 20 percent of such patients (6,9,14).

Of 38 women who had mastectomy for their minimally invasive carcinomas (a single focus of 2 mm or less or up to three invasive foci, none exceeding 1 mm), none had axillary node metastases, and none developed recurrences or metastases (18). The few other studies with a comparable, but not exactly the same definition of microinvasion and follow-up data, support the excellent prognosis for these patients (2,12,15,19,22). Since it is impossible for pathologists to routinely examine an entire sample exhaustively, it is quite possible that small foci of invasive carcinoma are missed, particularly in a setting of extensive in situ carcinoma. Given the absence of an ideal or optimal study and the limitations imposed by routine tissue sampling, microinvasion is best defined as the largest size (?1 mm, ?2 mm, ?5 mm) of one or more foci with the lowest acceptable level of risk (10 percent) for axillary lymph node metastases.

For management purposes, it is appropriate to sample the sentinel node for women with extensive and particularly high-grade DCIS/DIN, with or without minuscule foci of invasive carcinoma (9) diagnosed in a needle core biopsy and with mammographic confirmation of extent.

Several recent studies (using the AJCC definition of microinvasion) have found axillary lymph node metastases in 7.5 to 10.0 percent (7,10,10a,26) of women with DCIS and microinvasion. The metastases are often confined to the sentinel lymph node, and many are micrometastases. In many women, the sentinel node is the only involved node after complete axillary lymph node dissection (CAD). For those with positive sentinel nodes, the decision to proceed to CAD is not mandatory if the sentinel node shows micrometastatic disease, but this issue needs further assessment.

Since there is no universally accepted definition of microinvasion, a pathology report should provide the size of the largest focus of invasion along with the number of foci of invasion, noting any special studies utilized to arrive at the diagnosis (i.e., 1.3 mm, 2 foci, immunohistochemistry). Whole mounts or macrosections increase the chances of finding multiple foci of microinvasion.

REFERENCES

1. American Joint Committee on Cancer. AJCC cancer staging manual, 5th ed. Philadelphia: Lippincott-Raven; 1997:172-173.
2. Damiani S, Ludvikova M, Tomasik G, Bianchi S, Gown AM, Eusebi V. Myoepithelial cells and basal lamina in poorly differentiated in situ duct carcinoma of the breast. An immunohistochemical study. Virchows Arch 1999;434:227-234.
3. de Mascarel I, MacGrogan G, Mathoulin-Pelissier S, Soubeyran I, Picot V, Coindre JM. Breast ductal carcinoma in situ with microinvasion: a definition supported by a long-term study of 1248 serially sectioned ductal carcinomas. Cancer 2002;94:2134-2142.
4. Elston CW, Ellis IO, eds. Systemic pathology, 3rd ed, vol 3, the Breast. Edinburgh: Churchill Livingstone; 1998:242.
5. European Guidelines for Quality Assurance in Mammography Screening. Luxembourg: 2nd ed. Office for Official Publications of the European Communities; 1996.
6. Howat AJ, Armour A, Ellis IO. Microinvasive lobular carcinoma of the breast. Histopathology 2000;37:477-478.
7. Intra M, Zurrida S, Maffini F, et al. Sentinel lymph node metastasis in microinvasive breast carcinoma. Ann Surg Oncol 2003;10:1160-1165.
8. Kinne DW, Petrek JA, Osborne MP, Fracchia AA, DePalo AA, Rosen PP. Breast carcinoma in situ. Arch Surg 1989;124:33-36.
9. Klauber-DeMore N, Tan LK, Liberman L, et al. Sentinel lymph node biopsy: is it indicated in patients with high-risk ductal carcinoma-in-situ and ductal carcinoma-in-situ with microinvasion? Ann Surg Oncol 2000;7:636-642.
10. Le Bouedec G, de Lapasse C, Mishellany F, et al. [Ductal carcinoma in situ of the breast with microinvasion. Role of sentinel lymph node biopsy.] Gynecol Obstet Fertil 2007;35:317-322. [French]
10a. Le Bouedec G, Gimbergues P, Feillel V, Penault-Llorca F, Dauplat J. [In situ mammary duct carcinoma with microinvasion. Which axillary lymph node exploration?] Presse Med 2005;34:208-212. [French.]

11. Nemoto T, Castillo N, Tsukada Y, Koul A, Eckert KH Jr, Bauer RL. Lobular carcinoma in situ with microinvasion. J Surg Oncol 1998;67:41-46.

12. Padmore RF, Fowble B, Hoffman J, Rosser C, Hanlon A, Patchefsky AS. Microinvasive breast carcinoma: clinicopathologic analysis of a single institution experience. Cancer 2000;88:1403-1409.

13. Prasad ML, Hyjek E, Giri DD, Ying L, O'Leary JJ, Hoda SA. Double immunolabeling with cytokeratin and smooth-muscle actin in confirming early invasive carcinoma of the breast. Am J Surg Pathol 1999;23:176-181.

14. Prasad ML, Osborne MP, Giri DD, Hoda SA. Microinvasive carcinoma (T1mic) of the breast: clinicopathologic profile of 21 cases. Am J Surg Pathol 2000;24:422-428.

15. Rosner D, Lane WW, Penetrante R. Ductal carcinoma in situ with microinvasion: a curable entity using surgery alone without need for adjuvant therapy. Cancer 1991;67:1498-1503.

16. Schuh ME, Nemoto T, Penetrante RB, Rosner D, Dao TL. Intraductal carcinoma. Analysis of presentation, pathologic findings, and outcome of disease. Arch Surg 1986;121:1303-1307.

17. Schwartz GF, Feig SA, Rosenberg AL, Patchefsky AS, Schwartz AB. Staging and treatment of clinically occult breast cancer. Cancer 1984;53:1379-1384.

18. Silver SA, Tavassoli FA. Mammary ductal carcinoma in situ with microinvasion. Cancer 1998;82:2382-2390.

19. Silverstein MJ, Gierson ED, Colburn WJ, Rosser RJ, Waisman JR, Gamagami P. Axillary lymphadenectomy for intraductal carcinoma of the breast. Surg Gynecol Obstet 1991;172:211-214.

20. Solin LJ, Fowble BL, Yeh IT, et al. Microinvasive ductal carcinoma of the breast treated with breast-conserving surgery and definitive irradiation. Int J Radiat Oncol Biol Phys 1992;23:961-968.

21. Tavassoli F. Pathology of the breast, 2nd ed. Stamford, CT: Appleton & Lange/McGraw Hill; 1999.

22. Wong JH, Kopald KH, Morton DL. The impact of microinvasion on axillary node metastases and survival in patients with intraductal breast cancer. Arch Surg 1990;125:1298-1301.

23. Yang M, Moriya T, Oguma M, et al. Microinvasive ductal carcinoma (T1mic) of the breast. The clinicopathological profile and immunohistochemical features of 28 cases. Pathol Int 2003;53:422-428.

24. Yaziji H, Gown AM, Sneige N. Detection of stromal invasion in breast cancer: the myoepithelial markers. Adv Anat Pathol 2000;7:100-109.

25. Youngson BJ, Liberman L, Rosen PP. Displacement of carcinomatous epithelium in surgical breast specimens following stereotaxic core biopsy. Am J Clin Pathol 1995;103:698-702.

26. Zavagno G, Belardinelli V, Marconato R, et al. Sentinel lymph node metastasis from mammary ductal carcinoma in situ with microinvasion. Breast 2007;16:146-151.

7 STAGING OF BREAST CARCINOMA AND PROGNOSTIC AND PREDICTIVE INDICATORS

Staging is the assessment of a given tumor based on its anatomic extent. The breast cancer TNM staging system is based on the premise that the tumor progresses in extent and that progression is directly related to prognosis. Any approach to tumor staging incorporates the application of the most recent knowledge on the subject and, as such, there is a need to continuously update this knowledge in order to incorporate the latest scientific achievements, especially in this age of rapid technological advances. This is one of the reasons why Veronesi et al. (137) have proposed the "dynamic" TNM approach that is based on a "personalized" classification of each patient.

There are limitations in the ability to accurately stage breast cancer, such as the fact that breast cancer is not one type of tumor, but one that changes its biological behavior with grade, type, and anatomic extent. The currently recommended staging system for breast cancer is the one adopted in 2002 by the American Joint Committee on Cancer (AJCC) as well as the Union Internationale Contre le Cancer (UICC) (1). Similar to previous staging protocols, the present one is based on the features of the primary tumor (T), the extent of regional lymph node metastases (N), and the presence of distant metastases (M). The histopathologic confirmation of the diagnosis is mandatory.

Compared to the 1997 TNM staging system, the current system includes some changes. Micrometastases, tumor deposits greater than 0.2 mm but less than 2.0 mm in largest dimension that may have histologic evidence of malignant activity (defined broadly as proliferation and/or stromal reaction), are classified as pN1mi. They must be distinguished from isolated tumor cells (ITCs), defined as single cells or small clusters of cells not greater than 0.2 mm in largest dimension, usually with no histologic evidence of malignant activity (i.e., proliferation and/or stromal reaction). ITCs are classified as pN0

even if spotted in routine hematoxylin and eosin (H&E)-stained specimens. If ITCs are revealed by immunohistochemistry in H&E apparently negative lymph nodes, these are designated as pN0(i+). This point needs to be changed in the next version of the TNM system as now it seems that ITCs exist only if stained with a keratin antibody.

Identifiers are used to indicate sentinel lymph nodes and immunohistochemical and molecular techniques. If micrometastasis is detected only by immunohistochemistry, the case is designated as pN1mi(i+). Cases that are negative with histology and immunohistochemistry but are positive for metastases using reverse transcriptase-polymerase chain reaction (RT-PCR) are designated pN0(mol+). This is because there is no definitive genetic marker of malignancy as yet and false positive results can be obtained with this technique. When the classification is based only on sentinel lymph node dissection, the designation of sn (sentinel node) should be given. In cases where sentinel node dissection is followed by standard axillary lymph node dissection, the classification is based on the total result (axillary lymph node plus sentinel node dissection).

Lymph node status is now classified according to the number of involved nodes determined by H&E staining or by immunohistochemistry, including nodes with ITCs. Metastasis to the infraclavicular lymph nodes is classified as N3. Changes have been introduced in the classification of internal mammary nodes in which the microscopic involvement as detected by sentinel node dissection using lymphoscintigraphy only is classified as N1. Macroscopic involvement as detected by imaging studies (excluding lymphoscintigraphy) or by clinical examination is classified as N2 in the absence of, or N3 if it occurs in the presence of, metastases to the axillary lymph nodes. Also, metastases to the supraclavicular nodes are classified as N3 rather than M1 in the previous version.

123

Table 7-1

2002 TNM STAGING CLASSIFICATION[a]

Primary Tumor (T)

(Note: Definitions for classifying the primary tumor (T) are the same for the clinical and pathologic classification. If the measurement is made by physical examination, the examiner will use the major headings (T1, T2, or T3). If other measurements, such as mammographic or pathologic measurements are used, the subsets of T1 can be used. Tumors should be measured to the nearest 0.1 cm increment.)

TX Primary tumor cannot be assessed

T0 No evidence of primary tumor

Tis Carcinoma in situ

Tis Ductal carcinoma in situ (DCIS)

Tis Lobular carcinoma in situ (LCIS)

Tis Paget's disease of the nipple with no tumor (Paget's disease associated with a tumor is classified according to the size of the tumor.)

T1 Tumor 2 cm or less in greatest dimension

   T1mic Microinvasion 0.1 cm or less in greatest dimension

   T1a Tumor more than 0.1 cm but not more than 0.5 cm in greatest dimension

   T1b Tumor more than 0.5 cm but not more than 1 cm in greatest dimension

   T1c Tumor more than 1 cm but not more than 2 cm in greatest dimension

T2 Tumor more than 2 cm but not more than 5 cm in greatest dimension

T3 Tumor more than 5 cm in greatest dimension

T4 Tumor of any size with direct extension to (a) chest wall or (b) skin, only as described below

   T4a Extension to chest wall, not including pectoralis muscle

   T4b Edema (including peau d'orange) or ulceration of the skin of the breast, or satellite skin nodules confined to the same breast (all other skin involvement such as dimpling, nipple retraction, or any other change except those described under T4b and T4d, may occur in T1, T2, and T3 without changing the classification)

   T4c Both T4a and T4b

   T4d Inflammatory carcinoma

Regional Lymph Nodes (N)

Clinical

   NX Regional lymph nodes cannot be assessed (e.g., previously removed)

   N0 No regional lymph node metastasis

   N1 Metastasis to movable ipsilateral axillary lymph node(s)

   N2 Metastases in ipsilateral axillary lymph nodes fixed or matted, or in clinically apparent[b] ipsilateral internal mammary nodes in the absence of clinically evident axillary lymph node metastasis

   N2a Metastasis in ipsilateral axillary lymph nodes fixed to one another (matted) or to other structures

   N2b Metastasis only in clinically apparent[b] ipsilateral internal mammary nodes and in the absence of clinically evident axillary lymph node metastasis

   N3 Metastasis in ipsilateral infraclavicular lymph node(s) with or without axillary lymph node involvement, or in clinically apparent[b] ipsilateral internal mammary lymph node(s) and in the presence of clinically evident axillary lymph node metastasis, or metastasis in ipsilateral supraclavicular lymph node(s) with or without axillary or internal mammary lymph node involvement

   N3a Metastasis in ipsilateral infraclavicular lymph node(s)

   N3b Metastasis in ipsilateral internal mammary lymph node(s) and axillary lymph nodes

   N3c Metastasis in ipsilateral supraclavicular lymph node(s)

Pathologic (pN)

(Note: Classification is based on axillary lymph node dissection with or without sentinel lymph node dissection. Classification based solely on sentinel lymph node dissection without subsequent axillary lymph node dissection is designated (sn) for "sentinel node", i.e., pN0 (i+) (sn).

   pNX Regional lymph nodes cannot be assessed (e.g., previously removed, or not removed for pathologic study).

   pN0 No regional lymph node metastasis histologically, no additional examination for isolated tumor cells (ITC)

CLINICAL AND PATHOLOGIC STAGING

Clinical staging is used in some circumstances but is far less accurate than pathologic staging. Palpation, in general, overestimates tumor size when compared to pathologic measurement. The overall error rate in clinical lymph node assessment is remarkable: 48 percent of patients clinically classified T2N0 show histologic evidence of metastasis after surgery, while 41

Table 7-1 (Continued)

(Note: ITCs are defined as single tumor cells or small cell clusters not greater than 0.2 mm, usually detected only by immunohistochemical (IHC) or molecular methods but which may be verified on hematoxylin and eosin (H&E) stains; ITCs do not usually show evidence of malignant activity (e.g., proliferation or stromal reaction).

pN0(i-) No regional lymph node metastasis histologically, negative IHC

pN0(i+) No regional lymph node metastasis histologically, positive IHC, no IHC cluster greater than 0.2 mm

pN0(mol-) No regional lymph node metastasis histologically, negative molecular findings (with reverse transcription polymerase chain reaction [RT-PCR])

pN0(mol+) No regional lymph node metastasis histologically, positive molecular findings (RT-PCR)

pN1 Metastasis in 1 to 3 axillary lymph nodes, and/or in internal mammary nodes with microscopic disease detected by sentinel lymph node dissection but not clinically apparent[c]

pN1mi Micrometastasis (greater than 0.2 mm, none greater than 2.0 mm)

pN1a Metastasis in 1 to 3 axillary lymph nodes

pN1b Metastasis in internal mammary nodes with microscopic disease detected by sentinel lymph node dissection but not clinically apparent[c]

pN1c Metastasis in 1 to 3 axillary lymph nodes and in internal mammary lymph nodes with microscopic disease detected by sentinel lymph node dissection but not clinically apparent[c] (If associated with more than 3 positive axillary lymph nodes, the internal mammary nodes are classified as pN3b to reflect increased tumor burden)

pN2 Metastasis in 4 to 9 axillary lymph nodes, or in clinically apparent[b] internal mammary lymph nodes in the absence of axillary lymph node metastasis

pN2a Metastasis in 4 to 9 axillary lymph nodes (at least one tumor deposit greater than 2.0 mm)

pN2b Metastasis in clinically apparent[c] internal mammary lymph nodes in the absence of axillary lymph node metastasis

pN3 Metastasis in 10 or more axillary lymph nodes, or in infraclavicular lymph nodes, or in clinically apparent[b] ipsilateral internal mammary lymph nodes in the presence of 1 or more positive axillary lymph nodes; or in more than 3 axillary lymph nodes with clinically negative microscopic metastasis in internal mammary lymph nodes; or in ipsilateral supraclavicular lymph nodes

pN3a Metastasis in 10 or more axillary lymph nodes (at least one tumor deposit greater than 2.0 mm), or metastasis to the infraclavicular lymph nodes

pN3b Metastasis in clinically apparent[b] ipsilateral internal mammary lymph nodes in the presence of 1 or more positive axillary lymph nodes; or in more than 3 axillary lymph nodes and in internal mammary lymph nodes with microscopic disease detected by sentinel lymph node dissection but not clinically apparent[c]

pN3c Metastasis in ipsilateral supraclavicular lymph nodes

Distant Metastasis (M)

MX Distant metastasis cannot be assessed

M0 No distant metastasis

M1 Distant metastasis

[b]Data taken from AJCC cancer staging manual, 6th ed. New York: Springer; 2002.

[b]Clinically apparent = detected by imaging studies (excluding lymphoscintigraphy) or by clinical examination or grossly visible pathologically.

[c]Not clinically apparent = not detected by imaging studies (excluding lymphoscintigraphy) or by clinical examination.

percent of patients clinically classified T2N1 are T2N0 after histologic assessment (106).

Pathologic staging must include all data obtained by clinical staging. If the tumor is not totally excised and neoplastic cells are present at the resection margins, the lesion has to be coded as pTX. If surgery intervenes after neoadjuvant chemotherapy, hormonal therapy, immunotherapy, or radiation therapy, the prefix y is added to the code.

The entire text of the 2002 TNM staging classification is presented in Table 7-1.

PROGNOSTIC AND PREDICTIVE INDICATORS

The prognostic indicators in breast cancer are data obtained at the time of diagnosis that relate to the clinical outcome in the absence of adjuvant therapy. Predictive indicators are those related to the degree of response to the therapy administered. Therefore, some indicators can be of both prognostic and predictive value while others are one or the other. The value of any indicator depends on the impact on prognosis, on response to therapy, or both, and it is usually established after multivariate statistical tests.

In the 1999 consensus statement (52) of the College of American Pathologists, prognostic indicators were classified into three categories, of which the most relevant for prognosis was category 1. In a conference statement from the National Institutes of Health (NIH) consensus development panel, 2000 (39), accepted prognostic and predictive factors included age, lymph node status, size of tumor, pathologic grade, tumor type, and hormone receptor status.

Lymph Node Status

Axillary lymph node status has traditionally been regarded as the single most important prognostic indicator for disease-free and overall survival in patients with invasive carcinomas of the breast (52). Only 20 to 30 percent of patients with negative axillary lymph nodes develop recurrences within 10 years as opposed to 70 percent of patients with positive axillary lymph nodes.

The greater the number of positive axillary nodes, the worse the prognosis. In a study that included 24,740 patients with lesions under 20 mm (21), the 5-year survival rate was 93.3 percent if no axillary nodes were affected, 87.4 percent for those with 1 to 3 positive nodes, and 66 percent for those with 4 or more involved nodes. The same trend was seen for patients with tumors of 20 to 50 mm: 89 percent, 79.9 percent, and 58.7 percent, respectively. For those with neoplasms over 50 mm, the figures were 82 percent, 73 percent, and 45.5 percent, respectively. It was concluded that the size of the metastatic tumor burden as well as the presence of metastases is prognostically important (119). It also appears that there is an inverse linear relationship between survival and an increasing number of histologically positive axillary lymph nodes (87).

The level of nodal involvement also provides useful information. Metastasis at level III (see chapter 1 for the definition of axillary lymph node levels) of the axilla is less favorable than metastasis at lower levels (125).

Extracapsular extension is not yet a fully settled prognostic feature, but Hartveit (62) proposed that the presence of tumor cells in efferent vessels, located around the hilum, is a marker of poor prognosis in node-positive patients. The tumor grade (see later) does not change between the primary tumor and metastatic node disease (78).

To assess lymph node status, an adequate number of lymph nodes should be examined. The smaller the number of lymph nodes examined, the greater the likelihood of understaging the disease and of leaving residual involved lymph nodes in the axilla. Millis et al. (80) proposed that a median of 24 lymph nodes be examined in any axillary clearance, a number that "reflects the completeness of the surgery and the assiduousness of the pathologic examination." Various methods for improving the detection of metastases in lymph nodes, including the use of solvents to clear axillary fat, have been proposed. Little benefit has been demonstrated by using these methods (82), as most lymph nodes are easily detected by careful palpation of the specimen or by thin parallel slices of the axillary fat.

Still, 20 to 30 percent of patients with negative nodes subsequently develop metastatic disease. These figures have led to the search for other prognostic factors. One approach consists of studying negative nodes more carefully to find occult metastases. Micrometastases (tumor clumps 2 mm or smaller) are found in about 10 percent of "node negative" patients using H&E-stained step sections (50), a percentage that increases to 20 percent if immunohistochemistry is used (70). The prognostic significance of occult metastases is controversial and conflicting results are obtained in different studies. When multivariate analysis is used as a method of investigation, the presence of occult metastases is not found to be an independent predictor of survival (50,80). This led Millis et al. (79) to state that "the current evidence does not support the routine use of either multiple sections or immunohistochemistry for the detection of occult metastases in axillary clearance specimens."

The prognostic significance of morphologic changes present within the lymph nodes, such as sinus histiocytosis and capsular versus parenchymal localization of the metastasis, is still controversial.

Sentinel Lymph Node(s)

The definition of sentinel lymph node is based on the Halstedian theory (11) that presupposes a sequential and orderly spread of cancer cells from the primary tumor to the first node to receive lymphatic drainage from the tumor. Sentinel lymph node biopsy is a diagnostic test to establish the status of regional lymph nodes (76). This procedure was first clinically applied to stage malignant melanomas (23) and only later to axillary lymph nodes to stage breast cancer (129). While for melanomas this type of staging procedure is accepted as clinically useful in terms of feasibility, specificity, and false negative results, the same cannot be said for breast tumors (76). Not only is axillary sentinel node biopsy a recent test with consequent lack of standardized procedures (11,112), but the lymphatic drainage system of the breast is very complex. In one study (19), 5 percent of lesions located in the outer quadrants drained to internal mammary lymph nodes (IMCs), while 18 percent of tumors located in the inner or central quadrants drained to IMCs. Fourteen percent of IMC sentinel nodes were positive, indicating that internal mammary chain lymph nodes are an important step in breast cancer metastasis.

Many of the published studies on the usefulness of sentinel lymph node biopsy for breast cancer diagnosis and staging do not specify the false negative rate (the number of false negative biopsies compared to the number of patients with positive lymph nodes) (76). The site of introduction of the tracer (i.e., peritumoral, subcutaneous, subareolar, intradermal), the type of dye used, and the different radioactive probes employed are all issues that could lead to variable results and are not yet settled. A consensus (at least in Europe) has been reached on the high sensitivity and specificity of the results obtained when both tracers (dye and radioactive) are used together (11, 112). In the proceedings of a consensus conference on the role of sentinel lymph node biopsy in carcinoma of the breast held in April 2001 (115), it was stated that "until a surgeon documents his or her own experience with the procedure and consistently achieves a detection rate of greater than 90 percent and a false negative rate of less than 5 percent, he or she should perform a concomitant traditional axillary dissection." It was unfortunate that this statement was not followed by an agreement on how to train the surgeons, although in Germany and the United Kingdom there are ongoing "standardized sentinel node biopsy programmes" (11).

There is no agreement on the method of pathologic assessment of lymph nodes: in some institutions, frozen sections alone are routinely used (135); in others, frozen section is followed by analysis of paraffin-embedded tissue (129), while Lee et al. (70) advocates using paraffin-embedded tissue only. We think that the latter procedure is the safest, considering the 24 percent false negative rate obtained at frozen section examination by Veronesi et al. (135) and the substantial loss of nodal tissue in trimming when frozen sections are cut. Cochran (23), who has the longest experience with sentinel lymph node pathology, discourages the use of frozen sections because 1) the identification of small numbers of tumor cells is more accurate in well-fixed and stained sections; 2) critical diagnostic tissue is lost during the facing up of the frozen block when the permanent fixed material is processed; and 3) with radioactive tracer at least 24 hours are necessary to permit the isotope to decay to safe levels of radioactivity. Admittedly, Cochran's focus was on melanomas, but we think that these critical points are the same in breast tumors.

The optimal histopathologic workup for lymph node assessment is still a matter of debate. Cserni (27) found that central cross section of only a sentinel lymph node fails to detect metastases in 31 percent of patients while at least 45 steps are needed to attain a sensitivity of 100 percent. As stated by Lee et al. (70), in the absence of standardized guidelines, the more thorough the workup the better. The obvious (unrealistic) optimal pathologic examination is the embedding of all lymph nodes and serial section evaluation of the entire lymph node. Immunohistochemistry, using antikeratin antibodies, improves the diagnostic sensitivity by up to 20 percent, making the metastases easier to see (70). We feel that it is best to cut the lymph node perpendicular to the long axis, so as to better visualize the marginal sinuses, a view also shared by Lee et al. Micrometastases (i.e., pN1mi [i+]) should be identified since microfoci of cancer cells are associated with a 34 to 50 percent incidence of metastatic involvement in the remaining axillary lymph nodes (13,34,76). In a metaanalysis of 789 patients from 25 studies (30), axillary (nonsentinel) lymph node involvement was found in 19.8 percent of cases following the H&E diagnosis of micrometastases in a previously excised sentinel node. The percentage increases to 25 percent if sentinel node positivity is found after immuno-histochemistry, which also reveals ITCs. Only 9 percent of nonsentinel axillary lymph nodes have only ITCs on biopsy (28)

Distinguishing micrometastases from ITC is an "easy" task in theory, but is difficult in practice, as shown by the low kappa value (maximum kappa, 0.49) obtained by the several pathologists of the European Working Group for breast pathology screening who attempted to distinguish ITC from micrometastases using digital images (29).

The management of nonsentinel lymph nodes is variable. At one extreme is the 2005 recommendation of the Executive Committee of the breast section of the Royal Australasian College of Surgeons, which advised excision of nonsentinel lymph nodes in all positive cases (11). At the other extreme, Cady et al. (18) suggested that there are defined groups of patients with such low probability of nodal involvement that a positive sentinel lymph node biopsy can be neglected. These cases include small tumors of favorable histology, T1a and T1b tumors detected at mammography of low-grade histology, and older patients with estrogen receptor (ER)-positive tumors who would undergo hormonal treatment irrespective of nodal status.

Size of Tumor

Tumor size is one of the most reliable indicators of the presence of nodal metastases and survival rate. Tumors are smaller in populations screened by mammography than in unscreened patients (56): tumors less than 1 cm occurred in 16 percent of screened versus 3 percent of unscreened patients; tumors greater than 2 cm occurred in 26 percent of screened versus 52 percent of unscreened patients.

There is substantial agreement that the measurement should be a pathologic one. The gross measurement gives figures higher than the respective histologic measurement in 47 percent of cases, but the variation is of low clinical impact as judged by the similar 10-year actuarial rate of recurrence-free survival in both groups of patients (104). In the consensus statement by the College of American Pathologists (52), "the size of the tumor, as measured by gross examination, must

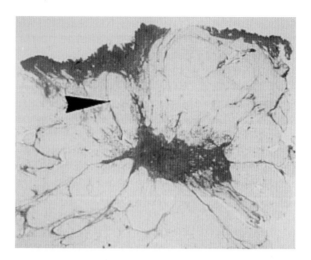

Figure 7-1

SIZE OF TUMOR ON LARGE SECTION

This large section is representative of a quadrant. The bulk of the lesion measures 2.7 cm, but, as shown by the arrow, there are thin neoplastic extensions far beyond the main mass. The latter were not evident to the naked eye. Therefore, the total gross and microscopic size of the tumor is much greater. (Fig. 20-7A from Silverstein MJ, Recht A, Lagios MD. Ductal carcinoma in situ of the breast, 2nd ed. Philadelphia: Lippincott; 2002:253.)

be verified by microscopic examination. If there is discrepancy...the microscopic measurement of the invasive component takes precedence."

There are several significant problems involved with tumor measurement. In a study undertaken by 23 European pathologists (121), a wide range in tumor size was observed in cases measured by histologic means. This study paralleled the results obtained by the United Kingdom (UK) National Breast Screening Programme (120). The main reasons for inconsistency appear to be: tumor asymmetry, poor circumscription, uncertainty about the inclusion of ductal carcinoma in situ (DCIS) extending beyond the invasive component, patients who have received multiple core biopsies resulting in the massive distortion of the tumor area and expansion of the gross tumor size by reactive changes within and around the tumor, and large tumors that require more than one paraffin block to be measured in toto. To obviate most of these inconsistencies, Foschini et al. (54) proposed the use of large (macro) sections (see Appendix) that in practice combine the advantages of gross and histologic examinations (fig. 7-1). Large sections are helpful for multifocal tumors as well (53); it is possible to measure each focus and provide an aggregated size.

A consensus has been achieved on the size of the invasive part as a prominent indicator for prognosis (52), but in the European Breast Screening Guidelines (44,120), apart from measuring the widest diameter of an invasive carcinoma, it is recommended that, if the invasive tumor is surrounded by DCIS, a second measurement should be provided inclusive of the whole neoplastic area.

In a long-term follow-up study, Rosen et al. (108) found that in patients with T1N0M0 tumors, the 20-year recurrence-free survival rate was 86 percent when the tumor was 1.0 cm or less, significantly better than the 69 percent for patients with tumors 1.1 to 2.0 cm. Size appears to be an independent prognostic factor (21) and shows a linear relationship with the number of positive lymph nodes (122). Accordingly, survival rates vary from 96 percent for patients whose tumors were less than 2 cm with no involved lymph nodes to 45.5 percent for patients with tumors 5 cm or larger with metastatic axillary lymph nodes (21,44,73,107).

Occult Carcinoma. *Occult carcinoma* is a clinical diagnosis that refers to nonpalpable, asymptomatic, and in some cases, not even mammographically demonstrable cancer presenting with palpable axillary metastases, or rarely, with distant metastases (109). To these cases are added those identified incidentally during reduction mammoplasty. Among 516 consecutive cases of reduction mammoplasty, 5 percent of cases showed DIN1, 3 percent showed LIN 1, and 1 case (0.2 percent) showed tubular carcinoma (37a). In a large series of patients with breast carcinoma, 0.35 percent presented with axillary lymph node metastases only (105). Enlargement of one or more axillary lymph nodes was the sole symptom among these patients.

Axillary lymph node enlargement does not necessarily indicate a metastasis from an ipsilateral carcinoma. Metastases represented the minority of cases (7 percent) in one series of enlarged lymph nodes, while inflammatory changes (69.5 percent of cases) and malignant lymphomas (14 percent of cases) were far more numerous (37).

Before accepting that the malignant changes in an enlarged axillary lymph node are the result of a metastasis from a clinically occult ipsilateral breast carcinoma, the following possibilities have to be taken into consideration. Metastases from carcinomas of lung, kidney, and ovary as well as malignant melanoma should be excluded. When an extramammary metastatic carcinoma has been excluded after a careful clinical and immunohistochemical workup, the possibility of a carcinoma located in the contralateral breast must be considered. This was the case in 6 of 42 patients in one series (4). This situation occurs especially after contralateral local recurrence. Rarely, a carcinoma arises in epithelial inclusions in axillary lymph nodes (48) or from the tail of the breast (6). If the lesion consists of a small cell neuroendocrine Merkel cell–like carcinoma, the primary tumor has to be searched for in the skin. In the absence of a skin primary, a rare Merkel cell–like carcinoma originating within the axillary lymph nodes should be considered (46). Finally, medullary type carcinoma in the axillary tail may resemble a metastasis in a lymph node.

Patients with metastases from an ipsilateral occult breast carcinoma range in age from 30 to 83 years. A positive family history is reported in nearly 50 percent of cases (105). A clinical abnormality in the ipsilateral breast is found in about 25 percent of patients and a mammographic abnormality is seen in up to 35 percent (109). In most patients, an invasive carcinoma is found, but 21 percent of patients in one series (109) had a noninvasive neoplastic lesion. In these cases, it is likely that the infiltrative portion of the carcinoma was minute and had not been detected. This series was composed mostly of referral and consultation cases that presumably were not worked up by a specialist in breast pathology. In fact, the proportion of patients in whom a primary tumor is found is closely related to the care taken to examine the breast specimen (6). Nevertheless, in rare instances, no primary tumor is found in the ipsilateral breast or anywhere else, in spite of very careful pathologic study.

In a series of patients who did not undergo mastectomy, the interval between the nodal enlargement and the detection of a clinical or mammographically visible breast anomaly was between 6 and 36 months (mean, 15 months)

(65). In these circumstances, there is general agreement that mastectomy is indicated (6). The 6-year postmastectomy survival rate of patients with occult lesions was the same, if not better, than a matched series of patients with stage II breast cancer who presented with palpable tumors (109).

Some cases reported as "occult" averaged 4 cm in size, ranging from 1 to 6 cm. This usually occurs in large dense breast tissue of young patients and in cases of invasive lobular carcinoma.

Incidental Carcinomas. By analogy with papillary thyroid cancer, *incidental carcinomas* are a special variant of occult carcinomas of the breast. This point has been well addressed by Nielsen et al. (88) in a study of 110 nonselected medicolegal autopsies of young and middle-aged women (20 to 54 years old) with no breast symptoms. In these cases, breast carcinomas were found in 22 (20 percent) patients: 2 invasive and 20 in situ carcinomas. This high incidence of incidental occult breast carcinoma may be the result of some fortuitous selection bias, but if this incidence is real, it indicates that, as in the thyroid, some tumors never progress to a clinical level and consequently are prognostically irrelevant.

Grade of Tumor

Pathologists have known for over a century that anaplasia and a high number of mitotic figures are often associated with aggressive breast tumor behavior (25). Over the years, several grading systems have been utilized to help determine prognosis. At present, the most widely used histologic grading system is the one proposed by Elston and Ellis (42). It has been recommended by the College of American Pathologists (52) and by the American Joint Committee on Cancer (2), and is used by the European Commission Working Group on Breast Screening Pathology (121). This grading system is also referred to as the Nottingham combined histologic grade, or modified Bloom and Richardson (16) histologic grade (B&R). Elston and Ellis added to the B&R precise criteria a semiquantitative evaluation of the percentage of glandular formation, the degree of nuclear pleomorphism, and a mitotic count based on the definition of a field area.

In the Elston and Ellis histologic grading system (42), glands are defined as structures having a central lumen. Quantitatively, all parts of a tumor are scored and the proportion occupied by glandular structures is assessed. A score of 1 point is allocated when more than 75 percent of the tumor contains glandular structures. Two points are given to tumors containing 10 to 75 percent of glands and 3 points to tumors with less than 10 percent of glandular structures.

Nuclear pleomorphism is assessed by comparing the size and shape of the neoplastic cells with normal cells contained within the tumor or adjacent to it. In the absence of normal cells, lymphocytes are used for comparative purposes (43). When the nuclei are of the same size and shape as in normal epithelium and have a regular profile and dispersed chromatin, 1 point is allocated. When nuclei are larger than normal, more vesicular with moderate variation in size and shape, and have "visible, usually single nucleoli" (43), 2 points are allocated. If there is a striking variation in nuclear size or larger size with prominent and often multiple nucleoli, 3 points are allocated.

Mitotic count is assessed as follows: the number of indisputable mitotic figures is counted per field area, in a minimum of 10 fields, at the periphery of the tumor where the proliferative activity is greatest. In order to standardize the count to a defined field area, a plot chart is provided by which different microscopes can be calibrated, since microscopes can vary up to six-fold (fig. 7-2) (43).

To obtain the tumor grade, the scores for each factor are added together, giving a total ranging from 3 to 9 points. The histologic grade (Nottingham combined histologic grade) recommended along with the TNM classification is: GX, grade cannot be assessed; G1, low combined histologic grade (favorable) (3 to 5 points); G2, intermediate combined histologic grade (6 to 7 points); and G3, high combined histologic grade (8 to 9 points). In heterogeneous tumors, such as mixed carcinomas, the least differentiated areas have to be assessed.

Immediate fixation is recommended as some authors have shown a decline in mitotic figures of up to 53 percent when the time lag between excision and fixation is 6 hours or more. The quicker the fixation, the better the tissue features are preserved. We feel that the decline of mitotic figures in these circumstances is

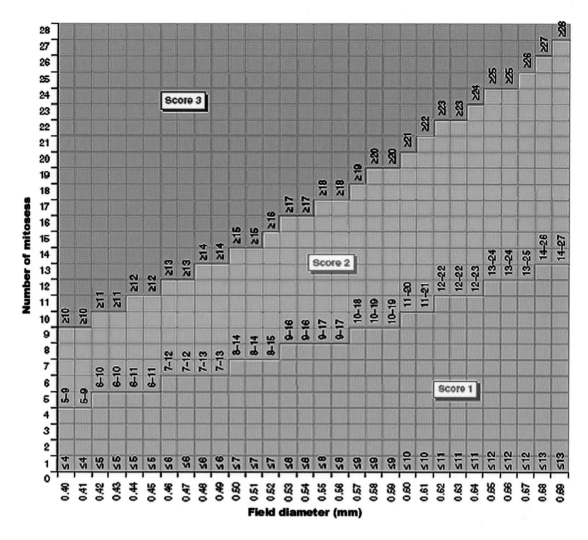

Figure 7-2

CALIBRATION OF MICROSCOPIC MAGNIFICATION

Aide-memoire to assist calibration of microscopic field diameter with mitotic frequency count grading cut-off points. (Fig. 49 from Pathology reporting of breast disease. NHSBSP Publication No. 58, Jan 2005:80. www.cancerscreening.nhs.uk.)

overemphasized since others (35) have found no substantial mitotic count change in the same period of delayed fixation.

Using the above grading criteria, Elston and Ellis (42) assessed the grade of tumor in 1,830 patients with breast cancer: 342 (19 percent) were grade 1, 631 (34 percent) grade 2, and 857 (47 percent) grade 3. The different grades are described in chapter 8.

There was a highly significant correlation between histologic grade and prognosis. The recurrence-free interval and overall survival are worse in patients with grade (G)3 tumors compared with those with G1 carcinomas. It has also been shown that grading, assessed by the above method, is an independent prognostic factor in multivariate analysis both for overall and disease-free survival in premenopausal and postmenopausal women (33). That grading is a powerful prognostic factor is abundantly clear from ample data in the literature. Despite the different grading systems used, the overall results point in one direction and indicate that patients with G1 carcinomas have a better prognosis than those with G3 tumors, which exhibit a more aggressive clinical course (25).

Contesso et al. (26) found that grading was more discriminating in terms of prognosis than the histologic subtype, a finding confirmed by Pereira et al. (93). The latter, in a multivariate analysis of 2,658 cases, found that grade was the most important independent factor in predicting survival. Grading is most effective in mixed type tumors, where histotyping has the lowest discriminating rate. Nevertheless, when the histologic type of carcinoma is included among the different factors considered, it is also an independent prognostic factor, although of less importance than grade. Pereira et al. rightly concluded that any carcinoma should be both typed and graded to define it more accurately.

Despite efforts to "induce a degree of discipline in pathologists" (43) with the use of strict criteria, reproducibility of grade is unsatisfactory. This is seen in intraobserver and interobserver studies and in both unicenter and multicenter studies (119). The largest multicenter consistency study on grade was undertaken by 250 pathologists under the auspices of the UK National Coordinating Group for Breast Screening Pathology (119). Kappa statistics of 0.36 for G1, 0.18 for G2, and 0. 21 for G3 carcinomas were obtained. Better, but still unsatisfactory results were obtained when "experts" assessed the tumors. Similar unsatisfactory results were obtained by 23 European pathologists from 12 countries who graded a series of invasive carcinomas (121): the kappa statistics were 0.56 for G1, 0.35 for G2, and 0.70 for G3 carcinomas. Unfortunately, no improvement in consistency was achieved in four different rounds of assessment. This indicates that, despite strict criteria, the weakness of the method is intrinsic.

A major weakness is the assessment of nuclear pleomorphism. This point was highlighted by Dunne and Going (38), who found that only 9 of 100 cases were given the same score by 17 pathologists in a multicenter study. G2 carcinomas are the most difficult to score based on nuclear pleomorphism, as shown by the data obtained in different multicenter studies where nuclear G2 tumors have the lowest kappa statistics, at most 0.35 (121).

The mitotic count is also difficult to assess. Tumors detected by screening programs are increasingly smaller and it is difficult to find the 10 high-power fields required to count mitoses.

In the future, the grading system may use the MIB1 labeling index which is not affected by delayed fixation of up to 12 hours (28) and correlates strongly with the number of mitotic figures in tumor cells (140).

In spite of all these "critical points," we think that for the present grade is one of the best histologic features we have for predicting prognosis. The prognostic impact of histologic grading is destined to decrease with the progressive reduction of the tumor size as a result of mammographic screening.

Combined Prognostic Indicators

The optimal integration of multiple prognostic indicators remains an unresolved issue. In a multivariate analysis of nine possible prognostic indicators in a series of 387 patients with primary breast cancer, three were shown to have a significant relationship to prognosis: tumor size, histologic grade, and lymph node status (64). From these, an index was devised, the Nottingham Prognostic Index, which stratifies patients into good, moderate, and poor prognostic groups. Galea et al. (55) demonstrated an annual mortality rate of 3 percent in the good, 7 percent in the moderate, and 30 percent in the poor prognostic groups. Another approach was followed by van Diest et al. (132) who combined the mitotic count, lymph node status, and tumor size to obtain a morphometric prognostic index.

Steroid Hormone Receptors (Estrogen and Progesterone Receptors)

Hormone receptor status is the only molecular marker included in category I among the prognostic factors accepted by the College of American Pathologists (52). It is such a powerful predictive indicator that it has led the NIH Consensus Development Panel of 2000 (39) to state that "adjuvant hormonal therapy should be offered only to women whose tumors express hormone receptor protein."

There are two types of estrogen receptor (ER). The one used in clinical practice (ERα) is codified by a gene located on chromosome 6q25.1; the other (ERβ) is codified by a gene located on chromosome 14q22-q24. Although there is evidence that the activity of estradiol depends on the relative expression of the two receptors

(120), in practice, only the alpha-receptor is clinically useful since beta-receptors are scanty and commercial ERβ antibodies are not readily available at the present (84). ERα is synthesized in the cytoplasm, translocates to the nucleus, and thereafter shuttles between the nucleus and cytoplasm. Two isoforms also exist for progesterone receptors (PRα and PRβ), both codified by a gene located on chromosome 1. The diagnostic methods currently available cannot distinguish between these two isoforms since the available antibodies (KD68, 1A6, 636) react against an N-terminal portion that is common to both.

Traditionally, cytosol assays were employed in the assessment of steroid receptors. Currently, the immunohistochemical approach that uses monoclonal antibodies is recommended by the American Society of Clinical Oncology for the assessment of ER and PR (10). The advantage of immunohistochemistry over cytosol assays is the visualization of the reaction, which gives information on individual neoplastic cells. The cytosol assays give numerical data on a lesion that has only been identified macroscopically and may have variable quantities of normal tissues admixed.

The immunohistochemical methods currently performed on paraffin-embedded tissue allow very small lesions to be studied. Monoclonal antibodies are also useful in sparsely cellular invasive carcinomas such as lobular neoplasms, in needle core biopsies, and in fine needle cytologic smears. The disadvantages of immunohistochemistry are that no information is provided on the functional state of the receptor, that there is an inability to provide a numerical value, and that the assessment of the stained nuclei is subjective and the interobserver reproducibility is moderate (kappa statistics: 0.57 for ER and 0.53 for PR in the most favorable scores) (99). Reproducibility is better when the levels of ER are high; in such cases, ER positivity is demonstrated in more than 80 percent of laboratories. This percentage drops to only 37 percent in low expression tumors (101).

With the aim of rendering the immunohistochemical data more objective, several semiquantitative scoring systems have been proposed (44,99). For the sake of simplicity, we report the percentage of positive cells to the nearest 10 percent. It should be noted, however, that a significant benefit from adjuvant endocrine treatment is observed in patients whose tumors contain 1 percent of ER-positive cells (41). Efforts to obtain objective data are maximized in several ways: by using a quality control scheme that includes external assessment procedures; by immediately fixing the tissue in neutral buffered formalin for a period ranging from 24 to 72 hours to optimize staining (138); by increasing the efficiency of the antigen retrieval step (102); by the correct selection of the antibody (101); by the inclusion of a positive normal control, possibly in the same slide; and finally, by using an automated technique rather than a manual technique (99).

Nuclear positivity has to be considered when assessing for hormone receptors. In normal menstrual breast, 10 to 15 percent of secretory cells in lobules and ducts stain for hormone receptors. The staining reaction of ER in the normal ductal or lobular epithelium is heterogeneous and strongly positive, weakly positive or negative nuclei are observed side by side (fig. 7-3A) (86).

Myoepithelial cells are negative for steroid receptors. Usually, cells that are positive for ER are also positive for PR, although ER positivity slightly decreases in the secretory phase of the cycle (119). Both receptors are far more abundant in prepuberal girls and in men. In female involuted lobules, immunostaining is seen in virtually all cells in the same lobule (119). Steroid receptors are seen in fibroadenomas, benign stromal spindle cell tumor (BSSCT), and pseudoangiomatous stromal hyperplasia (PASH) but not in fibromatosis (3,75). ER and PR are absent in apocrine epithelium, which expresses androgen receptors. Well-differentiated DCIS, ductal intraepithelial neoplasia grade 1 (DIN1), and lobular intraepithelial neoplasias (LIN) are consistently positive for ER and PR (fig. 7-3B,C) (17). Tubular, mucoid, invasive lobular, and invasive duct carcinomas with nuclear grade 1 are all positive for ER. On the contrary, medullary, apocrine, metaplastic, and high-grade carcinomas are negative (86). ER-negative and PR-positive carcinomas are rare, or, according to Nadji et al. (86), nonexistent.

Approximately 60 percent of invasive carcinomas are strongly positive for ER (fig. 7-3), 20 percent are weakly positive (and missed by the laboratories with insufficiently sensitive

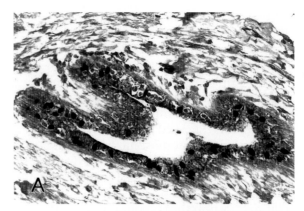

Figure 7-3

ESTROGEN RECEPTOR IMMUNOHISTOCHEMISTRY

A: Normal duct. Only some nuclei stain for estrogen receptor (ER).

B: Invasive lobular carcinoma. The majority of nuclei stain intensely for ER.

C: Invasive lobular carcinoma. ER positivity highlights the invasion of nerves.

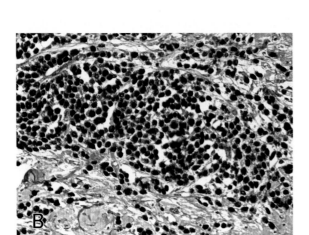

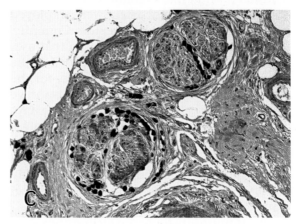

immunohistochemical techniques), and 20 percent are negative (127). At variance with these data, Nadji et al. (86) stated that the immunohistochemical reaction for ER is an all-or-none phenomenon. Positive nuclear staining for ER and PR was found in 75 percent and 55 percent, respectively, of 5,993 invasive carcinomas. In 92 percent of ER-positive cases, diffuse and intense nuclear staining was observed, while the remaining 8 percent of cases showed a focal ER reaction, interpreted as the result of inadequate fixation. Collins et al. (24) depicted a bimodal frequency distribution of immunohistochemically detected ER that was either completely negative or positive, with 70 percent or more immunoreactive cells. These conflicting results probably reflect technical problems, some of which arise from the use of different brands of antibodies.

Steroid receptor positivity in lymph node metastases parallels that of the primary tumor. Adjuvant endocrine therapy selects steroid receptor-negative cells, with the result that ER-negative lymph node metastases can be obtained

from ER-positive tumors (7). Positive cases show a heterogeneous pattern: islands of strongly positive cells lie adjacent to areas with little ER positivity or absence of ER (123). Well-differentiated invasive duct carcinomas and classic invasive lobular carcinomas are consistently positive, while neoplasms with reactive lymphocytic stroma are often negative (31,51,110).

Agreement between the results of the "new" immunohistochemistry and the "old" cytosol techniques is 70 to 90 percent. Current guidelines are interpreted in the light of immunohistochemical data, even though most of the data were generated by the "old" cytosol assays (10). About 30 percent of unselected patients respond to hormone therapy. Using a cytosol assay for ER, at most about 60 percent of patients with ER-positive tumors respond as opposed to about 10 percent of patients with ER-negative tumors (89). About 80 percent of patients with ER- and PR-positive tumors respond to hormone therapy while only 45 percent of patients with ER-negative, PR-positive tumors respond (89).

Androgen Receptors

Androgen receptors (AR) are members of a large nuclear receptor family that mediates the biologic actions of androgens. The *AR* gene is located on the X chromosome at Xq11-12. There is evidence that androgens stimulate the growth of human breast cancer cell lines (74). A perspective study involving a large cohort of premenopausal and postmenopausal women has indicated a role for androgens in the development of breast cancer (12,77). A direct relationship between invasive breast cancer and preoperative high serum androgen levels was demonstrated in both premenopausal and postmenopausal women.

In normal breast tissue, ARs, as revealed by nuclear positivity with immunohistochemistry, are present in the apocrine epithelium, which is negative for ERs and progesterone receptors (PRs) (47), and in nonapocrine epithelium, where nuclei stain in 10 to 40 percent of the total cell population (81).

Two series have reported ARs in 66 to 82 percent of DCIS/DIN lesions (81,103). Invasive duct carcinomas express AR in 56 to 60 percent of cases (81,103), and invasive lobular carcinomas immunoreact for AR in up to 87 percent of cases, including LCIS/LIN (103).

Most AR-positive cases show a low proliferative index (63 percent) and a low or intermediate histologic grade (G1-G2, 63.0 percent) (103). Positive immunoreactions for AR were observed in 46 and 76 percent of G3 invasive duct carcinomas and G3 DCIS lesions, respectively, by Moinfar et al. (81).

AR expression is frequently associated with ER (65.2 percent) and PR (66.9 percent) positivity (103), but a statistically significant association between ER, PR, and AR was found only in invasive lobular carcinomas, while no statistical correlation was found with grade and stage (103). ARs are equally present in HER2/neu-negative and -positive cases. Thirty-nine percent of G3 invasive breast carcinomas are AR and ER negative and 30.5 percent are ER and PR negative, HER2/neu positive (81). AR seems also to be a prognostic indicator in metastatic breast cancer since the median survival period after disease recurrence for patients with AR-expressing tumors is significantly longer compared to that for patients with AR-negative tumors (114).

The future will tell whether ARs are going to be a novel prognostic factor that will have the same remarkable impact as ER in terms of a new target for hormone therapy.

Vascular Invasion

Vascular invasion in the breast is not exclusive to malignant conditions and has also been described in association with benign proliferative conditions. In one study, infiltration of the intima of an artery by two-layered tubules, along with venous wall infiltration, was evident in 4 of 44 consecutive cases of sclerosing adenosis (45). Intravascular dislodgement of benign epithelium can follow fine needle aspiration or stereotactic procedures (145,146) and these cells can be transported passively to axillary lymph nodes after a biopsy (20). These findings have no impact on prognosis.

The opposite is true of neoplastic vascular invasion that in univariate analyses is strongly associated with lymph node status, tumor size, histologic grade (95), and nonstellate tumor border growth pattern (33). Vascular invasion is an independent prognostic indicator of both local recurrence and survival, especially in node-negative patients (13,22). Lymphatic and vascular channel invasion is included under the heading of category II in the classification of prognostic factors (52). This is probably because assessment of lymphatic and blood vessel invasion is a time-consuming exercise that is difficult to reproduce and results in significant interobserver variation. The frequency of lymphatic invasion in node-negative patients is highly variable, ranging in the literature from 8.8 to 36.0 percent (95). The same range of variation is seen for blood vessel invasion. In a large study in which 23 pathologists from 12 European countries examined 57 randomly selected patients with invasive carcinomas, complete agreement was reached in only 22 (39 percent) of the cases, with an overall low kappa score of 0.38 (121).

The exercise of separating invasion of lymphatics from invasion of blood vessels is difficult, and when it has been attempted, no prognostic difference was found (69). The view that it is not worth separating the two is very acceptable (95). Invasion of large vessels is not a diagnostic problem, however, assessment of small vessel invasion is. The determination of vascular or lymphatic invasion is aided by the following: 1) the spaces generated by retraction artifacts are difficult to distinguish from vascular lumens. As suggested by Sloane (119), tumor clumps separated from the stroma following shrinkage artifacts conform to the space in which they lie. Whether spaces are true artifacts is a matter of uncertainty since cases showing these have a higher incidence of lymph node metastasis (1a). It is possible that spaces represent expanded prelymphatic channels (see below); 2) fibrin clots and red blood cells, when present, are a reliable sign of vascular invasion; 3) the proximity of a putative lymphatic embolus to a neurovascular bundle is of help in diagnosing lymphatic invasion; and 4) some neoplastic emboli totally fill the lumens. When this occurs, DCIS is simulated (95). This is why vascular invasion is universally evaluated at the periphery of the neoplasm where is situ lesions are easier to recognize. Unfortunately, this has led to a virtual lack of information about the prognostic value of intratumoral vascular invasion. In cases simulating in situ carcinomas, immunohistochemistry using antibasal lamina antibodies, traditional endothelial markers such as factor VIII-related antigen, CD34, CD31, *Ulex europaeus* lectin (60), and ABH isoantigen can be useful (72). Nevertheless, obvious lymphatic spaces containing tumor cells are commonly negative for vascular markers (60), with the exception of the novel monoclonal antibody D2-40 (67), and studies of a large number of cases with antibodies for lymphatic endothelial cells are currently unavailable. The negative results with immunohistochemistry may also be due to direct destruction of the endothelial cell layer by enzymatic digestion of matrix proteins by the neoplastic cells, or simply, a true lack of expression of the antigens. This has led Hanau et al. (60) to state that vascular invasion cannot be ruled out by negative immunostaining for endothelial cell markers.

As a general rule, what we call vascular invasion is the equivalent of in transit metastases, as seen for instance in malignant melanomas. The neoplastic cells that are seen histologically are those that grow locally within vessels surrounding the tumor and do not necessarily migrate to lymph nodes. This is probably the reason why local recurrence is more frequent when vascular invasion is present. Single neoplastic cells that

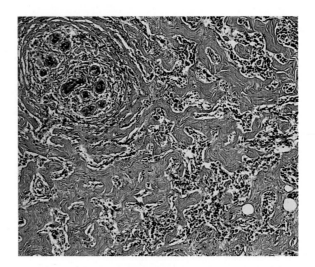

Figure 7-4

LYMPHOMA IN PRELYMPHATIC CHANNEL

In this primary lymphoma, the neoplastic cells float within channels that have a plexiform architecture. (Figs. 7-4 and 7-5 are from the same patient.)

float freely within the vessels and are revealed in the systemic blood by molecular marker assays (126) are not detected at the histologic level and are probably those that metastasize to distant sites. The fact that multifocal distribution of invasive lobular and ductal carcinomas is associated with a high frequency of lymphovascular invasion (42 percent) (128) is indirect proof of the possibility that some multifocal areas of invasion are related to intramammary in-transit metastases (53).

Prelymphatic System

Damiani et al. (32) reported three cases of malignant lymphoma and two of poorly differentiated carcinoma spreading and floating within open anastomosing spaces that formed a complex network of plexiform channels (figs. 7-4, 7-5). These superficially resembled artefactual stromal spaces. This network of channels consisted of spaces lined by attenuated CD34- and bcl-2-positive spindle cells, which dissected the dense fibrous stroma. In some parts of each lesion, the channels were slit-like in shape, with a narrow lumen, and lacked a recognizable cell bordering the lumens. Damiani et al. proposed that the neoplastic cells were spreading through the dilated "hidden prelymphatic channels" defined by Hartveit (63). Most of the time the latter

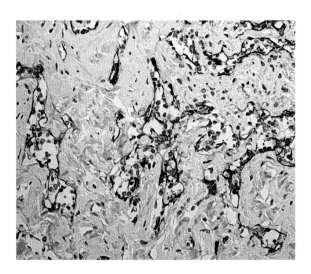

Figure 7-5

**IMMUNOHISTOCHEMISTRY OF
PRELYMPHATIC CHANNELS**

The cells that line the spaces are CD34 positive, but negative for factor VIII, CD31, D2-40, and *Ulex europaeus*.

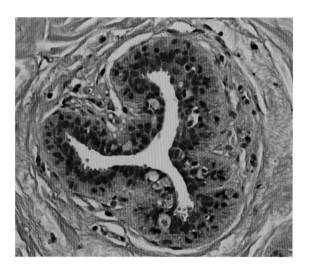

Figure 7-6

PERIDUCTAL PRELYMPHATIC CHANNELS

In normal breast, Hartveit prelymphatics surround the ducts. The clefted circumferential pattern can easily be overlooked as an artifact. (Figs. 7-6 and 7-7 are from the same patient.)

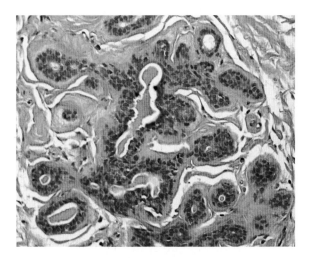

Figure 7-7

INTRALOBULAR PRELYMPHATIC CHANNELS

Hartveit spaces appear dilated and dissect the stroma of this normal lobule.

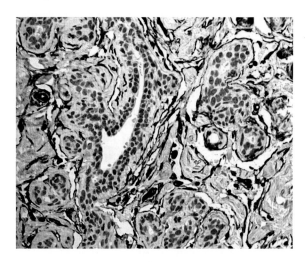

Figure 7-8

**IMMUNOHISTOCHEMISTRY OF
PRELYMPHATIC CHANNELS**

The cells that line the spaces stain for CD10 as well as CD34.

are virtual spaces, but depending on the need for drainage, their lumens are widened to form a complex labyrinth of lymphatics that permits quick communication between the breast stroma and the main lymphatic system. The spaces are mostly visualized in mammotome-obtained biopsies, are numerous around ducts, and dissect the stroma of the lobules (figs. 7-6, 7-7). The cells that line the spaces are modified fibroblasts positive with CD34 and CD10 (fig. 7-8) but are negative for the classic endothelial markers CD31, factor VIII, *Ulex europaeus*, and D2-40.

There is, therefore, an under-recognized pathway of "prelymphatic" spread that closely simulates artefactual stromal spaces. Hartveit

(63) suggested that tumor cells pass passively through the stromal prelymphatic channels and thus reach the lymphatic flow. There are no data in the literature on the prognostic importance of this phenomenon, but it is possible that the cases reported in the literature as having "probable vascular invasion" as the tumor "was seen in a space with the appearance of a vessel but without a clear endothelial layer" represent a condition very similar to the cases reported by Damiani et al. (32). The prognosis of these patients is similar to that of patients showing definite vascular invasion.

Angiogenesis

Angiogenesis, or neoangiogenesis, is the growth of new vessels within and around a neoplastic process. It is seen in invasive breast carcinomas mostly of high-grade malignancy (59), in inflammatory conditions of the breast (60), around poorly differentiated in situ carcinomas (DIN3), in metastatic lymph nodes, and in reactive lymph nodes adjacent to metastatic ones (71). Vascular proliferation is highlighted by immunohistochemistry with factor VIII, CD34, and CD31 (5,117,141). Weidner et al. (141) were the first to quantify tumor angiogenesis in breast carcinoma.

Although experimental evidence leaves little doubt that angiogenesis is necessary for tumor growth and metastatic dissemination, in practice, its correlation with prognosis has produced conflicting results. Angiogenesis has been placed in category III of prognostic factors (52). Claims that angiogenesis is a significant and independent prognostic indicator have been made by Weidner et al. (141) and several others. On the other hand, Axelsson et al. (5), who trained in Dr. Weidner's laboratory, did not find any prognostic indication with both univariate and multivariate analyses. The latter conclusion was reached by numerous other authors with the result that Sloane (120) stated that "there is insufficient evidence to recommend that microvessel density should form part of the routine histopathological assessment...." The reasons for inconsistent data are numerous: different methods of measurement (manual, semimanual, or computerized); low reproducibility of data among observers; different types of antibodies used; different areas counted (center or periphery of the tumor); the number of blocks studied per case; and the fact that angiogenesis is probably not the only factor that helps tumors grow (94). Invasive lobular carcinomas do not often express microvessel proliferation but metastasize all the same, via the prelymphatic labyrinth. Invasive lobular carcinomas have a lower expression of vascular endothelial growth factor (VEGF) than invasive duct carcinomas (71).

HER2/neu (c-erbB-2)

HER2/neu is a gene mapped on chromosome 17q12-21.32 that encodes a 185-kDa transmembrane protein showing 50 percent homology to the epidermal growth factor receptor. No molecular marker has undergone more studies and development in such a short period of time than HER2/neu. In 2000 it was classified in category II of prognostic factors by Fitzgibbons et al. (52) since its prognostic value is highly questionable (8,131). In the 2000 American Society of Clinical Oncology clinical practice guidelines, the routine use of HER2/neu overexpression for prognostic purposes was not recommended (10). Ross et al. (111) reviewed the literature concerning *HER2/neu*, which included 80 studies encompassing more than 25,000 patients, and found that most studies reported that *HER2/neu* amplification or overexpression was associated with poor outcome in patients with axillary lymph node metastases, but not in patients with tumor-negative lymph nodes. Data have progressively accumulated to the point that the 2007 American Society of Clinical Oncology practice guidelines (144) regarded HER2/neu as a prognostic factor, stating that HER2/neu overexpression/gene amplification was associated with a bad prognosis (high rate of recurrence and mortality) in patients with newly diagnosed breast cancer who were not receiving adjuvant systemic therapy.

The importance of *HER2/neu* was further revitalized following the observation that it is a predictive indicator for immunotherapy and choice of endocrine therapy and chemotherapy, especially after the demonstration that *HER2/neu* amplification is associated with a negative response to tamoxifen (85). *HER2/neu* was included among predictive markers in the 2007 American Society of Clinical Oncology practice guidelines (144). The presence of strong 3+ membrane immunohistochemical staining is associated with a response to trastuzumab (humanized monoclonal antibody) in several clinical trials, while 1+ or 2+ immunohistochemical staining, even in the presence of amplification, appears to result in a lesser degree of efficacy of trastuzumab (58).

The most widely used methods for revealing the *HER2/neu* oncogene are fluorescence in situ hybridization (FISH) and immunohistochemistry. FISH reveals gene amplification, while immunohistochemistry indicates protein overexpression. Both methods can be applied to formalin-fixed and paraffin-embedded tissues and although FISH seems slightly more sensitive (92).

The value of this marker is hampered by several factors, similar to those discussed above for steroid receptors. There is lack of standardization of the various methods and scoring systems used to detect the HER2/neu protein. There are more than 20 antibodies available with a sensitivity ranging from 6 to 60 percent (61). In addition, some antibodies bind to the intracellular domain (for instance CB11), while the humanized monoclonal antibody (trastuzumab) binds to the extracellular domain. It is also a matter of concern as to which signal should be regarded as positive in immunohistochemistry. Most of the data are based on membrane positivity on the assumption that strong membrane staining correlates with gene amplification (8). Nevertheless, it has been suggested that cytoplasmic positivity has prognostic/predictive value in tumors of the breast as well as in tumors of other organs (61). Several scoring systems have been developed both for FISH and immunohistochemistry, none of which has been tested adequately. The College of American Pathologists (52) recommends that each report contain every detail of the scoring system followed and the method employed (i.e., antibody used, antigen retrieval technique) (fig. 7-9).

Normal breast tissue does not stain for HER2/neu protein, although apocrine non-neoplastic cells can be decorated (116). LIN and grade 1 DCIS/DIN1 are also negative. On the other end of the spectrum, grade 3 DCIS/DIN3 is positive in over 80 percent of cases (8,9,131) and in virtually all cases associated with Paget's carcinoma

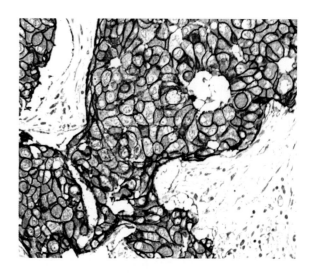

Figure 7-9

HER2/NEU IMMUNOHISTOCHEMISTRY

Strong (3+) membrane staining is obtained by anti-HER2/neu antibody (clone CB11, dilution 1:50; antigen retrieval: heat).

(68). In a study from 13 Australian laboratories on 1,536 carcinomas (15), unequivocal overexpression (3+ immunohistochemically with Hercep Test kit) was seen in 186 (12 percent) and equivocal results (2+) in 206 (13 percent). In this study, 97 percent of cases with unequivocal HER2/neu overexpression were invasive duct (NOS) carcinomas of histologic grade 2 to 3, while only 1 of 124 invasive lobular carcinomas (0.8 percent) was 3+ immunoreactive. None of the 49 "specific type" carcinomas were positive. Gene amplification was seen in 98 percent of cases that were 3+ but in only 23 percent of cases that were 2+. An unsatisfactory level of agreement (kappa 0.4) was obtained among pathologists when the slides were circulated.

Approximately 20 percent of current HER2/neu tests are said to be not accurate due to several technical, methodological, and interpretational pitfalls (144). To minimize variations in testing, stringent guidelines recommended by the American Association of Clinical Oncology (144) offer cultural and practical techniques for standardization. A specific recommendation is devoted to fixation requirements to ensure that pathology laboratories use 10 percent buffered formalin and fix breast excision specimens for 6 to 48 hours and core biopsies for at least 1 hour. An algorithm of positive, equivocal, and negative findings was recommended for both HER2/neu protein expression and gene amplification. Discordant results between immunohistochemistry and fluorescent in situ hybridization are low (about 4 percent of cases) and therefore both methods are interchangeable in 3+ positive and negative cases. Positive 3+ immunohistochemical cell surface protein expression is defined as uniform intense membrane staining of more than 30 percent of the invasive tumor cells. Positive FISH of amplified *HER2/neu* gene copy number is defined as an average of more than six gene copies/nucleus for test system, which does not include a control probe or a HER2/neu:CEP17 ratio of more than 2.2

Equivocal HER2/neu testing results should not exceed 15 percent of samples. An equivocal test shows complete membrane staining of 10 to 30 percent of invasive cells. Some equivocal cases have *HER2/neu* gene amplification in about 12 percent of cases and, therefore, additional testing using FISH is required. The latter shows equivocal results when HER2/neu:CEP17 ratios vary from 1.8 to 2.2. Patients with equivocal test results undergo treatment, a situation that makes pathologists wonder about the great deal of effort involved in offering tests irrelevant to treatment, which is administered irrespective of the results.

A negative immunohistochemical score of 0 or 1+ indicates that 10 percent of invasive cells have membrane staining. The guidelines are very detailed in many sections, and it is a pity that there is a lack of standardization of the cell count. It is not clear how many areas have to be studied to count positive cells in relation to the total neoplastic proliferation. This lack of standardization may also be the source of inconsistencies among different observers.

Genetic Portraits Using DNA Microarray

The present capacity to measure the expression of thousands of genes has led to the classification of novel groups of breast carcinomas that are also related to clinical outcome (124,130). The signature *BRCA1* gene mutation in patients with hereditary breast cancer has been established and can be distinguished from *BRCA2* carriers (133,142). Data are consistent with the finding that *BRCA1* mutant tumors are ER negative and have prominent stromal lymphoid stroma.

Sorlie et al. (124) analyzed 78 carcinomas by hierarchical clustering, separating the tumors into two branches. One branch was characterized by tumors with low or absent *ER* gene expression. This branch was divided into three subgroups. The basal cell subtype was characterized by cells having a high expression of cytokeratins (CK)5 and 17, in addition to laminin. This group of tumors had already been characterized and named as basaloid carcinomas by Jones et al. (66). A second subgroup was the HER2/neu subtype characterized by high expression of numerous genes of the *HER2* amplicon. The third group was composed of "normal" breast-like clusters containing many genes known to be expressed mainly by adipose tissue. The second branch was characterized by tumors with the highest expression of the *ERα* gene and was defined as the luminal/ER group. This group was further subdivided into three subgroups showing luminal-enriched genes. A highly significant difference was found in overall survival and relapse-free survival among patients with different subtypes, with patients in the basal-like group and the HER2 group displaying the shortest survival and relapse-free times.

Van de Vijver et al. (130) were able to define two groups that had strong independent prognostic significance with a Cox regression analysis based on the analysis of 70 genes in 295 patients. A poor prognostic gene signature was attached to 180 patients while 115 had a good prognostic signature. The mean overall 10-year survival rate was 54.5 percent for those with a poor survival signature and 94.5 percent for those with a good prognostic signature. The probability of remaining free from distant metastases was 59.6 percent and 85.2 percent, respectively. The independent predictive indicators of overall prognosis were a poor prognosis signature, the larger size of the tumor, and the nonuse of adjuvant chemotherapy. This suggests that genetic portraits might be used not only as prognostic indicators but also as a useful means of guiding adjuvant therapy in patients with node-positive and -negative breast tumors.

Using a different microarray platform, a gene expression signature of 76 genes was retrospectively found related to 286 patients with lymph node–negative breast cancer, who had not received adjuvant systemic therapy (139). The

76-gene profile consisted of 60 genes for patients positive for ER and 16 genes for ER-negative patients. This signature was highly informative in identifying patients who developed metastases within 5 years and may be a useful technique for the identification of patients at high risk of disease progression. It is difficult to compare these data to those presented above (130) because different microarray platforms were used, resulting in the overlap of only three genes between the two signatures. Although microarray data are very promising, their translation into clinical practice is still not fully applicable (100).

The reproducibility of data from different laboratories appears to be poor (100). To use the words of Reis-Filho (100), "although the results are promising, further optimization and standardization of the (various) techniques and properly designed clinical trials are required before using these techniques as reliable tools for clinical decisions." The possible scenario in which a patient has a tumor with a genotypic good signature, but established pathologic criteria of a poor prognosis, should be avoided.

Phenotypic Portraits Using Tissue Microarray

Along with the enthusiasm for the use of cDNA microarray, numerous papers have appeared using tissue microarray technology (TMA) in breast carcinomas in an attempt to obtain a phenotypic immunohistochemical portrait. The largest study available with TMA is based on 1,944 cases (40) which were studied with no fewer than six antibodies (for type of antibodies see below). This led to the establishment of four phenotypes.

The luminal phenotype consisted of 1,323 cases (71.4 percent of patients). These cases expressed luminal markers only (CK7/8, CK18, and CK19). The basal phenotype consisted of 15 patients (0.8 percent) whose tumors expressed one or more of the basal markers (CK5/6, CK14, and smooth muscle actin). A combined luminal and basal phenotype was observed in 508 patients (27.4 percent) whose tumors were positive for one or more of the luminal markers together with one or more of the basal markers. A null phenotype was observed in 6 patients (0.4 percent) whose tumors were negative for both luminal and basal markers. The luminal phenotype tumors were ER positive in 80.1 percent of the patients, the luminal and basal phenotype tumors were ER positive in 44.5 percent of patients (positivity in the luminal side), while the pure basal and null phenotypes were negative for ER. The expression of luminal markers was associated with better outcome, while expression of basal markers was associated with poor clinical behavior (1). TMA studies give more consistent results than cDNA microarray studies (98), but still they suffer from the lack of validation on a large number of cases.

Other Prognostic and Predictive Indicators

There are many other morphologic and molecular markers reported in the literature, but as yet, none with definite impact on prognosis and/or prediction of treatment efficacy (10,52). Some of the morphologic signs have been commented upon in the chapter on invasive duct carcinomas, NOS.

TREATMENT

The care of patients with breast cancer involves several disciplines and, at the moment, the general trend is to minimize breast treatment. This includes limited surgery (lumpectomy) (49,134) which allows conservation of the breast, sentinel node biopsy which avoids unnecessary removal of unaffected axillary lymph nodes (118), increased used of limited radiation therapy(118), and appropriate adjuvant therapy with tailored targeted therapies in individual patients (36,57,58).

To avoid improper management, guidelines for treatment have been published and periodically updated. The European guidelines for quality assurance in breast cancer screening and diagnosis (90), the St. Gallen conferences (58), and the international consensus conferences (118) periodically and systematically review the standard of care. In all of these, the role of pathology is in guiding the hands of surgeons, clinical oncologists, and radiotherapists.

Surgery. Surgery is used for both diagnostic and therapeutic purposes. The majority of both palpable or nonpalpable breast cancers receive a preoperative diagnosis using fine needle aspiration cytology (FNAC) or core biopsy (90,96,118). The advantages or disadvantages of FNAC over core biopsy are discussed in the Appendix. It appears that core biopsy is becoming more and more utilized due to microwave fast processing (97), which has minimized the length of processing time for this procedure. Frozen sections are justified only in cases in which definitive treatment is required in the same session (90). This can be done only when the lesion is macroscopically identified, the tissue is abundant enough to leave additional material for routine fixation, and the preoperative diagnosis had proven impossible (90).

Breast conserving treatment generally applies to small, unifocal, invasive carcinomas (up to an arbitrarily 4 cm determined size). It is intended to achieve local control of the disease, together with optimal breast cosmesis. It includes a combination of surgical procedures (quadrantectomy or excisional biopsy [lumpectomy]) that should have free margins of 1 cm (90), together with radiotherapy. The measurement of the margins (type and dimension) is matter of hot debate, and often agreement is difficult to reach, so that in some consensus conferences a measurement figure is not given, and free margins are accepted when they are "adequate" (118). The lack of agreement on these very important issues is due to the lack of conclusive data in the literature and to the anxiety of the physician for causing overtreatment to the patient. Radiation therapy should avoid the heart, lung, and contralateral breast.

Accelerated partial breast irradiation (APBI) is the delivery of radiation to a limited target volume (the surgical cavity plus the surrounding tissue) in a single treatment or at the most within a week. Although APBI schemes are becoming popular, especially in view of patient's convenience, no data are available on its long-term efficacy, nor from phase III trials (58).

The main aim of any breast cancer therapy is to contain the relapse rate of invasive breast cancer in the range of 1 to 2 percent per year (83) without exceeding 15 percent at 10 years (90).

Mastectomy. Mastectomy is considered if the size of the invasive tumor is larger than 5 cm, if there is extensive lymph node involvement (more than 4 lymph nodes), if there is noticeable vascular invasion, if the margins are involved, if there is skin or muscle invasion, or for patient preference. Mastectomy consists of removing all the breast tissue together with the skin and nipple/areolar complex (14,91). An

acceptable outcome is a chest wall relapse rate (of invasive carcinoma) of less than 10 percent after 10 years (90).

Chemotherapy. There is at the moment no consensus on the most appropriate sequence of therapy. Many institutions have adopted different approaches, despite the recommendation that chemotherapy should precede radiotherapy (58). Concurrent chemotherapy and radiation therapy appear feasible with cyclophosphamide, methotrexate, and fluorouracil as well as with tamoxifen, but antracycline-based regimens and taxans increase the risk of radiation-induced damage in normal tissue (58).

Patients have been stratified as endocrine responsive, of uncertain response, or unresponsive to endocrine management, depending on intense, moderate, or no expression of steroid hormone receptors (58). Risk categories have also been proposed (low, intermediate, and high risk) based on the absence or presence of node metastases; size and grade of tumors; absence or presence of peritumoral vascular invasion; *HER2/neu* gene either overexpressed or amplified; and age lower or higher than 35 years (58). Patients placed in the category of low risk and also included in the category of endocrine responsive are treated with endocrine therapy. On the contrary, chemotherapy alone (without endocrine treatment) is administered to high-risk, endocrine-nonresponsive patients (58). Although the St. Gallen guidelines (58) for postoperative adjuvant systemic therapies are based on evidence from clinical trials demonstrating reduction of relapse and increase of survival duration, long-term data currently are lacking.

When tumors are too large for breast conserving treatment, preoperative chemotherapy is advocated by some oncologists (113,143). A remission rate of 80 percent for women with primary breast cancer has been shown with different regimens and complete pathologic remission has been noted in 7 to 15 percent of patients (113,143). Unfortunately, these same trials have shown that there is no difference in survival among patients treated with preoperative or postoperative chemotherapy (113,143). An acceptable outcome would be one similar to breast cancer therapy: a relapse rate of 15 percent after 10 years.

REFERENCES

1. Abd El-Rehim DM, Pinder SE, Paish EC, et al. Expression of luminal and basal cytokeratins in human breast carcinoma. J Pathol 2004;203:661-671.

1a. Acs G, Dumoff KL, Solin LJ, Pasha T, Xu X, Zhang PJ. Extensive retraction artifact correlates with lymphatic invasion and nodal metastasis and predicts poor outcome in early stage breast carcinoma. Am J Surg Pathol 2007;31:129-140.

2. AJCC cancer staging manual, 6th ed. Greene FL, Page DL, Fleming IO, et al., eds. New York: Springer; 2002.

3. Anderson C, Ricci A, Pedersen CA, Cartun RW. Immunocytochemical analysis of estrogen and progesterone receptors in benign stromal lesions of the breast. Evidence for hormonal etiology in pseudoangiomatous hyperplasia of mammary stroma. Am J Surg Pathol 1991;15:145-149.

4. Ashikari R, Rosen PP, Urban JA, Senoo T. Breast cancer presenting as an axillary mass. Ann Surg 1976;183:415-417.

5. Axelsson K, Ljung BM, Moore DH 2nd, et al. Tumor angiogenesis as a prognostic assay for invasive ductal breast carcinoma. J Natl Cancer Inst 1995;87:997-1008.

6. Azzopardi JG, Ahmed A, Millis RR. Problems in breast pathology. Major Prob Pathol 1979;11:1-466.

7. Barnes DM, Hanby AM. Oestrogen and progesterone receptors in breast cancer: past, present and future. Histopathology 2001;38:271-274.

8. Barnes DM, Lammie GA, Millis RR, Gullick WL, Allen DS, Altman DG. An immunohistochemical evaluation of c-erbB-2 expression in human breast carcinoma. Br J Cancer 1988;58:448-452.

9. Bartkova J, Barnes DM, Millis RR, Gullick WJ. Immunohistochemical demonstration of c-erbB-2 protein in mammary ductal carcinoma in situ. Hum Pathol 1990;21:1164-1167.

10. Bast RC Jr, Ravdin P, Hayes DF, et al. 2000 update of recommendations for the use of tumor markers in breast and colorectal cancer: clinical practice guidelines of the American Society of Clinical Oncology. J Clin Oncol 2001;19:1865-1878.

11. Benson JR, della Rovere GO: Axilla Management Consensus Group. Management of the axilla in women with breast cancer. Lancet Oncol 2007;8:331-348.

12. Berrino F, Muti P, Micheli A, et al. Serum sex hormone levels after menopause and subsequent breast cancer. J Natl Cancer Inst 1996-88:291-296.

13. Bettelheim R, Penman HG, Thornton-Jones H, Neville AM. Prognostic significance of peritumoral vascular invasion in breast cancer. Br J Cancer 1984;50:771-777.

14. Bijker N, Rutgers EJ, Peterse JL, et al. Low risk of locoregional recurrence of primary breast carcinoma after treatment with a modification of the Halsted radical mastectomy and selective use of radiotherapy. Cancer 1999;85:1773-1781.

15. Bilous M, Ades C, Armes J, et al. Predicting the HER2 status of breast cancer from basic histopathology data: an analysis of 1500 breast cancers as part of the HER2000 International Study. Breast 2003;12:92-98.

16. Bloom HJ, Richardson WW. Histological grading and prognosis in breast cancer; a study of 1409 cases of which 359 have been followed for 15 years. Br J Cancer 1957;11:359-377.

17. Bobrow LG, Happerfield LC, Gregory WM, Springall RD, Millis RR. The classification of ductal carcinoma in situ and its association with biological markers. Semin Diagn Pathol 1994;11:199-207.

18. Cady B, Stone MD, Schuler JG, Thakur R, Wanner MA, Lavin PT. The new era in breast cancer: invasion, size and nodal development dramatically decreasing as a result of mammographic screening. Arch Surg 1996;131:301-308.

19. Carcoforo P, Sortini D, Feggi L, et al. Clinical and therapeutic importance of sentinel node biopsy of the internal mammary chain in patients with breast cancer: a single-center study with long-term follow-up. Ann Surg Oncol 2006;13:1338-1343.

20. Carter BA, Jensen RA, Simpson JF, Page DL. Benign transport of breast epithelium into axillary lymph nodes after biopsy. Am J Clin Pathol 2000;113:259-265.

21. Carter CL, Allen C, Henson DE. Relation of tumor size, lymph node status, and survival in 24,740 breast cancer cases. Cancer 1989;63:181-187.

22. Clemente CG, Boracchi P, Andreola S, Del Vecchio M, Veronesi P, Rilke FO. Peritumoral lymphatic invasion in patients with node-negative mammary duct carcinoma. Cancer 1992;69:1396-1403.

23. Cochran AJ. Surgical pathology remains pivotal in the evaluation of 'sentinel' lymph nodes. Am J Surg Pathol 1999;23:1169-1172.

24. Collins LC, Botero ML, Schnitt SJ. Bimodal frequency distribution of estrogen receptor immunohistochemical staining results in breast cancer: an analysis of 825 cases. Am J Clin Pathol 2005;123:16-20.

25. Contesso G, Jotti GS, Bonadonna G. Tumor grade as a prognostic factor in primary breast cancer. Eur J Cancer Clin Oncol 1989;25:403-409.

26. Contesso G, Mouriesse H, Friedman S, Genin J, Sarrazin D, Rouesse J. The importance of histologic grade in long-term prognosis of breast cancer: a study of 1,010 patients, uniformly treated at the Institut Gustave-Roussy. J Clin Oncol 1987;5:1378-1386.

27. Cserni G. Metastases in axillary sentinel lymph nodes in breast cancer as detected by intensive histopathological work up. J Clin Path 1999;52:922-924.

28. Cserni G, Amendoeira I, Apostolikas N, et al. Pathological work-up of sentinel lymph nodes in breast cancer. Review of current data to be considered for the formulation of guidelines. Eur J Cancer 2003;39:1654-1667.

29. Cserni G, Bianchi S, Boecker W, et al. Improving the reproducibility of diagnosing micrometastases and isolated tumor cells. Cancer 2005;103:358-367.

30. Cserni G, Gregori D, Merletti F, et al. Meta-analysis of non-sentinel node metastases associated with micrometastatic sentinel nodes in breast cancer. Br J Surg 2004;91:1245-1252.

31. Dadmanesh F, Peterse JL, Sapino A, Fornelli A, Eusebi V. Lymphoepithelioma-like carcinoma of the breast: lack of evidence of Epstein-Barr virus infection. Histopathology 2001;38:54-61.

32. Damiani S, Eusebi V, Peterse JL. Malignant neoplasms infiltrating "pseudoangiomatous" stromal hyperplasia of the breast: an unrecognized pathway of tumour spread. Histopathology 2002;41:208-215.

33. Davis BW, Gelber R, Goldhirsch A, et al. Prognostic significance of peritumoral vessel invasion in clinical trials of adjuvant therapy for breast cancer with axillary lymph node metastasis. Hum Pathol 1985;16:1212-1218.

34. den Bakker MA, van Weeszenberg A, de Kanter AY, et al. Non-sentinel lymph node involvement in patients with breast cancer and sentinel node micrometastasis; too early to abandon axillary clearance. J Clin Path 2002;55:932-935.

35. Di Tommaso L, Kapucuoglu N, Losi L, Trerè D, Eusebi V. Impact of delayed fixation on evaluation of cell proliferation in intracranial malignant tumors. Appl Immunohistochem Mol Morph 1999;7:209-213.

36. Dietel M, Sers C. Personalized medicine and development of targeted therapies: the upcoming challenge for diagnostic molecular pathology. A review. Virchows Arch 2006;448:744-755.

37. Dockerty MB, Gray HK, Pierce EH. Surgical significance of isolated axillary adenopathy. Ann Surg 1957;145:104-107.

37a. Dotto J, Kluk M, Geramizadeh B, Tavassoli FA. Frequency of clinically occult intraepithelial and invasive neoplasia in reduction mammoplasty specimens: a study of 516 cases. Int J Surg Pathol 2008;16:25-30.

38. Dunne B, Going JJ. Scoring nuclear pleomorphism in breast cancer. Histopathology 2001;39:259-265.

39. Eifel P, Axelson JA, Costa J, et al. National Institutes of Health Consensus Development Conference Statement: adjuvant therapy for breast cancer, November 1-3, 2000. J Natl Cancer Inst 2001;93:979-989.

41. Elledge RM, Osborne CK. Oestrogen receptors and breast cancer. Br Med J 1997;314:1843-1844.

42. Elston CW, Ellis IO. Assessment of histological grade. In: Elston CW, Ellis IO, eds. The breast. Edinburgh: Churchill Livingstone; 1998:365-384.

43. Elston CW, Ellis IO. Pathological prognostic factors in breast cancer. I. The value of histological grade in breast cancer: experience from a large study with long-term follow-up. Histopathology 1991;19:403-410.

44. Elston CW, Ellis IO, Goulding H, Pinder SE. Role of pathology in the prognosis and management of breast cancer. In: Elston CW, Ellis IO, eds. The breast, 3rd ed. Edinburgh: Churchill Livingstone; 1998:385-433.

45. Eusebi V, Azzopardi JG. Vascular infiltration in benign breast disease. J Pathol 1976;118:9-16.

46. Eusebi V, Capella C, Cossu A, Rosai J. Neuroendocrine carcinoma within lymph nodes in the absence of a primary tumor, with special reference to Merkel cell carcinoma. Am J Surg Pathol 1992;16:658-666.

47. Eusebi V, Damiani S, Losi L, Millis RR. Apocrine differentitation in breast epithelium. Adv Anat Pathol 1997;4:139-155.

48. Fechner RE. Mammary carcinoma arising in benign axillary epithelial lymph node inclusions. Histopathology 1989;14:434-435.

49. Fisher B, Anderson S, Bryant J, et al. Twenty-year follow-up of a randomized trial comparing total mastectomy, lumpectomy, and lumpectomy plus irradiation for the treatment of invasive breast cancer. N Engl J Med 2002;347:1233-1241.

50. Fisher ER, Palekar A, Rockette H, Redmond C, Fisher B. Pathologic findings from the National Surgical Adjuvant Breast Project (Protocol No. 4). V. Significance of axillary nodal micro- and macrometastases. Cancer 1978;42:2032-2038.

51. Fisher ER, Redmond CK, Liu H, Rockette H, Fisher B. Correlation of estrogen receptor and pathologic characteristics of invasive breast cancer. Cancer 1980;45:349-353.

52. Fitzgibbons PL, Page DL, Weaver D, et al. Prognostic factors in breast cancer. College of American Pathologists Consensus Statement 1999. Arch Pathol Lab Med 2000;124:966-978.

53. Foschini MP, Righi A, Cucchi MC, et al. The impact of large sections and 3D technique on the study of lobular in situ and invasive carcinoma of the breast. Virchows Arch 2006;448:256-261.

54. Foschini MP, Tot T, Eusebi V. Large-section (macrosection) histologic slides. In: Silverstein MJ, ed. Ductal carcinoma in situ of the breast, 2nd ed. Philadelphia: Lippincott Williams & Wilkins; 2002:249-254.

55. Galea MH, Blamey RW, Elston CE, Ellis IO. The Nottingham Prognostic Index in primary breast cancer. Breast Cancer Res Treat 1992;22:207-219.

56. Gibbs NM. Topographical and histological presentation of mammographic pathology in breast cancer. J Clin Pathol 1988;41:3-11.

57. Goldhirsch A, Glick JH, Gelber RD, Coates AS, Thurlimann B, Senn HJ. Meeting highlights: international expert consensus on the primary therapy of early breast cancer 2005. Ann Oncol 2005;16:1569-1583.

58. Goldhirsch A, Wood WC, Gelber RD, et al. Progress and promise: highlights of the international expert consensus on the primary therapy of early breast cancer 2007. Ann Oncol 2007;18:1133-1144.

59. Goulding H, Abdul Rashid NF, Robertson JF, et al. Assessment of angiogenesis in breast carcinoma: an important factor in prognosis? Hum Pathol 1995;26:1196-1200.

60. Hanau CA, Machera H, Miettinen M. Immunohistochemical evaluation of vascular invasion in carcinomas with five different markers. Appl Immunohistochem 1993;1:46-50.

61. Hanna W, Kahn HJ, Trudeau M. Evaluation of HER-2/neu(erbB-2) status in breast cancer: from bench to bedside. Mod Pathol 1999;12:827-834.

62. Hartveit F. Attenuated cells in breast stroma: the missing lymphatic system of the breast. Histopathology 1990;16:533-543.

63. Hartveit F. Paranodal vascular spread in breast cancer with axillary node involvement. J Pathol 1979;127:111-114.

64. Haybittle JL, Blamey RW, Elston CW, et al. A prognostic index in primary breast cancer. Br J Cancer 1982;45:361-366.

65. Jackson B, Scott-Conner C, Moulder J. Axillary metastasis from occult breast carcinoma: diagnosis and management. Am Surg 1995;61:431-434.

66. Jones C, Nonni AV, Fulford L, et al. CGH analysis of ductal carcinoma of the breast with basaloid/myoepithelial cell differentiation. Br J Cancer 2001;85:422-427.

67. Kahn HJ, Bailey D, Marks A. Monoclonal antibody D2-40, a new marker of lymphatic endothelium, reacts with Kaposi's sarcoma and a subset of angiosarcomas. Mod Pathol 2002;15:434-440.

68. Lammie GA, Barnes DM, Millis RR, Gullick WJ. An immunohistochemical study of the presence of c-erbB-2 protein in Paget's disease of the nipple. Histopathology 1989;15:505-514.

69. Lauria R, Perrone F, Carlomagno C, et al. The prognostic value of lymphatic and blood vessel invasion in operable breast cancer. Cancer 1995;76:1772-1778.

70. Lee AH, Ellis IO, Pinder SE, Barbera D, Elston CW. Pathological assessment of sentinel lymph-node biopsies in patients with breast cancer. Virchows Arch 2000;436:97-101.

71. Lee AH, Happerfield LC, Bobrow LG, Millis RR. Angiogenesis and inflammation in invasive carcinoma of the breast. J Clin Path 1997;50:669-673.

72. Lee AK, DeLellis RA, Wolfe HJ. Intramammary lymphatic invasion in breast carcinomas. Evaluation using ABH isoantigens as endothelial markers. Am J Surg Pathol 1986;10:589-594.

73. Linell F, Ljunberg O, Andersson I. Breast carcinoma. Aspects of early stages, progression and related problems. Acta Pathol Microbiol Scand Suppl 1980;(272):1-233.

74. Lippman M, Bolan G, Huff K. The effects of androgens and antiandrogens on hormone-responsive human breast cancer in long-term tissue culture. Cancer Res 1976;36:4610-4618.

75. Magro G, Bisceglia M, Michal M. Expression of steroid hormone receptors, their regulated proteins, and bcl-2 protein in myofibroblastoma of the breast. Histopathology 2000;36:515-521.

76. McMasters KM, Giuliano AE, Ross MI, et al. Sentinel lymph-node biopsy for breast cancer—not yet the standard of care. N Engl J Med 1998;339:990-995.

77. Micheli A, Muti P, Secreto G, et al. Endogenus sex hormones and subsequent breast cancer in premenopausal women. Int J Cancer 2004;112:312-318.

78. Millis RR, Barnes DM, Lampejo OT, Egan MK, Smith P. Tumor grade does not change between primary and recurrent mammary carcinoma. Eur J Cancer 1998;34:548-553.

79. Millis RR, Springall R, Lee AH, Ryder K, Rytina ER, Fentiman IS. Occult axillary lymph node metastases are of no prognostic significance in breast cancer. Br J Cancer 2002;86:396-401.

80. Millis RR, Springall RJ, Hanby AM, Ryder K, Fentiman IS. A high number of tumor free axillary lymph nodes from patients with lymph node negative breast carcinoma is associated with poor outcome. Cancer 2002;94:2307-2309.

81. Moinfar F, Okcu M, Tsybrovskyy O, et al. Androgen receptors frequently are expressed in breast carcinomas: potential relevance to new therapeutic strategies. Cancer 2003;98:703-711.

82. Morrow M, Evans J, Rosen PP, Kinne DW. Does clearing of axillary lymph nodes contribute to accurate staging of breast carcinoma? Cancer 1984;53:1329-1332.

83. Morrow M, Harris JR, Schnitt SJ. Local control following breast conserving surgery for invasive cancer: results of clinical trials. J Natl Cancer Inst 1995;87:1669-1673.

84. Mosselman S, Polman J, Dijkema R. ER beta: identification and characterization of a novel human estrogen receptor. FEBS Lett 1996;392:49-53.

85. Muss HB, Thor AD, Berry DA, et al. c-erbB-2 expression and response to adjuvant therapy in women with node-positive early breast cancer. N Engl J Med 1994;330:1260-1266.

86. Nadji M, Gomez-Fernandez C, Ganjei-Azar P, Morales AR. Immunohistochemistry of estrogen and progesterone receptors reconsidered: experience with 5,993 breast cancers. Am J Clin Pathol 2005;123:21-27.

87. Nemoto T, Vana J, Bedwani RN, Baker HW, McGregor FH, Murphy GP. Management and survival of female breast cancer: results of a national survey by the America College of Surgeons. Cancer 1980;45:2917-2924.

88. Nielsen M, Thomsen JL, Primdahl S, Dyreborg U, Andersen JA. Breast cancer and atypia among young and middle-aged women: a study of 110 medicolegal autopsies. Br J Cancer 1987;56:814-819.

89. NIH. Steroid receptors in breast cancer: an NIH Consensus Development Conference, Bethesda, Maryland, June 27-29, 1979. Cancer 1980;46:2759-2963.

90. O'Higgins N, Linos D, Blichert-Toft M, et al. Quality assurance guidelines for surgery. In: Perry N, Broeders M, de Wolf C, Tornberg S, Holland R, von Karsa L, eds. European guidelines for quality assurance in breast cancer screening and diagnosis, 4th ed. European Communities, Belgium 2006:315-334.

91. Overgaard M. Overview of randomized trials in high risk breast cancer patients treated with adjuvant systemic therapy with or without postmastectomy irradiation. Semin Radiat Oncol 1999;9:292-299.

92. Pauletti G, Dandekar S, Rong H, et al. Assessment of methods for tissue-based detection of the HER-2/neu alteration in human breast cancer: a direct comparison of fluorescence in situ hybridization and immunohistochemistry. J Clin Oncol 2000;18:3651-3664.

93. Pereira H, Pinder SE, Sibbering DM, et al. Pathological prognostic factors in breast cancer. IV: Should you be a typer or a grader? A comparative study of two histological prognostic features in operable breast carcinoma. Histopathology 1995;27:219-226.

94. Pezzella F, Harris AL, Gatter KC. Ways of escape: are all tumours angiogenic? Histopathology 2001;39:551-553.

95. Pinder SE, Ellis IO, Galea M, O'Rouke S, Blamey RW, Elston CW. Pathological prognostic factors in breast cancer. III. Vascular invasion: relationship with recurrence and survival in a large study with long-term follow-up. Histopathology 1994;24:41-47.

96. Pinder SE, Reis-Filho JS. Non-operative breast pathology. J Clin Path 2007;60:1297-1299.

97. Ragazzini T, Magrini E, Cucchi MC, Foschini MP, Eusebi V. The fast track biopsy (FTB): description of a rapid histology and immunohistochemistry method for evaluation of preoperative breast core biopsies. Int J Surg Pathol 2005;13:247-252.

98. Rakha EA, Putti TC, Abd El-Rehim DM, et al. Morphological and immunophenotypic analysis of breast carcinomas with basal and myoepithelial differentiation. J Pathol 2006;208:495-506.

99. Regitnig P, Reiner A, Dinges HP, et al. Quality assurance for detection of estrogen and progesterone receptors by immunohistochemistry in Austrian pathology laboratories. Virchows Arch 2002;441:328-334.

100. Reis-Filho JS, Westbury C, Pierga JY. The impact of expression profiling on prognostic and predictive testing in breast cancer. J Clin Path 2006;59:225-231.

101. Rhodes A, Jasani B, Balaton AJ, et al. Study of interlaboratory reliability and reproducibility of estrogen and progesterone receptor assay in Europe. Documentation of poor reliability and identification of insufficient microwave antigen retrieval time as a major contributory element of unreliable assay. Am J Clin Pathol 2001;115:44-58.

102. Rhodes A, Jasani B, Barnes DM, Bobrow LG, Miller KD. Reliability of immunohistochemical demonstration of oestrogen receptors in routine practice: interlaboratory variance in the sensitivity of detection and evaluation of scoring systems. J Clin Path 2000;53:125-130.

103. Riva C, Dainese E, Caprara G, et al. Immunohistochemical study of androgen receptors in breast carcinoma. Evidence of their frequent expression in lobular carcinoma. Virchows Arch 2005;447:695-364.

104. Rosen PP. Invasive duct carcinoma: assesmsment of prognosis, morpholigic prognostic marker, and tumor growth rate. In: Rosen PP, ed. Rosen's breast pathology, 2nd ed. Philadelphia: Lippincott Williams & Wilkins; 2001:325-364.

105. Rosen PP. Unusual clinical presentations of carcinoma. In: Rosen PP, ed. Rosen's book of pathology, 2nd ed. Philadelphia: Lippincott Williams & Wilkins; 2001:653-687.

106. Rosen PP, Fracchia AA, Urban JA. "Residual" mammary carcinoma following simulated partial mastectomy. Cancer 1975;35:739-747.

107. Rosen PP, Groshen S. Factors influencing survival and prognosis in early breast carcinoma (T1N0M0-T1N1M0). Assessment of 644 patients with median follow-up of 18 years. Surg Clin North Am 1990;70:937-962.

108. Rosen PP, Groshen S, Saigo PE, Kinne DW, Hellman S. A long-term follow-up study of survival in stage I (T1N0M0) and stage II (T1N1M0) breast carcinoma. J Clin Oncol 1989;7:355-366.

109. Rosen PP, Kimmel M. Occult breast carcinoma presenting with axillary lymph node metastases: a follow-up study of 48 patients. Hum Pathol 1990;21:518-523.

110. Rosen PP, Menendez-Botet CJ, Nisselbaum JS, et al. Pathological review of breast lesions analyzed for estrogen receptor protein. Cancer Res 1975;35:3187-3194.

111. Ross JS, Fletcher JA, Linette GP, et al. The Her-2/gene and protein in breast cancer 2003: biomarker and target therapy. Oncologist 2003;8:307-325.

112. Sandrucci S, Casalegno PS, Percivale P, Mastrangelo M, Bombardieri E, Bertoglio S. Sentinel lymph node mapping and biopsy for breast cancer: a review of the literature relative to 4791 procedures. Tumori 1999;85:425-434.

113. Sapunar F, Smith IE. Neoadjuvant chemotherapy for breast cancer. Ann Med 2000;32:43-50.

114. Schippinger W, Regitnig P, Dandachi N, et al. Evaluation of the prognostic significance of androgen receptor expression in metastatic breast cancer. Virchows Arch 2006;449:23-30.

115. Schwartz GF, Giuliano AE, Veronesi U. Consensus Conference Committee. Proceedings of the consensus conference on the role of sentinel lymph node biopsy in carcinoma of the breast, April 19-22, 2001, Philadelphia, Pennsylvania. Hum Pathol 2002;33:579-589.

116. Selim AA, El-Ayat G, Wells CA. Expression of c-erbB2, p53, Bcl-2, Bax, c-myc and Ki-67 in apocrine metaplasia and apocrine change within sclerosing adenosis of the breast. Virchows Arch 2002;441:449-455.

117. Siitonen SM, Haapasalo HK, Rantala IS, Helin HJ, Isola JJ. Comparison of different immuno-histochemical methods in the assessment of angiogenesis: lack of prognostic value in a group of 77 selected node-negative breast carcinomas. Mod Pathol 1995;8:745-752.

118. Silverstein MJ, Lagios MD, Recht A, et al. Image-detected breast cancer: state of the art diagnosis and treatment. Am Coll Surg 2005;201:586-597.

119. Sloane JP, Trott PA, Lakhani SR, eds. Biopsy pathology of the breast, 2nd ed. London: Oxford Univ. Press; 2001.

120. Sloane JP. Infiltrating carcinoma–morphological and molecular features of prognostic significance. In: Sloane JP, Trott PA, Lakhani SR, eds. Biopsy pathology of the breast, 2nd ed. London: Oxford Univ. Press; 2001:215-236.

121. Sloane JP, Amendoeira I, Apostolikas N, et al. Consistency achieved by 23 European pathologists from 12 countries in diagnosing breast disease and reporting prognostic features of carcinomas. European Commission Working Group on Breast Screening Pathology. Virchows Arch 1999;434:3-10.

122. Smart CR, Myers MH, Gloeckler LA. Implications from SEER data on breast cancer management. Cancer 1978;41:787-789.

123. Snead DR, Bell JA, Dixon AR, et al. Methodology of immunohistological detection of oestrogen receptor in human breast carcinoma in formalin-fixed, paraffin-embedded tissue: a comparison with frozen section methodology. Histopathology 1993;23:233-238.

124. Sorlie T, Perou CM, Tibshirani R, et al. Gene expression patterns of breast carcinomas distinguish tumor subclasses with clinical implications. Proc Natl Acad Sci USA 2001;98:10869-10874.

125. Sugg SL, Donegan WL. Staging and prognosis. In: Donegan WL, Spratt JS, eds. Cancer of the breast, 2nd ed. Philadelphia: Saunders; 2002:477-506.

126. Taback B, Chan AD, Kuo CT, et al. Detection of occult metastatic breast cancer cells in blood by multimolecular marker assay: correlation with clinical stage of disease. Cancer Res 2001;61:8845-8850.

127. Tavassoli FA. Pathology of the breast, 2nd ed. Stamford, CT: Appleton-Lange/McGraw Hill; 1999.

128. Tot T. Clinical relevance of the distribution of the lesions in 500 consecutive breast cancer cases documented in large format histologic sections. Cancer 2007;110:2551-2560.0

129. Turner RR, Ollila DW, Stern S, Giuliano AE. Optimal histopathologic examination of the sentinel lymph node for breast carcinoma staging. Am J Surg Pathol 1999;23:263-267.

130. van de Vijver MJ, He YD, van't Veer LJ, et al. A gene-expression signature as a predictor of survival in breast cancer. N Engl J Med 2002;347:1999-2009.

131. van der Vijver MJ, Peterse JL, Mooi WJ, et al. Neu-protein overexpression in breast cancer. Association with comedo-type ductal carcinoma in situ and limited prognostic value in stage II breast cancer. N Engl J Med 1988;319:1239-1245.

132. van Diest PJ, Baak JP. The morphometric prognostic index is the strongest prognosticator in premenopausal lymph node-negative and lymph node-positive breast cancer patients. Hum Pathol 1991;22:326-330.

133. van't Veer LJ, Dai H, van de Vijver MJ, et al. Gene expression profiling predicts clinical outcome of breast cancer. Nature 2002;415:530-536.

134. Veronesi U, Cascinelli N, Mariani L, et al. Twenty-year follow-up of a randomized study comparing breast-conserving surgery with radical mastectomy for early breast cancer. N Engl J Med 2002;347:1227-1232.

135. Veronesi U, Paganelli G, Galimberti V, et al. Sentinel-node biopsy to avoid axillary dissection in breast cancer with clinically negative lymph-nodes. Lancet 1997;349:1864-1867.

136. Veronesi U, Paganelli G, Viale G, et al. Sentinel lymph node biopsy and axillary dissection in breast cancer: results in a large series. J Natl Cancer Inst 1999;91:368-373.

137. Veronesi U, Viale G, Rotmesz N, Goldhirsch A. Rethinking TNM: breast cancer TNM classification for treatment decision-making and research. Breast 2006;15:3-8.

138. von Wasielewski R, Mengel M, Wiese B, Rudiger T, Muller-Hermelink HK, Kreipe H. Tissue array technology for testing interlaboratory and interobserver reproducibility of immunohistochemical estrogen receptor analysis in a large multicenter trial. Am J Clin Pathol 2002;118:675-682.

139. Wang Y, Klijn JG, Zhang Y, et al. Gene-expression profiles to predict distant metastasis of lymph-node negative primary breast cancer. Lancet 2005;365:671-679.

140. Weidner N, Moore DH 2nd, Vartanian R. Correlation of Ki-67 antigen expression with mitotic figure index and tumor grade in breast carcinomas using the novel "paraffin" reactive MIB1 antibody. Hum Pathol 1994;25:337-342.

141. Weidner N, Semple JP, Welch WR, Folkman J. Tumor angiogenesis and metastasis—correlation in invasive breast carcinoma. N Engl J Med 1991;324:1-8.

142. Wessels LF, van Welsem T, Hart AA, van't Veer LJ, Reinders MJ, Nederlof PM. Molecular classification of breast carcinomas by comparative genomic hybridization: a specific somatic genetic profile for BRCA1 tumors. Cancer Res 2002;62:7110-7117.

143. Wolff AC, Davidson NE. Primary systemic therapy in operable breast cancer. J Clin Oncol 2000;18:1558-1569.

144. Wolff AC, Hamond EH, Schwartz JN, et al. American Society of Clinical Oncology/College of American Pathologists guideline recommendations for human epidermal growth factor receptor 2 testing in breast cancer. J Clin Oncol 2007;25:118-145.

145. Youngson BJ, Cranor M, Rosen PP. Epithelial displacement in surgical breast specimens following needling procedures. Am J Surg Pathol 1994;18:896-903.

146. Youngson BJ, Liberman L, Rosen PP. Displacement of carcinomatous epithelium in surgical breast specimens following stereotaxic core biopsy. Am J Clin Pathol 1995;103:598-602.

8 MAJOR VARIANTS OF CARCINOMA

INVASIVE DUCT CARCINOMA, NOT OTHERWISE SPECIFIED

Definition. *Invasive duct carcinoma, not otherwise specified* (IDC, NOS) comprises a large heterogeneous group of tumors that fail to exhibit sufficient characteristics to achieve classification as a specific histologic type (World Health Organization, 2003). Synonyms include *infiltrating carcinoma with productive fibrosis* (70,95) and *invasive duct carcinoma of no special type* (73). The term "duct" is not indicative of origin from ducts, since most breast carcinomas arise in the terminal duct lobular unit (TDLU; see chapter 1); rather it reflects a variety of growth patterns and cell types.

Clinical Features. IDC, NOS constitutes the largest group of invasive carcinomas: 41 to 77 percent of invasive carcinomas reported in the literature (25,37). The main reason for such a wide range of incidence in different reports is because not all authors recognize or separate the mixed category of invasive carcinomas (i.e., a combination of duct NOS and specific type pattern) (25). A carcinoma is classified as IDC, NOS if the specific subtype comprises less than 10 percent of the total carcinoma and as mixed if the features of the specific type comprise 10 to 90 percent of the total neoplastic proliferation (91). Those who recognize the mixed category claim a better outlook for these patients. This view is arguable since a great difference in survival is unlikely when the special subtypes comprise 10 to 30 percent of the total neoplastic proliferation.

The majority of patients with IDC, NOS are between 50 and 69 years of age; in 6 percent, the tumor manifests before 39 years of age (37). Grade 3 (G3) carcinomas are seen in 65 percent of patients under 39 years of age, and in 38 percent of patients over 70 years (37), a trend seen also among Japanese patients who show a high proportion of androgen receptor (AR)-positive apocrine carcinomas (57).

Gross Findings. About 60 percent of IDC, NOS are discoid in shape (95) and have irregular edges that project into the surrounding fibrofatty tissue (38). The cut surface is depressed, hard, difficult to cut, and pink to gray with frequent yellow streaks of elastosis (fig. 8-1) (4). The rest of the tumors have macroscopically circumscribed borders (fig. 8-2, left), a cut surface that tends to bulge above the surrounding tissues, and a soft consistency with no yellow streaks of elastosis. After fine needle aspiration cytology (FNAC), the cut surface can be hemorrhagic (fig. 8-2, left). The circumscription is never sharp when submicroscopic techniques are employed and thin spicules of invasive tissue are usually seen projecting from the edge of the tumor (fig. 8-2, right).

Microscopic Findings. IDC, NOS lesions are so heterogeneous that no case is similar to the next. The variability from case to case is so great that the histology ranges from well-differentiated carcinomas with bland cytology to highly pleomorphic carcinomas (88). The neoplastic cells grow in sheets, cords, nests, trabeculae, and glands (fig. 8-3). In cases with a macroscopic irregular edge, the neoplastic cells extensively invade the surrounding tissue, including the perineural spaces, which appear invaded in up

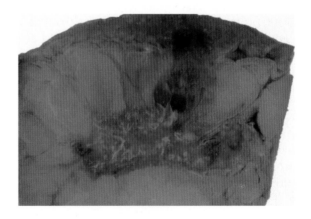

Figure 8-1

INVASIVE DUCT CARCINOMA

Yellow streaks are numerous in this invasive tumor. (Courtesy of Professor J.G. Azzopardi, London, England.)

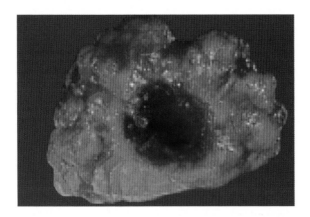 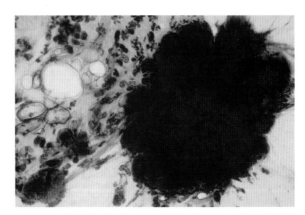

Figure 8-2

INVASIVE DUCT CARCINOMA

Left: The hemorrhagic surface of this circumscribed nodule is the result of a fine needle aspiration biopsy.

Right: Margins of invasive carcinoma that appear well-circumscribed to the naked eye, display thin invasive projections microscopically. (Courtesy of Dr. T. Tot, Falun, Sweden.)

to 27.8 percent of cases (38). The higher the grade, the more frequently the tumors show a central focus of fibrosis (54) surrounded by a cuff of neoplastic cells (fig. 8-3E).

The neoplastic cells react strongly and consistently for cytokeratin (CK)7, CAM5.2, and epithelial membrane antigen (EMA). A very high proportion of cases are positive for "luminal" CK7/8, 18, and 19 (98.3 percent, 88.7 percent, and 92.8 percent, respectively) (1). Virtually all invasive duct carcinomas are positive for E-cadherin (fig. 8-4) (1) and the decrease of immunohistochemical expression of this marker has been regarded as an independent indicator of poor prognosis in node-negative patients (9). S-100 protein is immunoreactive in up to 60 percent of cases while CK20, CK17, and CK14 are negative. When CK17, CK14, and actin (basal markers) appear positive in patches, the tumor is named *myoepithelial-rich invasive duct carcinoma*, which indicates that an ordinary invasive IDC, NOS is intermingled with patches of myoepithelial cell differentiation (18). The percentages of CK14- and smooth muscle actin-positive cells are 14 percent and 13 percent, respectively, in one study (2).

The central fibrotic focus present in some IDC, NOS lesions is characterized by myofibroblasts that are mostly abundant at the periphery. These are smooth muscle actin, calponin, desmin, and myosin heavy chain positive (10,41). In 20 percent of cases, the fibrotic focus contains

CD10-positive spindle cells, which are scattered throughout the fibrotic area or line the neoplastic cellular nests (59). The central fibrotic focus is negative for CD34 (5) and in this respect is different from the stroma of radial scars, which is consistently positive for this marker (80). Myofibroblasts are identified at the ultrastructural level by stress fibers (86), the most prominent ultrastructural finding (fig. 8-5).

Focal and/or diffuse elastosis is present in the central fibrous focus in up to 86 percent of invasive carcinomas (4). Focal elastosis is of two types. Periductal elastosis is mainly visible in the central core of the fibrous focus. It consists of a thick amorphous and/or fibrillar eosinophilic cuff that encircles duct epithelium that can be morphologically normal, hyperplastic, or replaced by carcinoma. To demonstrate elastosis, we routinely use Weigert's method (fig. 8-6) but orcein and specific antibodies to elastin elicit similar information. Vascular elastosis usually affects veins of all sizes, but not arteries. Perivenous elastosis can be so prominent that the lumen of the vessel is reduced to a narrow slit or even disappears, and the presence of remnants of endothelial cells can be proven only by immunohistochemistry for endothelial markers (fig. 8-7).

In most cases, periductal elastosis is more prominent, in other cases, periductal and vascular elastosis are present equally. Occasionally, vascular elastosis dominates (4). In addition to focal elastosis, many cases also show

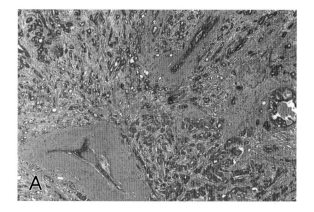

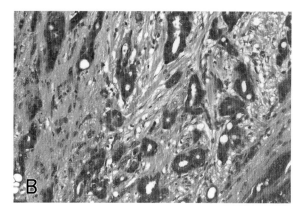

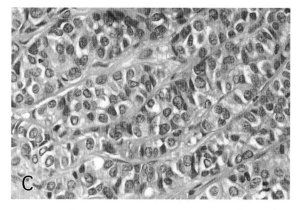

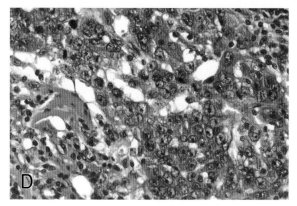

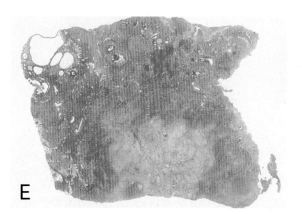

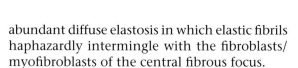

Figure 8-3

INVASIVE DUCT CARCINOMA

A: Invasive duct carcinoma, grade 1, forms glands. There is prominent periductal elastosis.

B: Glandular structures are immersed within cellular stroma.

C: In invasive duct carcinoma grade 2, prominent trabecular structures and solid nests are seen.

D: In invasive duct carcinoma grade 3, sheets of atypical cells have irregular nuclei and prominent nucleoli.

E: A central focus of fibrosis is surrounded by a cuff of neoplastic cells.

abundant diffuse elastosis in which elastic fibrils haphazardly intermingle with the fibroblasts/myofibroblasts of the central fibrous focus.

Studies have shown a positive correlation between the degree of elastosis and estrogen receptors (ER), older age, and tubular carcinoma (69,98). Elastosis is usually absent in mucoid and medullary carcinomas. Breast carcinomas metastatic to the lymph nodes, gastrointestinal tract, and pancreas occasionally show vascular elastosis (fig. 8-7D). Periductal and diffuse elas-

tosis can be seen in benign lesions such as duct ectasia, obliterative mastopathy (19), radial scar (30,50), and sclerosing adenosis (99). Vascular elastosis, on the contrary, is seen only occasionally in benign conditions. The stromal changes useful in differentiating the central fibrous foci of invasive carcinomas and the central fibrous core of radial scar are listed in Table 8-1.

There is general consensus, at least in carcinomas, that elastosis is induced by the neoplastic cells and that the abnormal elastic tissue

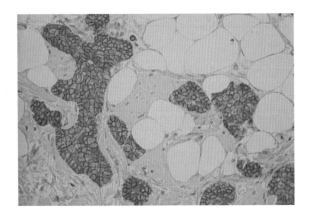

Figure 8-4

INVASIVE DUCT CARCINOMA

Invasive carcinomas of ductal type have E-cadherin-positive cell membranes.

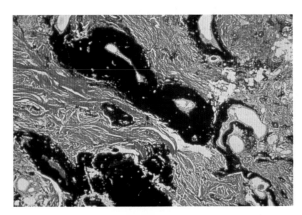

Figure 8-6

PERIDUCTAL ELASTOSIS

Periductal elastosis surrounds non-neoplastic epithelium (Weigert method).

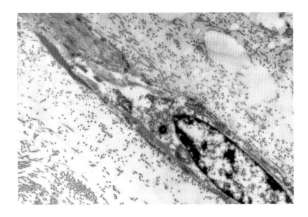

Figure 8-5

ULTRASTRUCTURE OF MYOFIBROBLASTS

An elongated myofibroblast is immersed in collagen fibers.

Table 8-1

STROMAL FEATURES OF INVASIVE DUCTAL CARCINOMA (IDC) NOS AND RADIAL SCAR

	IDC	Radial Scar
Periductal elastosis	+	+
Venous elastosis	+	very rare
Diffuse elastosis	+	+
CD34-positive cells	no	+
CD10-positive cells	20%	rare
Actin-positive cells	+	rare
Calponin-positive cells	rare	no
Myosin-positive cells	+	no

is synthesized by fibroblasts and smooth muscle cells (3). This can be proven by the observation of increased myoid proliferation in the walls of the veins at the ultrastructural level (figs. 8-8, 8-9). In the diffuse type of elastosis, myofibroblasts are immersed within elastotic material (fig. 8-10).

Necrosis is frequent in carcinomas, and was noted in 33 percent of IDC, NOS tumors in a large series (38). When central necrosis and fibrosis are abundant and the viable neoplastic cells show evidence of myoepithelial cell differentiation, there is a high risk of brain and lung metastases and of death from cancer independent of lymph nodal status and tumor size (100). FNAC procedures can also cause massive necrosis, especially in carcinomas with onco-cytic differentiation (15), similar to oncocytic tumors of the thyroid gland.

Calcifications are frequent and were found with the help of the von Kossa stain in about 60 percent of cases by Fisher et al. (38), an incidence that approximated that noted by clinical mammography by the same authors. Calcifications are observed in the stroma or in the neoplastic cells as granular, strongly basophilic precipitates or as laminar psammomatous bodies (3). If calcium is removed, the substance underlying the granular material is composed of nuclear DNA debris derived from necrotic cells. Proteinaceous mucoid material is in the background of the laminar calcifications, which are mostly seen within the lumens of neoplastic glands (40).

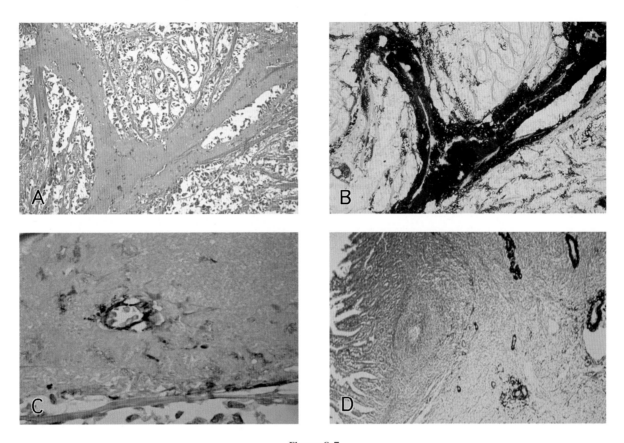

Figure 8-7

PERIVENOUS ELASTOSIS

A: The lumen of the vessel is obliterated.

B: Abundant elastic tissue is visible along the walls of this small vein (Weigert method).

C: Remnants of endothelial elements of this vein stain for CD31.

D: Perivenous elastosis is present in a small intestine metastasis from an invasive lobular carcinoma. (Courtesy of Professor J.G. Azzopardi, London, England.)

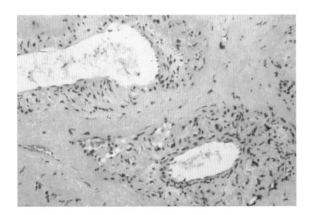

Figure 8-8

PERIVASCULAR ELASTOSIS

A proliferation of myoid cells is evident in the artery and vein walls.

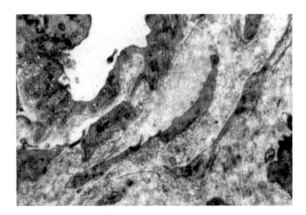

Figure 8-9

PERIVENOUS ELASTOSIS

Perivenous elastosis containing myoid cells.

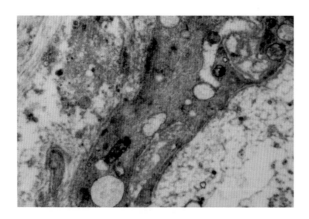

Figure 8-10

DIFFUSE TYPE OF ELASTOSIS

A myofibroblast surrounded by basal lamina is immersed in elastic tissue.

Ductal carcinoma in situ (DCIS) within the invasive carcinoma is a frequent finding and was found in 30 percent of cases in a large series (38). The grade is similar to the grade of the related invasive carcinoma (62), if the DCIS is classified according to Holland et al. (56). When the accompanying DCIS in an invasive carcinoma is extensive and forms at least 25 percent of the tumor, the lesion is termed *infiltrating duct carcinoma with extensive in situ component* and is regarded as a lesion leading to local recurrence in up to 25 percent of cases (55). This is probably because the extensive in situ component extends far beyond the excisional margins (90). Local recurrences are less frequent in cases with negative margins, independent of an extensive in situ component (48). The status of margins is far less important for recurrence if lumpectomy or quadrantectomy is followed by radiotherapy (36,101).

There are rare cases of invasive G3 carcinomas resembling grade 3 DCIS/ductal intraepithelial neoplasia (DIN)3 that are accompanied by the simultaneous presence of lymph node metastases. These cases have been labeled *infiltrating comedocarcinoma* (95) and are characterized by invasive tumors that histologically mimic a grade 3 DCIS/DIN3. In routine practice, the assessment of grade 3 DCIS/DIN3 by immunohistochemistry for the presence of the myoepithelial cell layer and basal lamina confirms the in situ nature of the lesion and minimizes the possible underdiagnosis of invasion (16). In the

premammographic era, these cases were more numerous than today, leading Stewart (95) to state that "comedocarcinoma is invariably infiltrating when its presence is discovered" and Sirtori and Talamazzi (89) to affirm that in situ carcinomas of the breast hardly exist. Taking these comments into account, it is fair to state that grade 3 DCIS/DIN3, especially when extensive, probably has invaded somewhere along its course. Before diagnosing and final sign out of such cases, they need to be carefully worked up, including additional sampling, deeper levels, and immunohistochemical assessment.

Cytologic Findings. FNAC of palpable IDC, NOS requires at least two needle passes to obtain diagnostic material. This minimizes false negative results, especially in sparsely cellular carcinomas.

Positive "obviously malignant" smears are characterized by: a background of necrotic debris and/or hemorrhage; neoplastic cells aggregated in many different configurations that vary from loose sheets with no evidence of polarization, to glandular structures, to nests (fig. 8-11A); poor cellular cohesion with numerous isolated neoplastic elements floating freely in the smear; one cell type only (i.e., carcinomatous cells) present in the smear (fig. 8-11B) since the observation of two cell types characterizes a benign process most of the time; large neoplastic cells with an altered nuclear to cytoplasmic ratio (fig. 8-11C); and nuclear irregularities and prominent nucleoli highlighted by the Papanicolaou stain.

Mitoses are rare. In this respect, the cytologic findings are different from the histologic findings since mitoses are easily found with the latter. The reason for this discrepancy is not clear, but may be because mitoses are blocked suddenly in a cytologic smear preparation where the cells are rapidly killed (90).

Cytologically, IDC, NOS should be distinguished from mucoid, tubular, and endocrine carcinomas, but we feel that a positive smear is often more than enough for a diagnosis. To press for a more specific diagnosis can lead to errors of interpretation.

The benign lesion that most frequently is mistaken for carcinoma is fibroadenoma. This is because the epithelial cells in fibroadenoma display large irregular nuclei with prominent nucleoli. The presence of two cell

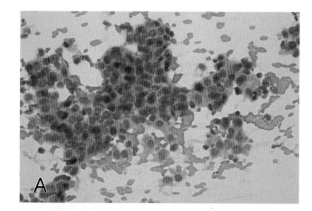

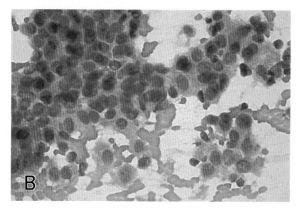

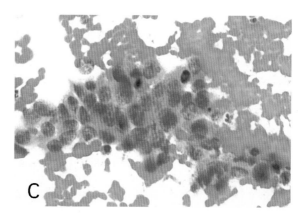

Figure 8-11

CYTOLOGY OF INVASIVE DUCTAL CARCINOMA

A: An irregular sheet of cohesive neoplastic cells is surrounded by isolated neoplastic elements.

B: One type of cell is present. The nuclei are slightly irregular and overlap, and the nuclear to cytoplasmic ratio is altered.

C: Irregular nuclei are immediately visible.

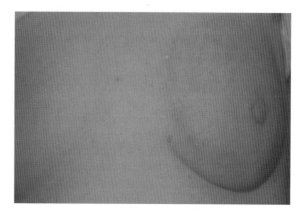

Figure 8-12

INFLAMMATORY CARCINOMA

The left breast is reddened and edematous. The patient noticed inflammatory changes 2 months earlier.

types (epithelial and myoepithelial cells) in fibroadenoma is the most useful criterion to distinguish it from carcinoma, which is composed of only one cell type. Myoepithelial cells are usually smaller than epithelial elements and show round to ovoid nuclei. They are observed around epithelial clumps and when occasionally observed in isolation, for unknown reasons, they are grouped together in pairs (90). In situ duct carcinomas can also display myoepithelial cells around neoplastic clumps. In these cases, the myoepithelial cells are never as numerous as in fibroadenomas.

The neoplastic cells ultrastructurally may show abundant cytoplasmic organelles. Microvilli are seen at the luminal borders or even in the intracytoplasmic lumens.

Treatment and Prognosis. See chapter 2 and Appendix.

INFLAMMATORY CARCINOMA

Definition. *Inflammatory carcinoma* (IC) is the designation of a prognostically ominous form of advanced invasive breast carcinoma, classified as T4d in the TNM classification. It

is characterized in its classic presentation by edema and reddening of the skin of the breast (fig. 8-12) and an underlying G3 IDC, NOS that diffusely permeates blood and lymphatic vessels, including those in subdermal and dermal locations. This type of presentation has been called *primary IC* as opposed to *secondary IC*; the latter is defined as recurrent carcinoma with inflammatory features (84).

Clinical Features. The incidence of IC varies from 1 to 10 percent of breast carcinomas, depending on the diagnostic criteria employed and the nature of the reporting center (general hospital versus referral center) (24,65). The median patient age is 57 years and up to 15 percent of the patients have bilateral involvement (11).

Clinically, there is an increase in the volume of the breast, which becomes tender and painful. Within a few weeks (median, 4 weeks [49]) the skin of the breast becomes warm and shows pink discoloration that soon changes into bright red. The redness initially tends to be prominent in the lower half of the breast, but eventually involves at least one third of the skin of the breast (49). Nipple retraction and crusting occur in 15 percent of patients; a breast nodule is palpable in 35 percent (49). Metastases are present in up to 30 percent of cases at presentation (11).

Skin thickening is usually evident on mammography. In most cases, this is the only evidence of a pathologic condition, together with a diffuse increase in parenchymal density.

Gross Findings. The breast either is diffusely involved or contains a single tumor that may be up to 12 cm in greatest dimension (84).

Microscopic Findings. IC consists of poorly differentiated G3 IDC that diffusely permeates vessels, including those localized in the subdermis and dermis. Lymphatics and small capillaries are dilated and the papillary dermis and reticular dermis are diffusely thickened by edema. A moderate degree of lymphoplasmacytic reaction can be seen within the edematous stroma. Dermal lymphatic invasion has been found in 50 to 80 percent of cases, although the importance of this histologic finding is questionable since outcome is similar in cases diagnosed only by clinical criteria (11).

Occult inflammatory carcinoma refers to cases showing diffuse lymphatic involvement by tumor emboli without evidence of the clinical signs that characterize usual IC. Patients with clinically diagnosed IC (regardless of histologic confirmation) have a disease-free rate at 5 years of 25 percent compared with 51 percent for patients with occult IC (2).

Histogenesis. The term "inflammatory" is a misnomer as no inflammatory changes are seen in IC. The blood vessel dilatation in the dermis and the consequent redness of the skin are not necessarily caused by the neoplastic emboli since these are lacking in some (admittedly a minority) cases. Therefore, vascular dilatation may depend on some paracrine factors produced by the tumor.

Treatment. The best treatment for patients with IC is still a matter of debate, but the general consensus is for adjuvant therapy. Before the introduction of adjuvant therapy, the survival rate of IC patients at 5 years was less than 5 percent; at present, since multimodality therapy was introduced, the survival rate at 5 years ranges from 25 to 45 percent (14).

INVASIVE LOBULAR CARCINOMA

Definition. *Invasive lobular carcinoma* (ILC) is an invasive carcinoma composed of noncohesive, E-cadherin-negative cells showing several architectural patterns. The cells are similar to those of lobular intraepithelial neoplasia (LIN).

Carcinomas that have mixed lobular and ductal NOS components are classified as lobular if the lobular component comprises more than 90 percent of the tumor, as mixed lobular if the ductal NOS component makes up 10 to 90 percent, and as ductal if the lobular component is less than 10 percent (91). Despite the absence of a single criterion that would consistently distinguish ILC from IDC, NOS (3,82), in practice pathologists identify ILC with a high level of consistency (kappa, 0.76) (92).

Clinical Features. Patients with ILC range in age from 26 to 86 years, with a peak around 50 years (96). The reported incidence varies from 0.7 to 14.7 percent of all invasive carcinomas depending on the criteria used (68). In most series, the incidence is about 10 percent of all invasive carcinomas (21), with a steady increase since 1977 in women over 50 years of age, probably because of the increase in estrogen and progestin replacement therapy (66).

Similar to other breast invasive carcinomas, 55 percent of women present with a mass. In about 10 percent of cases, minute nodules are palpable scattered throughout a large portion of the breast. In the remaining patients, a progressive unilateral enlargement and hardening

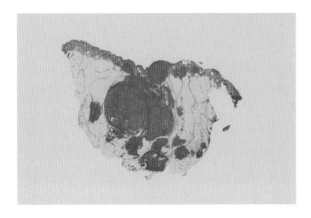

Figure 8-13

INVASIVE LOBULAR CARCINOMA

The pattern of growth is uninodular.

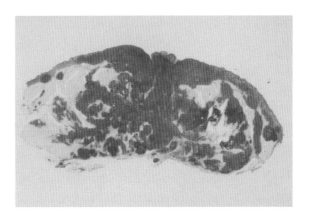

Figure 8-14

INVASIVE LOBULAR CARCINOMA

The pattern of growth is multinodular.

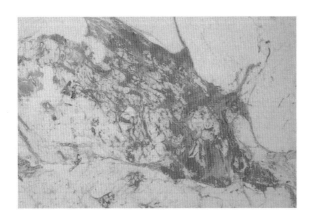

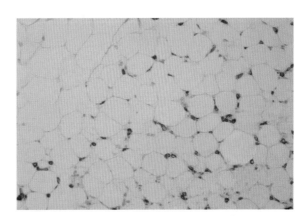

Figure 8-15

INVASIVE LOBULAR CARCINOMA

Left: The pattern of growth is diffuse, resembling a spiderweb. (Courtesy of Dr. T. Tot, Falun, Sweden.)
Right: Isolated cells are present within preexisting adipose tissue. The cells are positive for cytokeratin (CK) 7.

of the breast is the main symptom. The latter cases result in negative mammograms in up to 46 percent of patients who ultimately prove to have ILC (82). This is also one of the reasons for a high incidence (33 percent) of ILC among mammographically undetected interval cancers in breast screening programs (75).

Gross Findings. Macroscopy reflects the clinical signs. A nodule with irregular borders is seen in about 50 percent of cases. Micronodularity, described as multiple grains of sand, is infrequent (82), while in about 30 percent of cases no nodules are seen and the breast appears macroscopically normal, with only subtle thickening of the fibrous parenchyma.

Microscopic Findings. ILC assumes several patterns of growth (97). These are mostly appreciated with the use of macro (large) sections that facilitate the correlation between macroscopy and clinical findings (42). A unifocal mass (fig. 8-13) is present in about 40 percent of cases and ranges in size from 5 to 50 mm, with an average of 15.3 mm (97). Multifocal small nodules (fig. 8-14) are observed in about 10 percent of cases. It is difficult to determine the size of the tumor in multifocal cases and large sections are the best way to obtain an aggregated diameter.

A diffuse permeative pattern of growth, resembling a spiderweb (fig. 8-15, left), is seen in 38 percent of cases (97). Sparse neoplastic cells,

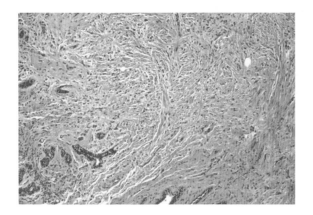

Figure 8-16

INVASIVE LOBULAR CARCINOMA

The stroma is desmoplastic.

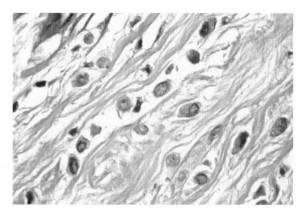

Figure 8-18

INVASIVE LOBULAR CARCINOMA: CLASSIC VARIANT

Neoplastic cells of classic invasive lobular carcinoma show a single file pattern. They appear to be located within an empty space.

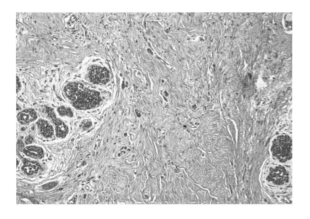

Figure 8-17

INVASIVE LOBULAR CARCINOMA

Sparse neoplastic cells are observed in preexisting stroma.

distributed over a vast area, invade the breast parenchyma and adipose tissue without destroying the preexisting tissue (fig. 8-15, right). These tumors are usually large and range from 11 to 70 mm (average, 37.6 mm).

There are cases with a combination of the above patterns. These cases represented 19 percent of the tumors in one series (97). They ranged in size from 11 to 60 mm, with an average of 30.5 mm.

Along with the different patterns of growth, two types of tumoral stroma are recognizable. In the nodular pattern, the stroma is exuberant, desmoplastic (fig. 8-16), and composed of numerous spindle fibroblasts/myofibroblasts that are smooth muscle actin and CD10 positive. Most of

these cells are negative for CD34. Elastosis of any type can be prominent. In the diffuse pattern of growth, the stroma resembles preexisting breast connective tissue dissected by the neoplastic cells (fig. 8-17). No neoangiogenesis is seen in these cases (63).

Histologic Variants. ILC has several histologic variants (68) that are often intermingled with one another. The predominant pattern (over 80 percent of tumor composition) determines the specific tumor type (21).

The Classic Variant. The classic variant has been recognized for a long time (35,68) and represents 3 percent of all invasive carcinomas (21). A diffuse growth pattern is typical of the classic variant, but occasionally, nodules are formed. The invasive cells are sparse and dissociated, and invade the mammary stroma in a single cell file fashion (fig. 8-18). Neoplastic cells also surround and invade the stroma of residual ducts in a concentric "targetoid" pattern (fig. 8-19). The fibrous septa of the adipose tissue are invaded and the neoplastic cells are frequently seen among adipocytes (fig. 8-20). When in single cell file arrangement, the neoplastic cells dissect the collagen in such a fashion that they seem located within spaces (fig. 8-21). Artifacts of fixation cannot be excluded as a cause of this pattern, but an alternative and plausible explanation is that neoplastic cells spread along the prelymphatic channels of Hartveit (17,53). This is consequent to the lack of cohesion of E-cadherin-negative ILC cells that

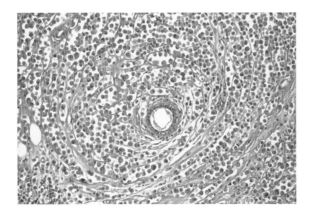 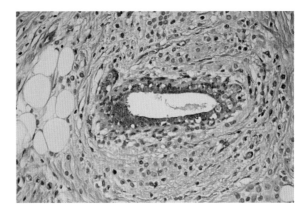

Figure 8-19

INVASIVE LOBULAR CARCINOMA: CLASSIC VARIANT

The neoplastic cells of the classic variant surround and invade the stroma of residual ducts in a concentric "targetoid" fashion.

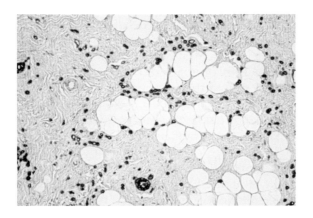 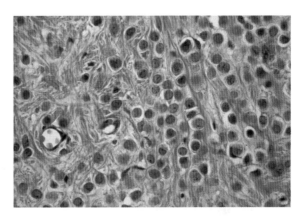

Figure 8-20

INVASIVE LOBULAR CARCINOMA: DIFFUSE GROWTH PATTERN, CLASSIC VARIANT

The tumor invades adipose tissue.

Figure 8-21

INVASIVE LOBULAR CARCINOMA: DIFFUSE GROWTH PATTERN, CLASSIC VARIANT

The cells show a single file type of invasion. They seem to spread along preexisting spaces.

find it "easy" to fall into, and "passively" spread along preexisting channels. This would explain why the noncohesive cells are arranged in single cell files and targetoid patterns as they find their way along thin lymphatic capillaries, similar to the single file lining of red blood cells in capillaries. In these cases the stroma shows very little inflammatory reaction, an indirect indication that it is an "innocent bystander." A similar phenomenon has been noticed in invasive duct carcinoma, NOS, in which the spaces are interpreted as retraction artifact (1b).

The infiltrating neoplastic cells of the classic variant, often referred to as bland or monoto-

nous, have round to ovoid nuclei that are occasionally indented (fig. 8-22). Chromatin is dispersed, the nuclear membrane is smooth, and one to two peripheral small nucleoli are visible. Mitoses and areas of necrosis are uncommon. A rim of cytoplasm is seen around mostly centrally located nuclei. The cytoplasm is pale eosinophilic and, in well-fixed specimens, exhibits intracytoplasmic lumens that have a central eosinophilic dot (fig. 8-23).

Ultrastructural studies have shown that the intracytoplasmic lumens are lined by microvilli (72). Gad and Azzopardi (47) found that the microlumens contain sialomucins. Intracytoplasmic

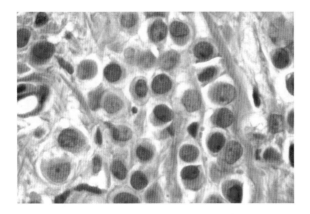

Figure 8-22

INVASIVE LOBULAR CARCINOMA: DIFFUSE GROWTH PATTERN, CLASSIC VARIANT

The cells have round to ovoid monotonous nuclei and small nucleoli. The nuclei are surrounded by a thin rim of cytoplasm.

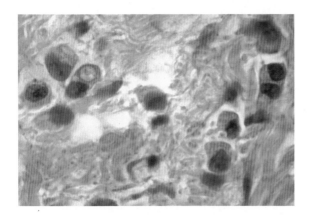

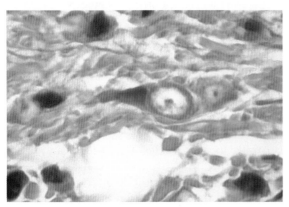

Figure 8-23

INVASIVE LOBULAR CARCINOMA

Intracytoplasmic lumens have a central eosinophilic dot.

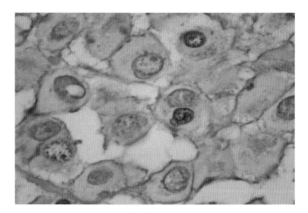

Figure 8-24

INVASIVE LOBULAR CARCINOMA

Intracytoplasmic lumens stain with Alcian blue.

lumens vary from 5 to 75 percent of the tumor. They are highlighted by Alcian blue, which creates a peripheral blue rim with a sharp outer margin. The central core of the globule usually stains faintly or not at all with Alcian blue, but it often shows strong periodic acid–Schiff (PAS) positivity (fig. 8-24) (47). Acidic mucins and EMA deposit along the microvillous surface of the intracytoplasmic lumens (33).

The neoplastic cells of the classic variant stain with luminal CK7 and CK8, the latter giving a perinuclear ring-like positivity (64). Estrogen and progesterone receptors (ER and PR) are positive in most cases, especially with the latest monoclonal antibodies (33,45). ARs are also positive in at least 80 percent of cases (81). C-erbB-2 and epithelial growth factor receptor (EGFR) are absent (78). P53 protein is seen in 3 percent and cathepsin D in 86 percent of cases (23).

FNAC leads to variably cellular smears ranging from those containing rare cells (a source of inadequate smears) to smears with numerous cells. These appear noncohesive. The neoplastic cells are of similar size, have round to indented nuclei, and have a small nucleolus. The cytoplasm is scanty and usually located at one pole of the cell (fig. 8-25). Intracytoplasmic lumens are often evident in a few cells.

The Loose Alveolar Variant. This variant was first identified by Martinez and Azzopardi (68) as loosely grouped neoplastic cells. It represented 1.8 percent of the invasive carcinomas in one series (21). The alveoli are of different sizes and are separated by thin to broad fibrous septa (fig.

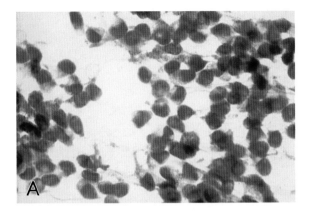

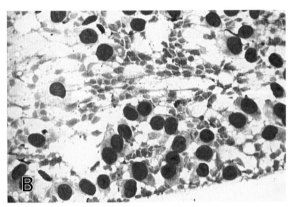

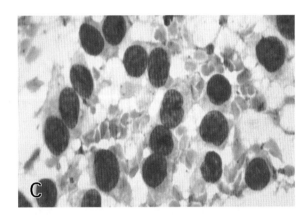

Figure 8-25

INVASIVE LOBULAR CARCINOMA: CLASSIC VARIANT

A: Noncohesive cells have the cytoplasm located at one pole (Papanicolaou stain).

B: Noncohesive cells are isolated and show scanty cytoplasm (B&C, Giemsa stain).

C: At higher magnification, nuclei appear monotonous, and have an altered nuclear to cytoplasmic ratio.

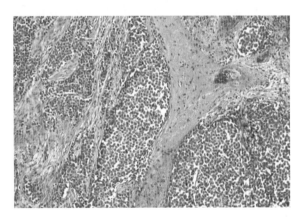

Figure 8-26

INVASIVE LOBULAR CARCINOMA: UNINODULAR PATTERN, LOOSE ALVEOLAR VARIANT

Alveoli are of different sizes, and separated by bands of dense collagen.

8-26). The neoplastic cells, in most cases, float freely within the alveoli and usually appear detached from the fibrous walls (fig. 8-27, left). The neoplastic cells are bland appearing, noncohesive especially on FNAC (fig. 8-27, right), have intracytoplasmic lumens (fig. 8-28), and display all the immunohistochemical changes of the classic variant. No necrotic areas are seen. ERs are positive in virtually all cases (87). This variant tends to evoke a desmoplastic stroma in which osteoclast-like giant cells can be found (77). The alveolar structures can be confluent, so as to simulate, at low-power magnification, a lymphomatous proliferation. The pattern of growth of this variant is mostly nodular.

The alveolar structures may be small, mimicking LIN. In these cases, the presence of myoepithelial cells at the periphery of the nests has to be excluded. The alveolar type ILC is simulated by duct carcinomas invading the fibers of the pectoral muscle.

The Tubulolobular Variant. This variant, described first by Fisher et al. (39), is discussed in chapter 9.

The Mixed Variant. This variant was categorized by Dixon et al. (21) and includes a mixture of the above patterns in which none is predominant. Eight such cases (0.7 percent of all invasive carcinomas) were observed in the series of Dixon et al., who also included in the same category

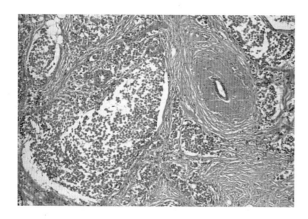
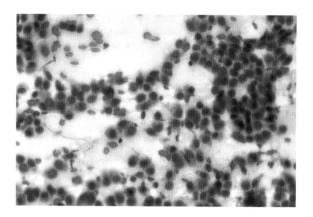

Figure 8-27

INVASIVE LOBULAR CARCINOMA: UNINODULAR PATTERN, LOOSE ALVEOLAR VARIANT

Left: The cells of alveoli appear detached from the fibrous walls and seem to float freely.
Right: Cytology shows noncohesive cells with monotonous nuclei.

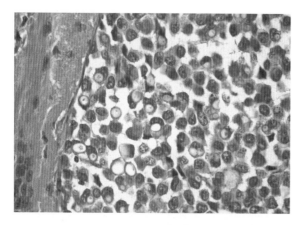

Figure 8-28

INVASIVE LOBULAR CARCINOMA: UNINODULAR PATTERN, LOOSE ALVEOLAR VARIANT

Noncohesive monotonous cells with intracytoplasmic lumens are seen.

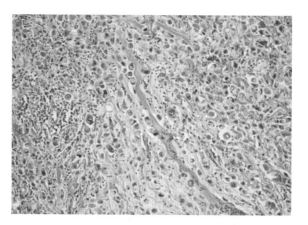

Figure 8-29

INVASIVE LOBULAR CARCINOMA: DIFFUSE PATTERN, WITH PLEOMORPHIC CYTOLOGY (INVASIVE PLEOMORPHIC LOBULAR CARCINOMA)

The cells are sparse and have irregular nuclei.

22 cases of pleomorphic lobular carcinoma, a specific variant that is discussed later.

LIN is associated with the above categories of ILC in 60 percent of cases and well-differentiated DCIS/DIN1 in 1.3 percent (21,40a).

Cytologic Variants. These variants have specific cytologic features. All may manifest within the different histologic variants.

Pleomorphic Variant. This variant represented 2.1 to 4.4 percent of invasive carcinomas in two different series (21,81). It affects female patients ranging in age from 24 to 94 years (mean, 57.5 years) (71). It assumes any pattern of growth.

There is parenchymal streaming of dissociated neoplastic cells in frequent single cell file or targetoid arrangements. The nuclei of these cells are often indented or even multilobated. A single prominent nucleolus is observed in nuclei that have sparse chromatin. Numerous hyperchromatic nuclei are seen in all cases. Mitoses vary from 1 to 3 per high-power field (31). The cytoplasm of the neoplastic cells is abundant, eosinophilic, and faintly granular. The cell shape varies from globoid to polygonal (fig. 8-29). Some cells have peripheral nuclei and resemble rhabdomyoblasts. The latter cases can

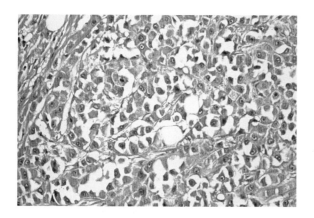
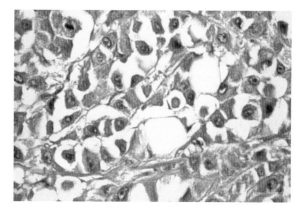

Figure 8-30

INVASIVE LOBULAR CARCINOMA: UNINODULAR PATTERN, LOOSE ALVEOLAR VARIANT WITH PLEOMORPHIC CYTOLOGY

The cells are noncohesive, and have abundant eosinophilic cytoplasm, irregular nuclei, and prominent nucleoli.

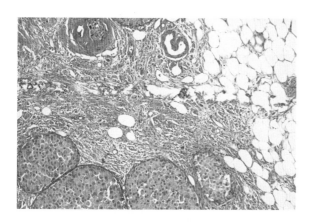
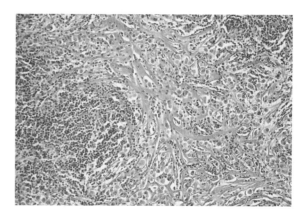

Figure 8-31

INVASIVE LOBULAR CARCINOMA: MULTINODULAR PATTERN, WITH PLEOMORPHIC CYTOLOGY

The in situ component is also formed by pleomorphic cells.

Figure 8-32

INVASIVE LOBULAR CARCINOMA: DIFFUSE PATTERN WITH PLEOMORPHIC CYTOLOGY

A lymphoid stromal reaction is seen.

be a source of confusion with rhabdomyosarcomas, especially when arranged (fortunately very rarely) in an alveolar pattern (fig. 8-30). LCIS is present in 45 to 60 percent of cases (31,71) and may be of the pleomorphic type (fig. 8-31) (46). Lymphoid infiltration is present in 70 percent of cases and occasionally is so intense (fig. 8-32) that the tumor resembles lymphoepithelial-like carcinoma (12).

Most cases are positive with the Alcian blue and PAS stains. They have intracytoplasmic lumens, as in the classic variant. In about 30 percent of cases, Alcian blue condenses at one cellular pole and forms a crescent (fig. 8-33) (31).

Apocrine differentiation, as confirmed by immunohistochemistry and in situ hybridization, is evident in 71 to 82 percent of cases (fig. 8-34) (6,71). Conflicting data exist in the literature concerning the presence of ERs and PRs. Rare cases were positive for ER and PR in one series (6) while 80 percent of cases were positive for ER and 90 percent for PR in another series (81). ARs are positive in 65 percent of cases (81). HER2/neu receptor is present in 53 percent of cases (43) and p53 in 48 percent (71).

Ultrastructurally, the apocrine neoplastic cells show osmiophilic granules and empty vesicles (27). Some cells also have a microvillous surface

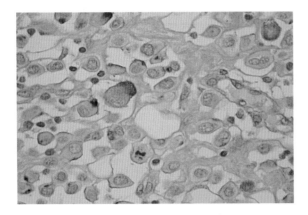

Figure 8-33

**INVASIVE LOBULAR CARCINOMA:
PLEOMORPHIC CYTOLOGY**

Alcianophilic staining is evident at one pole of the cell in a crescent-like fashion.

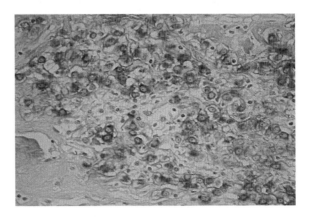

Figure 8-34

**INVASIVE LOBULAR CARCINOMA:
PLEOMORPHIC CYTOLOGY**

Apocrine differentiation is revealed by in situ hybridization for prolactin inducible protein (PIP) mRNA (PIP is synonymous with gross cystic disease fluid protein [GCDFP]-15).

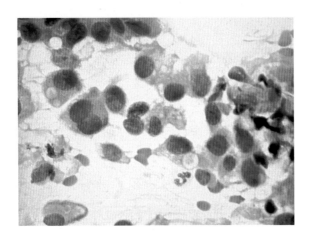

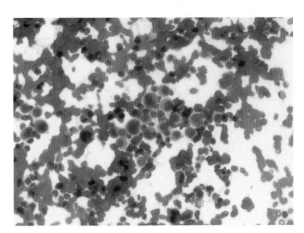

Figure 8-35

FINE NEEDLE ASPIRATION BIOPSY OF INVASIVE LOBULAR CARCINOMA WITH PLEOMORPHIC CYTOLOGY

Left: Nuclei are irregular, cells are multinuclear, and intracytoplasmic lumens are visible.
Right: Cells are of varying sizes.

at one pole of the cell, directly facing the collagen. This is the ultrastructural counterpart of the alcianophilic crescent seen with mucin stains. Noncohesive cells with irregular, often bilobated nuclei are seen by FNAC. Their cytoplasm is abundant, eosinophilic, and granular, and intracytoplasmic lumens are easily seen (fig. 8-35).

Apocrine Cell Variant. Rare cases with the architectural appearance of the classic and alveolar variants show cells with eosinophilic, granular cytoplasm and the immunohisto-

chemical features of apocrine cells. Nuclei are regular, bland, and ovoid, with prominent nucleoli. Mitoses are rare and necrosis is absent. These cases are frequently accompanied by LIN showing apocrine features (27).

Histiocytoid (Myoblastomatoid) Variant. The term histiocytoid carcinoma was coined by Hood et al. (58) to define metastatic mammary carcinomatous cells with foamy clear cytoplasm that resemble histiocytes. These cells are apocrine in nature and correspond to apocrine elements since they

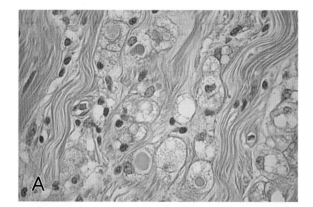

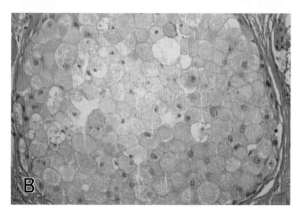

Figure 8-36

INVASIVE LOBULAR CARCINOMA: HISTIOCYTOID VARIANT

A: Foamy (histiocytoid) cytoplasm.

B: Lobular intraepithelial neoplasia (LIN) shows cells with a foamy (histiocytoid) appearance.

C: The foamy cytoplasm is positive for GCDFP-15.

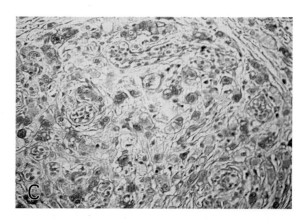

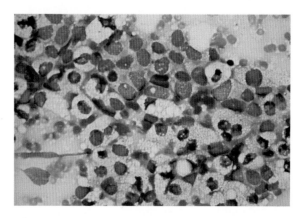

Figure 8-37

INVASIVE LOBULAR CARCINOMA: HISTIOCYTOID VARIANT

Fine needle aspiration shows cells with foamy cytoplasm that can be mistaken for inflammatory elements.

have large clear vesicles that store the secretory material, as seen ultrastructurally (28). Foamy apocrine epithelial cells are "nonspecific" in the sense that they can be seen in any type of apocrine carcinoma of ductal or lobular type (29), as well as in medullary carcinoma (32), and must be distinguished from histiocytes. The apocrine nature can only be ascertained with immunohistochemistry or in situ hybridization (13).

The term "histiocytoid" relates to the foaminess of the cytoplasm (fig. 8-36), which is abundant enough that the neoplastic cells resemble histiocytes; at low-power magnification as well as on FNAC, the tumor can be mistaken for an inflammatory reaction (fig. 8-37). In some cases, these cells display abundant granular eosinophilic cytoplasm and a granular cell tumor (myoblastoma) is mimicked, hence the term "myoblastomatoid carcinoma" (fig. 8-38) (29). Both these features are part of the spectrum of apocrine cell differentiation.

Histiocytoid carcinoma with lobular features was first reported by Walford and Ten Velden (102), who described two cases originally mis-

diagnosed as chronic sclerosing inflammation. Thirteen cases were subsequently reported (29): 2 cases were predominantly myoblastomatoid ILC; 3 were ILC with predominant histiocytoid features; 1 was histiocytoid, similar to an acinic

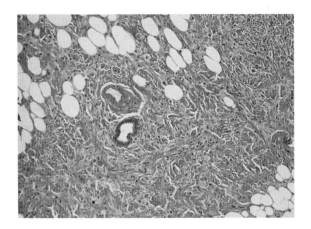
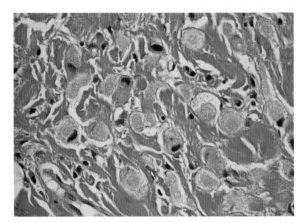

Figure 8-38

INVASIVE LOBULAR CARCINOMA: DIFFUSE PATTERN

The neoplastic cells have eosinophilic, granular (myoblastomatoid) cytoplasm.

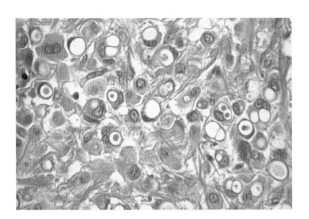
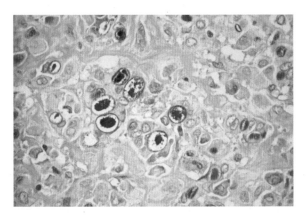

Figure 8-39

INVASIVE LOBULAR CARCINOMA: SIGNET RING CELL VARIANT

Left: The huge intracytoplasmic lumens result in a signet ring appearance.
Right: Alcian blue stains the border of the intracytoplasmic lumens. Periodic acid-Schiff (PAS) is positive in the eosinophilic dot.

cell carcinoma of the parotid gland; and 7 were histiocytoid/myoblastomatoid carcinomas with ductal qualities. These tumor cells had regular to slightly pleomorphic nuclei. They all proved to be apocrine in nature with immunohistochemistry and in situ hybridization.

Signet Ring Cell Variant. While focal signet ring cell differentiation is fairly common in ILC, cases with a predominance of signet ring cells are rare. There are two types of signet ring cells. One type is characterized by cells with nuclei dislodged and compressed to one pole of the cell by a large intracytoplasmic lumen. The mucin content in the intracytoplasmic lumen is very similar to

that seen in ordinary intracytoplasmic lumens (47) and the tumor cells have a similar microvillous structure (94). This type of signet ring cell is predominantly seen in ILC (fig. 8-39) and rarely noted in invasive duct carcinomas (26,79,94).

A second type of signet ring cell contains mucin synthesized and accumulated in the cisternae of the endoplasmic reticulum (52). A hyperchromatic nucleus is located at one pole of the cell. The cytoplasm is amphophilic and stains diffusely with either PAS or Alcian blue. This type of signet ring cell is predominantly seen in ductal carcinomas, but is rare in ILC (fig. 8-40) (52). It has been suggested that the presence

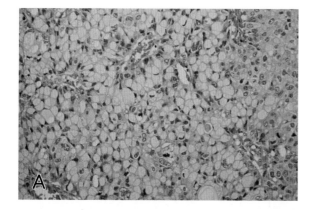

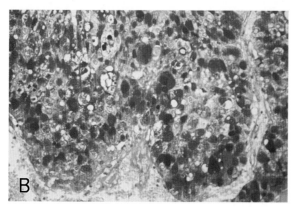

Figure 8-40

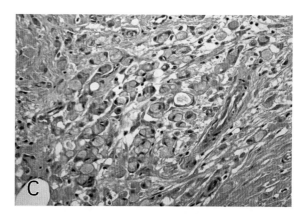

Figure 8-40

**INVASIVE DUCT CARCINOMA:
SIGNET RING CELL VARIANT**

A: Cohesive cells with amphophilic cytoplasm and signet ring features are present.

B: The signet ring cells are highlighted by the PAS stain.

C: Noncohesive signet ring cells in an invasive lobular carcinoma with a diffuse pattern of growth.

of 10 percent or more signet ring cells of both types is a poor prognostic factor for patients with stage 1 ILC (44).

Myoepithelial Cell Variant. This is the rarest variant. One case of single file invasive carcinoma with a diffuse pattern of growth was described by Cartagena et al. (8). The tumor displayed clear (probably glycogen rich) cytoplasm. A second case consisted of an in situ (actin rich/myoepithelial) lobular neoplasia associated with an invasive carcinoma showing a single file pattern. The neoplastic cells had clear cytoplasm that stained intensely for alpha-smooth muscle actin (93). Although this is a distinctive pattern, the cases reported are too limited and the possibility that this variant is a myoepithelial cell carcinoma mimicking ILC cannot be dismissed.

Other Variants. In 1975, six cases with a "confluent arrangement of cells in solid sheets" were considered a special variant of ILC (34). Patients with this variant have a worse survival rate, in both the short- and long-term, than patients with the other architectural variants of ILC (21). These cases are composed of sharply circumscribed

nests of uniform small cells, are sometimes E-cadherin positive (fig. 8-41), and display an endocrine nature (74). We believe that these E-cadherin-positive small cell carcinomas are endocrine carcinomas.

Differential Diagnosis. ILC should be distinguished from invasive duct carcinoma (Table 8-2).

Prognosis. No difference in survival is noted between patients with invasive duct and lobular carcinomas when matched for stage, but probably an advantage in disease-free survival is seen in patients with stage 1 ILC (20). Most of the recurrences occur in the vicinity of the primary tumor (85). The debate over whether ILC should be graded is an open question since most are grade 1 to 2 tumors while pleomorphic ILCs are grade 3. Therefore grade is intrinsic to the definition of the tumor. Pleomorphic (G3) ILCs are aggressive tumors that frequently metastasize to axillary lymph nodes and are lethal in 60 percent of patients (6,31,103). Pereira et al. (76) found that ILCs spanned all three grades. The 10-year survival rate ranged from 80 percent for

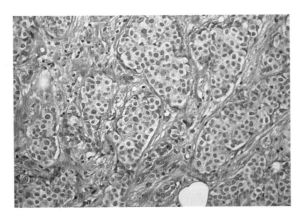 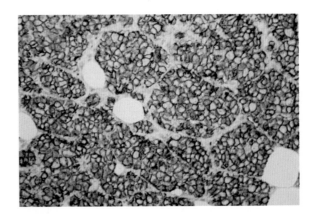

Figure 8-41

CONFLUENT PATTERN

Left: The cells are arranged in confluent solid sheets.
Right: The confluent pattern is an E-cadherin-positive invasive carcinoma showing endocrine differentiation.

Table 8-2

**REASONS TO DIFFERENTIATE INVASIVE LOBULAR CARCINOMA (ILC)
FROM INVASIVE DUCT CARCINOMA (IDC)**

ILC is often an occult carcinoma clinically and radiologically.

A rare familial cancer syndrome caused by a germline mutation in the E-cadherin gene links diffuse type gastric cancer and invasive lobular carcinomas (60). Sporadic ILC involves a somatic mutation in the E-cadherin gene.

ILC differs from IDC because there is no immunohistochemical evidence of E-cadherin.

ILC probably spreads "passively" through the prelymphatic system of Hartveit (53), a finding worthy of further investigation.

Very high positivity for ER, PR, and AR in ILC.[a]

ILC has a different pattern of metastasis than IDC. ILC metastasizes as sparse noncohesive cells, while metastatic IDC shows nests and glandular structures. ILC metastasizes more frequently (significant difference) than IDC to the leptomeninges, ovary, myometrium, stomach, and retroperitoneum (51). The spreading pattern recapitulates the features of the primary tumor making the distinction from a poorly differentiated carcinoma of the stomach very difficult, as both tumors have very similar features (and also might have a similar genetic profile). ER, PR, and AR immunocytochemical positivities favor a diagnosis of ILC of the breast. The identification of metastases in the bone marrow is enhanced by keratin immunohistochemistry as ILC displays cell sizes similar to that of hematopoietic cells, invades as single cells, does not incite tissue reaction, and occasionally, is associated with bone marrow granulomas (7,61,67).

Twenty percent of 103 patients with ILCs had synchronous or metachronous bilateral carcinoma, almost twice the likelihood of developing a contralateral carcinoma in patients with IDC (22), a finding confirmed by most authors (96).

[a]ER = estrogen receptor; PR = progesterone receptor; AR = androgen receptor.

those with G1 tumors to less than 50 percent for those with G3 tumors. The fact that patients with a diffuse growth pattern (i.e., large tumor size), more than three positive axillary lymph nodes, and a pleomorphic cytology (i.e., G3 tumors) have a high cancer-related death rate (97) recapitulates the general prognostic indicators of invasive duct carcinomas.

REFERENCES

1. Abd El-Rehim DM, Pinder SE, Paish EC, et al. Expression of luminal and basal cytokeratins in human breast carcinoma. J Pathol 2004;203:661-671.

1a. Acs G, Dumoff KL, Solin LJ, Pasha T, Xu X, Zhang PJ. Extensive retraction artifact correlates with lymphatic invasion and notal metastasis and predicts poor outcome in early stage breast carcinoma. Am J Surg Pathol 2007;31:129-140.

1b. Acs G, Lawton T, Rebbeck TR, LiVolsi VA, Zhang PJ. Differential expression of E-cadherin in lobular and ductal neoplasms of the breast and its biologic and diagnostic implications. Am J Clin Pathol 2001;115:85-98.

2. Amparo RS, Angel CD, Ana LH. Inflammatory breast carcinoma: pathological or clinical entity? Breast Cancer Res Treat 2000;64:269-273.

3. Azzopardi JG, Ahmed A, Millis RR. Problems in breast pathology. London: WB Saunders; 1979.

4. Azzopardi JG, Laurini RN. Elastosis in breast cancer. Cancer 1974;33:174-183.

5. Barth PJ, Ebrahimsade S, Ramaswamy A, Moll R. CD34+ fibrocytes in invasive ductal carcinoma, ductal carcinoma in situ, and benign breast lesions. Virchows Arch 2002;440:298-303.

6. Bentz JS, Yassa N, Clayton F. Pleomorphic lobular carcinoma of the breast: clinicopathologic features of 12 cases. Mod Pathol 1998;11:814-822.

7. Bitter MA, Fiorito D, Corkill ME, et al. Bone marrow involvement by lobular carcinoma of the breast cannot be identified reliably by routine histological examination alone. Hum Pathol 1994;25:781-788.

8. Cartagena N, Cabello-Inchausti B, Willis I, Poppiti R Jr. Clear cell myoepithelial neoplasm of the breast. Hum Pathol 1988;19:1239-1243.

9. Charpin C, Garcia S, Bonnier P, et al. Reduced E-cadherin immunohistochemical expression in node-negative breast carcinomas correlates with 10-year survival. Am J Clin Pathol 1998;109:431-438.

10. Chiavegato A, Bochaton-Piallat ML, D'Amore E, Sartore S, Gabbiani G. Expression of myosin heavy chain isoforms in mammary epithelial cells and in myofibroblasts from different fibrotic settings during neoplasia. Virchows Arch 1995;426:77-86.

11. Cole J, Kardinal CG. Locally advanced and inflammatory breast cancer. In: Donegan WL, Spratt JS, eds. Cancer of the breast, 5th ed. Philadelphia: Saunders; 2002:579-595.

12. Cristina S, Boldorini R, Brustia F, Monga G. Lymphoepithelioma-like carcinoma of the breast. An unusual pattern of infiltrating lobular cacinoma. Virchows Arch 2000;437:198-202.

13. Damiani S, Cattani MG, Buonamici L, Eusebi V. Mammary foam cells. Characterization by immunohistochemistry and in situ hybridization. Virchows Arch 1998;432:433-440.

14. Damiani S, Eusebi V. Gross and microscopic pathology. In: Donegan WL, Spratt JS, eds. Cancer of the breast, 5th ed. Philadelphia: Saunders; 2002:347-375.

15. Damiani S, Eusebi V, Losi L, D'Adda T, Rosai J. Oncocytic carcinoma (malignant oncocytoma) of the breast. Am J Surg Pathol 1998;22:221-230.

16. Damiani S, Ludvikova M, Tomasic G, Bianchi S, Gown AM, Eusebi V. Myoepithelial cells and basal lamina in poorly differentiated in situ duct carcinoma of the breast. An immunocytochemical study. Virchows Arch 1999;434:227-234.

17. Damiani S, Eusebi V, Peterse JL. Malignant neoplasms infiltrating "pseudoangiomatous" stromal hyperplasia of the breast: an unrecognized pathway of tumor spread. Histopathology 2002;41:208-215.

18. Damiani S, Riccioni L, Pasquinelli G, Eusebi V. Poorly differentiated myoepithelial cell rich carcinoma of the breast. Histopathology 1997;30:542-548.

19. Davies JD. Hyperelastosis, obliteration and fibrous plaques in major ducts of the human breast. J Pathol 1973;110:13-26.

20. DiCostanzo D, Rosen PP, Gareen I, Franklin S, Lesser M. Prognosis in infiltrating lobular carcinoma. An analysis of "classical" and variant tumors. Am J Surg Pathol 1990;14:12-23.

21. Dixon JM, Anderson TJ, Page DL, Lee D, Duffy SW. Infiltrating lobular carcinoma of the breast. Histopathology 1982;6:149-161.

22. Dixon JM, Anderson TJ, Page DL, Lee D, Duffy SW, Stewart HJ. Infiltrating lobular carcinoma of the breast: an evaluation of the incidence and consequence of bilateral disease. Br J Surg 1983;70:513-516.

23. Domagala W, Markiewski M, Kubiak R, Bartkowiak J, Osborn M. Immunohistochemical profile of invasive lobular carcinoma of the breast: predominantly vimentin and p53 protein negative, cathepsin D and estrogen receptor positive. Virchows Arch A Pathol Anat Histopathol 1993;423:497-502.

24. Ellis DL, Teitelbaum SL. Inflammatory carcinoma of the breast. A pathologic definition. Cancer 1974;33:1045-1047.

25. Elston CW, Ellis IO, Goulding H, Pinder SE. Role of pathology in the prognosis and management of breast cancer. In: Elston CW, Ellis IO, eds. The breast, 3rd ed. Edinburg: Churchill Livingstone; 1998:385-433.

26. Eltorky M, Hall JC, Osborne PT, el Zeky F. Signet-ring cell variant of invasive lobular carcinoma of the breast. Arch Pathol Lab Med 1994;118:245-248.

27. Eusebi V, Betts C, Haagensen DE Jr, Gugliotta P, Bussolati G, Azzopardi JG. Apocrine differentiation in lobular carcinoma of the breast: a morphologic, immunologic, and ultrastructural study. Hum Pathol 1984;15:134-140.

28. Eusebi V, Damiani S, Losi L, Millis RR. Apocrine differentiation in breast epithelium. Advances Anat Pathol 1997;4:139-155.

29. Eusebi V, Foschini MP, Bussolati G, Rosen PP. Myoblastomatoid (histiocytoid) carcinoma of the breast. A type of apocrine carcinoma. Am J Clin Pathol 1995;19:553-562.

30. Eusebi V, Grassigli A, Grosso F. [Breast scleroelastotic focal lesions simulating infiltrating carcinoma.] Pathologica 1976;68:507-518. [Italian.]

31. Eusebi V, Magalhaes F, Azzopardi JG. Pleomorphic lobular carcinoma of the breast: an aggressive tumor showing apocrine differentiation. Hum Pathol 1992;23:655-662.

32. Eusebi V, Millis RR, Cattani MG, Bussolati G, Azzopardi JG. Apocrine carcinoma of the breast. A morphologic and immunocytochemical study. Am J Pathol 1986;123:532-541.

33. Eusebi V, Pich A, Macchiorlatti E, Bussolati G. Morpho-functional differentiation in lobular carcinoma of the breast. Histopathology 1977;1:301-314.

34. Fechner RE. Histologic variants of infiltrating lobular carcinoma of the breast. Hum Pathol 1975;6:373-378.

35. Fechner RE. Infiltrating lobular carcinoma without lobular carcinoma in situ. Cancer 1972;29:1539-1545.

36. Fisher B, Anderson S, Bryant J, et al. Twenty-year follow-up of a randomized trial comparing total mastectomy, lumpectomy, and lumpectomy plus irradiation for the treatment of invasive breast cancer. N Engl J Med 2002;347:1233-1241.

37. Fisher CJ, Egan MK, Smith P, Wicks K, Millis RR, Fentiman IS. Histopathology of breast cancer in relation to age. Br J Cancer 1997;75:593-596.

38. Fisher ER, Gregorio RM, Fisher B, Redmond C, Vellios F, Sommers SC. The pathology of invasive breast cancer. A syllabus derived from findings of the National Surgical Adjuvant Breast Project (Protocol No. 4). Cancer 1975;36:1-85.

39. Fisher ER, Gregorio RM, Redmond C, Fisher B. Tubulolobular invasive breast cancer: a variant of lobular invasive cancer. Hum Pathol 1977;8:679-683.

40. Foschini MP, Fornelli A, Peterse JL, Mignani S, Eusebi V. Microcalcifications in ductal carcinoma in situ of the breast: histochemical and immunohistochemical study. Hum Pathol 1996;27:178-183.

40a. Foschini MP, Righi A, Cucchi MC, et al. The impact of large sections and 3D technique on the study of lobular in situ and invasive carcinoma of the breast. Virchows Arch 2006;448:256-261.

41. Foschini MP, Scarpellini F, Gown AM, Eusebi V. Differential expression of myoepithelial markers in salivary, sweat and mammary glands. Int J Surg Pathol 2000;8:29-37.

42. Foschini MP, Tot T, Eusebi V. Large-section (macrosection) histologic slides. In: Silverstein MJ, ed. Ductal carcinoma in situ of the breast, 2nd ed. Philadelphia: Lippincott Williams & Wilkins; 2002:249-254.

43. Frolik D, Caduff R, Varga Z. Pleomorphic lobular carcinoma of the breast: its cell kinetics, expression of oncogenes and tumour suppressor genes compared with invasive ductal carcinomas and classical infiltrating lobular carcinomas. Histopathology 2001;39:503-513.

44. Frost AR, Terahata S, Siegel RS, et al. The significance of signet ring cells in infiltrating lobular carcinoma of the breast. Arch Pathol Lab Med 1995;119:64-68.

45. Frost AR, Terahata S, Yeh IT, Siegel RS, Overmoyer B, Silverberg SG. An analysis of prognostic features in infiltrating lobular carcinoma of the breast. Mod Pathol 1995;8:830-836.

46. Frost AR, Tsangaris TN, Silverberg SG. Pleomorphic lobular carcinoma in situ. Pathology Case Reviews 1996;1:27-31.

47. Gad A, Azzopardi JG. Lobular carcinoma of the breast: a special variant of mucin-secreting carcinoma. J Clin Path 1975;28:711-716.

48. Gage I, Schnitt SJ, Nixon A. Pathologic margin involvement and the risk of recurrence in patients treated with breast-conserving therapy. Cancer 1996;78:1921-1928.

49. Haagensen CD. Diseases of the breast, 3rd ed. Philadelphia: W.B. Saunders; 1986.

50. Hamperl H. [Radial scars and obliterating mastopathy.] Virchows Arch A Pathol Anat Histopathol 1975;369:55-68. [German.]

51. Harris M, Howell A, Chrissohou M, Swindell RI, Hudson M, Sellwood RA. A comparison of the metastatic pattern of infiltrating lobular carcinoma and infiltrating duct carcinoma of the breast. Br J Cancer 1984;50:23-30.

52. Harris M, Wells S, Vasudev KS. Primary signet ring cell carcinoma of the breast. Histopathology 1978;2:171-176.

53. Hartveit E. Attenuated cells in breast stroma: the missing lymphatic system of the breast. Histopathology 1990;16:533-543.

54. Hasebe T, Tsuda H, Hirohashi S, et al. Fibrotic focus in invasive ductal carcinoma: an indicator of high tumor aggressiveness. Jpn J Canc Res 1996;87:385-394.

55. Hetelekidis S, Collins L, Silver B, et al. Predictors of local recurrence following excision alone for ductal carcinoma in situ. Cancer 1999;85:427-431.

56. Holland R, Peterse JL, Millis RR, et al. Ductal carcinoma in situ: a proposal for a new classification. Semin Diagn Pathol 1994;11:167-180.

57. Honma N, Sakamoto G, Akiyama F, et al. Breast carcinoma in women over age of 85: distinct histological pattern and androgen, oestrogen and progesterone receptor status. Histopathology 2003;42:120-127.

58. Hood CI, Font RL, Zimmerman LE. Metastatic mammary carcinoma in the eyelid with histiocytoid appearance. Cancer 1973;31:793-800.

59. Iwaya K, Ogawa H, Izumi M, Kuroda M, Mukai K. Stromal expression of CD10 in invasive breast carcinoma: a new predictor of clinical outcome. Virchows Arch 2002;440:589-593.

60. Keller G, Vogelsang H, Becker I, et al. Diffuse type gastric and lobular breast carcinoma in a familial gastric cancer patient with an E-cadherin germline mutation. Am J Pathol 1999;155:337-342.

61. Kettle P, Allen DC. Bone marrow granulomas in infiltrating lobular breast cancer. J Clin Path 1997;50:166-168.

62. Lampejo OT, Barnes DM, Smith P, Millis RR. Evaluation of infiltrating ductal carcinomas with a DCIS component: correlation of the histologic type of the in situ component with grade of the infiltrating component. Semin Diagn Pathol 1994;11:215-222.

63. Lee AH, Happerfield LC, Bobrow LG, Millis RR. Angiogenesis and inflammation in invasive carcinoma of the breast. J Clin Pathol 1997;50:669-673.

64. Lehr HA, Folpe A, Yaziji H, Kommoss F, Gown AM. Cytokeratin 8 immunostaining pattern and E-cadherin expression distinguish lobular from ductal breast carcinoma. Am J Clin Pathol 2000;114:190-196.

65. Levine PH, Steinhorn SC, Ries LG, Aron JL. Inflammatory breast cancer: the experience of the surveillance, epidemiology, and end results (SEER) program. J Natl Cancer Inst 1985;74:291-297.

66. Li CI, Anderson BO, Porter P, Holt SK, Daling JR, Moe RE. Changing incidence rate of invasive lobular breast carcinoma among older women. Cancer 2000;88:2561-2569.

67. Lyda MH, Tetef M, Carter NH, Ikle D, Weiss LM, Arber DA. Keratin immunohistochemistry detects clinically significant metastases in bone marrow biopsy specimens in women with lobular breast carcinoma. Am J Surg Pathol 2000;24:1593-1599.

68. Martinez V, Azzopardi JG. Invasive lobular carcinoma of the breast: incidence and variants. Histopathology 1979;3:467-488.

69. Masters JR, Millis RR, King RJ, Rubens RD. Elastosis and response to endocrine therapy in human breast cancer. Br J Cancer 1979;39:536-539.

70. McDivitt RW, Stewart FW, Berg JW. Tumors of the breast. Armed Forces Institute of Pathology: Washington; 1968.

71. Middleton LP, Palacios DM, Bryant BR, Krebs P, Otis CN, Merino MJ. Pleomorphic lobular carcinoma: morphology, immunohistochemistry, and molecular analysis. Am J Surg Pathol 2000;24:1650-1656.

72. Ozzello L. Ultrastructure of the human mammary gland. Path Annu 1971;6:1-59.

73. Page DL, Anderson TJ. Diagnostic histopathology of the breast. Edinburgh: Churchill Livingstone; 1987.

74. Papotti M, Macrì L, Finzi G, Capella C, Eusebi V, Bussolati G. Neuroendocrine differentiation in carcinomas of the breast: a study of 51 cases. Semin Diagn Pathol 1989;6:174-188.

75. Peeters PH, Verbeek AL, Straatman H, et al. Evaluation of overdiagnosis of breast cancer in screening with mammography: results of the Nijmegen programme. Int J Epidemiol 1989;18:295-299.

76. Pereira H, Pinder SE, Sibbering DM, et al. Pathological prognostic factors in breast cancer. IV: Should you be a typer or a grader? A comparative study of two histological prognostic features in operable breast carcinoma. Histopathology 1995;27:219-226.

77. Pettinato G, Manivel JC, Picone A, Petrella G, Insabato L. Alveolar variant of infiltrating lobular carcinoma of the breast with stromal osteoclast-like giant cells. Pathol Res Pract 1989;185:388-394.

78. Porter PL, Garcia R, Moe R, Corwin DJ, Gown AM. C-erbB-2 oncogene protein in in situ and invasive lobular breast neoplasia. Cancer 1991;68:331-334.

79. Raju U, Ma CK, Shaw A. Signet ring variant of lobular carcinoma of the breast: a clinicopathologic and immunohistochemical study. Mod Pathol 1993;6:516-520.

80. Ramaswamy A, Moll R, Barth PJ. CD34+ fibrocytes in tubular carcinomas and radial scars of the breast. Virchows Arch 2003;443:536-540.

81. Riva C, Dainese E, Caprara G, et al. Immunohistochemical study of androgen receptors in breast carcinoma. Evidence of their frequent expression in lobular carcinoma. Virchows Arch 2005;447:695-700.

82. Rosen PP. Invasive lobular carcinoma. In: Rosen PP, ed. Rosen's breast pathology, 2nd ed. Philadelphia: Lippincott Williams & Wilkins; 2001:627-652.

83. Rosen PP. Rosen's breast pathology, 2nd ed. Philadelphia: Lippincott Williams & Wilkins; 2001.

84. Rosen PP, Oberman HA. Tumors of the mammary gland. AFIP Atlas of Tumor Pathology, 3rd Series, Fascicle 7. Washington, DC: American Registry of Pathology; 1993.

85. Schnitt SJ, Connolly JL, Recht A, Silver B, Harris JR. Influence of infiltrating lobular histology on local tumor control in breast cancer patients treated with conservative surgery and radiotherapy. Cancer 1989;64:448-454.

86. Schurch W, Seemayer TA, Gabbiani G. The myofibroblast: a quarter century after discovery. Am J Surg Pathol 1998;22:141-147.

87. Shousha S, Backhous CM, Alaghband-Zadeh J, Burn I. Alveolar variant of invasive lobular carcinoma of the breast. Am J Clin Pathol 1986;85:1-5.

88. Silver SA, Tavassoli FA. Pleomorphic carcinoma of the breast: clinicopathological analysis of 26 cases of an unusual high-grade phenotype of ductal carcinoma. Histopathology 2000;36:505-514.

89. Sirtori C, Talamazzi F. [The intraductal carcinoma of the breast is never a carcinoma in situ.] Tumori 1967;53:641-644. [Italian.]

90. Sloane JP, Trott PA, LaKhani SM. Biopsy pathology of the breast, 2nd ed. London: Oxford Univ Press; 2001.

91. Sloane JP. Infiltrating carcinoma-pathological types. In: Sloane JP, ed. Biopsy pathology of the breast. London: Arnold; 2001:170-214.

92. Sloane JP, Amendoeira I, Apostolikas N, et al. Consistency achieved by 23 European pathologists from 12 countries in diagnosing breast disease and reporting prognostic features of carcinomas. Virchows Arch 1999;434:3-10.

93. Soares J, Tomasic G, Bucciarelli E, Eusebi V. Intralobular growth of myoepithelial cell carcinoma of the breast. Virchows Arch 1994;425:205-210.

94. Steinbrecher JS, Silverberg SG. Signet-ring cell carcinoma of the breast. The mucinous variant of infiltrating lobular carcinoma? Cancer 1976;37:828-840.

95. Stewart FW. Tumors of the breast. Washington, DC: AFIP; 1950.

96. Tavassoli FA. Pathology of the breast, 2nd ed. Stanford: Appleton-Lange; 1999.

97. Tot T. The diffuse type of invasive lobular carcinoma of the breast: morphology and prognosis. Virchows Arch 2003;443:718-724.

98. Tremblay G. Elastosis in tubular carcinoma of the breast. Arch Pathol 1974;98:302-307.

99. Tremblay G, Buell RH, Seemayer TA. Elastosis in benign sclerosing ductal proliferation of the female breast. Am J Surg Pathol 1977;1:155-159.

100. Tsuda H, Takarabe T, Hasegawa F, Fukutomi T, Hirohashi S. Large, central acellular zones indicating myoepithelial tumor differentiation in high-grade invasive ductal carcinomas as markers of predisposition to lung and brain metastases. Am J Surg Pathol 2000;24:197-202.

101. Veronesi U, Cascinelli N, Mariani L, et al. Twenty-year follow-up a randomized study comparing breast-conserving surgery with radical mastectomy for early breast cancer. N Engl J Med 2002;347:1227-1232.

102. Walford N, ten Velden J. Histiocytoid breast carcinoma: an apocrine variant of lobular carcinoma. Histopathology 1989;14:515-522.

103. Weidner N, Semple JP. Pleomorphic variant of invasive lobular carcinoma of the breast. Hum Pathol 1992;23:1167-1171.

9 CARCINOMAS OF LOW-GRADE MALIGNANCY

TUBULAR CARCINOMA

Definition. *Tubular carcinoma* (TC) is a low-grade (grade 1) invasive carcinoma composed of glands with open lumens that are lined by a single layer of monotonous cells (tubules). The tubules are of the same caliber throughout the tumor.

There is lack of consensus on the proportion of tubules required to establish the diagnosis of TC. There are studies in which no specific cut-off point is given (13,69), while others consider pure TC only those tumors composed 100 percent of tubules (26,35,149,154). Several authors (14,59,92,100) regard pure TC as those lesions with tubule formation of over 75 percent of the total neoplastic proliferation and mixed TC as those cases with the number of tubules below this figure. A proportion of tubules of 90 percent was the cut-off point adopted by Ellis et al. (40) for pure TC, who stated that their choice was a pragmatic one since it is unrealistic to expect 100 percent purity in a given tumor; tumors with a lesser proportion of tubules are placed in the mixed tubular category. The disparity over the cut-off point is relevant since, in general, the more tubules present in a tumor, the better the prognosis (111). A cut-off point of 90 percent is probably the best option since, as will be commented on later, patients with this proportion of tubules and a small lesion survive as long as the general population (37,103). A combined carcinoma requires that the second component comprise at least 10 percent of the tumor.

A noticeable exception to the 90 percent rule is the TC intermingled with invasive cribriform carcinoma. In this case, it is not as important to be strict on the proportion of tubularity since patients with cribriform carcinoma (described later) have the same prognostic outlook as those with TC (102).

Clinical Features. The incidence of TC varies from 0.8 to 8.0 percent of all breast cancers (13,37), depending on the criteria for tubularity adopted. The frequency of TC is much higher in patients screened mammographically (8 to19 percent) (106,113), and especially in patients with T1 cancer. Mammographically, TC is easily identified as small stellate areas, although it is often indistinguishable from radial scar (162).

Clinically, there are no specific manifestations. In most patients, a palpable lump is located at the periphery of the breast. It is present in the upper outer quadrant in 75 percent of patients (26), although it can originate in the lactiferous ducts just below the nipple (43).

TC is rarely seen in the male breast (152). The age of most female patients ranges from 23 to 79 years (153), with an average of 45 years in most series (159). Multicentric involvement in the ipsilateral breast is seen in 56 percent of patients, a history of bilateral mammary carcinoma is present in 38 percent, and a family history of mammary cancer in a first-degree relative is seen in 40 percent (81).

Gross Findings. The size of TC ranges from 0.2 to 5.0 cm (35,159), with an average of 1.3 cm (43). The majority are 1 cm or less, especially in those cases identified by mammography.

The lesions appear stellate; retraction of the surrounding tissue accentuates the radiating arms. The cut surface is gray-white and flecked with frequent elastotic yellow streaks (fig. 9-1). In about 30 percent of cases, there is an ill-defined area, which is seen as sclerotic stroma microscopically.

Microscopic Findings. TC has irregular margins that radiate, sometimes penetrating the adjacent adipose tissue (fig. 9-2). The neoplastic elements are arranged as glandular monolayered structures (tubules) with open lumens. The glands are usually of the same caliber but the size and shape of their lumens vary according to the plane of sectioning. The lumens appear round to ovoid, with their long axes at variable angles, rather than arranged parallel to one another. Most of the tubules display pointed ends (fig. 9-3).

The lumens frequently contain eosinophilic material. Alcian blue–positive intraluminal material was seen in 86 percent of a series of

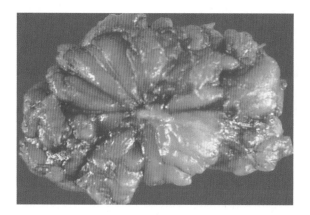

Figure 9-1

TUBULAR CARCINOMA

Small radiating tubular carcinoma (TC) with elastotic yellow streaks.

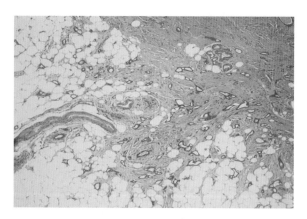

Figure 9-2

TUBULAR CARCINOMA

TC with irregular margins penetrates the adipose tissue.

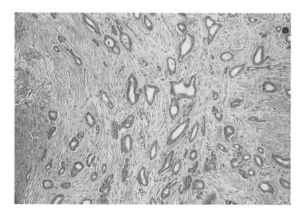

Figure 9-3

TUBULAR CARCINOMA

The size and shape of the glandular lumens of TC vary according to the plane of sectioning. Some tubules show pointed ends.

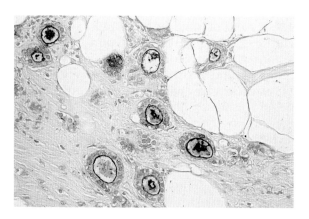

Figure 9-4

TUBULAR CARCINOMA

The lumens are filled by substances stainable with epithelial membrane antigen (EMA), which is also visible along the glycocalyx of tubules.

TCs (43). The quantity of mucosubstances present inside the lumens varies from case to case, from scanty at one extreme to abundant at the other. When the tubular lumens appear devoid of mucin, a thin rim of Alcian blue–positive material is seen coating the glycocalyx of the majority of the neoplastic tubules. Identical features are seen with epithelial membrane antigen (EMA) antibodies (fig. 9-4) (45). Occasional cases display cells with intracytoplasmic lumens containing Alcian blue– and periodic acid-Schiff (PAS)–positive mucosubstances in a target-like fashion, identical to that described by Gad and Azzopardi (57) in lobular carcinomas.

The glands are mostly formed by a single layer of cuboidal to columnar cells (tubules) with round to ovoid nuclei and small nucleoli. When ovoid, the long axis of the nucleus is oriented circumferentially. Mitoses are uncommon. The cytoplasm is eosinophilic and shows an irregular luminal surface in about 50 percent of cases and prominent cytoplasmic apical "snouts" in the rest of the cases (fig. 9-5). The neoplastic cells stain for cytokeratin (CK)7 and E-cadherin (fig. 9-6). They are negative for S-100 protein. Rarely, TC shows histologic, immunohistochemical, and molecular evidence of apocrine differentiation (fig. 9-7).

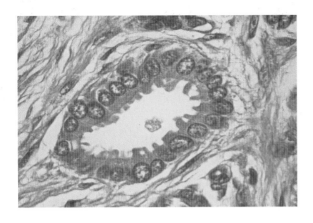

Figure 9-5

TUBULAR CARCINOMA

Prominent apical "snouts."

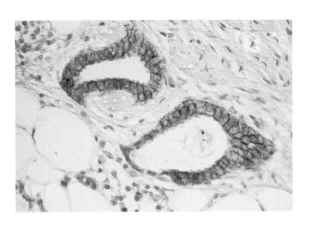

Figure 9-6

TUBULAR CARCINOMA

The cells of the tubules are outlined by E-cadherin.

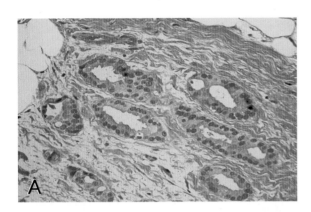

Figure 9-7

TUBULAR CARCINOMA

Apocrine TC (A) stains strongly for gross cystic disease fluid protein (GCDFP)-15 (B) and appears positive for prolactin inducible protein (PIP) mRNA (C).

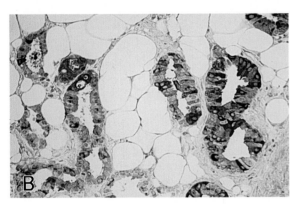

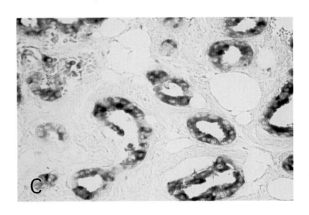

A basal lamina around the tubules is lacking, as confirmed by PAS negativity (53) and the lack of immunostaining for collagen IV and laminin (38,45). There is no evidence of basal lamina at the ultrastructural level (fig. 9-8) (42,43).

Myoepithelial cells are not present around the glands. This has been demonstrated by the lack of staining with antismooth muscle actin (fig. 9-9) (45), CK14, and calponin antisera. The lack of myoepithelial cells is also evident at the ultrastructural level (42,43).

The stroma is composed of plump fibroblasts immersed in Alcian blue–positive material (at pH 0.5) in about 70 percent of cases. In the

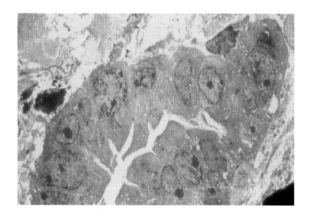

Figure 9-8

TUBULAR CARCINOMA

Ultrastructurally, the neoplastic tubules have a pointed microvillous surface and lack basal lamina. (Fig. 9 from Eusebi V, Betts CM, Bussolati G. Tubular carcinoma: a variant of secretory breast carcinoma. Histopathology 1979;3:415.)

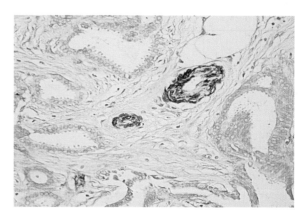

Figure 9-9

TUBULAR CARCINOMA

Myoepithelial cells are lacking in neoplastic tubules. Only the vascular walls are stained (smooth muscle actin).

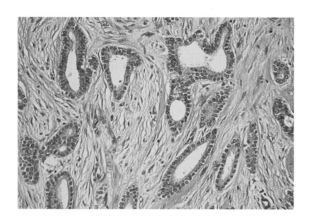

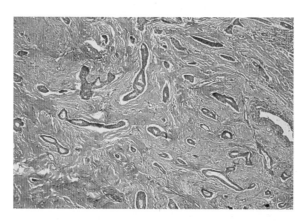

Figure 9-10

TUBULAR CARCINOMA

The stroma of TC is either desmoplastic (left) or sclerohyaline (right).

rest of the cases, the stroma is sclerohyaline (fig. 9-10).

Vascular, periductal, and stromal elastoses were observed in 60 percent of the cases in one series (43). The elastotic tissue stains strongly with Congo red, is digested by elastase, stains with orcein and the Verhoeff method, and ultrastructurally shows fibers consistent with elastic tissue (157). The elastotic tissue is irregularly scattered throughout the tumor and has no specific zone of distribution (fig. 9-11).

Calcifications are seen in up to 50 percent of the cases (149). These are present in the stroma or within the lumens, and are of laminar type (psammoma bodies). This type of calcification in breast is seen when calcium precipitates on acidic mucosubstances (54). Stromal lymphocytes are not part of the picture.

Ductal carcinoma in situ (DCIS)/ductal intraepithelial neoplasia (DIN) is present in about 65 percent of the cases (35). DCIS is of grade 1 (DIN1) and varies from flat epithelial atypia (50 percent of the cases) to micropapillary and cribriform (50). The in situ carcinoma component, in occasional cases, is very prominent, with the invasive neoplastic tubules constituting the

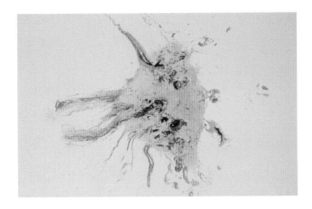

Figure 9-11

TUBULAR CARCINOMA

Vascular, periductal, and stromal elastoses are irregularly scattered throughout the tumor area (Verhoeff method).

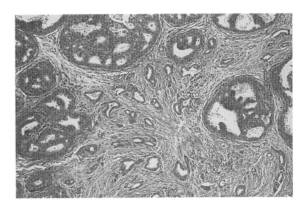

Figure 9-12

TUBULAR CARCINOMA

This is the only focus of TC in an extensive grade 1 ductal carcinoma in situ (DCIS)/ductal intraepithelial neoplasia (DIN1).

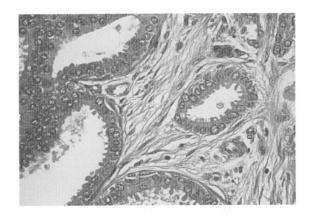

Figure 9-13

TUBULAR CARCINOMA

The cells composing the grade 1 DCIS/DIN1 and TC are identical.

minority of the total lesion, hidden among the neoplastic in situ glands (fig. 9-12). The cells that constitute the invasive neoplastic tubules are identical to the neoplastic elements that compose the in situ neoplasm (fig. 9-13). This indicates a common cell of origin, although no transition from the in situ lesion is demonstrable. Lobular intraepithelial neoplasia (LIN) is observed in up to 30 percent of the cases, sometimes in combination with the intraductal carcinoma (43).

Cytologically, cords, nests, and open glands constituted by one type of monotonous cell with round regular nuclei are seen in fine needle aspiration cytology (FNAC) specimens (fig. 9-14A-C). No myoepithelial cells are visible around these structures; rare isolated elements are evident in the smear. Intracytoplasmic lumens are readily seen (fig. 9-14D). The distinction from a benign scleroelastotic lesion (radial scar) can be difficult and the presence of myoepithelial cells around small cell nests supports the correct diagnosis. Usually, TC leads to abundant cytologic material, while scleroelastotic benign lesions often result in inadequate material.

TC is estrogen receptor (ER) and progesterone receptor (PR) positive, it has low Ki-67 nuclear labeling, and c-erbB-2 and epidermal growth factor receptor (EGFR) are negative (37). Few genetic alterations are present when compared with usual breast carcinomas. The chromosomal alterations seen in other types of carcinoma are not present in TC. This has led to TC be-

ing considered a genetically distinct group of carcinomas (91,165).

Histogenesis. Lobular carcinoma and TC are found in the same or opposite breast in about 30 percent of the cases (43), have a similarly high incidence of bilateral involvement, share similar histochemical and immunohistochemical properties, and at the ultrastructural level are constituted by neoplastic cells with an almost constant villous absorptive surface. These facts, combined with the tubulolobular carcinomas described by Fisher et al. (52) as having histologic and histochemical features of both invasive lobular carcinoma and TC (see below), have led some authors (43) to suggest

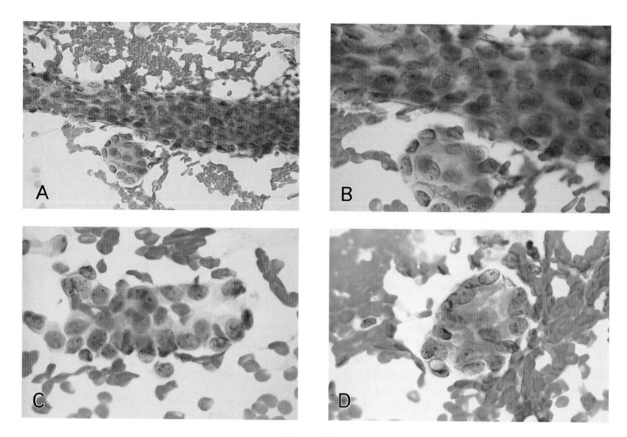

Figure 9-14

TUBULAR CARCINOMA

In a fine needle aspiration cytology (FNAC) specimen, TC shows cords, nests, and open glands of cohesive monotonous cells (A-C). An intracytoplasmic lumen is visible in D.

that TC is not a form of ductal carcinoma but a specialized E-cadherin–positive form of lobular carcinoma. This point is also addressed below in the description of tubulolobular carcinoma.

Linell (85) believes that TC arises in radial scars. This is not likely in the radial scars as originally defined by Hamperl (61). No evidence of supervening carcinoma is seen in patients with radial scars after long-term follow-up (2) and there is no evidence of an association between radial scars and carcinoma (96). Rare radial scars show intraepithelial and/or invasive well-differentiated carcinomas. This does not render radial scar a precancerous lesion since fibroadenoma or even normal breast can undergo cancerization.

It also has been suggested that TC is the earliest form of breast carcinoma, which then gives rise to other types of carcinoma (86). This view is suggested by observations that patients

with TC are younger than those with ordinary carcinoma and that mixed carcinomas are larger than pure TC. In the mixed form of TC, tubules are occasionally present in the center of the lesion. These observations may be the result of coincidence. In clinical practice, some cases of incompletely removed pure TC have recurred several times as such (43); this is an argument that contradicts the assumption that TC transforms into more aggressive forms in all cases.

Differential Diagnosis. The three conditions that most closely simulate TC are microglandular adenosis (20,123), low-grade adenosquamous (syringoid) carcinoma (161), and benign scleroelastotic lesions (radial scars) (46,61).

As depicted in Table 9-1, microglandular adenosis, in contrast to TC, shows small round glands invested by thin basal lamina. The glands are irregularly dispersed in a fibrofatty stroma. The cells that line the tubules are cuboidal with

Table 9-1

DIFFERENTIATING TUBULAR CARCINOMA (TC), MICROGLANDULAR ADENOSIS (MGA), AND LOW-GRADE ADENOSQUAMOUS CARCINOMA (LGA)

	TC	MGA	LGA
Architecture	Random	Random	Random
Glandular size	Small/medium	Small	Small/medium
Two cell types/myo-epithelial cells	No	No	Yes
Basal lamina	No	Yes	Yes
Desmoplastic stroma	Yes	No	Yes
Stromal lymphocytes	No	No	Yes
Elastosis	Yes	No	No
EMA[a]	Yes	No	+/−
Squamous cells	No	No	Yes
CIS	Frequent	No	No

[a]EMA = epithelial membrane antigen; CIS = in situ carcinoma.

Table 9-2

DIFFERENTIATING TUBULAR CARCINOMA (TC) AND RADIAL SCAR (RS)

	TC	RS
Zoning phenomenon	No	Yes
Glandular structures	Angulated	Entrapped
Myoepithelial cells	No	Yes
Luminal "snouts"	Yes	No
Basal lamina	No	Yes
Desmoplastic stroma	Frequent	No
Perivascular elastosis	Frequent	No
Periductal elastosis	Occasional	Constant
CIS[a]	Frequent	Rare
Epithelial hyperplasia	Occasional	Frequent

[a]CIS = in situ carcinoma.

clear cytoplasm and no luminal apical snouts. EMA and PR are negative (45), while S-100 protein is often positive (150).

Low-grade adenosquamous carcinoma also has angulated glands, but two layers of cells are easily seen (161). The outer layer is often actin rich (myoepithelial cells) (56) and the luminal elements show squamoid differentiation. In addition, frequent clumps of mature lymphocytes are seen in the stroma. A well-formed basal lamina is present.

Radial scars of the type first described by Hamperl (61) and Eusebi et al. (46) consist of a central core of fibroelastotic tissue surrounded at the periphery by hyperplastic epithelium (zoning phenomenon). The scleroelastotic central core is formed by obliterated ducts (33) where entrapped glands can be seen. These glands are present within the sclerotic ductal plaques and are encircled by myoepithelial cells. A basal lamina is also visible around them (Table 9-2).

Treatment and Prognosis. Patients with TC have an extremely good prognostic outlook, especially when compared with ordinary invasive carcinomas. The prognosis is influenced by tumor size, histology (pure versus mixed), and type of therapy.

A size of less than 10 mm is crucial for ascertaining an excellent prognosis. None of the 16 patients with tumors of 10 mm or less had nodal metastases compared with 5 of 15 patients presenting with larger tumors (103). In addition, no cases mammographically detected in another series had lymph node metastasis (81).

In one study, axillary lymph node metastases developed in 29 percent of patients with mixed TC, but in only 6 percent of patients with the pure type (above 90 percent tubularity) (35). Metaanalysis of 680 women with TC showed nodal metastases in 6 percent with pure TC compared with 25 percent with mixed TC (103). When the tubularity is less than 75 percent of the total neoplastic area, visceral metastases can be seen (111). If lymph node metastases occur, they appear in a maximum of three nodes. Often, the neoplastic metastatic tubules are either located within the capsule or in the lymph node parenchyma, and histologically, the features of the original tumor are repeated.

When small size is combined with pure histologic type, the survival of patients is similar to that of the general population (37). These cases are prognostically parallel to minute papillary carcinomas of the thyroid gland.

Incomplete excision leads to recurrence in 50 percent of the cases (35). Residual carcinoma was present in mastectomy specimens in 28 percent of patients with pure carcinoma and in 40 percent with mixed carcinoma. In a series of patients with T1N0 TC, treated with modified or radical mastectomy and followed for a median of 18 years, no recurrences were seen (126).

Simple mastectomy is considered appropriate due to the high incidence of multifocality in TC. A consensus is growing on sparing axillary lymph node dissection in women with small (less than 10 mm axis) TC (37,70,103,111) and in avoiding systemic adjuvant therapy (37).

TUBULOLOBULAR CARCINOMA

Definition. *Tubulolobular carcinoma* (TLC) is an invasive carcinoma that combines the features of classic invasive lobular carcinoma and TC (52).

Clinical Features. TLC comprised 1.4 percent of invasive mammary cancers in one series and was more frequent in patients 54 years of age or older (52). TLCs are smaller than ordinary invasive ductal carcinomas, but are the same size as TCs (59). They can be multifocal (29

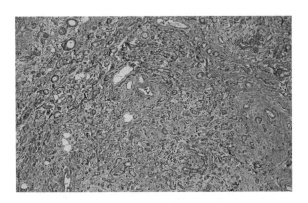

Figure 9-15

TUBULOLOBULAR CARCINOMA

Tubules intermingle with cells growing in a single file pattern.

percent of the cases); lymph node metastases are present in 60 percent of multifocal cases and in 33 percent of nonmultifocal cases.

Pathologic Findings. Histologically, tubular structures and features of invasive lobular carcinoma of single file type are seen together (fig. 9-15). The tubules are smaller and less angulated than in TC (144). Their nuclei are more often grade 2, as is the histologic grade. TLC contains more abundant mucin than invasive lobular carcinoma of ordinary type. The mucin is of acidic quality. E-cadherin outlines, as expected, the cytoplasm of the cells composing the tubules (79), but at variance with classic invasive lobular carcinomas, it is also evident along the cytoplasmic membranes of the cells showing the single cell pattern of invasion of lobular carcinoma (fig. 9-16). The stroma varies from loose to sclerotic, and perivenous and periductal elastosis are more frequent than in invasive lobular and ductal carcinomas of ordinary type. Ductal and lobular well-differentiated in situ carcinomas are present in 23 percent of the cases (52).

Treatment and Prognosis. Treatment failure is greater in patients with TLC than TC (17.4 versus 0 percent), while it is slightly better in those with TLC than with ordinary invasive lobular carcinoma (17.4 versus 25.4 percent). Whether this type of carcinoma is lobular or ductal in origin is a question that cannot be answered at present. These cases are probably the bridge that links invasive carcinomas showing acinar differentiation, where the mutation of the E-cadherin gene has not yet occurred (170).

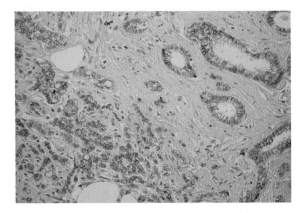

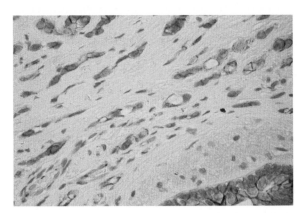

Figure 9-16

TUBULOLOBULAR CARCINOMA

All neoplastic cells are positive for E-cadherin, including the single file component.

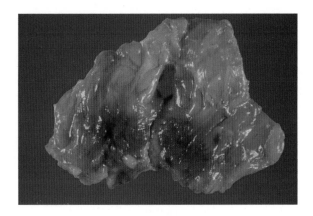

Figure 9-17

INVASIVE CRIBRIFORM CARCINOMA

Invasive "brown" cribriform carcinoma. (Courtesy of Dr. R. Holland, Nijmegen, the Netherlands.)

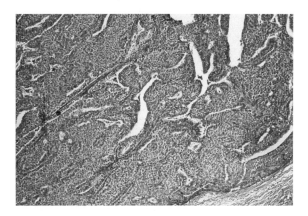

Figure 9-18

INVASIVE CRIBRIFORM CARCINOMA

Invasive cribriform carcinoma with pushing margins.

INVASIVE CRIBRIFORM CARCINOMA

Definition. *Invasive cribriform carcinoma* (ICC) is a low-grade (grade 1) invasive carcinoma nearly totally composed of a cribriform pattern of growth, similar to that seen with DCIS/DIN1.

The cribriform pattern (from Latin, cribrum, meaning sieve) is the most characteristic feature of these tumors. Carcinomatous nests or sheets of cohesive cells are perforated by small apertures, like a sieve.

The term was first introduced by Azzopardi (6), but the entity was fully delineated by Page et al. (102), who stated that the biologic behavior of ICC was strikingly similar to that of TC. These authors also questioned whether ICC and TC were indeed separate histologic types of breast carcinoma. There is no general consensus on the proportion of cribriform areas required to establish the diagnosis of ICC.

Classic (pure) ICC is defined as those cases in which the totality of the tumor proliferation is constituted by cribriform areas (102,163). The cut-off point of the cribriform proportion proposed by Elston and Ellis (41) is 90 percent; cases with less than 90 percent are designated as *mixed ICC*. Venable et al. (163) considered as mixed ICC those cases showing any proportion of infiltrating cribriform carcinoma intermingled with any other type of invasive carcinoma. Page et al. (102), on the contrary, included in the mixed group only those tumors "where more than 50 percent of the invasive component showed a cribriform pattern but areas of less well-differentiated invasive carcinoma were present." They therefore excluded from the mixed group those cases in which a TC was intermingled with an ICC. According to Page et al., when a TC is combined with an ICC, the case is considered pure TC if the tubularity is greater than 50 percent of the total neoplastic proliferation and pure (classic) ICC if the tubularity is lower than this.

Clinical Features. The incidence of ICC ranges from 0.8 to 3.6 percent of all breast carcinomas depending on the selection of patients: whether symptomatic or diagnosed via mammography. The average age of the 35 patients with classic (pure) ICC reported by Page et al. (102) was 53 years (range, 33 to 86 years), significantly younger than patients with the mixed type of ICC (average, 62 years; range, 39 to 85 years). In this study, the tumor was multifocal in 20 percent of cases and a contralateral carcinoma was present in 11 percent, one of which was TC.

Gross Findings. The tumors range from stellate to well circumscribed. Some are dark brown as a consequence of hemosiderin deposit in the stroma (*Holland brown tumor*) (fig. 9-17) (63).

Microscopic Findings. Microscopically, the cribriform invasive areas are very similar to those seen in grade 1 cribriform DCIS/DIN1, paralleling TCs that are architecturally and cytologically similar to the flat "clinging" grade 1 DCIS/DIN1 lesions often associated with the tumor.

The cribriform areas are large, with blunt, pushing margins (fig. 9-18) or are angulated. Numerous

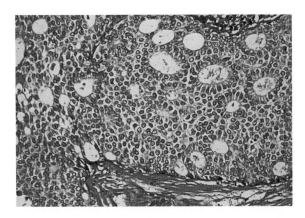

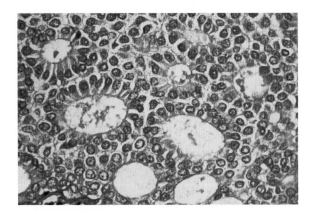

Figure 9-19

INVASIVE CRIBRIFORM CARCINOMA

The lumens are round and often of the same caliber, and the neoplastic cells are similar to one another (one type of cell).

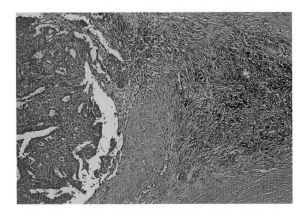

Figure 9-20

INVASIVE CRIBRIFORM CARCINOMA

Abundant hemosiderin accumulation is present in the absence of a previous FNAC.

lumens are present within carcinomatous nests or sheets, although solid areas are common. The lumens are mostly of the same caliber, round, and evenly spaced (fig. 9-19, left). The neoplastic cells are of one type throughout the lesion and have round to ovoid nuclei (nuclear grade 1 to 2) (fig. 9-19, right) (102). The cells are usually cuboidal but often their cytoplasm is columnar and oriented toward the center of the lumen (polarization).

Most of the neoplastic cells stain for CK7, while CK14 is absent. Mitoses are rare and the Ki-67 labeling index is very low. Most of the neoplastic cells are positive for ER, and in one study, 69 percent of cases were PR positive (163). C-erbB-2 is distinctly negative. Myoepithelial cells are absent

and, therefore, no actin-positive elements are seen. Alcianophilic mucosubstances are seen within the lumens.

The stroma is rich in fibroblasts or sclerotic, as in TC, and, in occasional cases, abundant hemosiderin accumulation is present (fig. 9-20). In some cases, stromal and intraluminal osteoclast-like giant cells are seen (63). Elastosis is not a feature of ICC.

In 80.0 percent of pure and in 62.5 percent of mixed ICCs, grade 1 DCIS/DIN1 is seen (102). Four of the six cases reported by Holland et al. (63) were associated with LIN, of which three also had an associated DCIS of well-differentiated flat (clinging) type (DIN1).

Ultrastructurally, only one type of cell is seen and no myoepithelial elements are present (63). The luminal spaces are lined by microvilli similar to those seen in the lumens of the glandular structures composing TC.

Differential Diagnosis. It is not easy to distinguish classic ICC, especially those cases showing blunt, pushing, large islands of growth from a purely cribriform grade 1 DCIS/DIN1. The entire lesion should be examined to distinguish the basal lamina and myoepithelial cells that are absent in ICC but remain as a residue in DCIS/DIN1.

Adenoid cystic carcinoma (ACC) is the lesion that most closely simulates ICC. In the recent past, the two terms (ACC and ICC) were used interchangeably (101). ICCs have distinctive features that allow a confident diagnosis. In particular, the one cell type, coupled with one type of space, the epithelial mucin content, and the presence of ERs are prominent features of ICC, which also lacks myoepithelial cells. The opposite is seen in ACC (see below).

Treatment and Prognosis. ICC is similar to TC in terms of prognosis and treatment. No patient with pure (classic) ICC has died of the disease (102,163). In one series, five patients (14 percent) presented with lymph node metastasis, but no more than three lymph nodes were involved (102,163). The cribriform structure was retained in the metastasis (102). Patients with mixed ICC, in contrast, have a higher incidence of axillary lymph node metastases (25 percent). Of 16 patients with mixed ICC, 2 had distant metastases at presentation; 37 percent died of disease in a period that averaged 12.5 years (102).

For the same reasons elaborated for TC, we feel that the best treatment is simple mastectomy for patients with pure ICC. These patients can be spared axillary lymph node dissection and adjuvant chemotherapy, at least as the first treatment option.

ADENOID CYSTIC CARCINOMA

Definition. *Adenoid cystic carcinoma* (ACC) is an epimyoepithelial carcinoma of low malignant potential that is histologically similar to the salivary gland counterpart. Other terms for this tumor are *carcinoma adenoides cysticum, adenocystic basal cell carcinoma,* and *cylindromatous carcinoma.*

Clinical Features. Although the first cases of ACC reported in the breast are attributed to Geschickter (58), the first accurate description is found in the first series of the Armed Forces Institute of Pathology (AFIP) Fascicle by Dr. F.W. Stewart (147), who noted the remarkable similarities between breast and salivary gland tumors. Stringent criteria should be adopted to avoid misclassifying lesions, as occurs in about 50 percent of the cases recorded by the Connecticut Tumor Registry (148). The literature published before 1979 was reviewed by Azzopardi (6) who accepted an incidence of 0.1 percent for these tumors. An identical incidence was reported by Lamovec et al. in 1989 (83), who found 6 examples of ACC among 5,994 consecutive cases of breast cancer.

Most of the cases arise in females, but occasional cases have been described in male patients (112). The age distribution ranges from 38 to 81 years, similar to that seen for ordinary breast

carcinomas, but anecdotal cases are reported outside this age range. ACC is equally distributed between the two breasts and in about 50 percent of patients, ACC is found in a subperiareolar region (6). The lesions may be painful or tender, and unexpectedly cystic. A discrete nodule is the most common presentation.

Gross Findings. Tumors vary from 0.7 to 12.0 cm, with an average of 3.0 cm. The lesions are circumscribed in most cases. Occasionally, pink, tan, or gray microcysts are evident (125).

Microscopic Findings. ACCs of the breast are similar to those of salivary glands, lung, and cervix (111a). Three basic patterns are seen: cribriform, trabecular-tubular, and solid (fig. 9-21). These patterns have been used by Ro et al. (119) to develop their grading system.

There are two types of "apertures" (spaces), mostly seen with the cribriform pattern. The first type, also referred to as pseudolumens (73), is the result of intratumoral invaginations of the stroma. This type of space is of variable shape, mostly round, and contains myxoid acidic stromal mucosubstances (fig. 9-22) that stain with Alcian blue (8) or straps of collagen with small capillaries (stromal spaces). In some cases, the stromal spaces are filled with hyaline collagen (fig. 9-22, bottom). Especially in the smallest spaces, the content is constituted by small spherules or cylinders of hyaline material. This material has been shown ultrastructurally and immunohistochemically to be basal lamina (16). A rim of laminin- and collagen IV-positive material outlines the spaces (fig. 9-23).

The second type of space is more difficult to see since it is less numerous and usually composed of small lumens. These spaces are genuine secretory glandular structures (glandular spaces) that contain eosinophilic granular secretion of neutral mucosubstances; they are positive for PAS after diastase digestion and for EMA (fig. 9-24) (8).

The dual structural pattern also reflects a dual cytologic cell component. One type of cell has scanty cytoplasm, a round to ovoid nucleus, and one to two nucleoli. This type of cell, referred to as a basaloid cell (83), comprises the bulk of the lesion and is also found lining the cribriform stromal spaces. The second type of cell lines true glandular lumens, is cuboidal to spindle shaped, and has eosinophilic cytoplasm and round nuclei similar to those of the basaloid cells. The

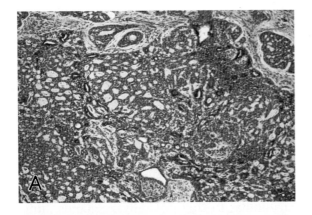

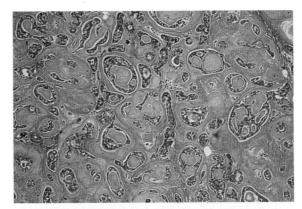

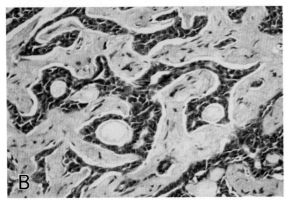

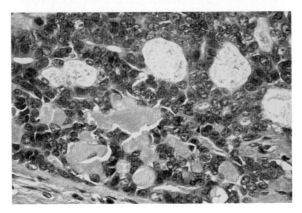

Figure 9-22

ADENOID CYSTIC CARCINOMA

Top: Stromal spaces may contain alcianophilic stromal type mucosubstances.

Bottom: The stromal spaces are filled by hyaline collagen.

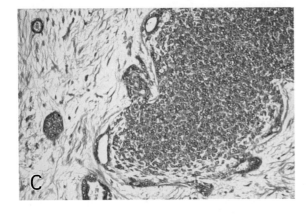

Figure 9-21

ADENOID CYSTIC CARCINOMA

A: Cribriform pattern.

B: Trabecular tubular pattern.

C: Solid pattern in which most of the cells are of one type.

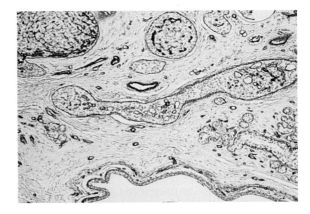

Figure 9-23

ADENOID CYSTIC CARCINOMA

The stromal spaces are outlined by collagen IV.

two cell types are different ultrastructurally and immunohistochemically as well.

Ultrastructurally, the basaloid cells have myoepithelial features, especially when located at

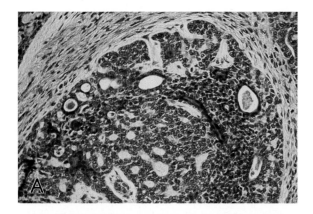

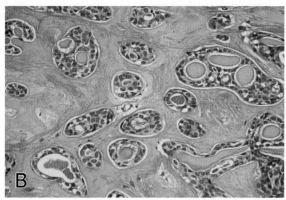

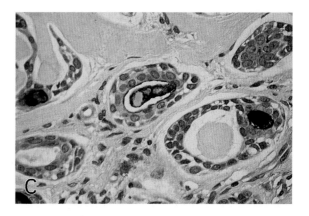

Figure 9-24

ADENOID CYSTIC CARCINOMA

The glandular spaces contain eosinophilic material (A) that is periodic acid–Schiff (PAS) positive after diastase digestion (B). The stroma is alcianophilic. EMA decorates secretory lumens (C).

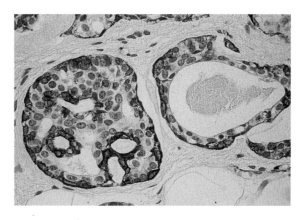

Figure 9-25

ADENOID CYSTIC CARCINOMA

Basaloid cells are positive for cytokeratin (CK) 14.

the interstitial surface that lines the pseudoglandular spaces (171). They have thin cytoplasmic filaments with points of focal condensation (169). These cells are positive for actin and myosin (4), and similar to salivary ACC, are positive for smooth muscle actin, calponin (111a), and CK14. Nevertheless, most basaloid cells are nondescript elements that ultrastructurally have filaments and organelles without specific features (77,151). This is also reflected at the immunohistochemical level: smooth muscle actin is often negative but the elements are vimentin (15) and CK14 positive (fig. 9-25).

The cells that line the glandular lumens are cuboidal to spindle shaped. When cuboidal, they have blunt microvilli along the luminal margins (secretory type). When spindle shaped, they show abundant tonofilaments together with blunt microvilli, meriting the designation of adenosquamous cell (151). The secretory type of cell is CK7 positive (fig. 9-26), while the adenosquamous cell is both CK7 and CK14 positive (111a). These cells can manifest squamous metaplasia, as seen in two of the cases reported by Lamovec et al. (83). Squamous metaplasia is relatively common in breast ACC, but is almost never seen in salivary gland ACC.

A third type of cell was seen in 14 percent of cases by Tavassoli and Norris (151). It is composed of sebaceous elements that in occasional cases can be numerous (fig. 9-27).

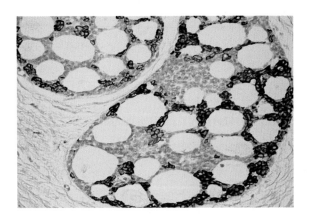

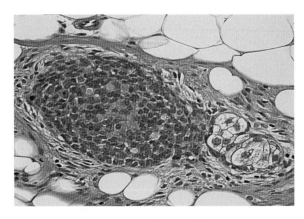

Figure 9-26

ADENOID CYSTIC CARCINOMA

Luminal cells are positive for CK7.

Figure 9-27

ADENOID CYSTIC CARCINOMA

Typical sebaceous cells are seen.

Figure 9-28

ADENOID CYSTIC CARCINOMA

In FNAC specimens, tubule-like structures of dissociated cells (A) and cylinders or globules of fibrillar interstitial material (B,C) are characteristic of adenoid cystic carcinoma (ACC). (Courtesy of Dr. J. Lamovec, Ljubljana, Slovenia.)

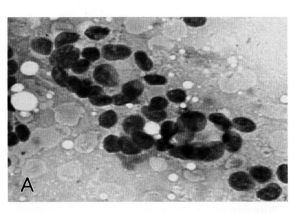

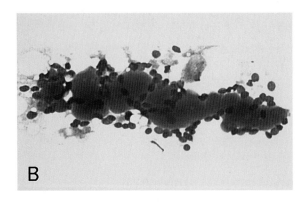

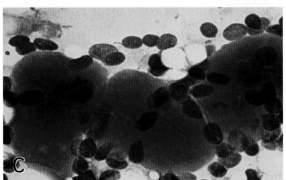

With occasional exceptions, ACC of the breast is devoid of ER, PR, and related proteins (119,158). Over 50 percent of the cases are c-kit positive while C-erbB-2 is consistently negative.

FNAC usually yields abundant material in which uniform, round to oval cells with regular nuclei are seen. Chromatin is finely granular and small nucleoli are evident. Sheets, small aggre-gates, or tubule-like structures are intermingled with dissociated cells. The Giemsa stain shows pink to red homogeneous or fibrillar globules, cylinders, or straps of interstitial material. These are surrounded by cells in a fashion reminiscent of stromal spaces (fig. 9-28). All these features have been regarded as characteristic of ACC in cytology smears (83).

ACC is generally composed of a central core of neoplastic cells, surrounded by areas of invasion, but a peripheral area of "ordinary" DCIS/DIN is not seen. The tumoral stroma varies from tissue similar to that seen in normal breast to desmoplastic, myxoid, or even extensive adipose tissue.

ACC has been seen in association with adenomyoepithelioma (160) and low-grade syringoid (adenosquamous) carcinoma (125), which suggests the existence of a close relationship among these epimyoepithelial tumors; these tumors probably all represent part of the same spectrum.

Differential Diagnosis. ACC has to be distinguished from collagenous spherulosis, a benign condition (21). In collagenous spherulosis, the collagenous spherules are encaseated within epithelial hyperplasia of usual type and rarely lobular neoplasia (138), the spaces are irregular and mostly located at the periphery of the glands, and no mucin is observed within lumens.

Cribriform carcinoma is the lesion that more closely simulates ACC (Table 9-3). Nevertheless, cribriform carcinoma is composed of a proliferation of one type of neoplastic cell only, and there are not two types of mucosubstances as seen in ACC. Also, ERs and PRs are abundant in cribriform carcinomas and absent in virtually all cases of ACC (158).

Treatment and Prognosis. ACC is a low-grade malignant tumor and is generally cured by simple mastectomy. Like its analogue in the salivary gland, breast ACC rarely spreads via the lymphatic system. Two cases only of metastasis to axillary lymph nodes have been reported (119,169). The cases that recur locally are the result of incomplete excision, although patients have been reported to survive even 16 years after the excision of the recurrence (110). The metastatic rate is about 10 percent, the lungs are frequently involved, and metastases can manifest in unexpected sites such as the kidney (24). Therefore, at present, no lymph node excision is indicated in ACC.

MUCINOUS CARCINOMA

Definition. *Mucinous carcinoma* (MC) is an invasive duct carcinoma of low malignant potential, characterized by neoplastic cells floating within extracellular mucins. Synonyms include

Table 9-3

DIFFERENTIATING INVASIVE CRIBRIFORM CARCINOMA (ICC) AND ADENOID CYSTIC CARCINOMA (ACC)

	ICC	ACC
Two types of spaces	No	Yes
Two cell types	No	Yes
Two types of mucin	No	Yes
Myoepithelial cells	No	Yes
Some spaces lined by BL[a]	No	Yes
CK7	Yes	Yes
CK14	No	Yes
Estrogen receptors	Yes	No
Adjacent in situ carcinoma	Yes	Rare
Associated TC	Possible	No

[a]BL = basal lamina; CK = cytokeratin; TC = tubular carcinoma.

colloid carcinoma, gelatinous carcinoma, and *mucoid carcinoma.*

MC is the breast tumor diagnosed with the highest level of consistency by pathologists because of its very striking appearance (144); a lack of agreement exists, however, in establishing its grade of purity. There are two views of the definition of purity. In one, a carcinoma is diagnosed as pure MC when at least 90 percent of the total neoplastic area exhibits neoplastic cells floating within extracellular mucins, and mixed when the mucinous component comprises 10 to 90 percent of the neoplastic lesion, with the remaining component constituted by ordinary invasive ductal carcinoma, not otherwise specified (NOS). Tumors containing less than 10 percent of mucinous area are classified according to the dominant invasive ductal component (39,48,144). Along the lines of Azzopardi's statement that "the more stringent the criteria in defining a pure mucinous carcinoma, the more favourable the prognosis" (6), several authors accept as pure MC only those cases composed of 100 percent mucinous features (11,18,76,98,115,135,155).

A related problem is the quantity of mucin required to establish the diagnosis of MC. Sometimes this is not an easy task, especially in cases that are not stained well; the mucin content goes unrecognized and histochemical stains are required to reveal it. The cut-off point for mucin

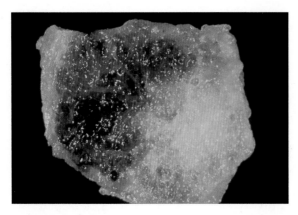 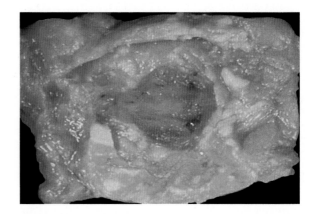

Figure 9-29

MUCINOUS CARCINOMA

Left: In type A mucinous carcinoma (MC), a prominent gelatinous surface is appreciated. (Courtesy of Professor G. Pettinato, Naples, Italy.)

Right: In type B MC, the cut surface of the tumor is nodular and translucent.

quantity required by Silverberg et al. (143) is 50 percent of the tumor volume; lower figures are required by others (33 percent [11] and 25 percent [155]).

For practical purposes, once an MC has been sampled extensively, anything close to 100 percent mucinous features in a given tumor is a great limit to its lethal potential. This is, as is seen later, one of the most important prognostic criteria for patients with MC. The quantity of mucin has much less importance, especially in terms of no correlation with lymph node metastases (76).

Clinical Features. The incidence of MC in the various series ranges from 0.8 to 5.3 percent of all breast carcinomas (40,143). This difference in incidence depends on the different diagnostic criteria used and whether pure and mixed forms are considered separately. The 1,221 patients with MC included in the San Antonio breast cancer data base represented 2.3 percent of all patients with breast cancer (37). Rasmussen et al. (115) reported an incidence of 2.0 percent, but this figure dropped to 0.9 percent when pure MCs were separated from mixed MCs. The ratio of pure versus mixed MC is also variable in different series and ranges from 4:1 to 1:1.2 (76,115).

MC rarely affects male patients. While there is no age difference between patients with the pure and mixed forms (3,48), MC, in general, occurs at an older age than ordinary invasive carcinomas. The median age varies from 62 to 68 years (37,155), which is significantly higher

than that of patients with NOS carcinomas. A family history of breast cancer was found in 11 percent of the patients reported by André et al. (3), who also found that 94 percent of their patients presented with a symptomatic nodule. Few lesions are detected by screening techniques since the older age of the patients often excludes them from screening programs (17).

Gross Findings. MC tends to have a well-circumscribed pushing border. Two distinct features are seen. In cases where there is more extracellular mucus than neoplastic cells, a pink gelatinous cut surface is appreciated, with frequent confluent hemorrhagic areas (fig. 9-29, left). In cases in which the neoplastic cellularity is more abundant than the extracellular mucus, the cut surface is nodular and translucent (fig. 9-29, right).

Tumor size ranges from 0.5 to 20.0 cm (126), but the mean size is 3.7 cm in most series (3). No statistically significant difference in size was seen when MC (pure and mixed) and NOS carcinomas were compared (76,135,155).

Microscopic Findings. Capella et al. (11) subdivided MC in two subtypes (A and B), with an intermediate type AB category. This subdivision, here adopted, is useful from diagnostic and histogenetic points of view, but it is not of prognostic relevance (135).

Type A MC. Type A MC has a greater content of extracellular mucin, ranging from 60 to 90 percent, than type B tumors (11). The neoplastic

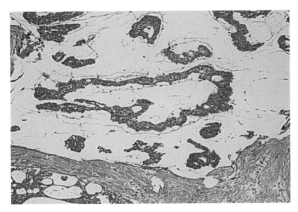
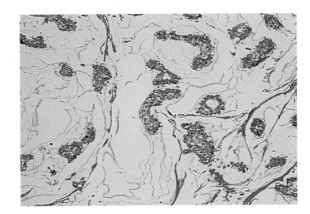

Figure 9-30

TYPE A MUCINOUS CARCINOMA

Ribbons and festoons in type A MC.

cells are arranged in rings, ribbons, and festoons (fig. 9-30). Some rings have small vessels in the center admixed with the mucus. These epithelial neoplastic structures seem to float within the mucus and, in some cases, are so scanty as to be overwhelmed by it. In most cases, the mucus pushes away the fibrous stroma at the periphery and appears to be in direct contact with it, without inducing any inflammatory reaction. Along the tumor stromal interface, in occasional cases, layers of neoplastic cells adhere to the collagen but myoepithelial cells and basal lamina are not seen. Vessels are hardly seen within the mucus.

The nuclei of the neoplastic cells are irregular, occasionally giant or bilobated, and range from grade 1 to 2 (fig. 9-31). The nucleoli are small and mitoses are not frequent. The cytoplasm is eosinophilic and hyaline, and occasionally foamy. No intracytoplasmic mucin is seen in these cells, a finding that led Tavassoli (149) to state that the neoplastic cells of MC "seem to produce the mucus predominantly for the purpose of exporting it to the extracellular space." This is mostly evidenced when the tumor is stained with Alcian blue or for EMA (MUC1) since the cytoplasm of the neoplastic cells remains unstained, with the exception of the subtle rim of the glycocalyx that invests the rings and festoons, indicating a sort of "inverted" polarity (fig. 9-32). MUC2, however, diffusely stains the cytoplasm and is credited for the benign clinical behavior of these tumors (1).

Occasionally, features of invasive micropapillary carcinoma and MC are present in the

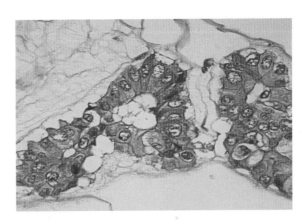

Figure 9-31

TYPE A MUCINOUS CARCINOMA

Type A MC is characterized by cells with irregular nuclei.

same tumor and the prognosis is related to the amount of MC areas present (87). The lack of MUC2 in invasive micropapillary carcinoma indicates the diversity of mucoid carcinomas (95). Ninety percent of MCs, irrespective of the type, are ER positive (142). In cases showing foamy cytoplasm, gross cystic disease fluid protein (GCDFP)-15 is localized, indicating apocrine differentiation.

Ultrastructurally, the features of type A MC are variable, depending on the degree of secretory activity. The cytoplasm is rich in organelles, mitochondria, well-developed Golgi complexes, vesicles of differing sizes, and mucin granules (49). Intermediate filaments are also present. The granules are oriented toward the outer

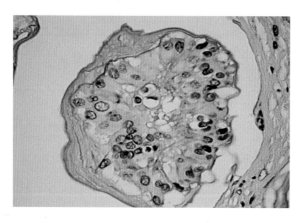
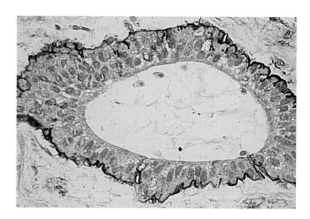

Figure 9-32

TYPE A MUCINOUS CARCINOMA

"Inverted" cellular polarity is shown by the Alcian blue (left) and EMA (right) stains.

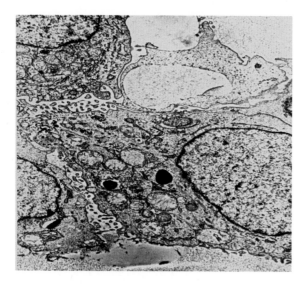
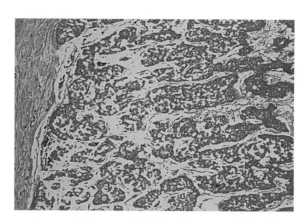

Figure 9-34

TYPE B MUCINOUS CARCINOMA

Numerous neoplastic elements are arranged in anasto-mosing sheets that "float" within mucus.

Figure 9-33

TYPE A MUCINOUS CARCINOMA

The stromal pole has a microvillous surface.

"stromal" pole where abundant microvilli are visible (inverted polarity) (fig. 9-33). The stroma contains deposits of secretory material, fibroblasts, and collagen fibers (6).

Type B MC. Type B MC has a mucin content that, in one series, ranged from 33 to 75 percent (11) and comprised 53 percent of all MC cases reported by Scopsi et al. (135). The neoplastic cells are arranged in rounded, ovoid, or elongated blunt-edged clumps, either isolated or confluent in anastomosing sheets floating within mucus (fig. 9-34). The neoplastic cells are

often seen in a palisading pattern at the edge of the clumps. Numerous vessels and fresh hemorrhage are seen within the extracellular mucus.

Necrosis has been recorded in up to 28 percent of cases (18). On occasion, most of the tumor is so necrotic, especially after FNAC, that the diagnosis is problematic. The nuclei are regular (usually grade 1), ranging from round to ovoid, with evident nucleoli. Mitoses are rare. The cytoplasm is eosinophilic and finely granular in most cases (fig. 9-35). Intracytoplasmic lumens, as seen in lobular carcinomas, are seen in a minority of cases, as are signet ring cells.

Ten of the 14 cases reported by Capella et al. (11) were argyrophilic, as were 12 of the 20 cases

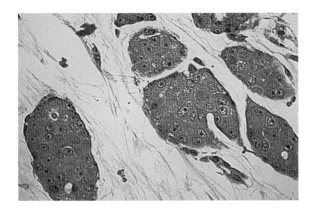

Figure 9-35

TYPE B MUCINOUS CARCINOMA

The nuclei of type B MC are regular and the cytoplasm appears granular and deeply eosinophilic.

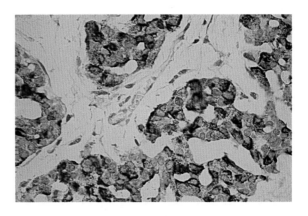

Figure 9-36

TYPE B MUCINOUS CARCINOMA

Chromogranin A stains numerous neoplastic cells.

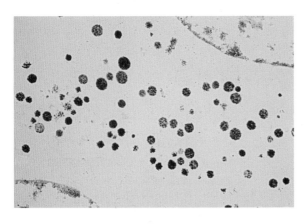

Figure 9-37

TYPE B MUCINOUS CARCINOMA

Ultrastructurally, silver precipitates on the granules (Grimelius stain). (Courtesy of Professor C. Capella, Varese, Italy.)

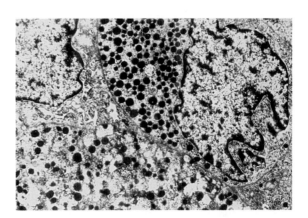

Figure 9-38

TYPE B MUCINOUS CARCINOMA

A heavily granulated endocrine cell is adjacent to an amphicrine cell that contains endocrine granules and large vescicles of finely reticulated mucin. (Fig. 8 from Capella C, Eusebi V, Mann B, Azzopardi JG. Endocrine differentiation in mucoid carcinoma of the breast. Histopathology 1980;4:623.)

reported by Scopsi et al. (135). The overall proportion of argyrophilic cells in type B MC varies from 10 to 100 percent. All the argyrophilic tumors contain cells that react with antibodies to chromogranins A and B (fig. 9-36). Argyrophilia and chromogranin A or B were also present in one case of type A MC, 50 percent of type AB MCs, and 4 of 23 mixed mucinous tumors (135). Coady et al. (22) found immunoreactive cells for carcinoembryonic antigen (CEA) in all type B tumors and S-100 protein in five of six tumors. Most attempts to localize specific hormones in type B MC have led to inconclusive results.

Ultrastructurally, argyrophilic type B MCs show highly dense, rounded to ovoid neuroendocrine granules. These are characterized by intense and diffuse, fine silver precipitates on the granule membrane when the cell is stained by the Grimelius method (fig. 9-37) (11). In some cases, the dominant cell is represented by amphicrine elements (amphi from ancient Greek, meaning both). These cells contain both endocrine granules and large vescicles of finely reticulated mucin (fig. 9-38). Amphicrine cells

191

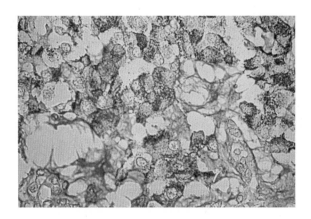

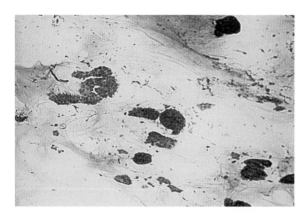

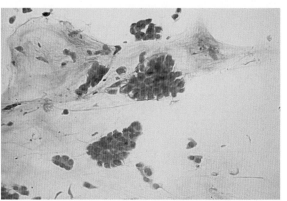

Figure 9-39

TYPE B MUCINOUS CARCINOMA

The Grimelius stain combined with Alcian blue highlights the amphicrine cells.

are also highlighted when the Grimelius stain (or chromogranin) is combined with Alcian blue (fig. 9-39). Intracytoplasmic lumens bordered by microvilli are also seen ultrastructurally.

Type AB MC. Tumors in this category represent 16 percent of the cases reported by Scopsi et al. (135). In these tumors, both subtypes are seen close to one another. Fifty percent of these are tumors that are argyrophil and chromogranin positive.

The qualitative mucin composition in all three variants of MC varies from 80.5 percent in cases in which mucin is predominantly acidic, to 13.0 percent in cases in which it is neutral, to 6.0 percent in cases in which both types are represented (3). In 30 percent of cases, the acidic mucins contain sulfomucins; sialomucins are present to a lesser extent (3). MUC1, present in normal mammary gland, is greatly decreased in MC cells, while MUC2 (intestinal) and MUC5 (bronchial) are greatly expressed (99). The same types of mucins are seen in mixed MC. The quality of the mucin is similar to that of mucinous carcinomas of the intestine (128,155).

Calcifications are observed in about 33 percent of cases (3), but most of them are present within DCIS/DIN lesions. DCIS/DIN, located at the periphery of the tumor, is a frequent finding with an observed incidence of 60 to 75 percent (48,126). The high incidence of DCIS/DIN has lead to the statement that "rarely one encounters a pure mucinous carcinoma with no apparent intraductal carcinoma" (126). The associated DCIS is well to intermediately differentiated

Figure 9-40

TYPE A MUCINOUS CARCINOMA

Top: FNAC shows clumps or festoons of cells with irregular nuclei immersed in a mucoid background.

Bottom: The neoplastic cells, arranged in a clump, show the secretory pole directed toward the exterior (inverted polarity).

(DIN1 and 2). In type A MC, it is flat (clinging), micropapillary, or cribriform. In type B lesions, DCIS/DIN shows regular nuclei and is solid, of the type defined as "solid papillary carcinoma" (89). The latter also shows neuroendocrine differentiation (11,48,89).

Cytologic Findings. FNAC of MC leads to abundant material in which mucus and clumps of monotonous cells are intermingled. Mucin must be distinguished from necrotic debris and interstitial fluid. In difficult cases, Alcian blue combined with PAS is a helpful stain.

Type A and B MCs can also be distinguished at the cytologic level (80). Type A MCs yield abundant mucin in which isolated cells and irregular clumps of cells with irregular nuclei are present (fig. 9-40). Argyrophilic/endocrine type B MCs have large cohesive nests of regular

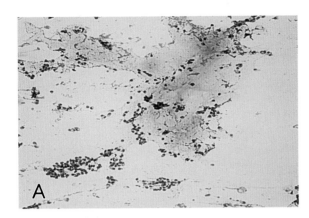

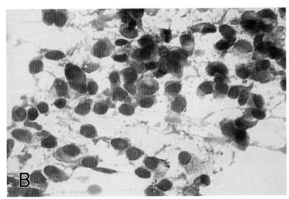

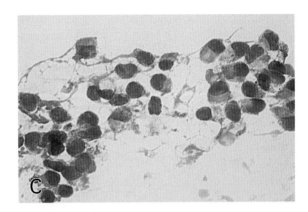

Figure 9-41

TYPE B MUCINOUS CARCINOMA

In a FNAC specimen (A), the cells are not cohesive (B) and are often plasmacytoid (C) with regular nuclei.

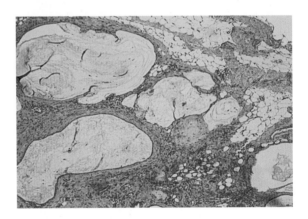

Figure 9-42

MUCOCELE-LIKE TUMOR

Abundant mucin is observed within enlarged ducts showing flat epithelium.

cells. Some neoplastic elements have a plasmacytoid appearance (fig. 9-41). No myoepithelial cell layer is seen at the periphery; staining by the Grimelius method and for chromogranin results in positive cells. Fibroadenomas with prominent myxoid stroma are excluded by the clinical history of a young patient. The distinction from a mucocele-like tumor and even from matrix-producing carcinoma is very difficult, if not impossible, cytologically.

Histogenesis. MC appears to be closely related to *mucocele-like tumors* (ML). The latter are multiple cysts lined by flat epithelium, and contain abundant mucin that frequently extrudes into the stroma (fig. 9-42) (124).

Several facts point to the relationship between these tumors. The 53 mucocele-like tumors reported by Hamele-Bena et al. (60) consisted of 12 cases of micropapillary atypical duct hyperplasia, 14 micropapillary and cribriform carcinomas, and 14 mucocele-like tumors with areas of MC. The other 13 cases contained duct hyperplasia or the cysts were lined by nondescript flattened epithelium. Of

seven mucocele-like tumors reported by Ro et al. (120), four were atypical duct hyperplasia and the other three had minute foci of MC. A case of mucocele-like tumors with atypical duct hyperplasia recurred a year later as MC (51). The mucin of mucocele-like tumors is identical to

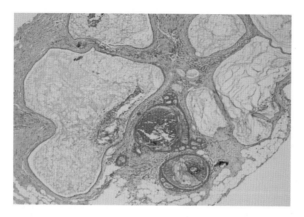 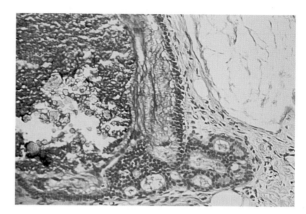

Figure 9-43

MUCOCELE-LIKE TUMOR

Left: In deeper sections of the case seen in figure 9-42, some lumens contain mucin as well as calcium deposits.
Right: Abundant granular calcium deposits are readily apparent within the lumen. A minute area of grade 1 cribriform DCIS/DIN1 is present.

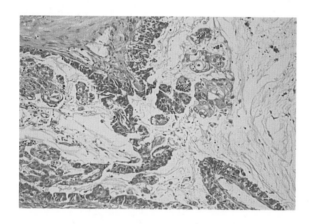

Figure 9-44

MUCINOUS CYSTOADENOCARCINOMA

Squamoid spherules float in mucus.

that seen in MC (120). Mucin-filled ducts are frequently present around or at a distance from the MC. Some of these are dilated and may show micropapillary DCIS/DIN (168). Finally, often a benign-appearing (flat epithelium) ML can hide a well-differentiated DCIS/DIN in deeper sections (fig. 9-43).

Overproduction of mucin by the neoplastic cells seems to detach these cells from the stroma, especially in cases with inverted polarity. The rings and festoons of epithelial neoplastic cells floating within the mucus of type A MC are probably the residue of cribriform structures and micropapillary processes.

Solid papillary carcinoma is a type of intraductal carcinoma with endocrine differentiation. It was described by Maluf and Koerner (89), who proposed that these lesions and type B MC are related based on several findings. The cells constituting solitary papillary carcinoma are round to ovoid with eosinophilic cytoplasm, very similar to the neoplastic elements seen in type B MC. Mucin, intracellular or extracellular, was present in 18 of the 20 solid papillary carcinomas in that study, although not to the same extent as seen in MC. Solid papillary carcinoma can be chromogranin positive. Of the 16 cases of solid papillary carcinoma harboring invasive carcinomas, 7 were pure and 4 were mixed type B MCs.

Differential Diagnosis. MC has to be distinguished from fibroadenoma with myxoid stroma, mucocele-like tumor, mucinous cystadenocarcinoma (75), matrix-producing carcinoma (166), and squamous cell carcinoma with prominent myxoid stroma (55).

Mucinous cystadenocarcinoma is a rare primary tumor of the breast. The original four cases reported appeared in patients younger than those with MC (average, 58 years). Mucinous cystadenocarcinomas are characterized by cystic spaces containing sulfated mucin, and lined by mucin-producing neoplastic elements that transform in the center of the cystic lumens into squamoid elements (fig. 9-44). The latter are not seen in ordinary MC. The histology of mucinous cystadenocarcinoma is very similar to that of MC of the ovary, which can be excluded, if not on clinical grounds, with immunohistochemistry. The mammary tumor is positive for CK7 but not CK20, a pattern not consonant with the ovarian tumor, which is characterized by CK20 positivity.

Matrix-producing carcinoma and squamous cell carcinoma with prominent myxoid stroma are both characterized by acidic stromal mucosubstances that are different from the mucin present in MC. In addition, the neoplastic cells of matrix-producing carcinoma are located at the periphery of the tumor. These cells are individually dispersed or arranged in small trabeculae or plexiform sheets, are frequently CK14 and smooth muscle actin positive, and chromogranin is not found in them. Positivity for CK14 and smooth muscle actin is not a feature of MC cells.

Squamous cell carcinomas with prominent myxoid stroma show elongated or globoid cells that are single or arranged in plexiform sheets (56). Occasional squamous pearls are observed. CK17 positivity is a feature of this tumor while it is not seen in MC.

Prognosis. As with most breast carcinomas, the prognosis is based on three factors. The first is the histologic type: patients with pure MC survive statistically longer than those with mixed MC, even after a long period of follow-up (21 years) (155); they have a better relapse-free survival rate (87 percent for those with pure MC and 54 percent for those with mixed MC at 10 years) (48); and they have fewer axillary lymph node metastases (48,76). The survival of patients with pure MC at 5 years is similar to that of the general population (37). In contrast, no difference in survival is seen between patients with mixed MC and those with ordinary invasive carcinoma (155).

The next factor is the size of the tumor: small pure MCs infrequently metastasize to lymph nodes. This is evident from the series of Andrè et al. (3) who did not find metastatic lymph nodes associated with T1 carcinomas. In MCs 1 cm or smaller, the incidence of node involvement was 4 percent in contrast to 19 percent for ordinary invasive carcinoma (37).

The last factor is the presence of lymph node metastases: in cases without node metastases no deaths are seen even on long-term follow-up (median, 20 years) (135). In a multivariate analysis of patients with MC, the single most important factor for predicting recurrence-free survival was

lymph node status (115). The histology of the metastases in pure MC is similar to that of the original tumor. In mixed MC, the metastatic appearance is similar to that of the nonmucoid component in most instances (48).

ENDOCRINE TUMORS

Endocrine tumors are neoplasms that are histologically characterized by a solid, trabecular, or glandular arrangement of cells, which may also form pseudorosettes or tubuloacinar structures. We have adopted the generic "old" World Health Organization (WHO) (146) definition of endocrine tumors in the belief that endocrine neoplasms of the breast are similar to those observed in other organs. A major advantage of this definition is the use of histologic criteria only. It is pertinent to note that the primary "carcinoid" tumors of the breast first reported by Cubilla and Woodruff (30) were recognized at frozen section, indicating that routine histology is vital for establishing the correct diagnosis.

No issue in breast pathology has raised so many "strident voices" as the acceptance of tumors with endocrine differentiation (88). One of the reasons for the strong opposition is the lack of a "normal" endocrine counterpart in the breast glandular tree. The presence of normal endocrine cells has been occasionally demonstrated along the ductular epithelium (10), but this occurrence is rare; no neuroendocrine cells were seen in a series of fetal and adult non-neoplastic mammary glands (164).

The nomenclature is also a cause of dispute. The term "carcinoid" introduced by Cubilla and Woodruff (30) in their seminal work was rejected by several authors (93,126). The latter believed that the term "carcinoma with neuroendocrine differentiation" was more precise to define these neoplasms.

Technology has played a major role in the dispute. When Cubilla and Woodruff (30) published their paper in 1977, they had available only silver precipitation techniques and electron microscopy. Some degree of nonspecificity was clearly present with both techniques (88). The lack of reliable results even with the Grimelius technique, which was at the time the technique of choice for evaluating endocrine differentiation, was pointed out by Papotti et al. (105), who found that the incidence of argyrophilic carcinomas in different series in the literature varies from 0 to 50 percent of cases. The lack of total reliability of the argyrophilic methods led Azzopardi et al. (7) to be very cautious in terms of nomenclature and to "...prefer the term of argyrophil carcinoma to carcinoid tumor on the basis of the existing evidence."

There were similar difficulties with the use of electron microscopy since dense core granules occur in normal nonendocrine epithelial resting mammary cells as well as during pregnancy and lactation (88). This led to fierce disputes (19) until it was shown that endocrine tumors of the breast are ultrastructurally heterogeneous. They are composed of no fewer than five different types of cells containing five types of granules, in which chromogranin A can be immunolocalized at the ultrastructural level (12). One tumor in the series reported by Capella et al. (12) had irregularly shaped granules resembling those of gastrointestinal enterochromaffin cells.

The conclusive evidence of endocrine differentiation in some breast carcinomas was obtained by the immunohistochemical localization of chromogranin A (10), chromogranin B (136), and synaptophysin (105). Neuron-specific enolase (NSE) is not used to establish the endocrine nature of a breast tumor because of its lack of specificity (93,129).

Raised levels of hormones such as calcitonin, adrenocorticotropic hormone (ACTH), norepinephrine, and parathyroid hormone have been sporadically documented in the plasma of patients with endocrine carcinoma (23,25,72). Ectopic production of neurotensin, ACTH, and serotonin was immunohistochemically localized to in situ and invasive endocrine tumors in isolated instances (12,29). ER is positive in 68 percent and PR in 45 percent of cases (132).

According to the WHO "old" criteria for endocrine tumors (146), four major categories can be recognized in the breast. These are described below.

Well-Differentiated Endocrine Tumor (Carcinoid)

Well-differentiated endocrine tumor is "an epithelial tumor of endocrine cells showing no or minimal atypia and growing in the form of small solid nests, trabeculae, gyriform cords, or, more rarely, pseudoglandular structures." If this definition of a tumor entirely composed of endocrine cells, as seen in carcinoid tumors of the gut, is applied stringently to breast neoplasms, then the breast counterpart is virtually nonexistent.

One well-differentiated endocrine tumor was mentioned in a textbook (122), four cases were alluded to in a large and highly selected series of endocrine breast tumors (133), and one case was diagnosed ultrastructurally (12). We have seen two cases, but a careful workup of both patients revealed a primary carcinoid located in the gut. Di Palma et al. (36) reported on a similar case and pointed out that metastasizing intestinal carcinoids can simulate a primary mammary carcinoma. Before accepting a carcinoid tumor as primary in the breast, a metastatic process has to be excluded.

Well-Differentiated Endocrine Carcinoma

Definition. *Well-differentiated endocrine carcinoma* is "a malignant epithelial tumor composed of endocrine cells showing mild to moderate atypia and growing in the form of solid nests and sheets, trabeculae, gyriform cords, or, less commonly, pseudoglandular structures." Most of the endocrine tumors reported in the breast belong to this category.

Endocrine carcinomas are composed of a heterogeneous mixture of endocrine and exocrine cells. The definition of "pure" endocrine carcinoma is a matter for debate since tumors containing 100 percent of demonstrable endocrine cells are virtually nonexistent.

Sapino et al. (133) proposed that "endocrine breast carcinomas are exclusively those tumors which express chromogranin A or B or synaptophysin in more than 50 percent of their cells." Miremadi et al. (93) were not in agreement with this view and used less stringent criteria. Their series of 99 patients with carcinoma with neuroendocrine differentiation included cases with only 5 percent neuroendocrine cells and none of their cases contained more than 50 percent of endocrine elements. Of the 91 tumors reported by Scopsi et al. (136), 44 contained cells with less than 10 percent endocrine differentiation.

The lack of uniform diagnostic criteria is reflected in the differences in incidence reported in the literature, which vary from 0.2 to 20.0 percent (30,93). Twenty percent is the reported incidence in a series of invasive breast carcinomas in men

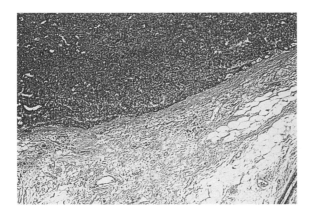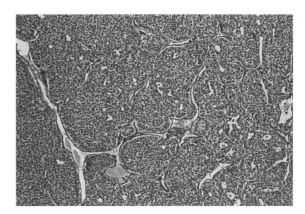

Figure 9-45

WELL-DIFFERENTIATED ENDOCRINE CARCINOMA

Compact nests of cohesive cells are seen.

(137). Despite the variation in criteria used for diagnosis, there is no significant association between the degree of endocrine differentiation and tumor size, stage, or prevalence of vascular invasion, nor significant difference in overall or disease-free survival rates between matched patients with tumors with and without endocrine differentiation (93,129,136).

Clinical Features. The age of reported patients ranges from 26 to 83 years, with a mean age of 47.5 years (30). A paraareolar lump is frequently observed, and four patients in one series had bloody nipple discharge. The tumor mass is frequently brown to red, depending on the amount of hemorrhage observed.

Grading. In general, the more numerous the endocrine cells, the better differentiated (grade [G] 1 to 2) the tumor is, with occasional exceptions. All 11 tumors in one series (136) containing over 80 percent of endocrine elements were G1 to 2 as opposed to tumors with less than 10 percent endocrine cells, which were G3. The prognosis of patients with endocrine carcinoma is strictly related to the tumor grade (129). Most endocrine tumors are of ductal type; a few are of the lobular variety and a confluent growth pattern (47) is the most frequent feature (105).

It is possible to recognize an endocrine tumor from the pattern of growth only in cases of well-differentiated (G1 to 2) carcinomas, while no specific pattern is shown by G3 tumors, which are recognized as such only with the use of special techniques. Pattern recognition was one of the main criteria used by Cubilla and Woodruff (30) and Azzopardi et al. (7) in their pioneer works.

Microscopic Findings. The most frequent pattern presented by well-differentiated endocrine carcinoma is a mostly circumscribed, cellular and cohesive neoplasm. These were also termed *carcinoid* (30), *type A neuroendocrine carcinoma* (105), *solid cohesive carcinoma*, and *low-grade insular ductal carcinoma* (88). The tumors grow in sheets, blunt nodules, or irregular compact nests of cohesive cells (fig. 9-45). At the edge of the neoplastic clumps, cells are often columnar, with elongated nuclei arranged toward the stroma to resemble palisades. These palisades of cells form a seam around the tumor clumps (fig. 9-46, left). Pseudorosettes are also a common feature. Columnar cells are orientated around a central blood vessel, with or without accompanying connective tissue (fig. 9-46, right). True glandular lumens are rare. Necrotic areas are absent.

The neoplastic cells of well-differentiated endocrine carcinoma have fine granular eosinophilic cytoplasm, are mostly round to polygonal, and have margins that vary from indistinct to moderately sharp. Some cells contain abundant intracellular mucin. Nuclei vary from ovoid to round, are either central or eccentric, and are uniform with a nuclear membrane that is sharply outlined. Chromatin is finely punctate and nucleoli are inconspicuous. Mitoses are few. The stroma is never abundant and appears highly vascular. Vessels are often dilated and engorged with blood, which results in the red-brown color of the tumor.

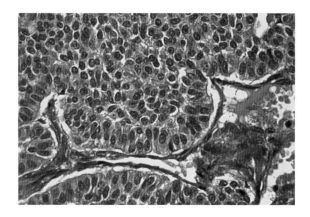
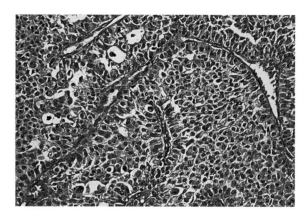

Figure 9-46

WELL-DIFFERENTIATED ENDOCRINE CARCINOMA

Cells are arranged in palisades at the edge of the clumps (left) and a pseudorosette is visible in the center (right).

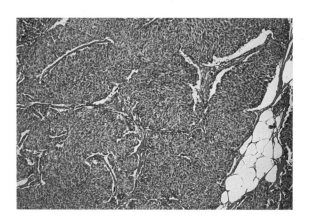
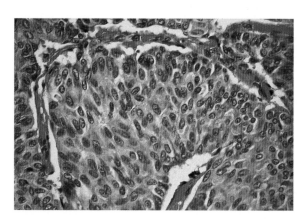

Figure 9-47

WELL-DIFFERENTIATED ENDOCRINE CARCINOMA

Most of the tumor is composed of spindle cells.

Most well-differentiated carcinomas are G2 lesions because of the rarity of glandular spaces. Some tumors, however, are so well differentiated that Scopsi et al. (136) and Sapino and Bussolati (129) scored them as G1 to 2 lesions, a grade that we feel does justice to this very low-grade tumor. Most patients survive longer that 10 years (131). Rare G3 tumors have the same pattern of growth but show irregular nuclei, numerous mitoses, and necrotic areas; these tumors are noticeably more aggressive (131).

Spindle cell endocrine carcinoma (127) is a rare variant of well-differentiated G1 to 2 endocrine carcinoma. The macroscopic and microscopic features are those of a well-circumscribed mass. The neoplastic cells are cohesive and spindle shaped (fig. 9-47). When sectioned in a transverse plane, those with eccentric nuclei appear vaguely plasmacytoid (127). The nuclei are ovoid to elongated and the cytoplasm of the neoplastic cells is eosinophilic and granular. In some cases, abundant mucin is present so as to suggest a close relationship with type B MC (90). These tumors are so well circumscribed as to simulate in situ endocrine carcinomas (E-DCIS/E-DIN), the features of which will be described in a separate section. Some cases are also close simulators of florid epithelial hyperplasia, a point emphasized by Azzopardi et al. (7).

Invasive spindle cell endocrine carcinomas lack the basal lamina and myoepithelial cells that characterize in situ lesions. These invasive

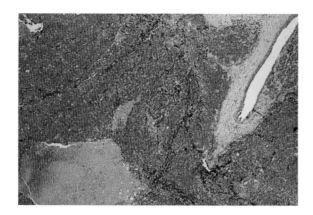 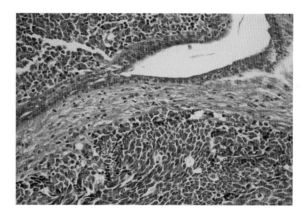

Figure 9-48

POORLY DIFFERENTIATED (SMALL CELL) ENDOCRINE CARCINOMA

Necrosis (left) and cells with dark nuclei without nucleoli (right) are seen.

tumors are composed mainly of one cell type that has abundant granular, eosinophilic, and chromogranin- and/or synaptophysin-positive cytoplasm, which are not features of epithelial hyperplasia (epitheliosis). The latter contains high molecular weight keratin (CK14)-positive elements (94), not found in endocrine carcinomas, which contain CK7-positive elements.

Solid papillary carcinoma is a tumor strictly related to spindle cell endocrine carcinoma. Papillary fronds are evident. The tumor is often in situ and is composed of spindle, plasmacytoid, and signet ring cells (89).

Cytologic Findings. FNAC of endocrine carcinomas shows specific features that allow a confident diagnosis (130). These include cell clusters with neat borders and single cells with a plasmacytoid appearance. Peripheral cytoplasmic granules are seen with the Giemsa stain. The spindle cell variant shows elongated cells with moderate pleomorphism that is reminiscent of atypical carcinoid tumors of the lung.

The presence of DCIS adjacent to the invasive component renders the diagnosis of primary endocrine carcinoma more confident. The incidence of intraductal carcinoma is difficult to obtain from the literature, but it is probably about 30 percent (152a).

Poorly Differentiated Endocrine Carcinoma–Small Cell Carcinoma

Poorly differentiated endocrine carcinoma is a malignant epithelial tumor showing highly atypical, small to intermediate sized cells with a high nucleocytoplasmic ratio, and poorly granular or agranular cytoplasm, which grows in the form of large, ill-defined solid aggregates, often with central necrosis, and diffuse cellular sheets. *Oat cell carcinoma* is included in this group.

Poorly differentiated endocrine carcinoma of the breast is a rare tumor and mainly reported as single cases. Patient age ranges from 43 to 70 years. Histologically, the tumors either are identical to oat cell carcinoma of the lung or resemble Merkel cell carcinoma of the skin (fig. 9-48). In 40 percent of cases, the small cell component intermingles with an invasive lobular or ductal carcinoma (140), a finding in keeping with the general rule that extrapulmonary poorly differentiated (small cell) endocrine carcinomas are frequently admixed with other tumor types (44).

DCIS was present in 8 of the 11 cases reported by Shin et al. (140). It was of small cell type in 5 and poorly differentiated in 3, of which one was associated with Paget cell carcinoma. Chromogranin and synaptophysin were positive in about 50 percent of the cases (fig. 9-49). Gastrin-releasing peptide was localized in 5 and calcitonin in 3 (104,140). ER and PR were positive in about 60 percent of cases (140). All 11 cases were E-cadherin positive (139), a finding that could not be corroborated in two cases of ours, which were E-cadherin negative.

The most important differential diagnosis with clinical impact is the distinction between primary and metastatic small cell carcinoma. Besides the clinical features, the most reliable

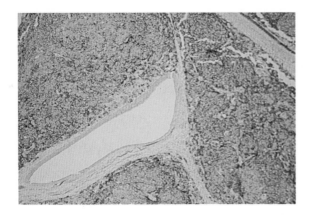

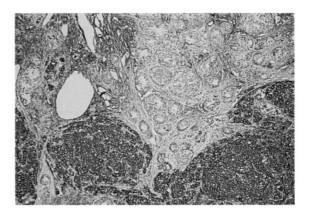

Figure 9-49

POORLY DIFFERENTIATED ENDOCRINE CARCINOMA

Synaptophysin-positive cells.

Figure 9-50

COMPOSITE EXOCRINE-ENDOCRINE CARCINOMA

The cells are partly positive for chromogranin A.

finding is the presence of DCIS/DIN within or near the tumor (104). The immunohistochemical detection of thyroid transcription factor 1 (TTF1), observed in 80 percent of cases of pulmonary oat cell carcinoma, is not helpful since it is also seen in about 20 percent of primary small cell carcinomas of breast (139). Merkel cell carcinoma of the skin can be separated from Merkel-like carcinomas of the breast as the latter lack CK20, which is a usual constituent of the skin neoplasms (5).

Axillary and widespread metastases are a feature of mammary small cell carcinoma. In spite of this, all 10 patients studied by Shin et al. (140) were alive at last follow-up which ranged from 3 to 35 months. The prognosis may not be as poor as previously believed, but this needs confirmation since three of four patients in a small series of small cell carcinomas of breast died within 15 months (104).

Mixed Exocrine-Endocrine Carcinoma

Mixed exocrine-endocrine carcinoma is "an epithelial tumor with a predominant exocrine component admixed with an endocrine component comprising at least one third of the entire tumor cell population." These lesions can show endocrine and exocrine components within the same cell (amphicrine), in an intimately admixed but individually separated cell (combined tumors), or in separated but adjacent tumor components (composite tumor) (fig. 9-50).

According to this definition, type B MC is such a tumor. Amphicrine cells, a mixture of endocrine

and exocrine elements (combined), or composite tumors in which types A and B carcinoma are adjacent are features frequently seen (34).

Endocrine carcinomas can also show apocrine differentiation (132). This type of exocrine differentiation can be present simultaneously in an endocrine cell, producing a novel type of amphicrine element. Of 21 such cases, 68 percent were G1; of these, 80 percent were positive for ARs. All patients with G1 tumors survived longer than 13 years, indicating once again that histologic grade is a powerful prognostic indicator.

MEDULLARY CARCINOMA

Definition. *Medullary carcinoma* is a poorly differentiated carcinoma with a plexiform architecture, intense lymphoid stroma, and microscopically well-circumscribed borders. Tubule formation is absent.

Clinical Features. The reported incidence is variable for this highly debated entity: a 5 to 7 percent incidence among all breast carcinomas was accepted by Tavassoli (149); less than 5 percent was accepted by Rosen (126). Typical medullary carcinoma accounted for less than 1 percent of all breast carcinomas according to Sloane (144). Only 26 cases were seen in 19 years at the Institute Gustave-Roussy by Rapin et al. (114), who stated that typical medullary carcinoma represented a very small fraction of the total infiltrating operable breast carcinomas.

The general consensus is that medullary carcinoma is overdiagnosed (114) because the

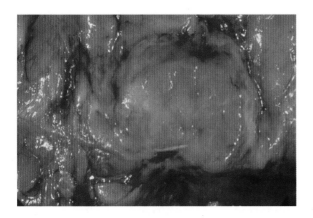

Figure 9-51

MEDULLARY CARCINOMA

Well-circumscribed nodularity is present. (Courtesy of Professor G. Pettinato, Naples, Italy.)

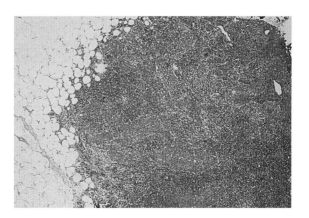

Figure 9-52

MEDULLARY CARCINOMA

Neoplastic cells with a plexiform architecture are immersed in a lymphoid stroma. Lymphoid elements penetrate the adipocytic septa for a short distance. This is a potential cause of disagreement when assessing circumscription.

criteria for its recognition are imprecise. Rosai (122) stated that he had "too often seen the term medullary carcinoma misused" and he "wondered whether medullary carcinoma constitutes a bona fide subtype of breast carcinoma as currently defined." It is not surprising that a low rate of intraobserver and interobserver agreement was obtained in multicenter studies (107,118,145). Among the various difficulties in diagnosis, is the lack of precise boundaries between medullary carcinomas and lymphoepithelioma-like carcinomas that are more frequent and have only recently been described in breast (31).

Most medullary carcinomas are discovered by palpation. Mammographically, they are well-circumscribed nodules that rarely show microcalcifications. The mean age of women with medullary carcinoma ranges from 45 to 54 years (126). Medullary carcinoma is unicentric in most of the patients and no predilection of site in breast parenchyma is seen. Bilateral carcinoma has been found in 3 to 18 percent of patients (126), further proof of the lack of precise diagnostic criteria. The contralateral carcinoma is usually infiltrating carcinoma NOS, with the medullary carcinoma tending to be the secondary tumor, appearing much later than nonmedullary carcinomas (8.8 versus 4.6 years) (117). Bilateral tumors are common when a family history is present. A history of maternal breast carcinoma is more frequent in patients with typical medullary carcinoma than a history of sibling breast carcinoma (117).

Gross Findings. Most medullary carcinomas do not exceed 2 cm, with the reported median size varying from 25 to 29 mm (84). The cut surface can be so well circumscribed (fig. 9-51) as to be confused with fibroadenoma (6) and can be bulging.

Classification. Ridolfi et al. (117) first attempted to introduce objective criteria for classifying medullary carcinoma. They defined *typical medullary carcinoma* as those tumors showing: growth in plexiform sheets ("syncytial" pattern) comprising over 75 percent of the total neoplastic area; complete microscopic circumscription (fig. 9-52); a moderate to marked stromal lymphoplasmacytic infiltrate; neoplastic cells with indistinct cytoplasmic borders and high nuclear grade (fig. 9-53); and a high mitotic rate (this criterion was added later [126]). They categorized tumors as *atypical medullary carcinomas* if they had the same quantity of plexiform sheets (75 percent), but exhibited no more than two of the following features: tumor margins showing focal or prominent infiltration; a mononuclear infiltrate that is mild or at the margins of the tumor; low-grade nuclei; and the presence of microglandular features. *Nonmedullary infiltrating carcinomas* are those having a plexiform sheet growth pattern of less than 75 percent or the presence of three or more of the above atypical features. The 75 percent cut-off is the point at which there is a significant difference

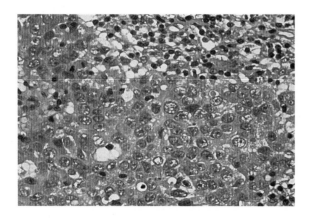

Figure 9-53

MEDULLARY CARCINOMA

Neoplastic cells have an "indistinct" cytoplasmic border.

in outcome in patients. Survival rates decrease when this growth pattern is less than 75 percent and the difference is even more conspicuous below 50 percent (126).

Attempts to simplify Ridolfi's classification resulted in three other classification schemes (108,149,167), all of which were variations on the theme. Lidang Jensen et al. (84) reclassified 60 breast carcinomas primarily diagnosed as medullary carcinoma according to three of the above classifications. Ridolfi's classification selected 13 patients who all survived longer than 10 years (117). It was found that Ridolfi's classification was more sensitive than Tavassoli's classification (149) and correlated better with survival than Pedersen's classification (108). If strict criteria are used, the risk of overdiagnosis or of undertreatment is minimized. Using Ridolfi's classification for typical medullary carcinoma, a small group of neoplastic lesions are isolated that do not exceed 2.9 cm in average size. Patients with these lesions have a statistically significant better survival rate than those with atypical medullary carcinoma and nonmedullary infiltrating carcinoma (see below).

The lack of agreement about the significance of separating medullary carcinoma and its variants from other breast tumors seemed to be mostly of academic interest (141) until it was found that many *BRCA1*-associated breast carcinomas have some of the features currently believed to be typical of medullary carcinoma. In a seminal paper that included 440 female

patients with familial breast cancer, Lakhani et al. (82) demonstrated by multifactorial analysis differences between sporadic breast cancers and cancers involving *BRCA1* and *BRCA2* mutations. The conclusion was that carcinomas showing *BRCA1* mutations exhibited higher mitotic counts, continuous pushing margins, and intense stromal lymphoid infiltrates than seen in sporadic (control) carcinomas. These three features are included in the definition of typical medullary carcinoma.

Medullary carcinoma patients have been shown to have up to 60 percent of *BRCA1* germline mutations, far higher than "ordinary" breast cancer cases (67). This excess was not found by Bermejo (83c), who stated that no significant standardized incidence ratio was seen for those with medullary carcinoma with the exception of patients whose mothers had ovarian cancer. Similar findings were obtained by Iau et al. (65) who studied 42 patients with medullary carcinoma unselected for family history. Therefore, it seems that medullary carcinomas are not an indication for *BRCA1* mutation in the absence of a significant family risk factor, but when risk factors are present, the corresponding tumor is very likely to be a medullary carcinoma.

Lakhani et al (82) also found that cancers associated with *BRCA2* mutations exhibited a higher score for tubule formation, a higher proportion of tumor perimeter with a continuous pushing margin, and a lower mitotic count than control cancers. These studies show that *BRCA2* cases are predominantly high-grade invasive ductal carcinomas of no special type that demonstrate no syncytial (plexiform) growth pattern, a mild lymphocytic infiltrate, consistent positivity for ER and CK8/18, and low positivity for CK14 (8a).

Microscopic Findings. Syncytium, from the Greek, means fusion of cells that consequently become multinucleated. It is unfortunate that the term syncytium has been employed in medullary carcinoma to indicate a structural type of growth. The ambiguity of the term is probably one of the reasons for the great diagnostic variability of this tumor among various observers. Pedersen et al. (108) regarded syncytial growth from a purely structural point of view as "broad interanastomosing sheets of tumour cells." Rosai (122) emphasized that "the large tumor cells grow in a syncytial fashion" and that sometimes they acquire a vague resemblance to syncytiotrophoblast. Most authors, including Ridolfi et al. (117), have included in the term both structure and cytology, stating that "syncytial growth features broad interanastomosing sheets of tumor cells with indistinct cell borders." We feel that the use of "syncytial growth" and of "indistinct borders" should be discontinued since they are subjective and vague terms and replaced by the descriptive term of plexiform architecture employed by Stewart in the first edition of the AFIP Fascicle (147) to indicate broad, interanastomosing sheets of tumor cells, as a more objective criterion.

Microscopic circumscription of margins is the feature most difficult to define and therefore the least reproducible criterion among the several studies published. We feel that the problem at the moment is not resolvable. If microscopic circumscription refers to the border of the infiltrating carcinoma, rather than to the periphery of the surrounding lymphoplasmacytic reaction, as stated by Rosen (126), then the vast majority of tumors with prominent plexiform finger-like projections cannot be considered circumscribed.

Medullary carcinomas express all the glandular type keratins, including CK19 (156). CK14 is found in up to 30.3 percent (67) and CK5 in up to 60 percent (120a) of typical medullary carcinomas but CK20 is negative (156). About 90 percent are negative for ER and all cases tested were aneuploid (156). A very low incidence of c-erbB-2 and a high incidence of p53 immunostaining have been reported (67,120a). P-cadherin stains up to 40 percent of cases (120a), epidermal growth factor receptor (EGFR) is positive in 70 percent, and smooth muscle actin is seen in 34.3 percent of cases (67). None of these findings is exclusive for medullary carcinoma, which has a similar profile to poorly differentiated invasive duct carcinoma but with less positivity for S-100 protein (122).

The distinction between medullary carcinoma and basal-like carcinoma is not yet settled. As stated in another section of this book, a comprehensive molecular profiling system using complementary cDNA expression arrays has led to the genetic identification of five groups of invasive carcinomas with different prognoses (109a,146a). Papers dealing with the phenotypic

definition of each of the five subtypes have proliferated, but the category that has attracted most attention is the basal-like subtype. Most authors agree that basal-like tumors are grade 3 invasive duct carcinomas (69a) that have a specific immunohistochemical profile consisting of ER and c-erbB-2 negativity and CK5/6 positivity (97). Among the several definitions of basal-like carcinoma, probably the most comprehensive is the one proposed by Livasy et al. (83a). According to these authors, morphologic features significantly associated with an invasive basal-like phenotype are grade 3, elevated mitotic count, geographic tumor necrosis, pushing margins of invasion, and stromal lymphocytic response. In addition, the most constant immunophenotype is negativity for ER and c-erbB-2 and positivity for vimentin, EGFR, CK8/18, and CK5/6. The basal-like phenotype has been reported to be characterized by poor clinical outcome (97,113a). Rodriguez-Pinilla et al. (120a) stated that 22 of 35 (62 percent) of their cases of sporadic invasive carcinoma with medullary features displayed a basal-like phenotype, which included lack of steroid receptors and c-erbB-2, but expression of CK5/6 and/or EGFR. The same conclusion was reached by Rakha et al. (113a) who found a predominant basal-like phenotype in 20 of 45 cases of medullary carcinoma.

While there are some similarities between a basal-like phenotype and medullary carcinoma in terms of pure morphology and immunohistochemical profile, the clinical outcome of the latter is far less ominous than that of "ordinary" basal-like carcinomas. It appears that immunohistochemistry per se does not indicate a specific clinical outlook as adenoid cystic carcinomas share the same immunohistochemical profile with basal-like carcinomas, but are among the least aggressive mammary tumors.

For the present, it is better to regard medullary carcinoma as a specific type of tumor that shares with basal-like carcinoma some morphologic and immunohistochemical features. If the theory of Azzopardi is true, i.e., medullary carcinoma is an in situ DCIS immersed within lymphoid stroma, then the similarity with basal-like carcinoma becomes closer. In fact, poorly differentiated DCIS/DIN3 lesions with an immunophenotype similar to medullary carcinoma and basal-like carcinoma have been reported (83b).

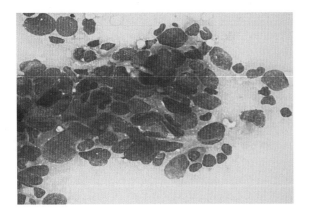

Figure 9-54

MEDULLARY CARCINOMA

FNAC specimen shows nonspecific pleomorphic elements. Background nuclear debris and lymphoid elements are visible.

The lymphoid stroma is composed of T lymphocytes intermingled with plasma cells. The production of immunoglobulin (Ig)A and IgG has been documented (64). The antigenic phenotypes of the lymphocytic infiltrate of medullary carcinoma and infiltrating ductal carcinoma are similar, however (9). Follicles with germinal centers and small granulomas may be present.

Nonspecific T lymphocytic lobulitis is frequently associated with medullary carcinoma and has to be distinguished from the benign lymphoepithelial lesions that accompany lymphoepithelioma-like carcinoma of the breast (see below) (31). The presence or absence of DCIS at the edge of a medullary carcinoma does not change the diagnosis (126).

Cytologic Findings. No specific cytologic features are seen other than smears rich in clumps of cells that can also be isolated. These cells have highly pleomorphic nuclei, intermingled with lymphoid elements. Abundant nuclear debris is present in the background (fig. 9-54). The cytologic findings have to be interpreted carefully when medullary carcinomas are located in the upper outer breast quadrant to avoid confusion with metastatic axillary lymph nodes.

Histogenesis. Typical medullary carcinoma, by definition, consists of a plexiform interconnected architecture, which is the prerequisite for the diagnosis. Whether this type of growth indicates mostly in situ neoplastic extension into lobular acini immersed in a dense lymphoid reactive stroma, as suggested by Azzopardi (6), has not been confirmed as yet. It is very difficult to confirm the presence of myoepithelial cells and basal lamina by immunohistochemistry in structures immersed in lymphoid stroma. Nevertheless, if Azzopardi's theory is verified, then the good prognosis of patients with typical medullary carcinoma is easily understood.

Treatment and Prognosis. Patients with medullary carcinoma have a good prognosis. The 10-year survival rates for patients with typical medullary carcinoma, atypical medullary carcinoma, and nonmedullary duct carcinoma are 84 percent, 74 percent, and 63 percent, respectively. The prognosis of the 26 patients with typical medullary carcinoma from Rapin's series (114) was much more favorable than that for the other two groups: a 10-year disease-free survival rate of 92 percent compared with 53 percent for those with atypical medullary carcinoma and 51 percent for those with nonmedullary duct carcinomas. The tumors in Rapin's study were small, measuring an average of 25 mm. Based on the results of the study, Rapin et al. suggested removal of only typical medullary carcinomas and suggested adjuvant therapy for patients with the other two types. Another study using Ridolfi's classification (84) found that all 13 patients with typical medullary carcinoma were alive at 10 years, while 29 percent and 39 percent of the 47 patients with atypical medullary carcinoma and nonmedullary carcinoma, respectively, died of their disease. The very similar prognosis between the last two groups of patients has led to the proposal to eliminate the atypical medullary carcinoma category.

Axillary lymph node metastases do not exceed three nodes in patients with typical medullary carcinoma (114). No patients with typical medullary carcinoma and axillary metastases died of their disease (117). The only prognostic factor for patients with medullary carcinoma appears to be the microscopic axillary lymph node status: 97.1 percent of patients with pN0 status survived with no evidence of disease at 10 years; in eight patients with axillary involvement, distant metastases appeared after a mean period of 20 months, and all patients died during the first 5 years after treatment (116). This corroborates Azzopardi's statement (6) that "if it [medullary carcinoma] kills, it kills more

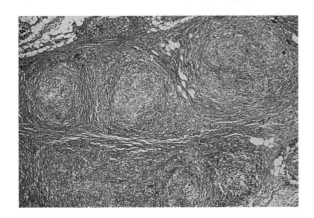

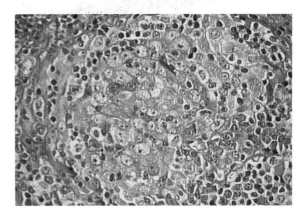

Figure 9-55

LYMPHOEPITHELIOMA-LIKE CARCINOMA

Left: Nodular growth pattern.
Right: The neoplastic elements are cohesive, have indistinct borders, and have an embryonal type of growth reminiscent of the Rigaud pattern.

rapidly. Tumors that prove fatal usually result in death within five years of operation."

LYMPHOEPITHELIOMA-LIKE CARCINOMA

Definition. *Lymphoepithelioma-like carcinoma* (LEC) is composed of undifferentiated malignant epithelial cells and a dense lymphoid stroma. The lesions in the breast are similar to those neoplasms seen in the nasopharynx.

The few reported cases have appeared in the recent literature (28,78,79a). This probably indicates that, in the past, similar cases were included in the medullary carcinoma group.

Clinical Features. The LECs reported to date have been in females from western countries, with exception of one Chinese patient. The age ranged from 43 to 69 years (median, 55 years). One patient had a family history of an established *BRCA1* mutation.

Microscopic Findings. Histologically, one LEC (31) had a Rigaud growth pattern (fig. 9-55) and five had a Schmincke pattern of growth (fig. 9-56). Lymphoid follicles with germinal centers were found in five cases. We have seen one case in which an intramammary lymph node metastasis was simulated (fig. 9-57); the lack of a marginal sinus and a capsule helped establish the correct diagnosis.

In all six cases reported by Dadmanesh et al. (31), benign epithelial cells lined ducts or the small ductules of lobules present at the edges of the lesions. The epithelial cells were surrounded

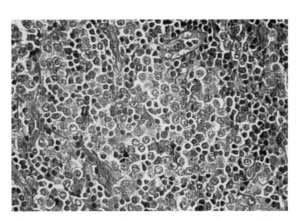

Figure 9-56

LYMPHOEPITHELIOMA-LIKE CARCINOMA

A Schmincke pattern of growth is seen, with single cells reminiscent of lobular carcinoma.

and infiltrated by lymphocytes and plasma cells. These structures mimic benign lymphoepithelial lesions (BLEL) as seen in other sites such as salivary glands (fig. 9-58). These BLEL-like features differ from the pure lymphocytic infiltrate seen around the ducts and in the lobules of medullary carcinoma, which shows no epithelial infiltration. At variance with LEC in other organs, Epstein-Barr virus (EBV) infection is not seen in the breast.

Differential Diagnosis. The lack of a plexiform growth pattern distinguishes LEC from medullary carcinoma. LECs are multinodular tumors that have an invasive border, features not compatible with medullary carcinoma.

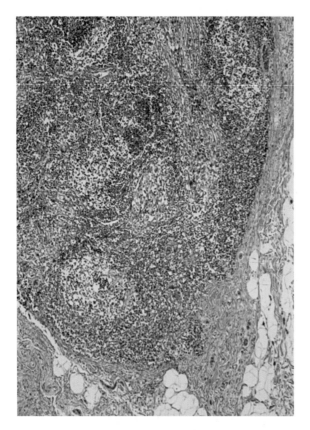

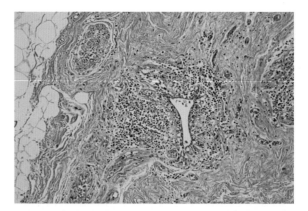

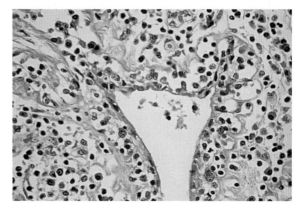

Figure 9-57

LYMPHOEPITHELIOMA-LIKE CARCINOMA

The circumscribed tumor has a lymphoid stroma with germinal centers, simulating an intramammary metastatic lymph node. No marginal sinus is present.

Figure 9-58

LYMPHOEPITHELIOMA-LIKE CARCINOMA

A lymphoepithelial lesion frequently accompanies this lesion. Lymphocytes and plasma cells are present within the glandular epithelium.

Treatment and Prognosis. Four patients with LEC were recurrence free after a median follow-up of 60 months (31). One patient presented with a contralateral LEC 3 years after the primary tumor was removed but was recurrence free 36 months after the second operation. The case reported by Kurose et al. (79a) led to nodal and lung metastases. Although the follow-up was short it was suggested that the good behavior observed in these high-grade tumors may be related to the close association of the malignant epithelium with the dense mononuclear infiltrate (31).

ACINIC CELL CARCINOMA

Definition. *Acinic cell carcinoma* (ACCA) is the breast counterpart of similar tumors that occur in the parotid gland and show acinic cell (serous) differentiation.

Clinical Features. The first case of ACCA of the breast was reported by Roncaroli et al. (121). The lesion is rare since only 15 cases have been reported since (32,109,134). Carcinomas showing serous secretion, and probably related to ACCA, have also been reported in the literature (66).

ACCA affects women between 20 and 80 years of age (mean, 53 years) (32,62). It presents as a palpable nodule ranging from 1 to 5 cm in size.

Pathologic Findings. The tumors vary from well-differentiated, and easily recognizable (fig. 9-59), to poorly differentiated and structurally solid, to microcystic lesions (fig. 9-60) (32,62,109). The case reported by Roncaroli et al. (121) showed comedo-like areas with a rim of microglandular structures at the periphery (figs. 9-61, 9-62).

The cells have abundant granular, amphophilic to eosinophilic cytoplasm that stains consistently with PAS after diastase digestion (fig. 9-63).

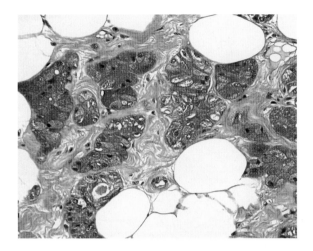

Figure 9-59

ACINIC CELL CARCINOMA

The neoplastic cells have abundant amphophilic to eosinophilic granular cytoplasm.

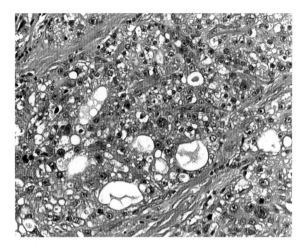

Figure 9-60

ACINIC CELL CARCINOMA: MICROCYSTIC ARCHITECTURE

The neoplastic cells have granular eosinophilic to clear cytoplasm. Nuclei are globoid with prominent nucleoli.

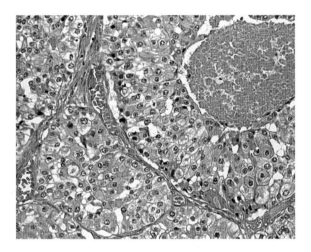

Figure 9-61

ACINIC CELL CARCINOMA: SOLID ARCHITECTURE

The neoplastic cells are clumped in solid nests. Comedo-like necrosis is observed.

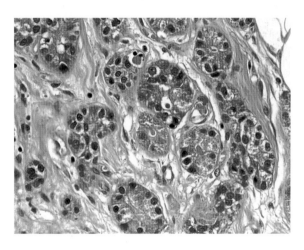

Figure 9-62

ACINIC CELL CARCINOMA: MICROGLANDULAR STRUCTURES

The neoplastic glands have one layer of cuboidal to columnar cells.

The granules may be large and coarse, and bright red (fig. 9-64). Neoplastic cells with clear "hypernephroid" cytoplasm are common (fig. 9-65). The nuclei are irregular, round to ovoid, with single nucleoli. The mitotic count varies and can be up to 15 mitoses per 10 high-power fields (32).

In almost all tumors reported, most of the cells stain intensely for salivary gland amylase (fig. 9-66), lysozyme (fig. 9-67), alpha-1-antichymotrypsin (fig. 9-68) (27,32,62) as well as EMA (fig. 9-69) and S-100 protein antisera (32,109). GCDFP-15 is focally positive. All tumors studied are consistently negative for ER, PR, and AR (109). In three cases so studied, the neoplastic cells showed cytoplasmic electron-dense, zymogen-like granules that measured from 0.08 to 0.9 mm (figs. 9-70, 9-71) (121,134).

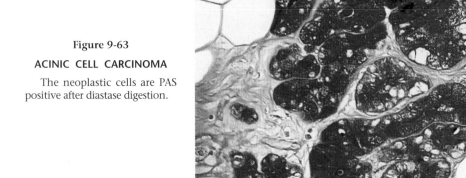

Figure 9-63

ACINIC CELL CARCINOMA

The neoplastic cells are PAS positive after diastase digestion.

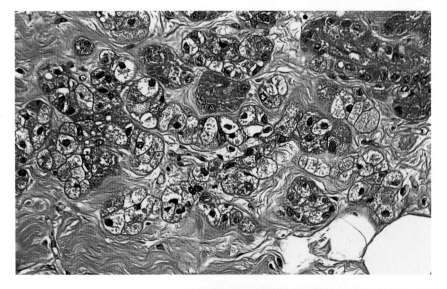

Figure 9-64

ACINIC CELL CARCINOMA

Some cytoplasmic granules are coarse and bright red.

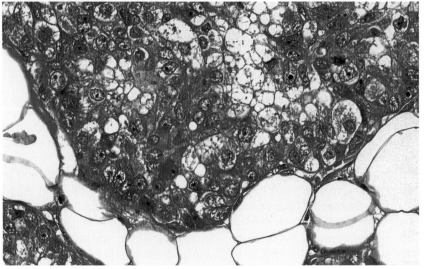

Figure 9-65

ACINIC CELL CARCINOMA

A hypernephroid pattern is seen.

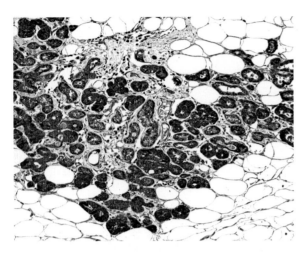

Figure 9-66

ACINIC CELL CARCINOMA

The neoplastic cells are positive for salivary gland amylase.

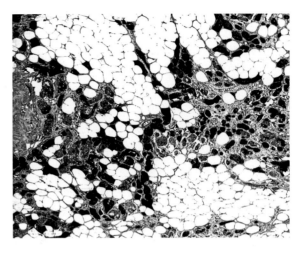

Figure 9-67

ACINIC CELL CARCINOMA

Strong positivity for lysozyme.

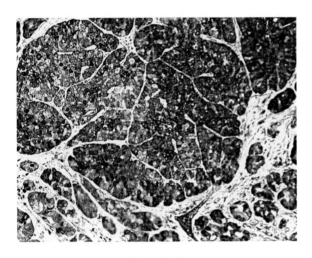

Figure 9-68

ACINIC CELL CARCINOMA

Alpha-1-antichymotrypsin stains the majority of cells.

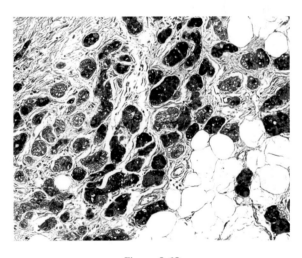

Figure 9-69

ACINIC CELL CARCINOMA

Most of neoplastic cells stain for EMA.

Histogenesis. Hirokawa et al. (62) reported on three cases of ACCA of the breast that superficially resembled secretory carcinoma. Nevertheless, the granularity of the cytoplasm and the hypernephroid features of the neoplastic cells of ACCA, coupled with immunocytochemical positivity for all the proteins present in the salivary gland counterpart, render the resemblance more apparent than real.

Treatment and Prognosis. None of the patients reported so far have died of tumor,

although follow-up was limited to a maximum of 10 years (mean, 3.3 years) (109). In three cases, axillary lymph nodes contained metastases. In three additional cases, recurrence and metastases manifested locally (32) in the liver (27) and lung (109). This led Schmitt et al. (134) to regard ACCA as a breast carcinoma variant with a good prognosis.

Treatment varies from lumpectomy to neoadjuvant chemotherapy and radical mastectomy (109).

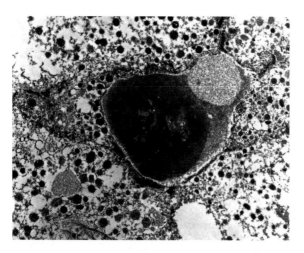

Figure 9-70

ACINIC CELL CARCINOMA

Numerous electron-dense granules are observed throughout the cytoplasm of most of the neoplastic cells.

ACCA Related to Microglandular Adenosis

A case of ACCA that merged with microglandular carcinoma was described by Kahan et al. (71), who suggested a close relationship between the two lesions. One of the typical features of ACCA is the presence of glandular structures similar to those of microglandular carcinoma, whose small glands have been interpreted as the malignant transformation of the small glands that compose microglandular adenosis (68). Koenig et al. (74) described four invasive carcinomas very similar to ACCA that were composed of cells showing cytoplasmic granularity; positivity for alpha-1-antichymotrypsin, lysozyme, antitrypsin, and S-100 protein; and negativity for ER and PR. These cases suggest that the association between microglandular adenosis and microglandular/acinic carcinoma is more than fortuitous, but difficult to judge from the different morphologic, immunohistochemical, and ultrastructural features that distinguish the two entities (Table 9-4) (45,74,134).

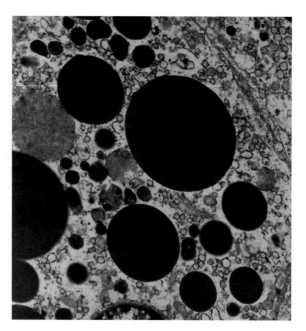

Figure 9-71

ACINIC CELL CARCINOMA

The granules vary greatly in size. (Fig. 7b from Roncaroli F, Lamovec J, Zidar A, Eusebi V. Acinic cell-like carcinoma of the breast. Virchows Arch 1996;429:73.)

Table 9-4

DIFFERENTIATING MICROGLANDULAR ADENOSIS (MGA) AND MICROGLANDULAR/ ACINIC CELL CARCINOMA (MAC/ACCA)

	MGA	MAC/ACCA
Regular nuclei	yes	no
One layer of cells	yes	+/–
Cuboidal cells	yes	+/–
Clear cytoplasm	yes	granular
Luminal content	eosinophilic	+/–
Basal lamina	yes	no
EMA[a]	no	yes
GCDFP-15	no	+/–
EM	empty cytoplasm	dense core granules

[a]EMA = epithelial membrane antigen; GCDFP = gross cystic disease fluid protein; EM = electron microscopy.

REFERENCES

1. Adsay NV, Merati K, Nassar H, et al. Pathogenesis of colloid (pure mucinous) carcinoma of exocrine organs. Coupling of gel-forming mucin (MUC2) production with altered cell polarity and abnormal cell-stroma interaction may be the key factor in the morphogenesis and indolent behavior of colloid carcinoma in the breast and pancreas. Am J Surg Pathol 2003;27:571-578.

2. Andersen JA, Gram JB. Radial scar in the female breast. A long term follow-up study of 32 cases. Cancer 1984;53:2557-2560.

3. André S, Cunha F, Bernardo M, Meneses e Sousa J, Cortez F, Soares J. Mucinous carcinoma of the breast: a pathologic study of 82 cases. J Surg Oncol 1995;58:162-167.

4. Anthony PP, James PD. Adenoid cystic carcinoma of the breast: prevalence, diagnostic criteria, and histogenesis. J Clin Path 1975;28:647-655.

5. Asioli S, Dorji T, Lorenzini P, Eusebi V. Primary neuroendocrine (Merkel cell) carcinoma of the nipple. Virchows Arch 2002;440:443-444.

6. Azzopardi JG. Problems in breast pathology. London: W.B. Saunders Company; 1979.

7. Azzopardi JG, Muretto P, Goddeeris P, Eusebi V, Lauweryns JM. "Carcinoid" tumours of the breast: the morphological spectrum of argyrophil carcinomas. Histopathology 1982;6:549-569.

8. Azzopardi JG, Smith OD. Salivary gland tumours and their mucins. J Path Bacteriol 1959;77:131-140.

8a. Bane AL, Beck JC, Bleiweiss I, et al. BRCA2 mutation-associated breast cancer exhibits a distinguishing phenotype based on morphology and molecular profiles from tissue microarrays. Am J Surg Pathol 2007;31:121-128.

9. Ben-Ezra J, Sheibani K. Antigenic phenotype of the lymphocytic component of medullary carcinoma of the breast. Cancer 1987;59:2037-2041.

10. Bussolati G, Gugliotta P, Sapino A, Eusebi V, Lloyd RV. Chromogranin-reactive endocrine cells in argyrophylic carcinomas ("carcinoids") and normal tissue of the breast. Am J Pathol 1985;120:186-192.

11. Capella C, Eusebi V, Mann B, Azzopardi JG. Endocrine differentiation in mucoid carcinoma of the breast. Histopathology 1980;4:613-630.

12. Capella C, Papotti M, Macrì L, Finzi G, Eusebi V, Bussolati G. Ultrastructural features of neuroendocrine differentiated carcinomas of the breast. Ultrastruct Pathol 1990;14:321-334.

13. Carstens PH. Tubular carcinoma of the breast. A study of frequency. Am J Clin Pathol 1978;70:204-210.

14. Carstens PH, Greenberg RA, Francis D, Lyon H. Tubular carcinoma of the breast. A long term follow up. Histopathology 1985;9:271-280.

15. Caselitz J, Becker J, Saifert G. Coexpression of keratin and vimentin filaments in adenoid cystic carcinoma of salivary glands. Virchows Arch A Pathol Anat Histopathol 1984;403:337-344.

16. Cheng J, Saku T, Okabe H, Furthmayr H. Basement membranes in adenoid cystic carcinoma. An immunohistochemical study. Cancer 1992;69:2631-2640.

17. Chinyama CN, Davies JD. Mammary mucinous lesions: congeners, prevalence and important pathological associations. Histopathology 1996;29:533-539.

18. Clayton F. Pure mucinous carcinomas of breast: morphologic features and prognostic correlations. Hum Pathol 1986;17:34-38.

19. Clayton F, Ordonez NG, Sibley RK, Hanssen G. Argyrophilic breast carcinomas: evidence of lactational differentiation. Am J Surg Pathol 1982;6:323-333.

20. Clement PB, Azzopardi JG. Microglandular adenosis of the breast—a lesion simulating tubular carcinoma. Histopathology 1983;7:169-180.

21. Clement PB, Young RH, Azzopardi JG. Collagenous spherulosis of the breast. Am J Surg Pathol 1987;11:411-417.

22. Coady AT, Shousha S, Dawson PM, Moss M, James KR, Bull TB. Mucinous carcinoma of the breast: further characterization of its three subtypes. Histopathology 1989;15:617-626.

23. Cohle SD, Tschen J, Smith FE, Lane M, McGavran MH. ACTH-secreting carcinoma of the breast. Cancer 1979;43:2370-2376.

24. Colome MI, Ro JY, Ayala AG, El-Naggar A, Siddiqui RT, Ordonez NG. Adenoid cystic carcinoma of the breast metastatic to the kidney. Journal of Urologic Pathology 1996;4:69-78.

25. Coombes RC, Easty GC, Detre SI, et al. Secretion of immunoreactive calcitonin by human breast carcinomas. Br Med J 1975;4:197-199.

26. Cooper HS, Patchefsky AS, Krall RA. Tubular carcinoma of the breast. Cancer 1978;42:2334-2342.

27. Coyne JD, Dervan PA. Primary acinic cell carcinoma of the breast. J Clin Path 2002;55:545-547.

28. Cristina S, Boldorini R, Brustia F, Monga G. Lymphoepithelioma-like carcinoma of the breast. An unusual pattern of infiltrating lobular carcinoma. Virchows Arch 2000;437:198-202.

29. Cross AS, Azzopardi JG, Krausz T, Van Noorden S, Polak JM. A morphological and immunocytochemical study of a distinctive variant of ductal carcinoma in situ of the breast. Histopathology 1985;9:21-37.

30. Cubilla AL, Woodruff JM. Primary carcinoid tumor of the breast. A report of eight patients. Am J Surg Pathol 1977;1:283-292.

31. Dadmanesh F, Peterse JL, Sapino A, Fornelli A, Eusebi V. Lymphoepithelioma-like carcinoma of the breast: lack of evidence of Epstein-Barr virus infection. Histopathology 2001;38:54-61.

32. Damiani S, Pasquinelli G, Lamovec J, Peterse JL, Eusebi V. Acinic cell carcinoma of the breast: an immunohistochemical and ultrastructural study. Virchows Arch 2000;437:78-81.

33. Davies JD. Hyperelastosis, obliteration and fibrous plaques in major ducts of the human breast. J Pathol 1973;110:13-26.

34. Del Vecchio M, Eusebi V. Tumors of the breast showing dual differentiation: a review. Intern J Surg Pathol 2004;12:345-350.

35. Deos PH, Norris HJ. Well-differentiated (tubular) carcinoma of the breast. A clinicopathologic study of 145 pure and mixed cases. Am J Clin Pathol 1982;78:1-7.

36. Di Palma S, Andreola S, Lombardi L, Colombo C. Ileal carcinoid metastatic to the breast. Report of a case. Tumori 1988;74:321-327.

37. Diab SG, Clark GM, Osborne CK, Libby A, Allred DC, Elledge RM. Tumor characteristics and clinical outcome of tubular and mucinous breast carcinomas. J Clin Oncol 1999;17:1442-1448.

38. Ekblom P, Miettinen M, Forsman L, Andersson LC. Basement membrane and apocrine epithelial antigens in differential diagnosis between tubular carcinoma and sclerosing adenosis of the breast. J Clin Path 1984;37:357-363.

39. Ellis IO, Galea M, Broughton N, Locker A, Blamey RW, Elston CW. Pathological prognostic factors in breast cancer. II. Histological type. Relationship with survival in a large study with long-term follow-up. Histopathology 1992;20:479-489.

40. Ellis IO, Pinder SE, Lee AH, Elston CW. Tumors of the breast. In: Fletcher CD, ed. Diagnostic histopathology of tumors, 3rd ed. Philadelphia: Churchill Livingstone; 2007:865-930.

41. Elston CW, Ellis IO. The breast, 2nd ed. Edinburgh: Churchill Livingstone; 1998.

42. Erlandson RA, Carstens HB. Ultrastructure of tubular carcinoma of the breast. Cancer 1973; 29:987-995.

43. Eusebi V, Betts CM, Bussolati G. Tubular carcinoma: a variant of secretory breast carcinoma. Histopathology 1979;3:407-419.

44. Eusebi V, Damiani S, Riva C, Lloyd RV, Capella C. Calcitonin free oat-cell carcinoma of the thyroid gland. Virchows Arch A Pathol Anat Histopathol 1990;417:267-271.

45. Eusebi V, Foschini MP, Betts CM, et al. Microglandular adenosis, apocrine adenosis, and tubular carcinoma of the breast. An immunohistochemical comparison. Am J Surg Pathol 1993;17:99-109.

46. Eusebi V, Grassigli A, Grosso F. [Breast sclero-elastotic focal lesions simulating infiltrating carcinoma.] Pathologica 1976;68:507-518. [Italian.]

47. Fechner RE. Histologic variants of infiltrating lobular carcinoma of the breast. Hum Pathol 1975;6:373-378.

48. Fentiman IS, Millis RR, Smith P, Ellul JP, Lampejo O. Mucoid breast carcinomas: histology and prognosis. Br J Cancer 1997;75:1061-1065.

49. Ferguson DJ, Anderson TJ, Wells CA, Battersby S. An ultrastructural study of mucoid carcinoma of the breast: variability of cytoplasmic features. Histopathology 1986;10:1219-1230.

50. Fernandez-Aguilar S, Simon P, Buxant F, Simonart T, Noel JC. Tubular carcinoma of the breast and associated intra-epithelial lesions: a comparative study with invasive low-grade ductal carcinomas. Virchows Arch 2005;447:683-687.

51. Fisher CJ, Millis RR. A mucocele-like tumour of the breast associated with both atypical ductal hyperplasia and mucoid carcinoma. Histopathology 1992;21:69-71.

52. Fisher ER, Gregorio RM, Redmond C, Fisher B. Tubulolobular invasive breast cancer: a variant of lobular invasive cancer. Hum Pathol 1977;8:679-683.

53. Flotte TJ, Bell DA, Greco MA. Tubular carcinoma and sclerosing adenosis: the use of basal lamina as a differential feature. Am J Surg Pathol 1980;4:75-77.

54. Foschini MP, Fornelli A, Peterse JL, Mignani S, Eusebi V. Microcalcifications in ductal carcinoma in situ of the breast. Hum Pathol 1996;27:178-183.

55. Foschini MP, Fulcheri E, Baracchini P, Ceccarelli C, Betts CM, Eusebi V. Squamous cell carcinoma with prominent myxoid stroma. Hum Pathol 1990;21:859-865.

56. Foschini MP, Pizzicannella G, Peterse JL, Eusebi V. Adenomyoepithelioma of the breast associated with low-grade adenosquamous and sarcomatoid carcinomas. Virchows Arch 1995;427:243-250.

57. Gad A, Azzopardi JG. Lobular carcinoma of the breast: a special variant of mucin-secreting carcinoma. J Clin Pathol 1975;28:711-716.

58. Geschickter CF. Diseases of the breast; diagnosis, pathology, teatment, 2nd ed. Philadelphia: JB Lippincott Co; 1945.

59. Green I, McCormick B, Cranor M, Rosen PP. A comparative study of pure tubular and tubulolobular carcinoma of the breast. Am J Surg Pathol 1997;21:653-657.

60. Hamele-Bena D, Cranor ML, Rosen PP. Mammary mucocele-like lesions. Benign and malignant. Am J Surg Pathol 1996;20:1081-1085.

61. Hamperl H. [Radial scars and obliterating mastopathy.] Virchows Arch A Pathol Anat Histopathol 1975;369:55-68. [German.]

62. Hirokawa M, Sugihara K, Sai T, et al. Secretory carcinoma of the breast: a tumour analogous to salivary gland acinic cell carcinoma? Histopathology 2002;40:223-229.

63. Holland R, van Haelst JM. Mammary carcinoma with osteoclast-like giant cells. Additional observations on six cases. Cancer 1984;53:1963-1973.

64. Hsu SM, Raine L, Nayak RN. Medullary carcinoma of the breast: an immunohistochemical study of its lymphoid stroma. Cancer 1981;48:1368-1376.

65. Iau PT, Marafie M, Ali A, et al. Are medullary breast cancers an indication for BRCA1 mutation screening? A mutation analysis of 42 cases of medullary breast cancer. Breast Cancer Res Treat 2004;85:81-88.

66. Inaji H, Koyama H, Higashiyama M, et al. Immunohistochemical, ultrastructural and biochemical studies of an amylase-producing breast carcinoma. Virchows Arch A Pathol Anat Histopathol 1991;419:29-33.

67. Jacquemier J, Padovani L, Rabayrol L, et al. Typical medullary breast carcinomas have a basal/myoepithelial phenotype. J Pathol 2005;207:260-268.

68. James BA, Cranor ML, Rosen PP. Carcinoma of the breast arising in microglandular adenosis. Am J Clin Pathol 1993:100;507-513.

69. Jao W, Recant W, Swerdlow MA. Comparative ultrastructure of tubular carcinoma and sclerosing adenosis of the breast. Cancer 1976;38:180-186.

69a. Jones C, Nonni AV, Fulford L, et al. CGH analysis of ductal carcinoma of the breast with basaloid/myoepithelial cell differentiation. Br J Cancer 2001;85:422-427.

70. Kader HA, Jackson J, Mates D, Andersen S, Hayes M, Olivotto IA. Tubular carcinoma of the breast: a population-based study of nodal metatases at presentation and of patterns of relapse. Breast J 2001;7:8-13.

71. Kahn R, Holtveg H, Nissen F, Holck S. Are acinic cell carcinoma and microglandular carcinoma of the breast related lesions? Histopathology 2003;42:195-196.

72. Kaneko H, Hojo H, Ishikawa S, Yamanouchi H, Sumida T, Saito R. Norepinephrine-producing tumors of bilateral breasts: a case report. Cancer 1978;41:2002-2007.

73. Kasami M, Olson SJ, Simpson JF, Page DL. Maintenance of polarity and a dual cell population in adenoid cystic carcinoma of the breast: an immunohistochemical study. Histopathology 1998;32:232-238.

74. Koenig C, Dadmanesh F, Bratthauer GL, Tavassoli FA. Carcinoma arising in microglandular adenosis: an immunohistochemical analysis of 20 intraepithelial and invasive neoplasms. Int J Surg Pathol 2000;8:303-315.

75. Koenig C, Tavassoli FA. Mucinous cystadeno-carcinoma of the breast. Am J Surg Pathol 1998;22:698-703.

76. Komaki K, Sakamoto G, Sugano H, Morimoto T, Monden Y. Mucinous carcinoma of the breast in Japan. A prognostic analysis based on morphologic features. Cancer 1988;61:989-996.

77. Koss LG, Brannan CD, Ashikari R. Histologic and ultrastructural features of adenoid cystic carcinoma of the breast. Cancer 1970;26:1271-1279.

78. Kumar S, Kumar D. Lymphoepithelioma-like carcinoma of the breast. Mod Pathol 1994;7:129-131.

79. Kuroda H, Tamaru J, Takeuchi I, et al. Expression of E-cadherin, alpha-catenin, and beta-catenin in tubulolobular carcinoma of the breast. Virchows Arch 2006;448:500-505.

79a. Kurose A, Ichinohasama R, Kanno H, et al. Lymphoepithelioma-like carcinoma of the breast. Report of a case with the first electron microscopic study and review of the literature. Virchows Arch 2005;447:653-659.

80. Kurosumi M, Era H, Sano Y, Kuwashima Y, Kishi K, Suemasu K, Higashi Y. Fine needle aspiration cytology of argyrophilic mucinous carcinoma of the male breast. Breast Cancer 1996;3:53-56.

81. Lagios MD, Rose MR, Margolin FR. Tubular carcinoma of the breast: association with multicentricity, bilaterality and family history of mammary carcinoma. Am J Clin Pathol 1980;73:25-30.

82. Lakhani SR, Jacquemier J, Sloane JP, et al. Multifactorial analysis of differences between sporadic breast cancers and cancers involving BRCA1 and BRCA2 mutations. J Natl Cancer Inst 1998;90:1138-1145.

83. Lamovec J, Us-Krasovec M, Zidar A, Kljiun A. Adenoid cystic carcinoma of the breast: a histologic, cytologic and immunohistochemical study. Semin Diagn Pathol 1989;6:153-164.

83a. Livasy CA, Karaca G, Nanda R, et al. Phenotypic evaluation of the basal-like subtype of invasive breast carcinoma. Mod Pathol 2006;85:422-427.

83b. Livasy CA, Perou CM, Karaca G, et al. Identification of a basal-like subtype of breast ductal carcinoma in situ. Hum Pathol 2007;38:197-204.

83c. Lorenzo Bermejo J, Hemminki K. Familial association of histology specific breast cancers with cancers at other sites. Int J Cancer 2004;109:430-435.

84. Jensen ML, Kiaer H, Andersen J, Jensen V, Melsen F. Prognostic comparison of three classifications for medullary carcinomas of the breast. Histopathology 1997;30:523-532.

85. Linell F. Radial scars of the breast and their significance for diagnosis and prognosis. Verh Dtsch Ges Pathol 1985;69:108-118.

86. Linell F, Ljunberg O, Andersson I. Breast carcinoma. Aspects of early stages, progression and related problems. Acta Pathol Microbiol Scand Suppl 1980;272:1-233.

87. Luna-More S, de los Santos F, Breton JJ. Estrogen and progesterone receptors, c-erbB-2, p53, and Bcl-2 in thirty-three invasive micropapillary breast carcinomas. Pathol Res Pract 1996;192:27-32.

88. Maluf HM, Koerner FC. Carcinomas of the breast with endocrine differentiation: a review. Virchows Arch 1994;425:449-457.

89. Maluf HM, Koerner FC. Solid papillary carcinoma of the breast. A form of intraductal carcinoma with endocrine differentiation frequently associated with mucinous carcinoma. Am J Surg Pathol 1995;19:1237-1244.

90. Maluf HM, Zukerberg LR, Dickersin GR, Koerner FC. Spindle cell argyrophilic mucin-producing carcinoma of the breast. Histological, ultrastructural and immunohistochemical studies of two cases. Am J Surg Pathol 1991;15:677-686.

91. Man S, Ellis IO, Sibbering M, Blamey RW, Brook JD. High levels of allele loss at the FHIT and ATM genes in non-comedo ductal carcinoma in situ and grade I tubular invasive breast cancers. Cancer Res 1996;56:5484-5489.

92. McDivitt RW, Boyce W, Gersell D. Tubular carcinoma of the breast. Clinical and pathological observations concerning 135 cases. Am J Surg Pathol 1982;6:401-411.

93. Miremadi A, Pinder SE, Lee AH, et al. Neuroendocrine differentiation and prognosis in breast adenocarcinoma. Histopathology 2002;40:215-222.

94. Moinfar F, Man Y, Lininger RA, Bodian C, Tavassoli FA. Use of keratin 34betaE12 as an adjunct in the diagnosis of mammary intraepithelial neoplasia-ductal type—benign and malignant intraductal proliferations. Am J Surg Pathol 1999;23:1048-1058.

95. Nassar H, Pansare V, Zhang H, et al. Pathogenesis of invasive micropapillary carcinoma: role of MUC1 glycoprotein. Mod Pathol 2004;17:1045-1050.

96. Nielsen M, Jensen J, Andersen JA. An autopsy study of radial scar in the female breast. Histopathology 1985;9:287-295.

97. Nielsen TO, Hsu FD, Jensen K, et al. Immunohistochemical and clinical characterization of the basal-like subtype of invasive breast carcinoma. Clin Canc Res 2004;10:5367-5374.

98. Norris HJ, Taylor HB. Prognosis of mucinous (gelatinous) carcinoma of the breast. Cancer 1965;18:879-885.

99. O'Connell JT, Shao ZM, Drori E, Basbaum CB, Barsky SH. Altered mucin expression is a field change that accompanies mucinous (colloid) breast carcinoma histogenesis. Hum Pathol 1998;29:1517-1523.

100. Oberman HA, Fidler WJ Jr. Tubular carcinoma of the breast. Am J Surg Pathol 1979;193:387-395.

101. Osborn DA. Morphology and the natural history of cribriform adenocarcinoma (adenoid cystic carcinoma). J Clin Path 1977;30:195-205.

102. Page DL, Dixon JM, Anderson TJ, Lee D, Stewart HJ. Invasive cribriform carcinoma of the breast. Histopathology 1983;7:525-536.

103. Papadatos G, Rangan AM, Psarianos T, Ung O, Taylor R, Boyages J. Probability of axillary node involvement in patients with tubular carcinoma of the breast. Br J Surg 2001;88:860-864.

104. Papotti M, Gherardi G, Eusebi V, Pagani A, Bussolati G. Primary oat cell (neuroendocrine) carcinoma of the breast. Virchows Arch A Pathol Anat Histopathol 1992;420:103-108.

105. Papotti M, Macrì L, Finzi G, Capella C, Eusebi V, Bussolati G. Neuroendocrine differentiation in carcinomas of the breast: a study of 51 cases. Semin Diagn Pathol 1989;6:174-188.

106. Patchefsky AS, Shaber GS, Schwartz GF, Feig SA, Nerlinger RE. The pathology of the breast cancer detected by mass population screening. Cancer 1977;40:1659-1670.

107. Pedersen L, Holck S, Schiodt T, Zedeler K, Mouridsen HT. Inter- and intraobserver variability in the histopathological diagnosis of medullary carcinoma of the breast, and its prognostic implications. Breast Cancer Res Treat 1989;14:91-99.

108. Pedersen L, Zedeler K, Holck S, Schiodt T, Mouridsen HT. Medullary carcinoma of the breast, proposal for a new simplified histopathological definition. Based on prognostic observations and observations on inter- and intraobserver variability of 11 histopathological characteristics in 131 breast carcinomas with medullary features. Br J Cancer 1991;63:591-595.

109. Peintinger F, Leibl S, Reitsamer R, Moinfar F. Primary acinic cell carcinoma of the breast: a case report with long-term follow-up and review of the literature. Histopathology 2004;45:645-646.

109a. Perou CM, Sorlie T, Eisen MB, et al. Molecular portraits of human breast tumours. Nature 2000;406:747-752.

110. Peters GN, Wolff M. Adenoid cystic carcinoma of the breast. Report of 11 new cases: review of the literature and discussion of biological behavior. Cancer 1982;52:680-686.

111. Peters GN, Wolff M, Haagensen CD. Tubular carcinoma of the breast. Clinical pathologic correlations based on 100 cases. Ann Surg 1981; 113:138-149.

111a. Pia-Foschini M, Reis-Filho JS, Eusebi V, Lakhani SR. Salivary gland-like tumours of the breast: surgical and molecular pathology. J Clin Pathol 2003;56:497-506.

112. Qizilbash AH, Patterson MC, Oliveira KF. Adenoid cystic carcinoma of the breast. Light and electron microscopy and a brief review of the literature. Arch Pathol Lab Med 1977;101:302-306.

113. Rajakariar R, Walker RA. Pathological and biological features of mammographically detected invasive breast carcinomas. Br J Cancer 1995;71:150-154.

113a. Rakha EA, El-Rehim DM, Paish C, et al. Morphological and immunophenotypic analysis of breast cacinomas with basal and myoepithelial differentiation. J Pathol 2006;208:495-506.

114. Rapin V, Contesso G, Mouriesse H, et al. Medullary breast carcinoma. A reevaluation of 95 cases of breast cancer with inflammatory stroma. Cancer 1988;61:2503-2510.

115. Rasmussen BB, Rose C, Christensen I. Prognostic factors in primary mucinous breast carcinoma. Am J Clin Pathol 1987;87:155-160.

116. Reinfuss M, Stelmach A, Mitus J, Rys J, Duda K. Typical medullary carcinoma of the breast: a clinical and pathological analysis of 52 cases. J Surg Oncol 1995;60:89-94.

117. Ridolfi RL, Rosen PP, Port A, Kinne D, Mikè V. Medullary carcinoma of the breast: a clinicopathologic study with 10 year follow up. Cancer 1977;40:1365-1385.

118. Rigaud C, Theobald S, Noel P, et al. Medullary carcinoma in the breast. A multicenter study of its diagnostic consistency. Arch Pathol Lab Med 1993;117:1005-1008.

119. Ro JY, Silva EG, Gallager HS. Adenoid cystic carcinoma of the breast. Hum Pathol 1987;18:1276-1281.

120. Ro JY, Sneige N, Sahin AA, Silva EG, del Junco GW, Ayala AG. Mucocele-like tumor of the breast associated with atypical ductal hyperplasia or mucinous carcinoma. Arch Pathol Lab Med 1991;115:137-140.

120a. Rodriguez-Pinilla SM, Rodriguez-Gil Y, Moreno-Bueno G, et al. Sporadic invasive breast carcinomas with medullary features display a basal-like phenotype: an immunohistochemical and gene amplification study. Am J Surg Pathol 2007;31:501-508.

121. Roncaroli F, Lamovec J, Zidar A, Eusebi V. Acinic cell-like carcinoma of the breast. Virchows Arch 1996;429:69-74.

122. Rosai J. Ackerman's surgical pathology, 8th ed. St. Louis: Mosby; 1996.

123. Rosen PP. Microglandular adenosis. A benign lesion simulating invasive mammary carcinoma. Am J Surg Pathol 1983;7:137-144.

124. Rosen PP. Mucocele-like tumors of the breast. Am J Surg Pathol 1986;10:464-469.

125. Rosen PP. Adenoid cystic carcinoma of the breast. A morphologically heterogeneous neoplasm. Path Annu 1989;24:237-254.

126. Rosen PP. Rosen's breast pathology, 2nd ed. Philadelphia: Lippincott Williams & Wilkins; 2001.

127. Ruffolo EF, Maluf HM, Koerner FC. Spindle cell endocrine carcinoma of the mammary gland. Virchows Arch 1996;428:319-324.

128. Saez C, Japon MA, Poveda MA, Segura DI. Mucinous (colloid) adenocarcinomas secrete distinct O-acylated forms of sialomucins: a histochemical study of gastric, colorectal and breast adenocarcinomas. Histopathology 2001;39:554-560.

129. Sapino A, Bussolati G. Is detection of endocrine cells in breast adenocarcinoma of diagnostic and clinical significance? Histopathology 2002;40:211-214.

130. Sapino A, Papotti M, Pietribiasi F. Diagnostic cytological features of neuroendocrine differentiated carcinoma of the breast. Virchows Arch 1998;433:217-222.

131. Sapino A, Papotti M, Righi L, Cassoni P, Chiusa L, Bussolati G. Clinical significance of neuroendocrine carcinoma of the breast. Ann Oncol 2001;12:115-117.

132. Sapino A, Righi L, Cassoni P, Papotti M, Gugliotta P, Bussolati G. Expression of apocrine differentiation markers in neuroendocrine breast carcinomas of aged women. Mod Pathol 2001;14:768-776.

133. Sapino A, Righi L, Cassoni P, Papotti M, Pietribiasi F, Bussolati G. Expression of the neuroendocrine phenotype in carcinomas of the breast. Semin Diagn Pathol 2000;17:127-137.

134. Schmitt FC, Ribeiro CA, Alvarenga S, Lopes JM. Primary acinic cell-like carcinoma of the breast —a variant with good prognosis? Histopathology 2000;36:286-289.

135. Scopsi L, Andreola S, Pilotti S, et al. Mucinous carcinoma of the breast. A clinicopathologic, histochemical, and immunocytochemical study with special reference to neuroendocrine differentiation. Am J Surg Pathol 1994;18:702-711.

136. Scopsi L, Andreola S, Pilotti S, et al. Argyrophilia and granin (chromogranin/secretogranin) expression in female breast carcinomas. Their relationship to survival and other disease parameters. Am J Surg Pathol 1992;16:561-576.

137. Scopsi L, Andreola S, Saccozzi R, et al. Argyrophilic carcinoma of the male breast. A neuroendocrine tumor containing predominantly chromogranin B (secretogranin I). Am J Surg Pathol 1991;15:1063-1071.

138. Sgroi D, Koerner FC. Involvement of collagenous spherulosis by lobular carcinoma in situ. Potential confusion with cribriform ductal carcinoma. Am J Surg Pathol 1995;19:1366-1370.

139. Shin SJ, DeLellis RA, Rosen PP. Small cell carcinoma of the breast. Additional immunohistochemical studies. Am J Surg Pathol 2001;25:831-832.

140. Shin SJ, DeLellis RA, Ying L, Rosen PP. Small cell carcinoma of the breast. A clinicopathologic and immunohistochemical study of nine patients. Am J Surg Pathol 2000;24:1231-1238.

141. Shousha S. Medullary carcinoma of the breast and BRCA1 mutation. Histopathology 2000;37:182-185.

142. Shousha S, Coady AT, Stamp T, James KR, Alaghband-Zadeh J. Oestrogen receptors in mucinous carcinoma of the breast: an immunohistological study using paraffin wax sections. J Clin Path 1989;42:902-905.

143. Silverberg SG, Kay S, Chitale AR, Levitt SH. Colloid carcinoma of the breast. Am J Clin Pathol 1971;55:355-363.

144. Sloane JP, Trott PA, Lakhani SR. Biopsy pathology of the breast, 2nd ed. London: Oxford Univ. Press; 2001.

145. Sloane JP, Amendoeira I, Apostolikas N, et al. Consistency achieved by 23 European pathologists from 12 countries in diagnosing breast disease and reporting prognostic features of carcinomas. European Commission Working Group on Breast Screening Pathology. Virchows Arch 1999;434:3-10.

146. Solcia E, Kloppel G, Sobin L. Histological typing of endocrine tumours, 2nd ed. WHO. Berlin: Springer; 2000.

146a. Sorlie T, Perou CM, Tibshirani R, et al. Gene expression patterns of breast carcinomas distinguish tumor subclasses with clinical implications. Proc Natl Acad Sci U S A 2001;98:10869-10874.

147. Stewart FW. Tumors of the breast. Washington, DC: AFIP; 1950.

148. Sumpio BE, Jennings TA, Merino MJ, Sullivan PD. Adenoid cystic carcinoma of the breast. Data from the Connecticut Tumor Registry and a review of the literature. Ann Surg 1987;205:295-301.

149. Tavassoli FA. Pathology of the breast, 2nd ed. Stamford: Appleton-Lange; 1999.

150. Tavassoli FA, Bratthauer GL. Immunohistochemical profile and differential diagnosis of microglandular adenosis. Mod Pathol 1993;6:318-322.

151. Tavassoli FA, Norris HJ. Mammary adenoid cystic carcinoma with sebaceous differentiation. A morphologic study of cell types. Arch Pathol Lab Med 1986;110:1045-1053.

152. Taxy JB. Tubular carcinoma of the male breast: report of a case. Cancer 1975;36:462-465.

152a. Taxy JB, Tischler AS, Insalaco SJ, Battifora H. "Carcinoid" tumor of the breast. A variant of conventional breast cancer? Hum Pathol 1981;12:170-179.

153. Taylor HB, Norris HJ. Well-differentiated carcinoma of the breast. Cancer 1970;25:687-692.

154. Tobon H, Salazar H. Tubular carcinoma of the breast. Clinical, histological and ultrastructural observations. Arch Pathol Lab Med 1977;101:310-316.

155. Toikkanen S, Kujari H. Pure and mixed mucinous carcinomas of the breast: a clinicopathologic analysis of 61 cases with long-term follow-up. Hum Pathol 1989;20:758-764.

156. Tot T. The cytokeratin profile of medullary carcinoma of the breast. Histopathology 2000;37:175-181.

157. Tremblay G. Elastosis in tubular carcinoma of the breast. Arch Pathol 1974;98:302-307.

158. Trendell-Smith NJ, Peston D, Shousha S. Adenoid cystic carcinoma of the breast: a tumor commonly devoid of oestrogen receptors and related proteins. Histopathology 1999;35:241-248.

159. Van Bogaert LJ. Clinicopathologic hallmarks of mammary tubular carcinoma. Hum Pathol 1982;13:558-562.

160. Van Dorpe J, De Pauw A, Moerman P. Adenoid cystic carcinoma arising in an adenomyoepithelioma of the breast. Virchows Arch 1998;432:119-122.

161. Van Hoeven KH, Drudis T, Cranor ML, Erlandson RA, Rosen PP. Low-grade adenosquamous carcinoma of the breast. A clinicopathologic study of 32 cases with ultrastructural analysis. Am J Surg Pathol 1993;17:248-258.

162. Vega A, Garijo F. Radial scar and tubular carcinoma. Mammographic and sonographic findings. Acta Radiol 1993;34:43-47.

163. Venable JG, Schwartz AM, Silverberg SG. Infiltrating cribriform carcinoma of the breast: a distinctive clinicopathologic entity. Hum Pathol 1990;21:333-338.

164. Viacava P, Castagna M, Bevilacqua G. Absence of neuroendocrine cells in fetal and adult mammary glands. Are neuroendocrine breast tumours real neuroendocrine tumours? Breast 1995;4:143-146.

165. Waldman FM, Hwang ES, Etzell J, et al. Genomic alterations in tubular breast carcinomas. Hum Pathol 2001;32:222-226.

166. Wargotz ES, Norris HJ. Metaplastic carcinoma of the breast. I. Matrix-producing carcinoma. Hum Pathol 1989;20:628-635.

167. Wargotz ES, Silverberg SG. Medullary carcinoma of the breast: a clinicopathological study with appraisal of current diagnostic criteria. Hum Pathol 1988;19:1340-1346.

168. Weaver MG, Abdul-Karim FW, Al-Kaisi N. Mucinous lesions of the breast. A pathological continuum. Pathol Res Pract 1993;189:873-876.

169. Wells CA, Nicoll S, Ferguson DJ. Adenoid cystic carcinoma of the breast: a case with axillary lymph node metastasis. Histopathology 1986;10:415-424.

170. Wheeler DT, Tai LH, Brathauer GL, Waldner DL, Tavassoli FA. Tubulolobular carcinoma of the breast: an analysis of 27 cases of a tumor with a hybrid morphology and immunoprofile. Am J Surg Pathol 2004;28:1587-1593.

171. Zaloudek C, Oertel YC, Orenstein JM. Adenoid cystic carcinoma of the breast. Am J Clin Pathol 1984;81:297-307.

10 UNCOMMON VARIANTS OF CARCINOMA

This chapter describes a variety of uncommon breast carcinomas with distinctive (special) morphologic patterns, even if their behavior is not always substantially different from the more common infiltrating ductal carcinomas. It is possible that once we discover the molecular alterations responsible for the specific morphologies of these lesions, we may be able to use alternative approaches to their management, improving survival and chances of cure.

METAPLASTIC CARCINOMA

Metaplastic carcinoma comprises a heterogeneous group of neoplasms generally characterized by an intimate admixture of adenocarcinoma with areas of spindle, squamous, chondroid, and osseous differentiation; the metaplastic spindle and squamous carcinomas may be present in pure form, without any recognizable adenocarcinoma component. Either purely epithelial or with a mesenchymal component, classification according to the apparent phenotype of the tumor is now required. If the tumor shows pure squamous differentiation, it is designated as squamous carcinoma. If the adenocarcinoma shows osseous differentiation, it is designated as such. Immunohistochemical confirmation is required for precise classification. The classification of metaplastic carcinomas into specific variants is illustrated in Table 10-1. More than one pattern of carcinoma and even melanoma may develop in these tumors (21a).

First described by Huvos et al. (12), the average age of the patients with metaplastic carcinoma, the clinical presentation, and the overall 5-year survival rate of 55 percent were similar to such findings in patients with regular infiltrating duct carcinoma. When patients with tumors showing spindle and squamous differentiation were combined in one group, they had a 63 percent 5-year survival rate and 56 percent of the women had axillary node metastases. Only 19 percent of patients with neoplasms showing osseous and chondroid differentiation had axil-

Table 10-1

CLASSIFICATION OF METAPLASTIC CARCINOMAS

Purely Epithelial Carcinoma
Squamous Carcinoma
  Large cell type, keratinizing or nonkeratinizing
  Squamous carcinoma with spindle cell metaplasia
    (with or without acantholytic changes)
Adenosquamous Carcinoma
  High grade
  Low grade
Adenocarcinoma with Spindle Cell Metaplasia

Mixed Epithelial and Mesenchymal Carcinoma
Carcinoma with chondroid differentiation
Carcinoma with osseous differentiation
Carcinoma with rhabdomyosarcomatous component
Carcinosarcoma

lary node metastases and their 5-year survival rate was 28 percent.

There is little information available on the efficacy of current therapies in the management of metaplastic carcinoma. Most studies that have addressed treatment of these lesions have not separated the subtypes, unfortunately. Rayson et al. (23) found that the 27 patients with metaplastic carcinomas diagnosed at the Mayo Clinic were more commonly (87 percent) node negative at presentation, and had a 3-year overall survival rate of 71 percent. About 50 percent of the women developed metastases, with a median disease-free survival period of 2.4 years; median survival after the development of metastases was 8 months. It was concluded that patients with metaplastic carcinoma, particularly those with metastatic disease, could be appropriate candidates for innovative therapeutic regimens since systemic therapy appeared to be less effective in their management. Based on a smaller number of cases, others have advocated that surgical and adjuvant therapy should follow the guidelines used for common breast cancers (1). In the experience of the European Institute of Oncology (17e), the overall survival rate of patients with metaplastic carcinoma was significantly

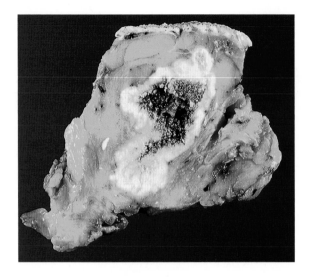

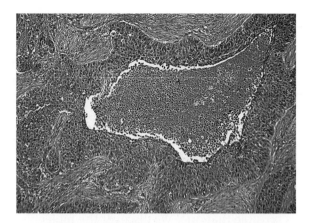

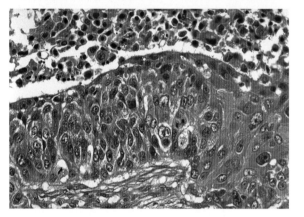

Figure 10-1

SQUAMOUS CARCINOMA

A typical sharply delineated lesion with a central cyst. (Courtesy of Dr. Okcu, Austria.)

Figure 10-2

SQUAMOUS CARCINOMA

Top: An irregularly shaped cyst is lined by moderately differentiated squamous epithelium.

Bottom: The cells lining the cyst are often moderately to well differentiated.

worse than that of a control group with poorly differentiated ductal carcinomas. There was no significant difference in the disease-free survival rate between the two groups, however.

PURE EPITHELIAL VARIANTS OF METAPLASTIC CARCINOMA

Squamous Carcinoma

Definition. *Squamous carcinoma* is composed exclusively of squamous cells, which may be keratinizing, nonkeratinizing, or spindled, and clearly not derived from the overlying skin or from other sites.

Clinical Features. Squamous carcinomas account for significantly less than 1 percent of all invasive breast carcinomas. Patients range in age from the late 20s to the mid 90s, with a mean age of 53 years (2–4,19,31,36). They present with a palpable mass that may get large enough to ulcerate through the skin. An origin from the overlying skin should be excluded. This can be difficult in cases in which large tumors become fixed to the skin or ulcerate through it. The mammographic presentation is a mass lesion. Calcification rarely occurs, and there are no specific mammographic findings (26).

Gross Findings. With a median size of 3 to 4 cm, more than half of these well-circumscribed

tumors are over 3 cm. Multiple and generally small cysts are apparent in larger tumors (fig. 10-1).

Microscopic Findings. Squamous carcinomas assume several phenotypes including large cell keratinizing, poorly differentiated, and less frequently, spindle cell and acantholytic types; some show a combination of patterns (4,5,9, 10,15,18,22,29,30). The tumor cells often proliferate around irregularly shaped, small cystic spaces (fig. 10-2). The most bland-appearing and well-differentiated cells often line the cystic spaces. As the tumor cells infiltrate the surrounding stroma, they become spindle shaped and lose their classic squamous features. A pronounced stromal reaction is often admixed with the spindled squamous carcinoma (figs. 10-3, 10-4). Some squamous carcinomas are

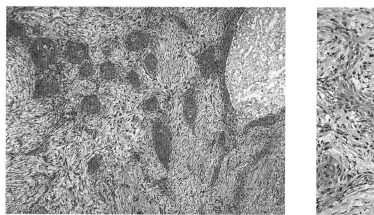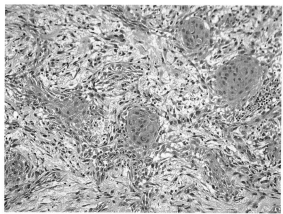

Figure 10-3

SQUAMOUS CARCINOMA

A pronounced stromal reaction is common in squamous carcinomas.

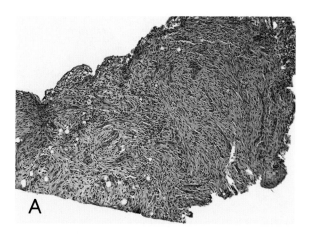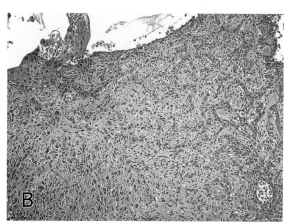

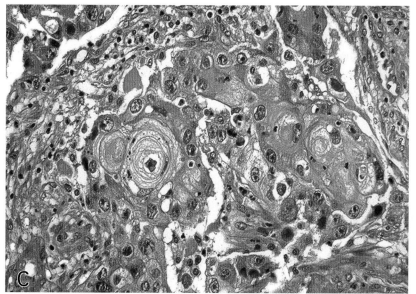

Figure 10-4

SQUAMOUS CARCINOMA

The spindle cell variant of squamous carcinoma in a core biopsy (A) is characterized by epithelioid cords (B) and a rare squamous nest (C).

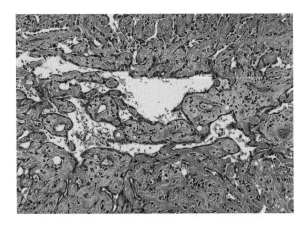
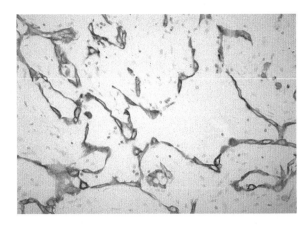

Figure 10-5

SQUAMOUS CARCINOMA, ACANTHOLYTIC TYPE

The tumor resembles angiosarcoma (left), but shows immunoreactivity with a variety of epithelial markers (right) (immunostain for kermix). (Fig. 10-6B,D from Tavassoli FA. Pathology of the breast, 2nd ed. Stamford, CT: Appleton & Lange/McGraw Hill; 1999:490.)

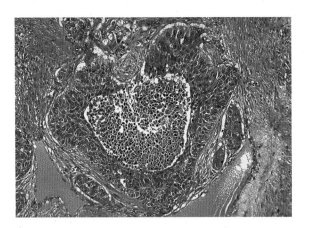
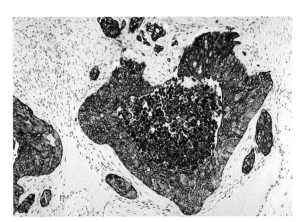

Figure 10-6

SQUAMOUS CARCINOMA

There is intense positivity with CK34betaE12.

less differentiated but contain keratin pearls. The acantholytic variant may be confused with an angiosarcoma. The positive reaction of the tumor cells with keratin and negative reaction with factor VIII or CD34 rules out the possibility of an angiosarcoma (fig. 10-5). The squamous differentiation is retained in the metastatic foci.

Cytologic Findings. It is possible to establish, or at least suggest, the possibility of a squamous carcinoma when atypical squamous cells are present in the cytology preparation (13,14, 20,21). When the atypia is subtle, or only well-differentiated squamous cells are identified, it is important to rule out reactive squamous

metaplasia. Reactive squamous metaplasia, with or without atypia, may develop around a biopsy cavity or aspiration site, around a subareolar abscess, and in duct ectasia (13,14,20,21,25).

Special Studies. The spindle cell and acantholytic variants require immunohistochemical confirmation of their epithelial nature, particularly when more typical areas of squamous differentiation are absent in the samples. The tumor cells are positive with kermix, high molecular weight cytokeratin (CK)34betaE12 (fig. 10-6), and p63, but negative for factor VIII or CD34 (5). Nearly all squamous carcinomas are negative for estrogen receptors (ERs), progesterone receptors

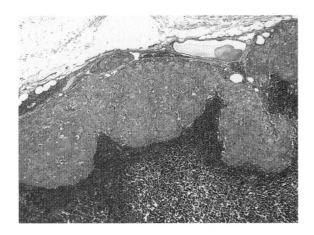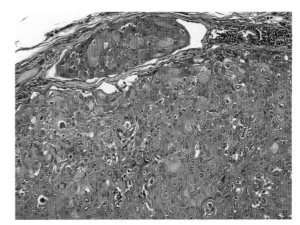

Figure 10-7

METASTATIC SQUAMOUS CARCINOMA

Squamous differentiation is retained in nodal metastases.

(PRs) (36), and Her2/neu. Of five cases with squamous and spindle cell metaplasia in one study, 72 percent had immunoreactivity with HER2/neu (1); a high proportion (69 percent) have 2+ expression of epithelial growth factor receptor (EGFR) (1a). In separate studies, it has been shown that 70 to 80 percent of metaplastic carcinomas overexpress EGFR (1a,17a,23a), but only 34 percent have *EGFR* gene amplification (23a). In another recent study, high *EGFR* copy number was noted secondary to aneusomy (22 percent) and amplification (4 percent) (10a).

Prognosis. As in other carcinomas, tumor size is of prognostic significance. Given the tumor size of over 5 cm in many cases, however, metastases to axillary nodes are relatively uncommon; approximately 10 to 15 percent of pure squamous carcinomas metastasize to axillary lymph nodes (23,36). The squamous morphology is retained in the axillary node metastases (fig. 10-7). Advanced tumor stage and lymph node involvement are associated with a more aggressive course, as anticipated. It has been suggested that the prognosis is similar to that of infiltrating ductal carcinomas for the first 9 years (17) and that at 5 years, it is no different from breast carcinomas in general (4). Among squamous carcinomas, the acantholytic variant may exhibit more aggressive behavior (5) and may be confused with angiosarcoma. A 5-year disease-free survival rate of 63 percent has been reported (36). Progression to an undifferentiated carcinoma may occur (18).

Adenosquamous Carcinoma

Definition. *Adenosquamous carcinomas* are composed of variable admixtures of adenocarcinoma and squamous carcinoma.

General Features. While focal squamous differentiation has been observed in 3.7 percent of infiltrating duct carcinomas (9), a prominent admixture of squamous carcinoma (10 percent or more) with infiltrating ductal carcinoma (fig. 10-8) is not common. The gross appearance of these generally ill-defined lesions varies depending on the amount of squamous differentiation, which manifests as pearly white nodules. The squamous component is often keratinizing and ranges from very well-differentiated keratinized areas to poorly differentiated nonkeratinized foci. The few reported cases have been aggressive, but behavior is generally a reflection of the degree of differentiation of the two components of the lesion.

Some have included infiltrating syringomatous tumor as a low-grade variant of adenosquamous carcinoma (fig. 10-9) (8,24,32); infiltrating syringomatous tumors have a tendency to recur because their infiltrative nature makes complete excision difficult, but there are no well-documented cases with metastasis. A mucoepidermoid carcinoma of breast morphologically similar to that of the salivary glands has also been reported (5).

Microscopic Findings. Adenosquamous carcinoma is composed of multiple ducts and

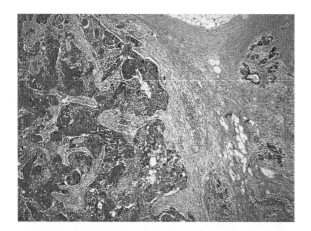

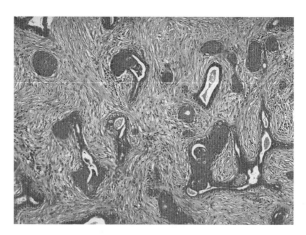

Figure 10-9

INFILTRATING SYRINGOMATOUS TUMOR

Considered a low-grade adenosquamous carcinoma by some, infiltrating syringomatous tumor is considered an adenoma by others since there are no well-documented cases with metastasis.

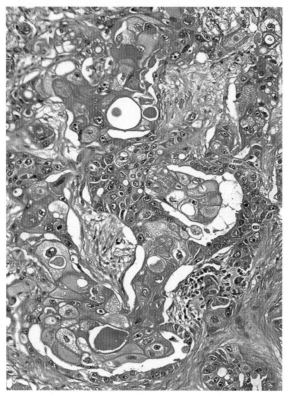

Figure 10-8

ADENOSQUAMOUS CARCINOMA

Infiltrating ductal carcinoma is admixed with areas of squamous differentiation.

the stroma surrounding the spaces. The stroma displays a prominent fibroblastic reaction to the invading tumor. The areas of squamous differentiation generally lack significant atypia or mitotic activity.

The histology of "low-grade adenosquamous carcinoma" is discussed in the section dealing with syringomatous tumors of the nipple (see chapter 15). Infiltrating syringomatous tumors within the breast proper display a prominent fibroblastic stroma and elongated infiltrating projections that often extend way beyond the main tumor mass, carrying with them the distinctive stroma. It is most likely the persistence of residual disease in these distant projections of the tumor that is responsible for local recurrences.

The squamous component is negative for both ER and PR. The positivity of the ductal carcinoma component for ER and PR depends on its degree of differentiation (24,32).

Adenocarcinoma with Spindle Cell Differentiation

Spindle cell differentiation occurs in pure adenocarcinomas (fig. 10-10), albeit rarely. The intraepithelial component of this lesion may also have a prominent spindle cell morphology, growing in a solid, papillary, or solid and cribriform pattern. To qualify as a spindle cell carcinoma (adeno or squamous), the spindle cells

cystic spaces lined by either a single layer of glandular epithelial cells, attenuated to well-developed squamous cells, or a combination of these cell types. The squamous component may form solid morules that protrude into the variably shaped spaces. They also form small nests or tubular arrangements as they invade

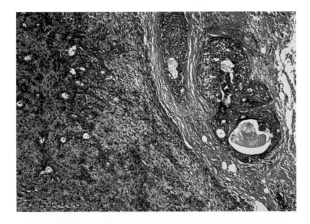

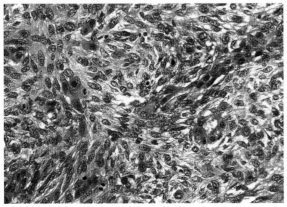

Figure 10-10

**ADENOCARCINOMA WITH
SPINDLE CELL DIFFERENTIATION**

The spindle cells in the solid nests are not squamous since they fail to react with CK34betaE12 or CK5/6.

should be positive for epithelial markers (kermix, CAM5.2, or 34betaE12), whether the cells appear bland or anaplastic. Spindled adenocarcinoma is generally negative for CK34betaE12 (7), while spindle cell squamous carcinoma is positive for this marker. Other studies have combined a variety of carcinomas with spindle cell differentiation, making it difficult to analyze the results (33).

We distinguish spindle cell carcinoma of myoepithelial origin from metaplastic spindle cell carcinoma of either squamous or glandular type. Probably many carcinomas referred to as "fibromatosis-like" carcinoma (11,28) and characterized by a low frequency of axillary lymph node metastases are spindle cell myoepithelial carcinomas (see chapter 11 and figs. 12-42 to 12-45). It is often possible to separate these

variants by thorough evaluation of the tumor on hematoxylin and eosin (H&E)-stained slides. Spindle cell squamous carcinoma nearly always has foci of recognizable squamous differentiation, although sometimes minuscule. Likewise, spindle cell adenocarcinomas have recognizable gland formation somewhere in the lesion. It is generally a myoepithelial carcinoma that is composed purely of spindle cells; emanation of the neoplastic spindle cells from the myoepithelial cell layer of the ductal structures at the periphery of the lesion can be identified somewhere in the tumor, helping to confirm the diagnosis.

If H&E-stained slides fail to provide definitive clues as to the nature of the lesion, positivity with CK7 indicates an adenocarcinoma since both squamous and myoepithelial carcinomas are negative for this marker. Unfortunately, distinguishing squamous cells from myoepithelial cells by immunohistochemistry is impossible since both have a nearly identical immunoprofile. It is possible that more specific markers will become available in the future to help simplify the separation of spindle cell squamous carcinoma from myoepithelial carcinoma; alternatively, squamous carcinomas may be of myoepithelial cell derivation.

MIXED EPITHELIAL/MESENCHYMAL VARIANTS OF METAPLASTIC CARCINOMA

Adenocarcinoma with Chondroid or Osseous Differentiation

General Features. Adenocarcinomas showing osseous or chondroid differentiation are generally reported together under the umbrella term of "matrix-producing carcinomas"; therefore, there is limited information on either as a separate entity. Chondroid and osseous differentiation occur focally in 0.2 percent of breast carcinomas (15,35). The tumors are generally well-circumscribed nodular masses that may become massive (up to 20 cm), resulting in nipple displacement and ulceration through the skin.

Mammographically, a well-delineated density, sometimes with a focally indistinct to spiculated margin and amorphous or coarse calcification, is the most typical presentation (27). Rarely, trabeculations reflecting osseous differentiation may occur and this feature is

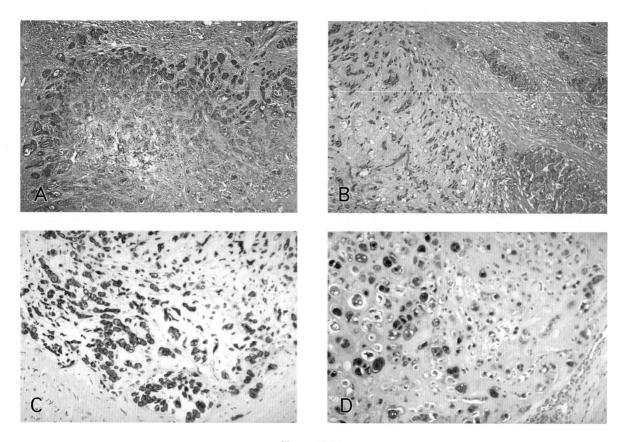

Figure 10-11

CARCINOMA WITH ABUNDANT CHONDROID DIFFERENTIATION

The adenocarcinoma forms a rim around the tumor (A). The chondroid areas have atypical nuclei (B). All tumor cells, including those clearly epithelial located at the periphery (C) and those in the chondroid area (D), immunoreact with epithelial markers (immunostain for kermix).

best appreciated on images at higher kilovoltage setting (6).

Gross Findings. Adenocarcinomas with chondroid differentiation are generally well-defined and firm. The cut surface has glistening areas corresponding to the foci of chondroid differentiation. Those with osseous differentiation are well-circumscribed masses that often exceed 3 cm in diameter and have a solid cut surface, sometimes with a gritty consistency.

Microscopic Findings. Microscopically, chondroid tumors consist of an infiltrating duct carcinoma sometimes admixed with areas of bland chondroid matrix. Other tumors appear as a predominantly chondroid mass with a rim of peripheral cellularity composed of cells with overlapping epithelial and chondroid features (fig. 10-11); some of these cells show clustered to tubular arrangements.

Osseous tumors are characterized by an admixture of adenocarcinoma (most often ductal type) with areas of benign osseous differentiation (fig. 10-12), some of which may be through enchondral ossification. The chondroid component of these tumors generally coexpresses epithelial and mesenchymal markers.

The metaplastic chondroid tumor cells are S-100 protein positive and simultaneously express kermix, but are negative for actin (29). From 0 to 33 percent of metaplastic carcinomas with chondroid differentiation are immunoreactive with HER2/neu (1,11a). For chondroid tumors, axillary lymph node metastases may or may not have the chondroid differentiation. The metastatic foci of osseous lesions either contain pure adenocarcinoma or display the mesenchymal component as well. Interestingly, a case of carcinoma with chondroid differentiation that metastasized to

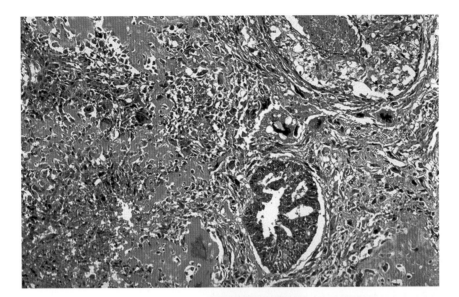

Figure 10-12

ADENOCARCINOMA WITH BENIGN-APPEARING OSSEOUS DIFFERENTIATION

Areas of osseous differentiation are often present in patches admixed with the epithelial elements of the carcinoma.

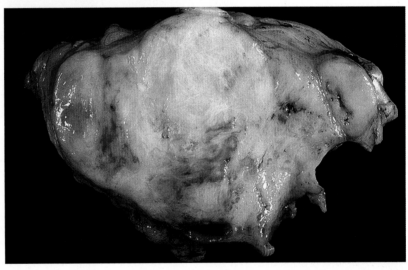

Figure 10-13

CARCINOSARCOMA

A solid, well-delineated large mass is the typical presentation.

the uterus closely mimicked a primary uterine mixed mesodermal tumor (29).

The tumor cells range from those rich in tonofilaments and desmosomal attachments to more rounded cells with short microvilli, abundant rough endoplasmic reticulum, prominent Golgi apparatus, and rare lipid droplets. The latter reflect the chondrocytic cells and are surrounded by a territorial matrix (29).

The adenocarcinoma component of these tumors is often high grade and lacks ER and PR expression. The osseous and chondroid elements are nearly always negative for ER, PR, and HER2/neu. In some cases, however, the adenocarcinoma is well to moderately differentiated and may express both ER and PR.

Prognosis. Tumor stage is the best-known prognostic indicator for these tumors, similar to the more common types of infiltrating carcinoma. In patients with carcinomas with chondroid and osseous metaplasia, the 5-year survival rate has ranged from 28 to 68 percent (11a,12,15,35). Recurrences develop within 2.5 years of initial diagnosis (35); among patients with recurrent disease, 89 percent die within 4 years. Given the rarity of this lesion, not much is known about optimal therapy.

Carcinosarcoma

Neoplasms with a true sarcomatous component admixed with carcinoma (figs. 10-13, 10-14) are essentially biphasic and should be referred to as

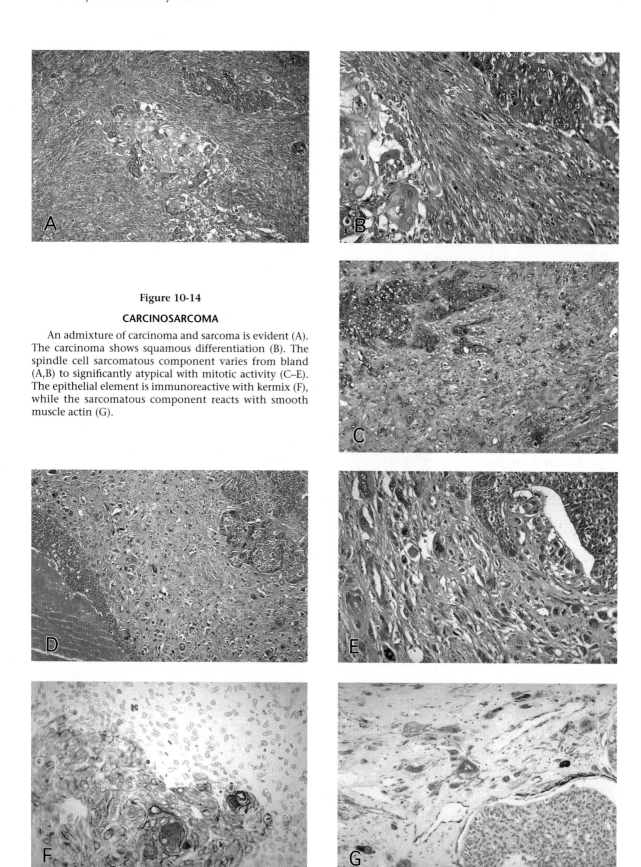

Figure 10-14

CARCINOSARCOMA

An admixture of carcinoma and sarcoma is evident (A). The carcinoma shows squamous differentiation (B). The spindle cell sarcomatous component varies from bland (A,B) to significantly atypical with mitotic activity (C–E). The epithelial element is immunoreactive with kermix (F), while the sarcomatous component reacts with smooth muscle actin (G).

carcinosarcomas regardless of their mode of origin (29,34). The epithelial component is generally an infiltrating duct carcinoma, but may show predominant or pure squamous differentiation (34). The sarcomatous component ranges from a nonspecific sarcoma to rare rhabdomyosarcoma. The sarcomatous component in these tumors does not display epithelial features immunohistochemically or ultrastructurally. Metastases may contain either or both components.

Molecular analysis of a small number of cases by assessment of microsatellites for loss of heterozygosity (LOH) has shown a similar LOH profile in the carcinomatous and sarcomatous components, with additional alterations in the sarcomatous component. This finding supports clonality and suggests derivation of the sarcomatous component through cumulative alterations beyond those present in the carcinomatous elements and supports the conversion hypothesis as a multistep mechanism for the histogenesis of carcinosarcomas (16,37).

Transcriptional profiling using half-a-genome oligonucleotide microarrays has been utilized to compare metaplastic breast carcinoma (the carcinosarcoma variant judging from the images) with infiltrating ductal carcinoma (17b). This comparison has shown upregulation of extracellular matrix–related genes and the downregulation of epithelial-related genes in the carcinosarcomas, accounting for some of the morphologic findings.

From 19 to 26 percent of carcinosarcomas metastasize to axillary lymph nodes and 21 percent metastasize to distant sites (34). Axillary node metastases are not as common as anticipated from the large size of many of these tumors. As in other more common mammary carcinomas, the stage of the tumor is a crucial prognostic factor. The overall 5-year survival rate for patients with carcinosarcomas is 49 percent; when separated by tumor stage, the survival for patients with stage 1 tumors is 100 percent, for stage 2, 63 percent, and for stage 3, only 35 percent (34).

APOCRINE CARCINOMA

Definition. *Apocrine carcinoma* is composed of cells with abundant pink, granular cytoplasm, prominent nucleoli, and the immunohistochemical features of apocrine cells evident in over 90 percent of the cells.

General Features. Strictly defined, apocrine carcinomas account for less than 1 percent of all mammary carcinomas (50), but a wide range of 0.3 to 4.0 percent has been reported in the literature based on variable definitions of the tumor (48,59,63). Focal apocrine differentiation is common and has been noted in 30 percent of usual breast carcinomas (58). When basing the diagnosis of apocrine carcinoma on immunoreactivity with gross cystic disease fluid protein (GCDFP)-15, the reported incidence has varied from 12 (48) to 72 percent (72). It should be noted, however, that GCDFP-15 expression is not specific to apocrine differentiation and occurs in a wide variety of mammary carcinomas. When the diagnosis of apocrine differentiation has been based on immunoreactivity with zinc alpha-2-glycoprotein, at least 36 percent of 145 breast carcinomas evaluated were positive (40). This study found no impact of apocrine metaplasia on ER and PR status, casting doubt on the validity of the criteria used by the authors for apocrine differentiation; a vast majority of apocrine cells (benign or malignant) are negative for ER and PR.

Clinical Features. Apocrine carcinomas are not significantly different from nonapocrine carcinomas in their clinical and gross pathologic presentations or mammographic features (51). Apocrine carcinomas have been observed in women 19 to 86 years of age (59,63), although at least one report has suggested that apocrine carcinoma occurs more frequently in elderly women (63). Mammographically, most apocrine carcinomas present as opacities often associated with microcalcifications (51). Occasionally, unusually mixed patterns of microcalcification have been noted in the intraepithelial component of apocrine carcinomas (55).

Histogenesis. Whether apocrine carcinomas develop through a metaplastic process or from native apocrine cells of the type noted in fetal breast tissue (71) is not known with certainty. It is also possible that apocrine lesions of the breast develop from both routes. Transition from metaplastic apocrine cells through the proliferation of relatively uniform-appearing cells or by acquisition of variable cytologic atypia is evident adjacent to some apocrine carcinomas (49,54,73). While most apocrine carcinomas are ductal in nature, lobular carcinomas with apocrine differentiation also occur (47). Interestingly, the

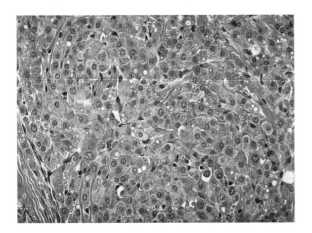
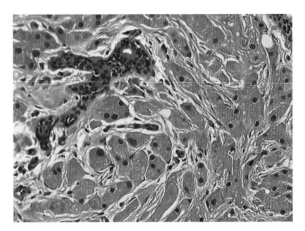

Figure 10-15

APOCRINE CARCINOMA

The cells have abundant granular, eosinophilic cytoplasm and round nuclei with prominent nucleoli.

latter are E-cadherin negative, while the ductal apocrine lesions are E-cadherin positive.

Microscopic Findings. The architectural appearance of invasive apocrine carcinoma ranges from isolated cells forming cords (lobular carcinomas) to tubules and solid aggregates (ductal type carcinomas). In the intraepithelial phase, the pattern is most frequently that of high-grade ductal carcinoma in situ grade 3 (DCIS, grade 3)/ductal intraepithelial neoplasia 3 (DIN3) with necrosis, but low-grade DCIS/DIN1, as well as lobular patterns, may occur.

Cytologic Findings. Atypical apocrine cells in cytology preparations suggest apocrine carcinoma, but they may also indicate simply the atypical apocrine differentiation that can be found in a variety of settings (41,52,64). When the specimen displays significant cellularity, nuclear overlapping, pleomorphism, or marked nuclear atypia and cellular debris, the likelihood of carcinoma increases significantly (74). Nucleoli are prominent in both benign metaplastic apocrine cells as well as those of apocrine carcinoma; as such, the presence of nucleoli does not help in the diagnosis. Furthermore, apocrine carcinomas may have bland cytologic features, compounding difficulties in diagnosing apocrine malignancy in cytology preparations (64)

It is foremost the morphologic appearance of apocrine carcinoma, associated with its distinctive immunoprofile, that sets it apart from other types of mammary carcinoma. Apocrine carcinomas are composed predominantly of large cells with abundant granular, eosinophilic cytoplasm and have mostly round to ovoid nuclei with prominent nucleoli (fig. 10-15); the granules are periodic acid-Schiff (PAS) positive after diastase digestion. A small proportion show transition from typical granular apocrine cells to a prominent population of cells containing numerous microvacuoles resembling sebaceous cells; this cell type is designated as sebocrine. The nuclei in the sebocrine cells are identical to those in the typical apocrine cells, but may appear more pyknotic and lack nucleoli. Other cells have cytologic features that may result in their misinterpretation as a granular cell tumor or a fibrohistiocytic tumor; these have been designated as myoblastomatoid (histiocytoid) carcinomas (see chapter 8) (46).

Mitotic activity is highly variable. These carcinomas show a range of grades.

Immunophenotype and Ploidy. Because of the variable criteria used for the interpretation of apocrine differentiation, there are conflicting results reported in the literature concerning the immunoprofile of apocrine carcinomas for ER, PR, and androgen receptor (AR) (48,61,63,70). When rigid criteria are applied, apocrine cells, whether benign or malignant, are generally positive for GCDFP-15, ER-beta, and AR (fig. 10-16), but are negative for bcl-2 protein, ER-alpha (the commonly used antibody), and PR (54a,54b,69). Immunohistochemical analysis of 102 apocrine lesions (benign and malignant) showed negative immunoreactivity for ER and

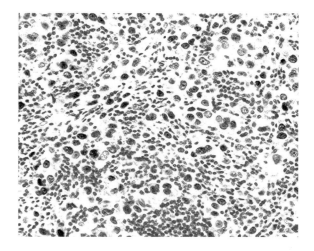

Figure 10-16

**APOCRINE CARCINOMA METASTATIC
TO AXILLARY LYMPH NODE**

Positivity for androgen receptor is seen.

PR in 98 percent, whereas, 94 percent of benign lesions and 72 percent of malignant lesions were positive for AR (70). Among intraepithelial apocrine neoplasias (DCIS), 97 percent were AR positive, while 62 percent were p53 positive; ER was negative in 94 percent of cases and PR was negative in 97 percent (56). Another study noted 17 percent immunoreactivity for ER and PR along with 25 percent positivity for bcl-2 among 24 apocrine carcinomas (59).

Although positivity for GCDFP-15 is characteristic of apocrine cells (60), it is not specific to apocrine carcinomas. The common expression of GCDFP-15 in a variety of breast carcinomas is the basis of using this antibody to support a breast origin for metastatic carcinomas of unknown primary site. While 75 percent of breast carcinomas with apocrine histology are positive for GCDFP-15, up to 90 percent of infiltrating lobular carcinomas are also positive (45,63). Furthermore, 23 percent of phenotypically nonapocrine carcinomas are also GCDFP-15 positive.

Apocrine cells, whether benign or malignant, are intensely immunoreactive with prolactin-inducible protein (PIP)/GCDFP-15. Detection of the mRNA for PIP/GCDFP-15 may be a more precise method for defining apocrine differentiation (65).

Even though most apocrine carcinomas are ER negative by immunohistochemical assess-

ment, they do have the ERmRNA (39) and the problem appears to be in the production of the protein. Apocrine carcinomas show immunoreactivity for carcinoembryonic antigen (CEA) in up to 47 percent of cases (56,68). Apocrine carcinomas are immunoreactive for p53 in 68.2 percent of cases; the proportion of positive lesions increases to 84.6 percent for high nuclear grade tumors (62).

Ploidy in apocrine carcinomas is dependent on the tumor grade. A diploid DNA content has been noted among benign metaplastic cells and low-grade intraductal carcinomas (DIN1) (44,66), whereas poorly differentiated apocrine carcinomas are aneuploid in 96 percent of cases (66).

Molecular Findings. Molecular studies comparing apocrine hyperplasia (6 cases), in situ carcinoma (DIN1-3) (25 cases), and invasive carcinoma (11 cases) have found a higher frequency of LOH in invasive carcinomas (30 to 50 percent) compared to in situ carcinomas (DIN1-3) (23 to 33 percent) and no LOH among the few hyperplastic lesions. The loci most frequently showing LOH were on chromosomes 17p13 (*Tp53*), 3p25 (*VHL*), 1p35-336 (*NB*), and 16p13 (*PKD1/TSC2*) (57). By comparative genomic hybridization (CGH), the mean number of alterations for invasive apocrine carcinomas was 14.8 compared to 10.2 for in situ carcinoma and 4.1 for hyperplasia; the CGH findings suggest that some apocrine hyperplasias are also clonal (53).

Ultrastructural Findings. Apocrine cells have numerous mitochondria, some with incomplete cristae, osmiophilic secretory granules, empty vesicles (48), and a variety of intracytoplasmic organelles (45,63,67,73).

Differential Diagnosis. The typical apocrine carcinoma with granular, eosinophilic cytoplasm may be confused with granular cell tumors, while the sebocrine variant may be mistaken for a histiocytoid carcinoma or a histiocytic process. A myoblastomatoid (histiocytoid) variant has also been described that may simulate fibrohistiocytic and granular cell tumors (46). Immunostaining with antibodies against keratin easily distinguishes apocrine carcinoma since both granular cell tumors and histiocytic lesions are negative while apocrine carcinomas are positive for cytokeratins.

Apocrine carcinoma should be distinguished from oncocytic carcinomas, which rarely

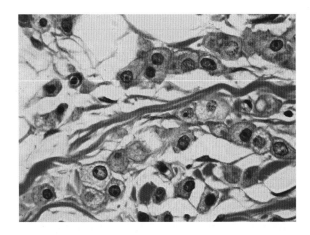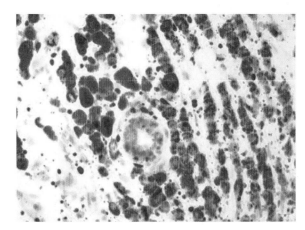

Figure 10-17

LIPID-RICH CARCINOMA

Left: The cytoplasm of the tumor cells contains numerous microvesicles.
Right: Abundant intracytoplasmic lipid is seen in nearly all the tumor cells with the oil red-O stain.

develop in the breast. The latter are GCDFP-15 negative, but show intense positivity with an antimitochondrial antibody (42). Oncocytic carcinomas have abundant mitochondria at the ultrastructural level.

Prognosis. There is no significant difference in the survival of patients with invasive apocrine carcinomas compared with those with non-apocrine carcinomas (38,43,47,68a). Novel therapeutic approaches targeted to specific molecular alterations in the near future may change survival statistics.

LIPID-RICH CARCINOMA

Definition. In the breast, *lipid-rich carcinoma* is composed of large cells with abundant neutral lipids present within 90 percent of the tumor. The term lipid-rich carcinoma has been used to refer to a heterogeneous group of tumors characterized by the presence of at least some cells that contain clear to vacuolated cytoplasm.

General Features. While 75 percent of breast carcinomas contain variable amounts of intracytoplasmic lipids when histochemical stains are used on frozen section specimens (77), very few show an abundance of intracytoplasmic lipids in 90 percent or more of the cells, a feature also detectable on H&E-stained sections due to cytoplasmic distension by microvacuoles. Because of this variation in the lipid content of cancer cells and depending on the stringency of criteria used, the reported incidence of lipid-rich carcinoma

varies from 0.8 percent in a study using Sudan III to stain frozen sections (85) to less than 1 to 6 percent in reports relying on the presence of foamy or clear cytoplasm on conventional H&E-stained sections (75,80,82). Some pathologists have preferred the designation of *lipid-secreting carcinoma* (84) for these tumors. Lipid-rich carcinomas have been reported among women on neuroleptic drugs for severe psychiatric disorders (81). These medications release prolactin, resulting in increased fatty synthetase activity and milk protein synthesis; this is manifested by galactorrhea clinically and pregnancy-like lactational changes in the in situ (intraepithelial) components of the carcinoma (81).

Clinical Features. Occurring predominantly in women 33 to 81 years of age, lipid-rich carcinoma has also been reported in a 55-year-old male (79). The majority of patients present with a palpable mass. The tumor varies in size from 1.2 to 15.0 cm (85).

Gross Findings. The cut surface of lipid-rich carcinoma is indistinguishable from ordinary infiltrating duct carcinoma.

Microscopic Findings. The hallmark of this tumor is the presence of cells with abundant microvacuolated, foamy or clear cytoplasm admixed with cells that simply have abundant pink cytoplasm (fig. 10-17); a vast majority of the cells contain neutral lipids (77,80). Rarely, they have areas with chondroid differentiation (83). The tumor generally assumes the pattern of an

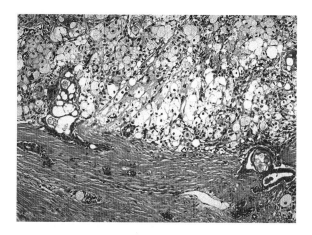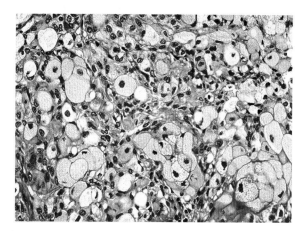

Figure 10-18

SEBACEOUS CARCINOMA

Left: The tumor has an expansile margin.

Right: The sebaceous cells are abundant and have eccentric nuclei surrounded by clear to finely vacuolated cytoplasm. The nuclei vary in size and shape.

infiltrating ductal carcinoma, and may be associated with either ductal or lobular intraepithelial neoplasia (75,80). Many of the tumors are high grade. While the tumor cells may contain alpha-lactalbumin and lactoferritin, they are generally devoid of mucins (85). An occasional cell may have fat globule membrane antigen (85). On aspiration cytology, the presence of atypical cells with large and small cytoplasmic lipid droplets has been reported (76). The few cases assessed for ER and PR have been negative (85). The tumor cells contain numerous lipid droplets and a well-developed Golgi apparatus (76,78).

Differential Diagnosis. Lipid-rich carcinoma most closely resembles apocrine carcinoma, particularly apocrine tumors with dominant sebocrine and histiocytoid cytology. The difference between the two is probably a reflection of the amount of intracytoplasmic lipid. A thorough assessment of the immunoprofile of apocrine and lipid-rich carcinomas may show more of a kinship between the two groups and may identify a functionally and therapeutically related or distinct group of tumors with overlapping morphology.

Prognosis. Given the heterogeneity of the reported cases and the relatively short period of follow-up available in many cases, the true behavior of this tumor is not well known. Nonetheless, many appear to be high-grade carcinomas (77). Lymph node metastases were present in 11 of 12 patients in one series (80).

SEBACEOUS CARCINOMA

Definition. *Sebaceous carcinoma* is a carcinoma with prominent sebaceous differentiation. There should be no evidence of origin from cutaneous adnexal sebaceous glands.

Clinical Features. Described in women ranging in age from 45 to 62 years, mammary sebaceous carcinoma is extremely rare, with only three cases described (88).

Gross Findings. Large and sharply delineated, the tumors range in size from 7.5 to 20.0 cm. The cut surface is uniformly solid, firm, and bright yellow or white, with patches of yellow discoloration, depending on the amount of sebaceous differentiation.

Microscopic Findings. The tumor is composed of lobules and nests, some of which are centrally infarcted. The lobules or nests are composed of a solid proliferation of large cells with abundant clear to foamy cytoplasm and round nuclei that display mild pleomorphism (fig. 10-18). Focally, hyperchromatic nuclei are noted, but these are sparse. The cytoplasm has a microvacuolated appearance. Smaller ovoid to spindle cells with eosinophilic cytoplasm and no vacuolization are often present at the periphery of the nests. Mitotic figures are present in some lobules, but are more common among the nonvacuolated cells, although they are few even among these cells. Morules of keratinizing squamous epithelium are seen in many lobules;

these cells appear very well differentiated and lack atypia or mitotic activity.

Involvement of the overlying skin or continuity with skin adnexal structures is not identified even after exhaustive sampling of the tumor. Both the overlying skin and the subjacent adnexal structures appear normal. The tumor cells have a distinct sebaceous appearance and contain intracytoplasmic lipid. The three tumors assessed for hormone receptors have shown immunoreactivity for PR in all; two were ER positive.

Differential Diagnosis. The entities in the differential diagnosis of sebaceous carcinoma are primary skin adnexal carcinoma, lipid-rich carcinoma, apocrine carcinoma with a prominent sebocrine cell population, and more remotely, liposarcoma. The absence of: 1) any skin involvement and 2) continuity with or engulfment of sebaceous glands, suggests a primary mammary sebaceous carcinoma.

Lipid-rich carcinoma infiltrates the mammary tissue like regular infiltrating duct carcinoma, with irregular cell clusters and cords rather than the compact lobulated pattern observed in sebaceous carcinoma. Furthermore, the vacuolization of the lipid-rich cells is of a much more subtle nature, to the point that it can be easily overlooked unless the tumor is examined at higher magnification. Many cells in both apocrine and lipid-rich carcinomas retain an eosinophilic cytoplasmic appearance. The formation of squamous morules, noted in some sebaceous carcinomas, has not been observed in either apocrine or lipid-rich carcinomas. Sebaceous differentiation is also seen in adenoid cystic carcinomas (see chapter 9).

The more remote possibility of a liposarcoma may be suggested in needle aspiration specimens or needle biopsies when the overall architecture of the tumor is not apparent and the sampling may pick up only the most vacuolated of the cells in the tumor. Again, the nesting architecture, the epithelial arrangements, the presence of squamous morules, and the absence of any lipoblasts rule out this possibility.

Since cases of sebaceous carcinoma of the eyelid have been reported following radiotherapy for cavernous hemangioma of the face, one may conclude that radiation therapy may have a role in the development of sebaceous carcinomas (86,87). Sebaceous differentiation has not been noted among carcinomas that recur following the increasing use of radiotherapy in the management of breast carcinomas, however.

SECRETORY CARCINOMA

Definition. *Secretory carcinoma* is a rare and distinctive type of carcinoma characterized by the presence of large amounts of intracellular and extracellular secretory material and composed of cells with granular eosinophilic or amphophilic cytoplasm.

General Features. Accounting for significantly less than 0.1 percent of all breast carcinomas (90,103), secretory carcinoma was originally described in 1966 by McDivitt and Stewart (105) who saw seven examples of this carcinoma, all in children. They therefore designated the tumor as "juvenile" carcinoma. In these seven children, the neoplasms had less aggressive behavior and the patients had a better prognosis than those with usual breast carcinoma. Hence, a conservative surgical approach (local excision) was advocated. Subsequently, isolated case reports and a series described axillary lymph node metastasis, local recurrences, and distant metastases; also, the tumor was observed in adults (107,114,115). It was, therefore, recommended that the descriptive term "secretory" carcinoma replace the older designation of "juvenile" carcinoma (115). About 20 secretory carcinomas have been reported in young boys and adult male patients (92,97,102,103,108,116).

Clinical Features. Patients range in age from 3 to over 80 years (89,95,105,107,110,115,117a). The tumor often presents as a solitary, discrete nodule; rarely, multicentric disease has been reported (109). In younger women, this nodular presentation is clinically mistaken for a fibroadenoma. A subareolar location is common in prepubertal girls and male patients given the presence of mammary tissue in that region. Mammographically, the tumor has a well-delineated outline with marginal irregularities (113).

Gross Findings. Ranging in size from less than 1 to over 10 cm, secretory carcinoma appears well delineated and often lobulated. Rarely, it is associated with bloody nipple discharge (100). The cut surface is solid and varies from gray-white to yellow-tan.

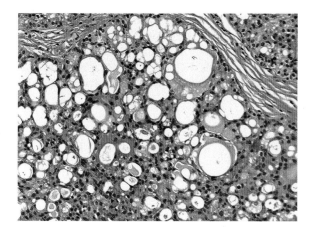 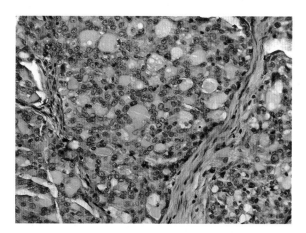

Figure 10-19

SECRETORY CARCINOMA

Abundant secretory material in seen in the small extracellular spaces. The tumor cells are uniform, with minimal cytologic atypia and inconspicuous mitotic figures. These tumors often have a pushing margin.

Microscopic Findings. Secretory carcinoma is characterized by the presence of abundant intracellular and extracellular secretory material in a neoplasm composed of a relatively uniform population of cells with round, bland nuclei and inconspicuous nucleoli (fig. 10-19). Mitotic activity is minimal. The tumor cells may have eosinophilic, amphophilic, or clear cytoplasm; many contain intracytoplasmic lumens.

The tumor cells may grow as solid masses separated by fibrous septa, surround minuscule spaces, or form larger cystic spaces. The eosinophilic secretory material stains with PAS and often retracts from the surrounding cells. Some cells have a vacuolated or signet ring cell appearance. A rare example of multicentric invasive carcinoma has been reported (109). Associated intraepithelial lesions often display similar secretory features. Recurrences and metastases retain the classic secretory pattern.

Cytologic Findings. Because of its distinctive morphology, the diagnosis of secretory carcinoma is possible on generous aspirates and definitely on needle core biopsies. Cytologically, rounded aggregates of mucoid material with cohesive sheets of tumor cells that assume a grape-like configuration are distinctive features of secretory carcinoma (91,93,94,96,108,112).

Immunoprofile and Special Studies. Most tumors are negative for ER both immunohistochemically and by biochemical methods (94,95,97,103,104,106,111,113); more than half of the cases are positive for PR (97,100,106,116). At least seven tumors recently evaluated by the author (FT) were all negative for HER2/neu. The few tumors evaluated by flow cytometry have been diploid or near diploid, with low S-phase fractions (103,106). The secretory material is immunoreactive with alpha-lactalbumin (90,93,97,103); the neoplastic cells are positive with S-100 protein (97,99,103) and CEA (97,99). The few cases that have been evaluated for immunoexpression of the lysozyme, alpha-1-antitrypsin, have been positive (99).

Molecular Findings. LOH was not detected at 17p13 among the 10 cases evaluated, whereas 46 percent of infiltrative duct carcinomas studied had LOH at this locus (104). Also, only one of the 10 cases had a *p53* mutation compared to a 35 to 50 percent frequency for infiltrating duct carcinomas. Comparative genomic hybridization has revealed recurrent gains of chromosomes 8q and 1q along with loss of 22q (93a). A single chromosomal translocation manifested by *ETV6-NTRK3* gene fusion has been proposed as a primary event in the development of secretory carcinoma; *ETV6-NTRK3* gene fusion was confirmed in 92 percent of 13 cases evaluated (117).

Ultrastructural Findings. Ultrastructurally, the hallmark of the tumor is the presence of variably sized intracytoplasmic lumens containing secretory material; microvillous cytoplasmic processes protrude into the spaces. The intracytoplasmic lumens fuse to form microcystic spaces. The cells are attached to one another by desmosomes and tight junctions, and surround extracellular spaces filled with secretory material (115).

Differential Diagnosis. Because of its frequently well-delineated nature, secretary carcinoma is often clinically mistaken for a fibroadenoma, particularly when it occurs in adolescent females. The microscopic appearance, however, is quite distinctive. Because of the presence of abundant secretory material, frequent circumscription, and occurrence in women of reproductive years, secretory carcinoma may be also mistaken for a lactating adenoma. A lactating adenoma is composed of a compact proliferation of distinct, individual tubules lined by epithelial and myoepithelial cells; such tubules with both epithelial and myoepithelial cell layers are absent in secretory carcinoma.

Treatment and Prognosis. While in many cases, secretory carcinoma behaves as a low-grade cancer, a more aggressive course is manifested in rare patients, particularly in those over 20 years of age. Recurrences may develop 6 and 8 years following both local excision and modified radical mastectomy, respectively (105–107), but may develop a couple of decades after an excisional biopsy (107). Lymph node metastases occur in about 15 percent of both children and adults (101–103,110,115).

Local excision with follow-up is recommended for children; conservation of the breast bud to the extent feasible is often attempted in prepubertal girls. The tumor should be treated as any other carcinoma based on its stage and low-grade morphology when it occurs in patients older than 20 years of age. Due to the small number of cases, the efficacy of radiation and chemotherapy has not been established for secretory carcinoma; since radiotherapy may inhibit normal mammary development, prudence in its administration for premenarchal girls is advised. No response was noted to chemotherapy used for management of pulmonary metastases in a 27-year-old woman who died 2.5 years after presentation with metastatic disease (98).

CLEAR CELL (GLYCOGEN-RICH) CARCINOMA

Definition. *Clear cell (glycogen-rich) carcinoma* is a lesion in which 90 percent or more of its neoplastic cells contain abundant clear cytoplasm.

Clinical Features. Clear cell (glycogen-rich) carcinoma is a rare tumor, accounting for 1 to 3 percent of all mammary carcinomas (119,120,122,123). The clinical presentation is similar to that of usual ductal carcinoma. Patients' median age is 57 years.

Gross Findings. Clear cell carcinomas are 1 to 8 cm in size. The gross features do not differ significantly from those of usual infiltrating duct carcinoma.

Microscopic Findings. Characterized by an infiltrative pattern and composed of mainly solid nests, or irregular clusters with tubule or papillary formations, the tumor cells (round, polygonal, or columnar) have sharply defined margins and clear or finely granular cytoplasm (figs. 10-20–10-22); the granules reflect PAS-positive and diastase-labile glycogen (119,120,126–128). The nuclei are small, hyperchromatic, and irregular in shape; occasional tiny nucleoli are seen. The intraepithelial component may show a pure clear cell composition or a cribriform or solid growth pattern, and rarely exceeds grade 2 DCIS/DIN2; frequently, clear cells and nonclear cells are admixed in the intraepithelial areas. An abrupt transition from normal ductal epithelium to columnar clear cells with centrally located nuclei is evident in adjacent ducts in some tumors.

Cytologically, glycogen-rich clear cells are identifiable on aspirates. Their presence is a clue to the diagnosis, but they are not always distinctive enough to predict the clear cell nature of the lesion (124).

Clear cell carcinomas vary in their expression of ER, PR, and HER2/neu. Many are ER and PR positive, but HER2/neu negative, but ER and PR negative, HER2/neu positive tumors occur as well (126a).

Differential Diagnosis. Clear cell carcinomas should be distinguished from two generally benign lesions, adenomyoepithelioma and clear cell hidradenoma. This distinction has significant implications in the management of the tumor. Both clear cell hidradenoma and adenomyoepithelioma are composed of two cell types, in contrast to the single cell population of clear cell carcinoma; this is the most easily identifiable difference. The clear cells of adenomyoepithelioma are immunoreactive for markers of myoepithelial cells (S-100 protein, p63, CD10, smooth muscle actin, calponin, caldesmon,

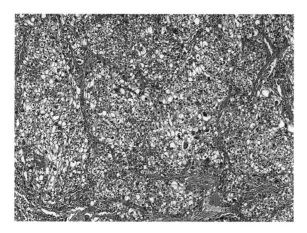

Figure 10-20

CLEAR CELL CARCINOMA

The typical clear cell carcinoma forms large nests composed of round to polyhedral cells with abundant clear cytoplasm. The nuclei appear hyperchromatic, with minimal to moderate atypia and pleomorphism.

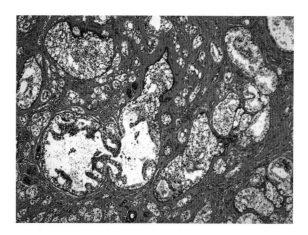

Figure 10-21

CLEAR CELL CARCINOMA

The invasive cells grow in small clusters and form tubular structures between ducts distended by the intraepithelial component.

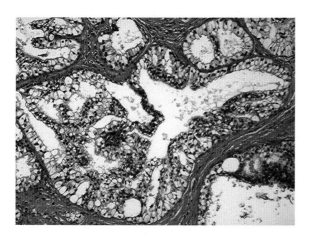

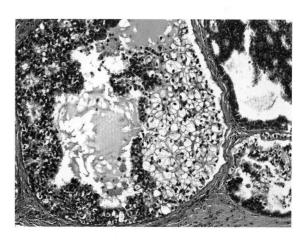

Figure 10-22

CLEAR CELL CARCINOMA: INTRAEPITHELIAL COMPONENT

The intraepithelial component of clear cell carcinoma assumes a variety of patterns including an admixture with nonclear cell phenotypes.

and others), while clear cell carcinoma generally shows no immunoreactivity with most myoepithelial cell markers except occasionally for S-100 protein, but is positive for GCDFP-15 (125). Hidradenomas are also often positive for S-100 protein. Clear cell myoepithelial tumors are positive for actin, p63, and CD10, but may be negative for CK34betaE12.

Another lesion that should be distinguished from clear cell carcinoma is the clear cell "sugar" cell tumor, a tumor showing differentiation to-

ward a putative perivascular epithelioid cell tumor (PECOMA). Only two examples of this lesion have been described in the breast (118,121); as is typical of PECOMAs, the neoplastic cells are immunoreactive with HMB45 and Melan-A, but show no immunoreactivity with antibodies to actins, S-100 protein, cytokeratins (CAM5.2 and AE1/AE3), desmin, and ER. The tumor cells in one of the two reported cases were positive for actin (118).

It is important to rule out the possibility of a metastatic clear cell (i.e., renal cell) carcinoma.

The clinical history is most crucial in this aspect, particularly when there is a solitary mammary nodule without an intraepithelial component. Immunoreactivity of the tumor cells for vimentin favors a renal cell carcinoma, as does the presence of multiple nodules; the presence of a solitary nodule with clear cell DCIS/DIN and immunoreactivity for GCDFP-15 favor a primary mammary clear cell carcinoma.

Other carcinomas in the differential diagnosis are lipid-rich and histiocytoid carcinomas. Lipid-rich carcinoma has abundant intracytoplasmic lipids not found in clear cell carcinoma.

Prognosis. The rarity of clear cell carcinoma precludes absolute statements concerning its behavior and prognosis. Judging from both recent studies and older series, the overall prognosis of patients with clear cell carcinoma is similar to, or worse than, that for conventional infiltrating duct carcinoma; this may be in part due to failure of clear cell carcinomas to respond to currently available therapies that are basically directed at conventional infiltrating duct carcinomas.

While some reports have noted no significant difference in the clinical behavior of clear cell carcinoma and usual infiltrating duct carcinoma (121), others have noted a higher frequency of axillary node metastases in clear cell carcinomas (122) and have suggested a more aggressive behavior for these tumors (124,126). A recent series of 20 patients with a higher proportion of smaller tumors found axillary node metastases in 35 percent of the cases (124a).

CARCINOMA WITH OSTEOCLASTIC GIANT CELLS

Definition. *Carcinoma with osteoclastic giant cells* includes mammary carcinomas with a variety of morphologic patterns (ductal and lobular) with multinucleated, osteoclastic giant cells dispersed mainly within the stroma, but also within the lumens of some ductal spaces. The stroma of the tumor is typically reactive, fibroblastic, and hypervascular, with extravasated red blood cells.

Clinical Features. Comprising 0.5 to 1.2 percent of all breast carcinomas (135,136), breast carcinomas with osteoclastic giant cells occur in patients of a wide age range. The average age at diagnosis is in the early to mid-fifties (129,136,138,141), but the tumor occurs from the 3rd to the 9th decades of life. The clinical

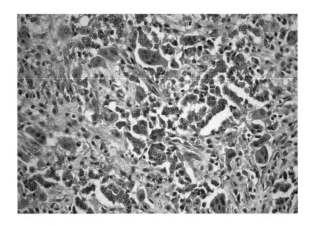

Figure 10-23

CARCINOMA WITH OSTEOCLASTIC GIANT CELLS

Multiple osteoclastic giant cells surround small clusters of invasive carcinoma.

presentation is similar to that of breast carcinomas in general.

It has been postulated that chemotactic factors elaborated by the cancer cells are responsible for the migration of monocytes and the formation of osteoclastic giant cells; angiogenic factors probably induce the stromal hypervascularity typical of this carcinoma (129,138). The giant cells also react with a variety of antibodies to macrophages, leading to the conclusion that the giant cells reflect macrophages with osteoclastic activity.

Mammographically, the tumor is well-circumscribed, resulting in its misinterpretation as a benign cyst or fibroadenoma (135,140).

Gross Findings. Ranging in size from less than 1 cm to 10 cm, a majority of the tumors are 1.5 to 3.0 cm in size. The most striking feature is the hemorrhagic to tan-brown appearance of the well-demarcated solitary mass, although some may be highly infiltrative and multinodular.

Microscopic Findings. A variety of ductal and lobular breast carcinomas may show a prominent population of osteoclastic giant cells (figs. 10-23, 10-24). The usual carcinoma is an infiltrating duct carcinoma, including invasive cribriform carcinoma (see chapter 9) (133,135,136,138,141). The giant cells are often evident in a reactive, fibroblastic, hypervascular stroma, but may be present admixed with, and often embracing, the epithelial cells (141). In

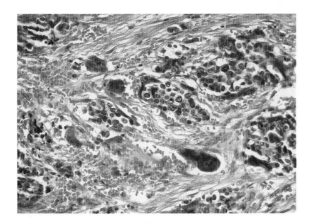

Figure 10-24

CARCINOMA WITH OSTEOCLASTIC GIANT CELLS

Stromal vascularity with extravasated red blood cells may be prominent.

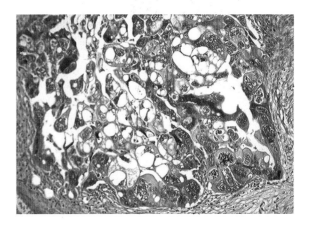

Figure 10-25

CARCINOMA WITH CHORIOCARCINOMATOUS FEATURES

Large tumor giant cells that resemble syncytiotrophoblasts surround mononucleated tumor cells in a distribution similar to the biphasic pattern of choriocarcinoma.

addition to the reactive stroma, there are often extravasated red blood cells within an infiltrate of lymphocytes admixed with mononucleated and binucleated histiocytes, some of which contain hemosiderin. The giant cells and the reactive stroma are often also evident in recurrences and metastases, supporting the belief that it is the elaboration of substances by the tumor cells that attracts the infiltrate and initiates the changes (141). When an associated intraepithelial component is present, it generally has a cribriform or solid pattern. While osteoclastic giant cells are occasionally present even in the intraepithelial component, they are most numerous in the invasive area.

The giant cells are acid phosphatase, nonspecific esterase, and lysozyme positive and immunoreactive with KP1/CD68. The giant cells are generally negative for ER and PR, cytokeratins, EMA, actin, and S-100 protein (141). These features, along with the absence of any epithelial features at the ultrastructural level, support a histiocytic type giant cell (130,132,135,137–139,141). While overall, low levels of ER and high levels of PR have been noted among these carcinomas (131,135,141), variations in ER and PR expression are a reflection of the variety of carcinomas that may be associated with a giant cell stromal reaction. On cytology preparations, a hypercellular aspirate showing an admixture of malignant cells with osteoclastic giant cells and erythrocytes is characteristic of carcinoma with osteoclastic giant

cells (131,139,140,142). The osteoclastic giant cells should be distinguished from the bizarre epithelial tumor giant cells that are diffusely immunoreactive for cytokeratin and EMA (134).

Treatment and Prognosis. Axillary lymph node metastases have been reported in one third of the cases. Distant metastases to a variety of sites including the eye and liver also have been reported (115,129,141). Following mastectomy and axillary node dissection, the 5-year survival rate is nearly the same or slightly better than that of women with ordinary infiltrating duct carcinomas. The behavior is most likely a reflection of the grade and subtype of the carcinoma and the tumor stage at presentation. While the reported cases have been treated mainly by mastectomy, current approaches to the treatment of breast carcinoma of similar stage should be considered for these lesions in the future.

BREAST CARCINOMA WITH CHORIOCARCINOMATOUS FEATURES

This variant of breast carcinoma contains syncytiotrophoblast-like multinucleated giant cells. The giant cells show immunoreactivity with human chorionic gonadotropin (HCG).

While expression of HCG has been noted in 12 to 18 percent of mammary carcinomas of all types, a morphology simulating the biphasic morphology of choriocarcinoma, with multinucleated syncytiotrophoblastic type cells surrounding nests of mononucleated cells and focal expression of HCG by mainly the multinucleated cells, is rare (fig. 10-25).

This is an extremely rare variant of breast carcinoma, with less than 10 cases observed (143–146). The three cases observed by one of the authors of this Fascicle were all in postmenopausal woman and were high-grade carcinomas. The tumor should be distinguished from metastatic choriocarcinoma, a lesion that occurs mainly in young women of child-bearing age. It is important to inquire about and exclude a prior history of chemotherapy, which may induce similar cytologic alterations but without the immunoexpression of HCG. Not much is known about the behavior or effective treatment of this rare tumor.

MELANOTIC CARCINOMA

While a variety of melanocytic lesions, including both primary and metastatic malignant melanoma and blue nevus, occur in the breast, there are also rare breast carcinomas that produce melanin pigment. Melanin-producing breast carcinomas should be distinguished from breast carcinomas that phagocytize melanin when they extend to the skin of the nipple in the form of Paget's disease (147–149,153), those that incorporate pigmented dendritic cells into the tumor (156), and those that are pigmented due to phagocytosis of lipofuscin. The few reported cases have occurred in women 34 to 72 years of age (151,152,157,159).

Ranging in size from 2.0 to 5.5 cm, and solid or partially cystic, the cut surface of these tumors often has black pigmentation either in a diffuse or patchy distribution. Microscopically, the tumor is composed of poorly cohesive round cells with abundant intracytoplasmic pigment admixed with nested and alveolar areas composed of round, oval, and spindle tumor cells devoid of pigmentation (fig. 10-26). The nonpigmented areas have the appearance of a poorly differentiated carcinoma and show immunoreactivity for epithelial markers, while the pigmented areas react with HMB45 and vimentin; both components may be immunoreactive with S-100 protein (150–152,154,159). The pigment stains with Fontana-Masson and is removed with melanin bleach (KMnO4).

In addition to the presence of melanin pigment on light microscopy, melanosomes and

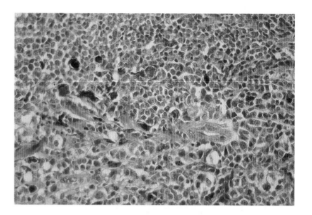

Figure 10-26

MELANOTIC CARCINOMA

Melanin-containing cells are dispersed in patches throughout the carcinoma.

premelanosomes can be identified in the tumor cells at the ultrastructural level. The two components (pigmented and nonpigmented elements) in one case were evaluated for loss of heterozygosity (LOH) with 37 microsatellite markers; there was no difference in the pattern of LOH in the two components (151).

These tumors should be distinguished from primary malignant melanoma of the skin. Melanomas show no immunoreactivity with epithelial markers, but are positive for HMB45 and S-100 protein.

At least half of the few recorded cases have metastasized to the axillary lymph nodes; the metastases may show patches of pigmentation as well. At least two patients have died from metastatic carcinoma (151,155); the follow-up on the remaining patients has been very short (1 to 2 years).

BASAL-LIKE BREAST CARCINOMAS

Gene expression profiling (GEP) of tumors offers the opportunity to classify tumors at a genomic level into subclasses of potential prognostic significance. GEP performed on complementary (c)DNA has been advanced as a potentially more powerful and/or independent predictor than traditional clinicopathologic factors (188). Its potential impact on the management of breast cancer has been debated and reviewed in detail (162,164,164a,175,187).

Using an intrinsic gene set and a hierarchical clustering method, breast tumors are classified

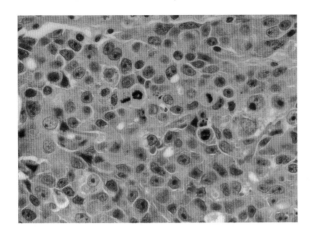 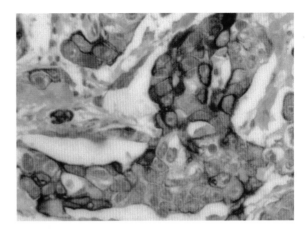

Figure 10-27

BASAL-LIKE BREAST CARCINOMA

Left: These tumor are generally poorly differentiated infiltrating duct carcinomas, not otherwise specified, with high nuclear grade and numerous mitotic figures.

Right: These tumor show variable degrees of positivity for CK5/6.

into subgroups with significantly different gene expression profiles. The subgroups include normal breast-like, luminal epithelial A, luminal epithelial B, HER2+, and basal types (175). The tumors that comprise the basal type generally cluster genes characteristically expressed in normal breast basal/myoepithelial cells, and are immunoreactive for CK5/6 and CK17. *Basal-like breast carcinomas* (BLBCs), as defined by GEP, have been found to be associated with comparatively worse overall and disease-specific survival rates compared to most other molecular subtypes (177,186). It has been suggested that the poor survival after breast cancer among BRCA1 carriers (particularly among women with lymph node negative disease) is attributable to the basal cancer phenotype (165).

Currently, BLBCs are defined by GEP and immunohistochemical features. As the former modality has not achieved widespread application in the routine clinical setting, most studies have defined BLBC immunohistochemically (160, 167,168,171,173,174,180). However, there is currently no international consensus on the precise complement of markers that define a BLBC. Most authors have included in their definitions, at least in part, immunopositivity for CK5 or CK 5/6 (160,163,166,168–170, 172,176,179,181–185,189).

To qualify as BLBC, some have specifically required lack of immunoreactivity for hormonal

receptors ER, PR, and HER2/neu (triple negative) (166,168,169,172,183,184), whereas others do not have this requirement. The differing definitions undoubtedly affect the proportion of cancers that are classified as basal-like and may be masking biologically relevant subclasses.

A major potential source of ambiguity in published studies on BLBC is that, with rare exceptions, most provide no explanation of how the immunostains were interpreted regarding the requisite percentage or intensity of staining. In the absence of such specification, it is not clear whether 1, 5, 10, 50, or more percent positive cells should be present in a tumor in order to designate it as BLBC and whether different levels of positivity correlate with any aspect of the tumor behavior.

The classic BLBC is a poorly differentiated infiltrating duct carcinoma, not otherwise specified (IDC-NOS) (fig. 10-27) (178). These carcinomas generally have high nuclear grade, poor tubule formation, numerous mitotic figures, and geographic necrosis, features typical of a poorly differentiated carcinoma.

Using immunohistochemical criteria, varying proportions of a wide spectrum of histologic subtypes may be classified as basal-like. Most notably, these include metaplastic carcinoma and traditional myoepithelial-type malignancies such as adenoid cystic carcinoma, myoepithelial carcinoma, and low-grade adenosquamous carcinoma. "Medullary" carcinomas seem to be a unique subtype, which by GEP analysis cluster with the basal IDC-NOS lesions (161), but, contrary to the aggressive behavior of BLBC, have a decidedly more favorable prognostic profile. Interestingly, IDC-NOS lesions that are GEP-defined as basal-like share some morphologic characteristic with "typical" and "atypical medullary" carcinomas, including high nuclear grade, tumor circumscription, and peritumoral lymphocytic infiltrates (171). The precise nature of the relationship between these putative distinct entities will require further study.

It appears that BLBCs, especially those defined as such based on their immunoprofile, are more heterogeneous phenotypically and biologically than anticipated from the GEP studies. The authors believe that just as there are carcinomas with highly variable morphologic and biologic behavior derived from the luminal epithelial cells, there is also a spectrum of carcinomas with different phenotypes, and functional and biologic characteristics derived from, or differentiating toward, the basal, myoepithelial, and stem cell populations of the mammary duct system (164). There is already substantial evidence in support of this spectrum at the morphologic and immunophenotypic level. Characterization of the gene expression profiles of these varieties is required for optimization of treatment modalities. Future characterization of mammary carcinoma stem cells will likely provide the much-needed explanation for many of the persistent ambiguities observed in BLBCs.

REFERENCES

Metaplastic Carcinoma

1. Bellino R, Arisio R, D'Addato F, et al. Metaplastic breast carcinoma: pathology and clinical outcome. Anticancer Res 2003:23:669-673.

1a. Bossuyt V, Fadare O, Martel M, et al. Remarkably high frequency of EGFR expression in breast carcinomas with squamous differentiation. Int J Surg Pathol 2005;4:319-327.

2. Cardoso F, Leal C, Meira A, et al. Squamous cell carcinoma of the breast. Breast 2000;9:315-319.

3. Chen KT. Fine needle aspiration cytology of squamous carcinoma of the breast. Acta Cytol 1990;34:664-668.

4. Eggers JW, Chesney TM. Squamous cell carcinoma of the breast: a clinicopathologic analysis of eight cases and review of the literature. Hum Pathol 1984;15:526-531.

5. Eusebi V, Lamovec J, Cattani MG, Fedeli F, Millis RR. Acantholytic variant of squamous cell carcinoma of the breast. Am J Surg Pathol 1986;10:855-861.

6. Evans HA, Shaughnessy EA, Nikiforov YE. Infiltrating ductal carcinoma of the breast with osseous metaplasia: imaging findings with pathologic correlation. AJR Am J Roentgenol 1999;172:1420-1422.

7. Farshid G, Moinfar F, Meredith DJ, Peiterse S, Tavassoli FA. Spindle cell ductal carcinoma in situ. An unusual variant of ductal intraepithelial neoplasia that simulates ductal hyperplasia or a myoepithelial proliferation. Virchows Arch 2001;439:70-77.

8. Ferrara G, Nappi O, Wick MR. Fine-needle aspiration cytology and immunohistology of low-grade adenosquamous carcinoma of the breast. Diagn Cytopathol 1999;20:13-18.

9. Fisher ER, Palekar AS, Gregorio RM, Paulson JD. Mucoepidermoid and squamous cell carcinomas of breast with reference to squamous metaplasia and giant cell tumors. Am J Surg Pathol 1983;7:15-27.

10. Gersell DJ, Katzenstein AL. Spindle cell carcinoma of the breast. A clinicopathologic and ultrastructural study. Hum Pathol 1981;12:550-561.

10a. Gilbert JA, Goetz MP, Reynolds CA, et al. Molecular analysis of metaplastic breast carcinoma: high EGFR copy number via aneusomy. Mol Cancer Ther 2008;7:944-951.

11. Gobbi H, Simpson JF, Borowsky A, Jensen RA, Page DL. Metaplastic breast tumors with a dominant fibromatosis-like phenotype have a high risk of local recurrence. Cancer 1999;85:2170-2180.

11a. Gwin K, Bossuyt V, Tavassoli FA. Breast carcinomas with chondroid differentiation. Mod Pathol 2008;21(Suppl 1):4A-396A.

12. Huvos AG, Lucas JC Jr, Foote FW Jr. Metaplastic breast carcinoma. Rare form of mammary cancer. NY State J Med 1973;73:1078-1082.

13. Jebsen PW, Hagmar BM, Nesland JM. Metaplastic breast carcinoma. A diagnostic problem in fine needle aspiration biopsy. Acta Cytol 1991;35:396-402.

14. Johnson TL. Kini SR. Metaplastic breast carcinoma: a cytopathologic and clinical study of 10 cases. Diagn Cytopathol 1996;14:226-232.

15. Kaufman MW, Marti JR, Gallager HS, Hoehn JL. Carcinoma of the breast with pseudosarcomatous metaplasia. Cancer 1984;53:1908-1917.

16. Kung FY, Tse GM, Lo KW, Law BK, Chang AR, Chen MH. Metachronous bilateral mammary metaplastic and infiltrating duct carcinomas: a molecular study for clonality. Hum Pathol 2002;33:677-679.

17. Lafreniere R, Moskowitz LB, Ketcham AS. Pure squamous cell carcinoma of the breast. J Surg Oncol 1986;31:113-119.

17a. Leibl S, Moinfar F. Metaplastic breast carcinomas are negative for Her-2 but frequently express EGFR (Her-1): potential relevance to adjuvant treatment with EGFR tyrosine kinase inhibitors? J Clin Pathol 2005;58:700-704.

17b. Lien HC, Hsiao YH, Lin YS, et al. Molecular signatures of metaplastic carcinoma of the breast by large-scale transcriptional profiling: identification of genes potentially related to epithelial-mesenchymal transition. Oncogene 2007;26:7859-7871.

17c. Luini A, Aguilar M, Gatti G, et al. Metaplastic carcinoma of the breast, an unusual disease with worse prognosis: the experience of the European Institute of Oncology and review of the literature. Breast Cancer Res Treat 2007;101:349-353.

18. Miura H, Taira O, Hiraguri S, Maeda J, Kato H. Recurrent squamous cell carcinoma of the breast with undifferentiated features: report of a case. Surg Today 2002;32:891-895.

19. Moisides E, Ahmed S, Carmalt H, Gillett D. Primary squamous cell carcinoma of the breast. ANZ J Surg 2002;72:65-67.

20. Motoyama T, Watanabe H. Extremely well differentiated squamous cell carcinoma of the breast. Report of a case with a comparative study of an epidermal cyst. Acta Cytol 1996;40:729-733.

21. Ng WK, Kong JH. Significance of squamous cells in fine needle aspiration cytology of the breast. A review of cases in a seven-year period. Acta Cytol 2003;47:27-35.

21a. Noske A, Schabe M, Pahl S, et al. Report of a metaplastic carcinoma with multidirectional differentiation: an adenoid cystic carcinoma, a spindle cell carcinoma and melanoma. Virchows Arch 2008. [Epub ahead of print.]

22. Oberman HA. Metaplastic carcinoma of the breast. A clinicopathologic study of 29 patients. Am J Surg Pathol 1987;11:918-929.

23. Rayson D, Adjei AA, Suman VJ, Wold LE, Ingle JN. Metaplastic breast cancer: prognosis and response to systemic therapy. Ann Oncol 1999;10:413-419.

23a. Reis-Filho JS, Pinheiro C, Lambros MB, et al. EGFR amplification and lack of activating mutations in metaplastic breast carcinomas. J Pathol 2006;209:445-453.

24. Rosen PP. Ernsberger D. Low-grade adenosquamous carcinoma. A variant of metaplastic mammary carcinoma. Am J Surg Pathol 1987;11:351-358.

25. Saad RS, Silverman JF, Julian T, Clary KM, Surgis CD. Atypical squamous metaplasia of seromas in breast needle aspirates from irradiated lumpectomy sites: a potential pitfall for false-positive diagnoses of carcinoma. Diagn Cytopathol 2002;26:104-108.

26. Samuels TH, Miller NA, Manchul LA, DeFreitas G, Panzarella T. Squamous cell carcinoma of the breast. Can Assoc Radiol J 1996;47:177-182.

27. Shin HJ, Kim HH, Kim SM, et al. Imaging features of metaplastic carcinoma with chondroid differentiation of the breast. AJR Am J Roentgenol 2007;188:691-696.

28. Sneige N, Yaziji H, Mandavilli SR, et al. Low-grade (fibromatosis-like) spindle cell carcinoma of the breast. Am J Surg Pathol 2001;25:1009-1016.

29. Tavassoli FA. Classification of metaplastic carcinoma of the breast. Pathol Annu 1992;27:89-119.

30. Tayeb K, Saadi I, Kharmash M, et al. [Primary squamous cell carcinoma of the breast. Report of three cases.] Cancer Radiother 2002;6:366-368. [French.]

31. Toikkanen S. Primary squamous cell carcinoma of the breast. Cancer 1981;48:1629-1632.

31a. Tot T. Eccrine ductal and acrosyringeal differentiation of the breast epithelium—a lesion associated with some metaplastic breast carcinomas. Virchows Arch 2006;449:565-571.

32. Van Hoeven KH, Drudis T, Cranor ML, Erlandson RA, Rosen PP. Low-grade adenosqamous carcinoma of the breast. A clinicopathologic study of 32 cases with ultrastructural analysis. Am J Surg Pathol 1993;17:248-258.

33. Wargotz ES, Deos P, Norris HJ. Metaplastic carcinomas of the breast. II. Spindle cell carcinoma. Hum Pathol 1989;20:732-740.

34. Wargotz ES, Norris HJ. Metaplastic carcinoma of the breast. III. Carcinosarcoma. Cancer 1989;64:1490-1499.

35. Wargotz ES, Norris HJ. Metaplastic carcinoma of the breast. I. Matrix-producing carcinoma. Hum Pathol 1989;20:628-635.

36. Wargotz ES, Norris HJ. Metaplastic carcinoma of the breast. IV. Squamous cell carcinoma of ductal origin. Cancer 1990;65:272-276.

37. Zhuang Z, Lininger RA, Man YG, Albuquerque A, Merino MJ, Tavassoli FA. Identical clonality of both components of mammary carcinosarcoma with differential loss of heterozygosity. Mod Pathol 1997;10:354-362.

Apocrine Carcinoma

38. Abati AD, Kimmel M, Rosen PP. Apocrine mammary carcinoma. A clinicopathologic study of 72 cases. Am J Clin Pathol 1990;94:371-377.

39. Bratthauer GL, Lininger RA, Man YG, Tavassoli FA. Androgen and estrogen receptor mRNA status in apocrine carcinomas. Diagn Mol Pathol 2002;11:113-118.

40. Bundred NJ, Walker RA, Everington D, White GK, Stewart HJ, Miller WR. Is apocrine differentiation in breast carcinoma of prognostic significance. Br J Cancer 1990;62:113-117.

41. Carter D, Rosen PP. Atypical apocrine metaplasia in sclerosing lesions of the breast: a study of 51 cases. Mod Pathol 1991;4:1-5.

41a. Celis JE, Gromova I, Gromov P, et al. Molecular pathology of breast apocrine carcinomas: a protein expression signature specific for benign apocrine metaplasia. FEBS Lett 2006;580:2935-2944.

42. Damiani S, Eusebi V, Losi L, D'Adda T, Rosai J. Oncocytic carcinoma (malignant oncocytoma) of the breast. Am J Surg Pathol 1998;22:221-230.

43. D'Amore ES, Terrier-Lacombe MJ, Travagli JP, Friedman S, Contesso G. Invasive apocrine carcinoma of the breast: a long term follow-up study of 34 cases. Breast Cancer Res Treat 1988;12:37-44.

44. De Potter CR, Eeckhout I, Schelfhout AM, Geerts ML, Roels HJ. Keratinocyte induced chemotaxis in the pathogenesis of Paget's disease of the breast. Histopathology 1994;24:349-356.

45. Eusebi V, Betts CM, Haagensen DE, Gugliotta P, Bussolati G, Azzopardi JG. Apocrine differentiation in lobular carcinoma of the breast. A morphologic, immunologic, and ultrastructural study. Hum Pathol 198415:134-140.

46. Eusebi V, Foschini MP, Bussolati G, Rosen PP. Myoblastomatoid (histiocytoid) carcinoma of the breast. A type of apocrine carcinoma. Am J Surg Pathol 1995;19:553-562.

47. Eusebi V, Magalhaes F., Azzopardi AG. Pleomorphic lobular carcinoma of the breast: an aggressive tumour showing apocrine differentiation. Hum Pathol 1992;23:655-662.

48. Eusebi V, Millis RR, Cattani MG, Bussolati G, Azzopardi JG. Apocrine carcinoma of the breast. A morphologic and immunocytochemical study. Am J Pathol 1986;123:532-541.

49. Foote FW Jr, Stewart FW. A histologic classification of carcinoma of the breast. Surgery 1946;19:74-99.

50. Frable WJ, Kay S. Carcinoma of the breast. Histologic and clinical features of apocrine tumors. Cancer 1968;21:756-763.

51. Gilles R, Lesnik A, Guinebretiere JM, et al. Apocrine carcinoma: clinical and mammographic features. Radiology 1994;190:495-497.

52. Johnson TL, Kini SR. The significance of atypical apocrine cells in fine-needle aspirates of the breast. Diagn Cytopathol 1989;5:248-254.

53. Jones C, Damiani S, Wells D, Chaggar R, Lakhani SR, Eusebi V. Molecular cytogenetic comparison of apocrine hyperplasia and apocrine carcinoma of the breast. Am J Pathol 2001;158:207-214.

54. Higginson JF, McDonald JR. Apocrine tissue, chronic cystic mastitis and sweat gland carcinoma of the breast. Surg Gynecol Obstet 1949;88:1-10.

54a. Honma N, Takubo K, Akiyama F, et al. Expression of oestrogen receptor-beta in apocrine carcinomas of the breast. Histopathology 2007;50:425-433.

54b. Honma N, Takubo K, Arai T, et al. Comparative study of monoclonal antibody B72.3 and gross cystic disease fluid protein-15 as markers of apocrine carcinoma of the breast. APMIS 2006;114:712-719.

55. Kopans DB, Nguyen PL, Koerner FC, et al. Mixed form, diffusely scattered calcifications in breast cancer with apocrine features. Radiology 1990;177:807-811.

56. Leal C, Henrique R, Monteiro P, et al. Apocrine ductal carcinoma in situ of the breast: histologic classification and expression of biologic markers. Hum Pathol 2001;32:487-493.

57. Lininger RA, Zhuang Z, Man Y, Park WS, Emmert-Buck M, Tavassoli FA. Loss of heterozygosity is detected at chromosomes 1p35-36 (NB), 3p25 (VHL), 16p13 (TSC2/PKD1), and 17p13 (TP53) in microdissected apocrine carcinomas of the breast. Mod Pathol 1999;12:1083-1089.

58. Losi L, Lorenzini R, Eusebi V, Bussolati G. Apocrine differentiation in invasive carcinoma of the breast. Applied Immunohistochemistry 1995;3:91-98.

59. Matsuo K, Fukutomi T, Hasegawa T, Akashi-Tanaka S, Nanasawa T, Tsuda H. Histological and immunohistochemical analysis of apocrine breast carcinoma. Breast Cancer 2002;9:43-49.

60. Mazoujian G, Pinkus GS, Davis S, Haagensen DE Jr. Immunohistochemistry of a gross cystic disease fluid protein (GCDFP-15) of the breast. A marker of apocrine epithelium and breast carcinomas with apocrine features. Am J Pathol 1983;110:105-112.

61. Miller WR, Telford J, Dixon JM, Shivas AA. Androgen metabolism and apocrine differentiation in human breast cancer. Breast Cancer Res Treat 1985;5:67-73.

62. Moriya T, Sakamoto K, Sasano H, et al. Immunohistochemical analysis of Ki-67, p53, p21 and p27 in benign and malignant apocrine lesions of the breast: its correlation to histologic findings in 43 cases. Mod Pathol 2000:13:13-18.

63. Mossler JA, Barton TK, Brinkhous AD, McCarty KS, Moylan JA, McCarty KS Jr. Apocrine differentiation in human mammary carcinoma. Cancer 1980;46:2463-2471.

64. Ng WK. Fine needle aspiration cytology of apocrine carcinoma of the breast. Review of cases in a three-year period. Acta Cytol 2002;46:507-512.

65. Pagani A, Sapino A, Eusebi V, Bergnolo P, Bussolati G. PIP/GCDFP-15 gene expression and apocrine differentiation in carcinomas of the breast. Virchows Arch 1994;425:459-465.

66. Raju U, Zarbo RJ, Kubus J, Schultz DS. The histologic spectrum of apocrine breast proliferation: a comparative study of morphology and DNA content by image analysis. Hum Pathol 1993;24:173-181.

67. Roddy HJ, Silverberg SG. Ultrastructural analysis of apocrine carcinoma of the human breast. Ultrastruct Pathol 1980;1:385-393.

68. Shousha S, Bull TB, Southall PJ, Mazoujian G. Apocrine carcinoma of the breast containing foamy cells. An electron microscopic and immunohistochemical study. Histopathology 1987;11:611-620.

68a. Tanaka K, Imoto S, Wada N, Sakemura N, Hasebe K. Invasive apocrine carcinoma of the breast: clinicopathologic features of 57 patients. Breast J 2008;14:164-168.

69. Tavassoli FA, Jones MW, Majeste RM, Bratlhauer GL, O'Leary TJ. Immunohistochemical staining with monoclonal Ab B72.3 in benign and malignant breast disease. Am J Surg Pathol 1990;14:128-133.

70. Tavassoli FA, Purcell CA, Bratthauer GL, Man Y. Androgen receptor expression along with loss of bcl-2, ER and PR expression in benign and malignant apocrine lesions of the breast: implications for therapy. Breast J 1996;2:261-269.

71. Viacava P, Naccarato AG, Bevilacqua G. Apocrine epithelium of the breast: does it result from metaplasia? Virchows Arch 1997;431:205-209.

72. Wick MR, Lillemoe TJ, Copland GT, Swanson PE, Manivel JC, Kiang DT. Gross cystic disease fluid protein-15 as a marker for breast cancer: immunohistochemical analysis of 690 human neoplasms and comparison with alpha-lactalbumin. Hum Pathol 1989;20:281-287.

73. Yates AJ, Ahmed A. Apocrine carcinoma and apocrine metaplasia. Histopathology 1988;13:228-231.

74. Yoshida K, Inoue M, Furuta S, et al. Apocrine carcinoma vs apocrine metaplasia with atypia of the breast. Use of aspiration biopsy cytology. Acta Cytol 1996;40:247-251.

Lipid-Rich Carcinoma

75. Aboumrad MH, Horn RC Jr, Fine G. Lipid-secreting mammary carcinoma. Report of a case associated with Paget's disease of the nipple. Cancer 1963;16:521-525.

76. Aida Y, Takeuchi E, Shinagawa T, et al. Fine needle aspiration cytology of lipid-secreting carcinoma of the breast: a case report. Acta Cytol 1993;37:547-551.

77. Fisher ER, Gregorio R, Kim WS, Redmond C. Lipid in invasive cancer of breast. Am J Clin Pathol 1977;68:558-561.

78. Kurebayshi J, Izuo M, Ishida T, Kurosumi M, Kawai T. Two cases of lipid-secreting carcinoma of the breast: case reports and an electron microscopic study. Jpn J Clin Oncol 1988;18:249-254.

79. Mazzella FM, SieberSC, Braza F. Ductal carcinoma of male breast with prominent lipid-rich component. Pathology 1995;27:280-283.

80. Ramos CV, Taylor HB. Lipid-rich carcinoma of the breast. A clinicopathological analysis of thirteen examples. Cancer 1974;33:812-819.

81. Tsubura A, Hatano T, Murata A, et al. Breast carcinoma in patients receiving neuroleptic therapy. Morphologic and clinicpathologic features of thirteen cases. Acta Pathol Jpn 1992;42:494-499.

82. Van Bogaert LJ, Maldague P. Histologic variants of lipid-secreting carcinoma of the breast. Virchows Arch A Pathol Anat Histol 1977;375:345-353.

83. Varga Z, Robl C, Spycher M, Burger D, Caduff R. Metaplastic lipid-rich carcinoma of the breast. Pathol Int 1998;48:912-916.

84. Vera-Sempere F, Llombart-Bosch A. Lipid-rich versus lipd-secreting carcinoma of the mammary gland. Pathol Res Pract 1985;190:553-558.

85. Wrba F, Ellinger A, Reiner G, Spona J, Holzner JH. Ultrastructural and immunohistochemical characteristics of lipid-rich carcinoma of the breast. Virchows Arch A Pathol Anat Histopathol 1988;413:381-385.

Sebaceous Carcinoma

86. Rao NA, Hidayat AA, McLean IW, Zimmerman LE. Sebaceous carcinomas of the ocular adnexa: a clinicopathologic study of 104 cases, with five-year follow-up data. Hum Pathol 1982;13:113-122.

87. Schlernitzauer DA, Font RI. Sebaceous gland carcinoma of the eyelid. Arch Ophthalmol 1976;94:1523-1525.

88. Tavassoli FA. Pathology of the breast, 2nd ed. Stamford, CT: Appleton and Lange/McGraw Hill; 1999:555-558.

Secretory Carcinoma

89. Akhtar M, Robinson C, Ali MA, Godwin JT. Secretory carcinoma of the breast in adults. Light and electron microscopic study of three cases with review of the literature. Cancer 1983; 51:2245-2254.

90. Botta G, Fessia L, Ghiringhello B. Juvenile milk protein secreting carcinoma. Virchows Arch A Pathol Anat Histopathol 1982;395:145-152.

91. D'Amore ES, Maisto L, Gatteschi MB, Toma S, Canavese G. Secretory carcinoma of the breast. Report of a case with fine needle aspiration biopsy. Acta Cytol 1986;30:309-312.

92. De Bree E, Askoxylakis J, Giannikaki E, Chroniaris N, Sanidas E, Tsiftsis DD. Secretory carcinoma of the male breast. Ann Surg Oncol 2002;9:663-667.

93. de la Cruz Mera A, de la Cruz Mera E, Leston JS, de Agustin de Agustin P. Secretory carcinoma of the breast. Acta Cytol 1994;38:968-969.

93a. Diallo R, Tognon C, Knezevich SR, Sorensen P, Poremba C. Secretory carcinoma of the breast: a genetically defined carcinoma entity. Verh Dtsch Ges Pathol 2003;87:193-203.

94. Dominguez F, Riera JR, Junco P, Sampedro A. Secretory carcinoma of the breast. Report of a case with diagnosis by fine needle aspiration. Acta Cytol 1992;36:507-510.

95. Ferguson TB, McCarty KS Jr, Filston HC. Juvenile secretory carcinoma and juvenile papillomatosis: diagnosis and treatment. J Pediatr Surg 1987;22:637-639.

96. Gupta K, Lallu SD, Fauck R, Simpson JS, Wakefield SJ. Needle aspiration cytology, immunohistochemistry, and electron microscoy in a rare case of secretory carcinoma of the breast in an elderly woman. Diagn Cytopathol 1992;8:388-391.

97. Hartman AW, Magrish P, Carcinoma of breast in children. Case report: six-year-old boy with adenocarcinoma. Ann Surg 1955;141:792-797.

98. Herz H, Cooke B, Goldstein D. Metastatic secretory breast cancer. Non-responsiveness to chemotherapy: case report and review of literature. Ann Oncol 2000;11:1343-1347.

99. Hirokawa M, Sugihara K, Sai T, et al. Secretory carcinoma of the breast: a tumour analogous to salivary gland acinic cell carcinoma. Histopathology 2002;40:223-229.

100. Izumi J, Komaki K, Hirokawa M, Masuda E, Monden Y. Secretory carcinoma of the breast with a cystically dilated intraductal component: report of a case. Surg Today 2003;33:110-113.

101. Karl SR, Ballantine TV, Zaino R. Juvenile secretory carcinoma of the breast. J Pediatr Surg 1985;20:368-371.

102. Krausz T, Jenkins D, Grontoft O, Pollack DJ, Azzopardi JG. Secretory carcinoma of the breast in adults; emphasis on late recurrence and metastasis. Histopathology 1989;14:25-36.

103. Lamovec J, Bracko M. Secretory carcinoma of the breast: light microscopical, immunohistochemical and flow cytometric study. Mod Pathol 1994;7:475-479.

104. Maitra A, Tavassoli FA, Albores-Saavedra J, et al. Molecular abnormalities associated with secretory carcinomas of the breast. Hum Pathol 1999;30:1435-1440.

105. McDivitt RW, Stewart FW. Breast carcinoma in children. JAMA 1996;195:388-390.

106. Mies C. Recurrent secretory carcinoma in residual mammary tissue after mastectomy. Am J Surg Pathol 1993;17:715-721.

107. Oberman HA. Secretory carcinoma of the breast in adults. Am J Surg Pathol 1980;4:465-470.

108. Pohar-Marinsek Z, Golouh R. Secretory breast carcinoma in a man diagnosed by needle aspiration biopsy. A case report. Acta Cytol 1994;38:446-450.

109. Richard G, Hawk JC 3rd, Baker AS Jr, Austin RM. Multicentric adult secretory breast carcinoma: DNA flow cytometric findings, prognostic features, and review of the world literature. J Surg Oncol 1990;44:238-244

110. Rosen PP, Cranor ML. Secretory carcinoma of the breast. Arch Pathol Lab Med 1991;115:141-144.

111. Serour F, Gilad A, Kopolovic J, Krispin M. Secretory breast cancer in childhood and adolescence: report of a case and review of the literature. Med Pediatr Oncol 1992;20:341-344.

112. Shinagawa T, Tadokoro M, Kitamura H, Mizuguchi K, Kushima M. Secretory carcinoma of the breast. Correlation of aspiration cytology and histology. Acta Cytol 1994;38:909-914.

113. Siegel JR, Karcnik TJ, Hertz MB, Gelman H, Baker SR. Secretory carcinoma of the breast. Breast J 1999;5:204-207.

114. Sullivan JJ, Mayee HR, Donald KJ. Secretory (Juvenile) carcinoma of the breast. Pathology 1977;9:341-346.

115. Tavassoli FA, Norris HJ. Secretory carcinoma of the breast. Cancer 1980;45:2404-2413.

116. Titus J, Sillar RW, Fenton LE. Secretory breast carcinoma in a 9-year-old boy. Aust N Z J Surg 2000;70:144-146.

117. Tognon C, Knezevich SR, Huntsman D, et al. Expression of ETV6-NTRK3 gene fusion as a primary event in human secretory breast carcinoma. Cancer Cell 2002;2:367-376.

117a. Yaqoob N, Kayani N, ul Hasan SH. Painless breast lump in an elderly woman. Secretory breast carcinoma in an elderly woman. Arch Pathol Lab Med 2006;130:1073-1074.

Clear Cell Carcinoma

118. Damiani S, Chiodera P, Guaragni M, Eusebi V. Mammary angiomyolipoma. Virchows Arch 2002;440:551-552.

119. Dina R, Eusebi V. Clear cell tumors of the breast. Semin Diagn Pathol 1997;14:175-182.

120. Fisher ER, Tavares J, Bulatao IS, Sass R, Fisher B. Glycogen-rich, clear cell breast cancer: with comments concerning other clear cell variants. Hum Pathol 1985;16:1085-1090.

121. Govender D, Sabaratnam RM, Essa AS. Clear cell 'sugar' tumor of the breast. Another extrapulmonary site and review of the literature. Am J Surg Pathol 2002;26:670-675.

122. Hayes MM, Seidman JD, Ashton MA. Glycogen-rich clear cell carcinoma of the breast. A clinicopathologic study of 21 cases. Am J Surg Pathol 1995;19:904-911.

123. Hull MT, Warfel KA. Glycogen-rich clear cell carcinomas of the breast. A clinicopathologic and ultrastructural study. Am J Surg Pathol 1986;10:553-559.

124. Kern SB, Andera L. Cytology of glycogen-rich (clear cell) carcinoma of the breast. A report of two cases. Acta Cytol 1997;41:556-560.

124a. Kuroda H, Sakamoto G, Ohnisi K, Itoyama S. Clinical and pathological features of glycogen-rich clear cell carcinoma of the breast. Breast Cancer 2005;12:189-195.

125. Shirley S, Escoffery CT, Titus IP, Williams EE, West AB. Clear cell carcinoma of the breast with immunohistochemical evidence of divergent differentiation. Ann Diagn Pathol 2002;6:250-256.

126. Sorensen FB, Paulsen SM. Glycogen-rich clear cell carcinoma of the breast: a solid variant with mucus. A light microscopic, immunohistochemical and ultrastructural study of a case. Histopathology 1987;11:857-869.

126a. Takekawa Y, Kubo A, Morita T, et al. Histopathological and immunohistochemical findings in a case of glycogen-rich clear cell carcinoma of the breast. Rinsho Byori 2006;54:27-30.

127. Toikkanen S, Joensuu H. Glycogen-rich clear-cell carcinoma of the breast: a clinicopathologic and flow cytometric study. Hum Pathol 1991;22:81-83.

128. Varga Z, Caduff R. Glycogen-rich carcinomas of the breast display unique characteristics with respect to proliferation and the frequency of oligonucleosomal fragments. Breast Cancer Res Treat 1999;57:215-219.

Carcinoma with Osteoclastic Giant Cells

129. Agnantis NT, Rosen PP. Mammary carcinoma with osteoclast-like giant cells. A study of eight cases with follow-up data. Am J Clin Pathol 1979;72:383-389.

130. Athanasou NA, Wells CA, Quinn J, Ferguson DP, Heryat A, McGee JO. The origin and nature of stromal osteoclast-like multinucleated giant cells in breast carcinoma: implications for tumor osteolysis and macrophage biology. Br J Cancer 1989;59:491-498.

131. Bertrand G, Bidabe MC, Bertrand AF. [Breast carcinoma with multinucleated reactive stromal giant cells.] Arch Anat Cytol Pathol 1982;30:5-9. [French.]

132. Factor SM, Biempica L, Ratner I, Ahujak K, Biempica S. Carcinoma of the breast with multinucleated reactive stromal giant cells. A light and electron microscopic study of two cases. Virchows Arch A Pathol Anat Histol 1977;374:1-12.

133. Fisher ER, Palekar AS, Gregorio RM, Paulson JD. Mucoepidermoid and squamous cell carcinomas of breast with reference to squamous metaplasia and giant cell tumors. Am J Surg Pathol 1983;7:15-27.

134. Gupta RK. Aspiration cytodiagnosis of a rare carcinoma of breast with bizarre malignant giant cells. Diagn Cytopathol 1996;15:66-69.

135. Holland R, Van Haelst VJ. Mammary carcinoma with osteoclast-like giant cells. Additional observations on six cases. Cancer 1984;53:1963-1973.

136. Ichijima K, Kobashi Y, Ueda Y, Matsuo S. Breast cancer with reactive multinucleated giant cells: report of three cases. Actal Pathol Jpn 1986;36:449-457.

137. McMahon RF, Ahmed A, Connolly CE. Breast carcinoma with stromal multinucleated giant cells: a light microscopic, histochemical and ultrastructural study. J Pathol 1986;150:175-179.

138. Nielsen BB, Kiaer HW. Carcinoma of the breast with stromal multinucleated giant cells. Histopathology 1985;9:183-193.

139. Phillipson J, Ostrzega N. Fine needle aspiration of invasive cribriform carcinoma wth benign osteoclastlike giant cells of histiocytic origin. A case report. Acta Cytol 1994;38:479-482.

140. Takahashi T, Moriki T, Hiroi M, Nakayama H. Invasive lobular carcinoma of the breast with osteoclast-like giant cells: a case report. Acta Cytol 1998;42:734-741.

141. Tavassoli FA, Norris HJ. Breast carcinoma with osteoclast-like giant cells. Arch Pathol Lab Med 1986;110:636-639.

142. Volpe R, Carbone A, Nicalo G, Santi L. Cytology of the breast carcinoma with osteoclast-like giant cells. Acta Cytol 1983;27:184-187.

Breast Cancer with Choriocarcinomatous Features

143. Giannotti Filho O, Miiji LN, Vainchenker M, Gordan AN. Breast cancer with choriocarcinomatous and neuroendocrine features. Sao Paulo Med J 2001;119:154-155.

144. Murata T, Ihara S. Breast cancer with choriocarcinomatous features: a case report with cytopathological details. Pathol Int 1999;49:816-819.

145. Resetkova E, Sahin A, Ayala AG, Sneige N. Breast carcinoma with choriocarcinomatous features. Ann Diagn Pathol 2004;8:74-79.

146. Saigo PE, Rosen PP. Mammary carcinoma with "choriocarcinomatous" features. Am J Surg Pathol 1981;5:773-778.

Melanotic Carcinoma

147. Azzopardi JG, Eusebi V. Melanocytic colonization and pigmentation of breast carcinoma. Histopathology 1977;1:21-30.
148. Culberson JD, Horn RC. Paget's disease of the nipple: review of 25 cases with special reference to melanin pigmentation of "Paget cells." A.M.A. Arch Surg 1956;72:224-231.
149. Fernandez-Figueras MT, Puig L, Casanova JM, Musulen E, Matias-Guiu X, Navas-Paslacios JJ. Pigmented epidermotropic ductal carcinoma of the breast in a male. Ultrastructural evidence of melanocyte colonization and melanin transfer to the tumor. J Cutan Pathol 1995;22:176-180.
150. Lloreta-Trull J, Ordonez NG, Mackay B. Pigmented carcinoma of the breast: an ultrastructural study. Ultrastruct Pathol 2000;24:109-113.
151. Nobukawa B, Fujii H, Hirai S, et al. Breast carcinoma diverging to aberrant melanocytic differentiation: a case report with histopathologic and loss of heterozygosity analyses. Am J Surg Pathol 1999;23:1280-1287.
152. Padmore RF, Lara JF, Ackerman DJ, et al. Primary combined malignant melanoma and ductal carcinoma of the breast: a report of two cases. Cancer 1996;78:2515-2525.
153. Poiares-Baptista A, de Vasconcelos AA. Cutaneous pigmented metastasis from breast carcinoma simulating malignant melanoma. Int J Dermatol 1988;27:124-125.
154. Romanelli R, Toncini C. Pigmented papillary carcinoma of the male breast. Tumori 1986;72:105-108.
155. Ruffolo EF, Koerner FC, Maluf HM. Metaplastic carcinoma of the breast with melanocytic differentiation. Mod Pathol 1997;10:592-596.
156. Saitoh K, Saga K, Okazaki M, Maeda K. Pigmented primary carcinoma of the breast: a clinical mimic of malignant melanoma. Br J Dermatol 1998;139:287-290.
157. Sau P, Solis J, Lupton GP, James WD. Pigmented breast carcinoma. A clinical and histologic simulator of malignant melanoma. Arch Dermatol 1989;125:536-539.
158. Shin SJ, Kanomata N, Rosen PP. Mammary carcinoma with prominent cytoplasmic lipofuscin granules mimicking melanocytic differentiation. Histopathology 2000;37:456-459.
159. Yen H, Florentine B, Kelly LK, Bu X, Crawford J, Martin SE. Fine-needle aspiration of a metaplastic carcinoma with extensive melanocytic differentiation: a case report. Diagn Cytopathol 2000;23:46-50.

Basal-Like Breast Cancers

160. Banerjee S, Reis-Filho JS, Ashley S, et al. Basal-like breast carcinomas: clinical outcome and response to chemotherapy. J Clin Pathol 2006;59:729-735.
161. Bertucci F, Finetti P, Cervera N, et al. Gene expression profiling shows medullary breast cancer is a subgroup of basal breast cancers. Cancer Res 2006;66:4636-4344.
162. Brenton JD, Carey LA, Ahmed AA, Caldas C. Molecular classification and molecular forecasting of breast cancer: ready for clinical application? J Clin Oncol 2005;23:7350-7360.
163. Collett K, Stefansson IM, Eide J, et al. A basal epithelial phenotype is more frequent in interval breast cancers compared with screen detected tumors. Cancer Epidemiol Biomarkers Prev. 2005;14:1108-1112.
164. Fadare O, Tavassoli FA. The phenotypic spectrum of basal-like breast cancers: a critical appraisal. Adv Anat Pathol 2007;14:358-373.
164a. Fadare O, Tavassoli FA. Clinical and pathologic aspects of basal-like breast cancers. Nat Clin Pract Oncol 2008;5:149-159.
165. Foulkes WD, Brunet JS, Stefansson IM, et al. The prognostic implication of the basal-like (cyclin E high/p27 low/p53+/glomeruloid-microvascular-proliferation+) phenotype of BRCA1-related breast cancer. Cancer Res 2004;64:830-835.
166. Fulford LG, Easton DF, Reis-Filho JS, et al. Specific morphological features predictive for the basal phenotype in grade 3 invasive ductal carcinoma of breast. Histopathology 2006;49:22-34.
167. Jacquemier J, Padovani L, Rabayrol L, et al. Typical medullary breast carcinomas have a basal/myoepithelial phenotype. J Pathol 2005:207:260-268.
168. Kim MJ, Ro JY, Ahn SH, Kim HH, Kim SB, Gong G. Clinicopathologic significance of the basal-like subtype of breast cancer: a comparison with hormone receptor and Her2/neu-overexpressing phenotypes. Hum Pathol 2006;37:1217-1226.
169. Kusinska R, Potemski P, Jesionek-Kupnicka D, Kordek R. Immunohistochemical identification of basal-type cytokeratins in invasive ductal breast carcinoma—relation with grade, stage, estrogen receptor and HER2. Pol J Pathol 2005;56:107-110.
170. Laakso M, Loman N, Borg A, Isola J. Cytokeratin 5/14-positive breast cancer: true basal phenotype confined to BRCA1 tumors. Mod Pathol 2005;18:1321-1328.
171. Livasy CA, Karaca G, Nanda R, et al. Phenotypic evaluation of the basal-like subtype of invasive breast carcinoma. Mod Pathol 2006;19:264-271.

172. Matos I, Dufloth R, Alvarenga M, Zeferino LC, Schmitt F. p63, cytokeratin 5, and P-cadherin: three molecular markers to distinguish basal phenotype in breast carcinomas. Virchows Arch 2005;447:688-694.

173. Nielsen TO, Hsu FD, Jensen K, et al. Immunohistochemical and clinical characterization of the basal-like subtype of invasive breast carcinoma. Clin Cancer Res 2004;10:5367-5374.

174. Palacios J, Honrado E, Osorio A, Diez O, Rivas C, Benitez J. Re: Germline BRCA1 mutations and a basal epithelial phenotype in breast cancer. J Natl Cancer Inst 2004;96:712-714.

175. Perou CM, Sorlie T, Eisen MB, et al. Molecular portraits of human breast tumors. Nature 2000;406:747-752.

176. Potemski P, Kusinska R, Watala C, Pluciennik E, Bednarek AK, Kordek R. Prognostic relevance of basal cytokeratin expression in operable breast cancer. Oncology 2005;69:478-485.

177. Rakha EA, El-Rehim DA, Paish C, et al. Basal phenotype identifies a poor prognostic subgroup of breast cancer of clinical importance. Eur J Cancer 2006;42:3149-3156.

178. Rakha EA, El-Sayed ME, Green AR, Lee AH, Robertson JF, Ellis IO. Prognostic markers in triple-negative breast cancer. Cancer 2006;109:25-32.

179. Rakha EA, Putti TC, Abd El-Rehim DM, et al. Morphological and immunophenotypic analysis of breast carcinomas with basal and myoepithelial differentiation. J Pathol 2006;208:495-506.

180. Reis-Filho JS, Milanezi F, Steele D, et al. Metaplastic breast carcinomas are basal-like tumors. Histopathology 2006;49:10-21.

181. Ribeiro-Silva A, Ramalho LN, Garcia SB, Brandao DV, Chahud F, Zucoloto S. p63 correlates with both BRCA1 and cytokeratin 5 in invasive breast carcinomas: further evidence for the pathogenesis of the basal phenotype of breast cancer. Histopathology 2005;47:458-466.

182. Ribeiro-Silva A, Ribeiro do Vale F, Zucoloto S. Vascular endothelial growth factor expression in the basal subtype of breast carcinoma. Am J Clin Pathol 2006;125:512-518.

183. Rodriguez-Pinilla SM, Sarrio D, Honrado E, et al. Prognostic significance of basal-like phenotype and fascin expression in node-negative invasive breast carcinomas. Clin Cancer Res 2006;12:1533-1539.

184. Rodriguez-Pinilla SM, Sarrio D, Honrado E, et al. Vimentin and laminin expression is associated with basal-like phenotype in both sporadic and BRCA1-associated breast carcinomas. J Clin Pathol 2007;60:1006-1012.

185. Siziopikou KP, Cobleigh M. The basal subtype of breast carcinomas may represent the group of breast tumors that could benefit from EGFR-targeted therapies. Breast 2007;16:104-107.

186. Sorlie T, Perou CM, Tibshirani R, et al. Gene expression patterns of breast carcinomas distinguish tumor subclasses with clinical implications. Proc Natl Acad Sci U S A 2001;98:10869-10874.

187. Sorlie T. Molecular classification of breast tumors: toward improved diagnostics and treatments. Methods Mol Biol 2007;360:91-114.

188. van 't Veer LJ, Dai H, van de Vijver MJ, et al. Gene expression profiling predicts clinical outcome of breast cancer. Nature 2002;415:530-536.

189. van de Rijn M, Perou CM, Tibshirani R, et al. Expression of cytokeratins 17 and 5 identifies a group of breast carcinomas with poor clinical outcome. Am J Pathol 2002;161:1991–1996.

11 MYOEPITHELIAL LESIONS

Myoepithelial cells are a normal component of the mammary duct system and form a natural boundary, which together with the basement membrane, separate the epithelial cells from the surrounding stroma. Myoepithelial cells may give rise to myoid cells in "stromo-epithelial" lesions (14). Several mammary lesions are either derived from or composed of a dominant to pure population of myoepithelial cells. These include adenoid cystic carcinoma, the rare mixed tumor or pleomorphic adenoma (benign or malignant), myoepitheliosis, adenomyoepithelioma (benign or with a variety of malignant elements), and myoepithelioma of the benign or malignant (myoepithelial carcinoma) type. Adenoid cystic carcinoma is discussed in chapter 9, while pleomorphic adenoma is described in chapter 2. In this section, the focus is on the remaining lesions.

IMMUNOHISTOCHEMICAL PROFILE OF MYOEPITHELIAL CELLS

The normal, proliferative, and neoplastic myoepithelial cells have an immunoprofile that is significantly different from that of epithelial cells (2,3,21,25,29–32,37a,40–42,45,48,49,55,56,59–61). In the normal state, they display variable immunoreactivity with muscle-specific actin, alpha-smooth muscle actin, calponin, vimentin, S-100 protein, maspin, smooth muscle myosin-heavy chain, p63, and rarely, glial fibrillary acidic protein, but are negative for desmin. They are strongly reactive with cytokeratin (CK) 14; high molecular weight CK34betaE12 containing CK1, CK5, CK10, and CK14; and CD10. A faint to absent reaction is seen with CAM5.2 (CK8/18); the reaction of myoepithelial cells with kermix (AE1/AE3/LP34) is substantially weaker than the reaction simultaneously evident in the overlying epithelial cells. The reaction with each of these markers is probably related to the functional status of the cells. The immunoreactivity for all the markers noted above, but one, is cytoplasmic; p63 displays a nuclear reaction (42,61). The normal and neo-plastic myoepithelial cells are consistently negative for estrogen receptor (ER) and progesterone receptor (PR). See chapter 1 for an additional discussion of myoepithelial cells.

Cell lines derived from benign myoepithelial tumors express high levels of active angiogenic inhibitors including thromboplastin-1, tissue inhibitor of metalloproteinase-1 (TIMP-1), and soluble basic fibroblast growth factor (bFGF) receptors; they express very low levels of angiogenic factors (38). The cells respond to hypoxia by increasing hypoxia inducible factor-1alpha (HIF-1α), but only minimally increasing vascular endothelial growth factor (VEGF) and inducible nitric oxide synthetase (iNOS) steady state mRNA levels (38). The proliferating myoepithelial cells may accumulate abundant extracellular matrix devoid of angiogenesis but contain bound angiogenic inhibitors (38).

MYOEPITHELIOSIS

Definition. *Myoepitheliosis* is a multifocal, often microscopic proliferation of myoepithelial cells growing into and/or around small ducts and ductules, mainly in the region of terminal duct lobular unit (TDLU). The periductal variant is often associated with sclerosis and falls within the spectrum of sclerosing adenosis; this variant is not generally included among studies of myoepithelial lesions.

Clinical Features. When the nodular sclerosing adenosis variant is excluded, myoepitheliosis rarely presents as a palpable mass, but is commonly an incidental finding or presents as an area of parenchymal distortion on mammography. Patients with myoepitheliosis range in age from 22 to 87 years (55,56).

Gross Findings. Myoepitheliosis generally appears as a firm, irregular area within the biopsy, but a distinct mass is rarely observed.

Microscopic Findings. The lesion is characterized by a proliferation of spindled to cuboid cells growing into multiple ducts (figs. 11-1, 11-2). The proliferating cells are spindle shaped,

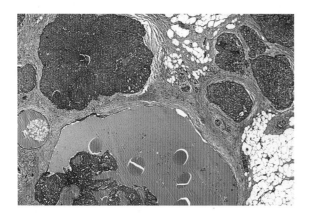

Figure 11-1

MYOEPITHELIOSIS

Multiple ducts are filled by a solid proliferation of spindled myoepithelial cells.

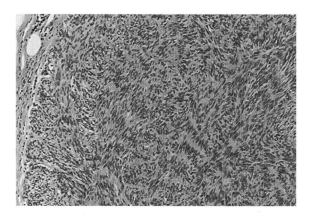

Figure 11-2

MYOEPITHELIOSIS

Nuclear palisading is evident in one duct.

sometimes assuming a prominent palisading pattern, and display varied nuclear shapes, sometimes with longitudinal nuclear grooves resembling transitional cells. Most lesions lack atypia or mitotic activity; when rare atypia and mitotic activity are present, the lesion is designated as *atypical myoepitheliosis*.

Differential Diagnosis. It is imperative to distinguish benign intraductal myoepitheliosis from the spindle cell variant of intraductal carcinoma (ductal intraepithelial neoplasia [DIN] of the spindle cell type) (18). The epithelial lesions are often found in continuity with the cribriform pattern, at least focally, and show intense immunoreactivity with CK7 and CAM5.2; they may show focal positivity with chromogranin, but are negative for smooth muscle actin, calponin, p63, and CD10. Immunostaining for S-100 protein is not reliable for separating epithelial and myoepithelial cells since some mammary epithelial cells also express S-100 protein. Spindle cell ductal carcinoma in situ (DCIS)/spindle cell DIN1-2 is generally negative for CK34betaE12, whereas most myoepithelial lesions are positive for this marker. Also, myoepithelial lesions are positive with CK5/6 (cocktail), as well as CK14, while epithelial carcinomas, with the exception of those rare cases with squamous or "basal" differentiation, are generally negative.

Treatment and Prognosis. Complete excision is generally curative when lesions lack atypia or mitotic activity. The potential for

the development of recurrences or an invasive process should be considered in atypical lesions, in which case complete excision becomes particularly crucial.

ADENOMYOEPITHELIOMA

Definition. *Adenomyoepithelioma* (AME) is a composite tumor with a predominant and generally solid proliferation of phenotypically variable myoepithelial cells around small epithelial-lined spaces. The epithelial, myoepithelial, or both components may become malignant (*malignant adenomyoepithelioma*).

Credited with the first description of mammary AME, Hamperl (24) also noted the varied phenotypes of the myoepithelial cells. The current classification of mammary myoepithelial lesions (Table 11-1) incorporates the many varieties of observed lesions formed by myoepithelial cells, either pure or admixed with epithelial cells. Over 150 AMEs have been reported (1,5,7,8,14,15,17,20,23,24,28,29,31,34,36,36a, 38a,40,44,48,50,51,54–56,59,60,62).

Clinical Features. Patients, predominantly female, range in age from 26 to 82 years, with a median age of 62 years (1,7,9,28,31,36,40,44, 55,59,60,62). Rare tumors have been reported in the male breast (5,54). Rarely associated with tenderness, AME presents as a palpable tumor, which may be massive and fungating. Women with myoepithelial lesions have been predominantly Caucasian, but Asian and black women are also affected. Mammographically, AME manifests as

Table 11-1

CLASSIFICATION OF MYOEPITHELIAL LESIONS[a]

Myoepitheliosis
Intraductal
Periductal (sclerosing adenosis)

Adenomyoepithelioma
Benign
Malignant[b]/Malignancy arising in adenomyo-
epithelioma
Myoepithelial carcinoma arising in an adenomyo-
epithelioma
Epithelial carcinoma[b] arising in an adenomyo-
epithelioma
Malignant epithelial and myoepithelial components
Sarcoma arising in adenomyoepithelioma
Carcinosarcoma arising in adenomyoepithelioma

Myoepithelioma
Benign
Malignant myoepithelioma (myoepithelial carcinoma)

[a]Adapted from data in references 55, 56, and 56a.
[b]Specify the subtype in parenthesis.

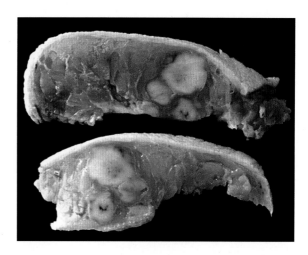

Figure 11-3

ADENOMYOEPITHELIOMA

The cut surface shows several solid, well-delineated, firm white nodules in a recurrent adenomyoepithelioma (AME).

a well-circumscribed density that may contain microcalcifications (5,7,14,44,54,56).

Gross Findings. AMEs are sharply delineated, rounded nodules. They range in size from less than 1 to 10 cm, with a median of 2.5 cm even when they recur (fig. 11-3). The solid cut surface is pink to tan with rare cystic and papillary areas and generally a firm, rubbery consistency. Hemorrhage and necrosis are rarely observed (5,15,17,28,31,36,55). AME generally manifests as a solitary mass or a dominant mass with significantly smaller satellite nodules.

Microscopic Findings. Microscopically, AMEs are highly varied, ranging in appearance from lesions with totally benign features to those with distinctively malignant features; the former are discussed under benign AMEs, while those with aggressive features are discussed under malignant AMEs. Sebaceous and apocrine metaplasia may develop in the epithelial cells, while osseous and chondroid metaplasia may develop in the myoepithelial component; squamous differentiation may develop as well, often emanating from the myoepithelial cells.

Benign AME. Well-delineated and often encapsulated, benign AMEs are characterized by a proliferation of layers or sheaths of myoepithelial cells around epithelial-lined spaces. The tumor may display a spindle cell, tubular, or most often, lobulated growth pattern (55,56).

The *spindle cell type* of benign AME assumes a solid or papillary architecture that often occludes distended duct-like spaces. Many are entirely intraductal lesions (fig. 11-4). Although invariably present, epithelial-lined spaces may be sparse within the spindle cell areas, resulting in frequent confusion with a leiomyoma. A storiform pattern may develop among the proliferating spindle cells.

Ill-defined and lacking encapsulation, the *tubular variant* is characterized by a compact collection of rounded tubules lined by a single layer of epithelial cells and multiple layers of myoepithelial cells (fig. 11-5). There is no significant atypia, but up to 3 mitotic figures per 10 high-power fields may be evident among the myoepithelial cells. While a tubular adenoma may resemble this lesion, it is generally sharply circumscribed and lacks the myoepithelial proliferation typical of this composite tumor.

Sometimes surrounded by a partial to complete thick fibrous capsule, the *lobulated variant* is composed of solid nests of clear, eosinophilic, or hyaline (plasmacytoid) myoepithelial cells proliferating around compressed epithelial-lined spaces (figs. 11-6, 11-7). Fibrous connective tissue septa of varying thickness divide the lesion into rounded nests or smaller lobules. Some tumors are composed purely of clear cells, but others show a pink to amphophilic cytoplasm, or rarely, a hyaline, plasmacytoid pattern. Mitotic activity

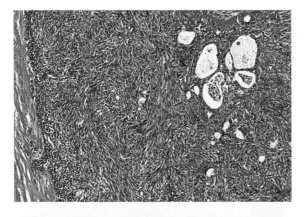

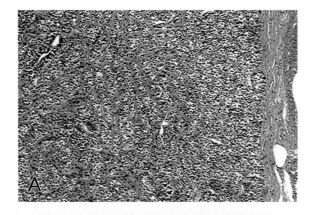

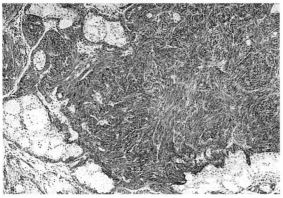

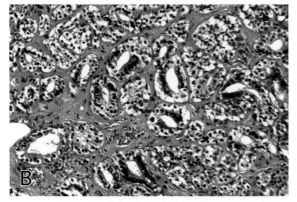

Figure 11-4

SPINDLE CELL ADENOMYOEPITHELIOMA

Top: A solid proliferation of spindled myoepithelial cells surrounds spaces lined by epithelial cells.

Bottom: Immunostain for S-100 protein decorates the proliferating myoepithelial cells.

is generally in the range of 1 to 2 mitotic figures per 10 high-power fields among the proliferating myoepithelial cells. Massive central infarction and hyaline degeneration are observed in some tumors. Calcification is evident in a third of the tumors. Satellite nodules, often identical to the main lesion, are seen adjacent to the lobulated variant in some cases, reflecting intraductal extension of the lesion.

Malignant AME/Malignancy arising in AME. Among the over 150 AMEs reported, about 40 have been considered to be malignant or potentially malignant (1,7,10,17,20,28,29,37a,38a,40, 46,48,50,51,55,59). An additional 19 have been reported in abstract form only (Hermmann M, Tavassoli FA, unpublished data, 2008). Either the epithelial, myoepithelial, or both components of an AME may give rise to a carcinoma, while

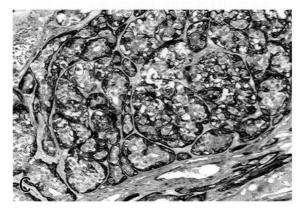

Figure 11-5

ADENOMYOEPITHELIOMA, TUBULAR TYPE

A: A compact aggregate of tubules is seen, many with compressed lumens.

B: Many tubules have prominent or pure myoepithelial cells; a luminal epithelial cell layer is apparent in some tubules.

C: The myoepithelial cells are positive for actin.

the background lesion retains its adenomyoepitheliomatous appearance (7,20,28,29,48,55,59). On extremely rare occasions, even the supportive stroma and vessels give rise to a malignancy (such as fibrosarcoma or angiosarcoma).

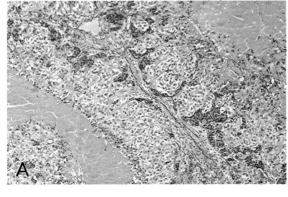

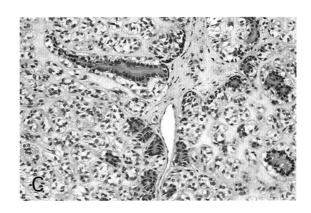

Figure 11-6

ADENOMYOEPITHELIOMA, LOBULATED TYPE

A: Each lobule shows central infarction, with sheaths of myoepithelial cells (lighter stained) proliferating around compressed, irregularly shaped and often obliterated epithelial-lined spaces.

B,C: The cytoplasm may be amphophilic (B) or clear (C). (B is fig. 8B from Tavasolli FA. Myoepithelial lesions of the breast. Myoepitheliosis, adenomyoepithelioma, and myoepithelial carcinoma. Am J Surg Pathol 1991;15:561.)

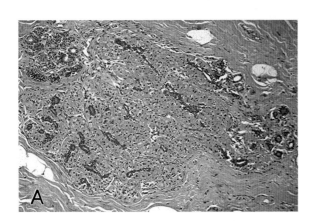

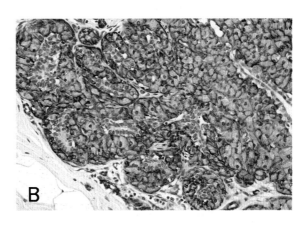

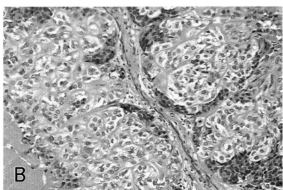

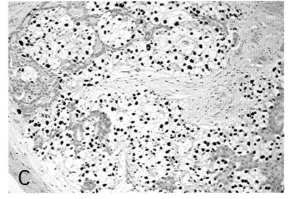

Figure 11-7

ADENOMYOEPITHELIOMA

A: In its early stages of development, the epithelial-lined spaces are compressed by proliferating myoepithelial cells.

B,C: The myoepithelial cells show cytoplasmic positivity with actin (C) and nuclear positivity with p63 (B).

Figure 11-8

MALIGNANCY ARISING IN ADENOMYOEPITHELIOMA

A: Infiltrating clusters composed of epithelial and myo-epithelial cells (simulating infiltrating epitheliosis) emanate from a space within an AME. (Fig. 15-20B from Tavassoli FA. Pathology of the breast, 2nd ed. Stamford, CT: Appleton & Lange/McGraw Hill; 1999:782.)

B: Metastatic tumor in a lymph node is composed of both epithelial and myoepithelial cells.

C: Calponin decorates a rim of myoepithelial cells around the epithelial cells in the lymph node.

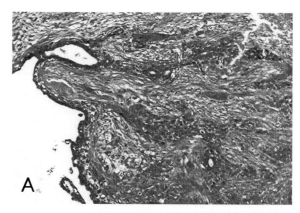

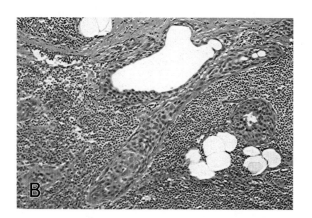

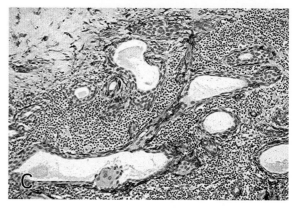

Most malignant alterations appear as focal lesions arising within a classic benign AME (fig. 11-8), but rare cases seem to be malignant de novo in the form of diffuse moderate atypia and abundant mitotic activity among the myoepithelial cells. Once mitotic activity exceeds 3 mitoses per 10 high-power fields, the lesion acquires the potential for local recurrence. The potential for distant metastasis probably increases with increasing mitotic activity. The aggressive myoepithelial cells may assume a spindle configuration, sometimes with clear cytoplasm, and develop into nodules resembling myofibroblastic lesions. Definitive criteria for malignancy include: invasion of the surrounding tissues, overgrowth of myoepithelial cells with moderate (more than 3 mitoses per 10 high-power fields) mitotic activity, and severe cytologic atypia.

In addition, distinctive patterns of carcinoma, such as myoepithelial carcinoma, adenoid cystic carcinoma, or carcinoma with chondroid differentiation, have been observed. A variety of epithelial-derived carcinomas also occur in this setting (Hermmann M, Tavassoli FA, unpublished data, 2008;38a,55,56). Rarely, both components develop into either separate malignancies or a single malignant infiltrative process composed of angulated tubules lined by both epithelial and myoepithelial cells (48,55). Multilabeling is useful for determining the immunophenotype of the lesion (37a).

Cytologic Findings. Aspiration cytology yields a cellular sample with a biphasic cell population that may be mistaken for a phyllodes tumor (34,36). There are clusters and sheets of benign epithelial cells admixed with clumps of bland-looking oval to spindle cells (fig. 11-9). The latter reflect the myoepithelial cells and have oval nuclei with fine chromatin, inconspicuous nucleoli, and scanty amphophilic cytoplasm (9). The cytoplasm may develop an elongated myoid, fibrillary appearance or may be so scant as to give the cells the appearance of naked nuclei.

Ultrastructural Findings. The ultrastructural features of AME depend on the myoepithelial and epithelial phenotypes present in the tumor. The hallmark of the myoepithelial cell is the presence of myofibrils with dense bodies, pinocytotic vesicles, desmosomes or tight junctions, and a patchy basement membrane. Pinocytotic vesicles are sparse

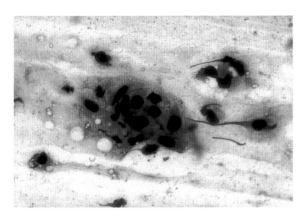

Figure 11-9

ADENOMYOEPITHELIOMA

Cytologically, clusters of predominantly myoepithelial cells dominate, occasionally surrounding one or more epithelial cells.

in the clear cell variant of myoepithelial cells. A complex meshwork of multilayered basement membrane surrounds the nests of myoepithelial cells (25,45,55,59,60). The epithelial cells lack pinocytotic vesicles or myofibrils; they display tonofilaments, variable amounts of secretory droplets, and desmosomal attachments.

Differential Diagnosis. The tubular variant of AME should be distinguished from a tubular adenoma; the latter has myoepithelial cells that are generally inconspicuous in contrast to the myoepithelial proliferation typical of an AME. Furthermore, tubular adenoma is generally a very well-circumscribed lesion, whereas tubular AME is partially circumscribed to poorly delineated, with the tubules extending between normal mammary structures.

The lobulated and spindle cell variants of AME should be distinguished from a mixed tumor. Mixed tumors generally have prominent areas of chondroid and/or osseous differentiation. When the spindle cell population is dominant and depending on the plane of section, such lesions may appear as pure myoepithelioma or smooth muscle tumors.

Treatment and Prognosis. A majority of mammary AMEs are benign (36a,55). Some, particularly those with the tubular pattern, may develop multiple recurrences (53,55,60). The tubular variant typically has an ill-defined boundary or demarcation, with the pathologic tubules often extending into and blending with the adjacent normal ducts. This feature could lead to incomplete excision and subsequent recurrence of the tumor.

At least 25 of the over 150 reported patients with AME had locally recurrent disease; the number of recurrences varied from 1 to 6 and recurrences or metastases occurred within 4 months to 23 years of the initial diagnosis (7,20, 29,40,44,48,51,55,59,62). In view of the presence of microscopic satellite nodules around many lobulated AMEs, some recurrences may actually reflect progression of residual disease. Factors with prognostic significance include invasive margins, overgrowth of the myoepithelial cells with increased mitotic activity, and severe cytologic atypia.

Malignant AMEs are generally low-grade neoplasms, but high-grade lesions do occur. Most of the rare patients with metastases have had an AME with a malignant myoepithelial or epithelial component. Metastases have been documented mainly in tumors 2 cm in diameter or larger and have been documented in up to 40 percent of malignant AMEs, generally as distant metastases (Hermmann M, Tavassoli FA, unpublished data, 2008). The lungs are a common site for metastatic disease, but metastases to the brain, jaws, and lymph nodes also develop. The metastases may be pure and composed of spindled myoepithelial cells or consist of both the epithelial and myoepithelial components. The myoepithelial elements dominate in advanced stage tumors as well as in recurrent or metastatic lesions. At least two women died from brain metastases. One had multiple recurrences followed by brain and lung metastases, with eventual death from the brain metastases (35); the tumor cells showed more than 10 mitotic figures per 10 high-power fields as well as focal cytologic anaplasia.

The treatment of benign AME is directed at complete excision of the lesion. Excision of a rim of uninvolved breast tissue is particularly important for those AME lesions with satellite nodules, infiltrative margins, and other aggressive features. When a distinctive carcinoma or sarcoma is present, appropriate therapy should be directed at these components. Although experience with radiation therapy is limited, it does not appear to be beneficial and it may possibly be associated with adverse effects since the four patients who died of their disease in one study had all received radiation therapy as a component of their management (Hermmann M, Tavassoli FA, unpublished data, 2008). In view of the tendency to metastasize to the lungs, baseline chest X rays and follow-up evaluation of lung fields are necessary.

MYOEPITHELIOMA

Pure spindle cell tumors of myoepithelial origin resemble smooth muscle tumors (6,12,43,58). Myoid and spindle cell transformations of myoepithelial cells occur most often in the setting of sclerosing adenosis and papillary lesions growing within ducts (58). The so-called muscular and myoid hamartomas may also have a myoepithelial origin (13), but these would qualify better as AME with an adipose tissue component. At least some benign myoepitheliomas are suboptimally sampled AMEs with myoepithelial cell overgrowth. Several benign myoepitheliomas have been reported (6,12,43).

Distinguishing myoepithelioma from pure smooth muscle tumors can be difficult. The immunoreactivity with high molecular weight cytokeratins (CK14, CK34betaE12) favors a myoepithelial lesion. Smooth muscle tumors may also show positivity with some cytokeratin markers (kermix, CAM5.2), however.

MALIGNANT MYOEPITHELIOMA (MYOEPITHELIAL CARCINOMA)

Definition. *Malignant myoepithelioma*, also termed *myoepithelial carcinoma*, is an infiltrating tumor composed purely of myoepithelial cells (predominantly spindled) with identifiable mitotic activity and sometimes prominent central hyalinization. Emanation of the spindle cells from the myoepithelial cell layer is evident in these tumors.

Clinical Features. Patients with malignant myoepithelioma range in age from 25 to 81 years, with a mean of 54 years. Similar to invasive ductal carcinoma, a palpable mass or an area of parenchymal density on mammography is the common presentation (16,25,30,33,39,45,46,52,55–57).

Gross Findings. Characterized by a wide size range (1 to 21 cm), malignant myoepithelioma is generally well-defined with focal marginal irregularity; some are stellate in shape. The cut surface appears firm, rubbery, and gray-white.

Foci of necrosis and hemorrhage are seen in the larger tumors. Nodular areas of hyalinization are sometimes observed even in smaller tumors.

Microscopic Findings. Microscopically, malignant myoepithelioma is a solitary lesion, characterized by an infiltrating proliferation of predominantly spindle cells, often with focal patches of more cuboidal epithelioid cells that lack significant atypia. Mitotic activity does not exceed 3 to 4 mitotic figures per 10 high-power fields. The spindled neoplastic cells appear to emanate from the myoepithelial cells of ductules entrapped in the periphery of the lesion (fig. 11-10), establishing the myoepithelial origin of the lesion. Aggregates of collagen, corresponding to the grossly visible hyalinized nodules, may be evident. Most reported cases have been purely invasive (16,33,55,56), but a prominent intraductal component or extension into ducts and lobules occurs (45,49,52,53,55,56).

Immunohistochemical Findings. At least some of the cells immunoreact with kermix (AE1/AE3/LP34); faint and often focal positivity may be observed with CAM5.2, CK34betaE12, p63, and CD10 are generally positive in the neoplastic cells, while calponin and smooth muscle actin are generally positive in the associated proliferating stromal myofibroblasts. Neoplastic myoepithelial cells often lose the expression of calponin and smooth muscle actin.

Ultrastructural Findings. Malignant myoepithelioma is composed purely of elongated or spindle-shaped myoepithelial cells dispersed in a collagenous stroma. The cells display pinocytotic vesicles, subplasmalemmal myofibrils with dense bodies, thick aggregates of often perinuclear tonofilaments, and patchy basal lamina; the quantity and distribution of these organelles vary in different cells. Tight and intermediate junctions attach the cytoplasmic processes of these cells; true desmosomes are rare (25,45,55).

Molecular Findings. By comparative genomic hybridization, myoepithelial carcinomas show relatively fewer molecular changes (2.1 changes) compared to ductal epithelial carcinomas (8.6 changes). The most common alterations are losses at 16q, 17p, 11q, and 16p- regions, also commonly deleted in ductal epithelial carcinomas, suggesting a common stem cell origin (26).

Differential Diagnosis. The differential diagnosis of malignant myoepithelioma includes

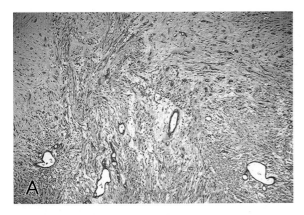

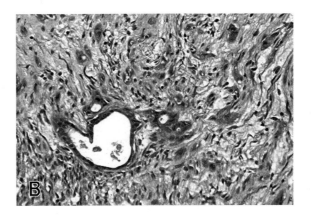

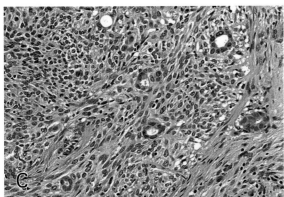

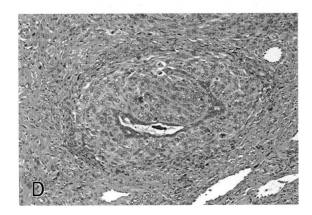

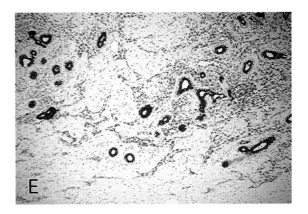

Figure 11-10

MALIGNANT MYOEPITHELIOMA
(MYOEPITHELIAL CARCINOMA)

A: An irregularly shaped mass is composed of spindle cells with what appears as entrapped tubules at its periphery.

B,C: The neoplastic spindle cells appear to emanate from the myoepithelial cell layer.

D: The myoepithelial cell layer is clearly hyperplastic around some of the peripheral tubules; the invasive cells often emanate from these hyperplastic layers.

E: AE1/AE3/LP34 intensely stains the epithelial cells lining the spaces. The proliferating myoepithelial cells are lighter stained.

spindle squamous carcinoma, poorly differentiated myoepithelial cell-rich sarcomatoid carcinoma, fibromatosis, and basically any of a variety of proliferative myofibroblastic lesions. The presence of a dominant nodule with irregular and shallow infiltration at the margins is helpful in distinguishing this lesion from fibromatosis and myofibroblastic tumors. Immunohistochemistry (Table 11-2) is often necessary in making the distinction between the variety of spindle lesions that occur in the breast; rarely electron microscopy may be required to confirm the

myoepithelial nature of a lesion. Since both myoepithelial and squamous carcinomas are immunoreactive with CK34betaE12, CK14, and p63, these markers are not helpful in distinguishing a spindle squamous carcinoma from a myoepithelial carcinoma. Therefore, emanation from themyoepithelial cell layer is required for designating a lesion as myoepithelial carcinomas. Squamous and myoepithelial carcinomas are most likely related. In our opinion, most of "fibromatosis-like" carcinomas (22) of the breast are malignant myoepithelial carcinomas and

257

Table 11-2

IMMUNOPROFILE OF VARIOUS SPINDLE CELL TUMORS OF THE BREAST[a]

Tumor	SMA[b]	Calponin	S-100	CK903	CAM5.2	ER	Desmin	CD34	HMB45	p63/CD10
Myoepithelioma	+/–	+/–	+	++	+/–	–	–	–	–	+
Spindle cell carcinoma	–	–	–	++	+	+/–	–	–	–	–/+
Smooth muscle tumors	+	+/–	–	–	+/–	+/–	+	–	–	–
Myofibroblastic lesions	+	+/–	+/–	–	–	–	–[c]	+	–	–
Melanoma	–	–	+	–	–	–	–	–	+	N/A

[a]Adapted from Table 15-2 from reference 56.
[b]SMA = smooth muscle actin; ER = estrogen receptor.
[c]Occasional cells may show immunoreactivity depending on the type of desmin used.

should be separated from the rare spindle cell adenocarcinomas of epithelial origin (see also chapter 10, Metaplastic Carcinomas).

Treatment and Prognosis. Local recurrence and distant metastases have been documented in malignant myoepithelioma, but death due to the carcinoma is rare (10,33). Metastases are blood-borne and dissemination occurs more frequently to the lungs and brain. Metastases to axillary lymph nodes were present at diagnosis in a 72-year-old woman who developed bone and cerebral metastases 28 months later (55). The follow-up period in some of the reported cases is short, varying from 3 to 32 months, however. Complete excision with uninvolved margins is required; this may necessitate mastectomy for large lesions. Sentinel node assessment would be prudent. Evaluation of lung fields is essential.

COMPARISON OF BREAST AND SALIVARY GLAND LESIONS

Given the longer recognition of combined epithelial and myoepithelial lesions in the salivary glands, it is natural to make comparisons of mammary and salivary gland lesions (4) and recommend the consideration of a homogeneous terminology for the same tumor occurring at various sites (47). The question, however, is what terminology is more appropriate. Lesions morphologically similar to AME are designated as epithelial-myoepithelial carcinoma when encountered in the salivary glands. There are substantial morphologic, and to some extent, clinical similarities among the tumors at the two sites. Death from even malignant AME is rare in the breast. The high frequency of lymph

node involvement in salivary gland AMEs may result from contiguity and close proximity of the nodes to the salivary glands.

The issue of homogeneous terminology is of great importance. It would be of interest to correlate the possible association of specific features of the lesion (increased mitotic activity among the myoepithelial cells, infiltrating margins) to aggressive behavior among the salivary gland epithelial-myoepithlelial carcinomas. There are clearly AMEs with a wide variety of morphologically aggressive features that range from focal atypia and sometimes minimally increased mitotic activity among the myoepithelial cells to those with clear-cut or distinctive carcinomas arising within them. It would seem illogical to equate all these lesions that display aggressive morphologic features with those totally devoid of such features by designating the entire group of lesions as epithelial-myoepithelial carcinomas. The terminology used in this chapter is far more logical for the breast. Perhaps attempts should be made to separate the salivary gland tumors that are more likely to behave aggressively on the basis of morphologic features as well.

Little is known about the molecular and genetic alterations in mammary myoepithelial lesions. The assessment of these aspects may shed some light on the differences in the behavior of morphologically similar tumors occurring in the breast and salivary glands (4).

CARCINOMA WITH MYOEPITHELIAL FEATURES

A few examples of carcinoma with myoepithelial differentiation have been described (11,19,28), based on the presence of relatively focal to diffuse immunostaining for CK14 and variable immunoreactivity for smooth muscle actin, caldesmon, and calponin. Interestingly, the immunoreactivity with CK14 is quite similar to that observed with the high molecular weight cytokeratin cocktail 34betaE12 in intraductal hyperplasia/low-risk DIN lesions and in about 10 percent of DCIS/DIN1-3 lesions (37). It is possible that these invasive carcinomas reflect the invasive counterpart of intraductal hyperplasia/ low-risk DIN. The reaction for the mesenchymal markers reported in these cases is most probably a reflection of a reaction in the supportive stroma that can be difficult to separate from the carcinoma component. Alternatively, at least some of these CK14-positive cells may reflect squamous differentiation among epithelial cells and have no direct relationship to a derivation from a myoepithelial cell population.

REFERENCES

1. Ahmad AA, Heller DS. Malignant adenomyoepithelioma of the breast with malignant proliferation of epithelial and myoepithelial elements. A case report and review of the literature. Arch Pathol Lab Med 2000;124:632-636.

2. Barbarschi M, Pecciarini L, Cangi MG, et al. p63, a p53 homologue, is a selective nuclear marker of myoepithelial cells of the human breast. Am J Surg Pathol 2001;25:1054-1060.

3. Bassler R, Katzer B. Histopathology of myoepithelial (basocellular) hyperplasias in adenosis and epitheliosis of the breast demonstrated by the reactivity of cytokeratins and S100 protein. An analysis of heterogenic cell proliferations in 90 cases of benign and malignant breast diseases. Virchows Arch A Pathol Anat Histopathol 1992;421:435-442.

4. Bennett AK, Mills SE, Wick MR. Salivary-type neoplasms of the breast and lung. Semin Diagn Pathol 2003;20:279-304.

5. Berna JD, Arcas I, Ballester A, Bas A. Adenomyoepithelioma of the breast in a male. AJR Am J Roentgenol 1997;169:917-918.

6. Bigotti G, DiGiorgio CG. Myoepithelioma of the breast: histologic, immunologic and electromicroscopic appearance. J Surg Oncol 1986;32:58-64.

7. Bult P, Verwiel JM, Wobbes T, Kooy-Smits MM, Biert J, Holland R. Malignant adenomyoepithelioma of the breast with metastasis in the thyroid gland 12 years after excision of the primary tumor. Case report and review of the literature. Virchows Arch 2000;436:158-166.

8. Cameron HM, Hamperl H, Warambo W. Leiomyosarcoma of the breast originating from myothelium (myoepithelium). J Pathol 1974;114:89-92

9. Chang A, Bassett L, Bose S. Adenomyoepithelioma of the breast: a cytologic dilemma. Report of a case and review of the literature. Diagn Cytopathol 2002;26:191-196.

10. Chen PC, Chen CK, Nicastri AD, Wait RB. Myoepithelial carcinoma of the breast with distant metastasis and accompanied by adenomyoepitheliomas. Histopathology 1994;24:543-548.

11. Damiani S, Riccioni L, Pasquinelli G, Eusebi V. Poorly differentiated myoepithelial cell rich carcinoma of the breast. Histopathology 1997;30:542-548.

12. Dardick I. Myoepithelioma: definitions and diagnostic criteria. Ultrastruct Pathol 1995;19:335-345.

13. Daroca PJ Jr, Reed RJ, Love GL, Krause SD. Myoid hamartomas of the breast. Hum Pathol 1985;16:212-219.

14. Di Tommaso L, Pasquinelli G, Damiani S. Smooth muscle cell differentiation in mammary stromoepithelial lesions with evidence of a dual orign: stromal myofibroblasts and myoepithelial cells. Histopathology 2003;42:448-456.

15. Erlandson RA. Benign adenomyoepithelioma of the breast. Ultrastruct Pathol 1989;13:307-314.

16. Erlandson RA, Rosen PP. Infiltrating myoepithelioma of the breast. Am J Surg Pathol 1982;6:785-793.

17. Eusebi V, Casadei GP, Bussolati G, Azzopardi JG. Adenomyoepithelioma of the breast with a distinctive type of apocrine adenosis. Histopathology 1987;11:305-315.

18. Farshid G, Moinfar F, Meredith DJ, et al. Spindle cell ductal carcinoma in situ. An unusual variant of ductal intra-epithelial neoplasia that simulates ductal hyperplasia or a myoepithelial proliferation. Virchows Arch 2001;439:70-77.

19. Foschini MP, Eusebi V. Carcinomas of the breast showing myoepithelial cell differentiation. A review of the literature. Virchows Arch 1998;432:303-310.

20. Foschini MP, Pizzicannella G, Peterse JL, Mignani S, Eusebi V. Adenomyoepithelioma of the breast associated with low-grade adenosquamous and sarcomatoid carcinomas. Virchows Arch 1995;427:243-250.

21. Gillett CE, Bobrow LG, Millis RR. S100 protein in human and mammary tissue—immunoreactivity in breast carcinomas including Paget's disease of the nipple, and value as a marker of myoepithelial cells. J Pathol 1990;160:19-24.

22. Gobbi H, Simpson JF, Borowsky A, Jensen RA, Page DL. Metaplastic breast tumors with a dominant fibromatosis-like phenotype have a high risk of local recurrence. Cancer 1999;85:2170-2182.

23. Gupta RK, Dowle CS. Immunocytochemical study in a case of adenomyoepithelioma of the breast. Diagn Cytopathol 1998;18:468-470.

24. Hamperl H. The myothelia (myoepithelial cells). Normal state, regressive changes, hyperplasia, tumors. Curr Top Pathol 1970;53:194-198.

25. Jolicoeur F, Seemayer TA, Babbiani G, et al. Multifocal, nascent, and invasive myoepithelial carcinoma (malignant myoepithelioma) of the breast: an immunohistochemical and ultrastructural study. Int J Surg pathol 2002;10:281-291.

26. Jones C, Foschini MP, Chaggar R, et al. Comparative genomic hybridization analysis of myoepithelial carcinomas of the breast. Lab Invest 2000;80:831-836.

27. Jones C, Nonni AV, Fulford L, et al. CGH analysis of ductal carcinoma of the breast with basaloid/myoepithelial cell differentiation. Br J Cancer 2001;85:422-427.

28. Kiaer H, Nielsen B, Paulsen S, Sorensen IM, Dyreborg U, Blichert-Toft M. Adenomyoepithelial adenosis and low-grade malignant adenomyoepithelioma of the breast. Virchows Arch A Pathol Anat Histopathol 1984;405:55-67.

29. Kurashina M. Fine-needle aspiration cytology of benign and malignant adenomyoepithelioma: report of two cases. Diagn Cytopathol 2002;26:29-34.

30. Kuwabara H, Uda H. Clear cell mammary malignant myoepithelioma with abundant glycogens. J Clin Pathol 1997;50:700-702.

31. Laforga JB, Aranda FI, Sevilla F. Adenomyoepithelioma of the breast: report of two cases with prominent cystic changes and intranuclear inclusions. Diagn Cytopathol 1998;19:55-58.

32. Lakhani SR, Chaggar R, Davies S, et al. Genetic alterations in "normal" luminal and myoepithelial cells of the breast. J Pathol 1999;189:496-503.

33. Lakhani SR, O'Hare MJ, Monaghan P, Winehouse J, Gazet JC, Sloane JP. Malignant myoepithelioma (myoepithelial carcinoma) of the breast: a detailed cytokeratin study. J Clin Pathol 1995;48:164-167.

34. Lee WY. Fine needle aspiration cytology of adenomyoepithelioma of the breast: a case indistinguishable from phyllodes tumor in cytological findings and clinical behavior. Acta Cytol 2000;44:488-490.

35. Loose JH, Patchefsky AS, Hollander IJ, Lavin LS, Cooper HS, Katz SM. Adenomyoepithelioma of the breast. A spectrum of biologic behavior. Am J Surg Pathol 1992;16:868-876.

36. McCluggage WG, McManus DI, Caughley LM. Fine needle aspiration (FNA) cytology of adenoid cystic carcinoma and adenomyoepithelioma of breast: two lesions rich in myoepithelial cells. Cytopathology 1997;8:31-39.

36a. McLaren BK, Smith J, Schuyler PA, Dupont WD, Page DL. Adenomyoepithelioma: clinical, histologic and immunohistologic evaluation of a series of related lesions. Am J Surg Pathol 2005;29:1294-1299.

37. Moinfar F, Man YG, Lininger RA, Bodian C, Tavassoli FA. Use of keratin 34BE12 as an adjunct in the diagnosis of mammary intraepithelial neoplasia-ductal type—benign and malignant intraductal proliferations. Am J Surg Pathol 1999;23:1048-1058.

37a. Nga ME, Lim KH, Tan EY, Chan P, Tan SY, Walford N. Malignant adenomyoepithelial tumor of the breast: multi-immunolabeling technique and detailed immunophenotypic study. Appl Immunohistochem Mol Morphol 2008;16:100-104.

38. Nguyen M, Lee MC, Wang JL, et al. The human myoepithelial cell displays a multifaceted anti-angiogenic phenotype. Oncogene 2000;19:3449-3359.

38a. Oka K, Sando N, Moriya T, Yatabe Y. Malignant adenomyoepithelioma of the breast with matrix production may be compatible with one variant of matrix producing carcinoma. A case report. Pathol Res Pract 2007;599-604.

39. Prasad AR, Zarbo RJ. Myoepithelial carcinoma of the breast: a clinicopathologic study of 18 cases. Mod Pathol 2000;13:46A.

40. Rasbridge SA, Millis RR. Adenomyoepithelioma of the breast with malignant features. Virchows Arch 1998;432:123-130.

41. Reis-Filho JS, Milanezi F, Silva P, Schmitt FC. Maspin expression in myoepithelial tumors of the breast. Pathol Res Pract 2001;197:817-821.

42. Reis-Filho JS, Schmitt FC. Taking advantage of basic research: p63 is a reliable myoepithelial and stem cell marker. Adv Anat Pathol 2002;9:280-289.

43. Rode L, Nesland JM, Johanessen JV. A spindle cell breast lesion in a 54-year-old woman. Ultrastruct Pathol 1986;10:421-425.

44. Rosen PP. Adenomyoepithelioma of the breast. Hum Pathol 1987;18:421-425.

45. Schurch W, Potvin C, Seemayer TA. Malignant myoepithelioma (myoepithelial carcinoma) of the breast: an ultrastructural and immunohistochemical study. Ultrastruct Pathol 1985;8:1-11.

46. Seifert G. Are adenomyoepithelioma of the breast and epithelial-myoepithelial carcinoma of the salivary glands identical tumors? Vichows Arch 1998;433:285-287.

47. Shiraishi , Nakayama T, Fukutome K, Watanabe M, Murata T. Malignant myoepithelioma of the breast metastasizing to the jaw. Virchows Arch 1999;435:520-523.

48. Simpson RH, Cope N, Skalova A, Michal M. Malignant adenomyoepithelioma of the breast with mixed osteogenic, spindle cell, and carcinomatous differentiation. Am J Surg Pathol 1998;22:631-636.

49. Soares J, Tomasic G, Bucciarelli E, et al. Intralobular growth of myoepithelial cell carcinoma of the breast. Virchows Arch 1994;425:205-210.

50. Sugano I, Nagao T, Tajima Y, et al. Malignant adenomyoepithelioma of the breast: a non-tubular and matrix-producing variant. Pathol Int 2001;51:193-199.

51. Takahashi II, Tashiro H, Wakasugi K, et al. Malignant adenomyoepithelioma of the breast. A case with distant metastases. Breast Cancer 1999;6:73-77.

52. Tamai M. Intraductal growth of malignant mammary myoepithelioma. Am J Surg Pathol 1992;16:1116-1125.

53. Tamai M, Nomura K, Hiyama H. Aspiration cytology of malignant intraductal myoepithelioma of the breast. A case report. Acta Cytol 1994;38:435-440.

54. Tamura G, Monma N, Suzuki Y, Satodate R, Abe H. Adenomyoepithelioma (myoepithelioma) of the breast in a male. Hum Pathol 1993;24:678-681.

55. Tavassoli FA. Myoepithelial lesions of the breast. Myoepitheliosis, adenomyoepithelioma, and myoepithelial carcinoma. Am J Surg Pathol 1991;15:554-568.

56. Tavassoli, FA. Myoepithleial lesions. Pathology of the breast, 2nd ed. Stamford, CT: Appleton & Lange/McGraw Hill; 1999:763-791.

56a. Tavassoli FA, Soares J. Myoepithelial lesions. In: Tavassoli FA, Devilee P, eds. Pathology and genetics of tumors of the breast and female genital organs. World Health Organization Classification of Tumors. Lyon: IAPS Press; 2003.

57. Thorner PS, Kahn HJ, Baumal R, et al. Malignant myoepithelioma of the breast. An immunohistochemical study by light and electron microscopy. Cancer 1986;57:745-750.

58. Toth J. Benign human mammary myoepithelioma. Virchows Arch A Pathol Anat Histopathol 1977;374:263-269.

59. Trojani M, Guiu M, Trouette H, De Mascarel I, Cocquet M. Malignant adenomyoepithelioma of the breast. An immunohistochemical, cytometric and ultrastructural study of a case with lung metastases. Am J Clin Pathol 1992;98:598-602.

59a. Van Dorpe J, de Pauw A. Adenoid cystic carcinoma arising in an adenomyoepithelioma of the breast. Virchows Arch 1998;432:119-122.

60. Weidner N, Levine JD. Spindle-cell adenomyoepithelioma of the breast. A microscopic, ultrastructural, and immunocytochemical study. Cancer 1988;62:1561-1567.

61. Werling RW, Hwang H, Yaziji H, Gown AM. Immunohistochemical distinction of invasive from noninvasive breast lesions: a comparative study of p63 versus calponin and smooth muscle myosin heavy chain. Am J Surg Pathol 2003;27:82-90.

62. Young RH, Clement PB, Adenomyoepithelioma of the breast. A report of three cases and review of the literature. Am J Clin Pathol 1988;89:308-314.

12 BENIGN SOFT TISSUE LESIONS

STROMAL CHANGES SIMULATING MALIGNANCY

Multinucleated Stromal Giant Cells

Multinucleated stromal giant cells were described in 1979 by Rosen (94) as an unusual benign microscopic stromal change that in one instance had been interpreted as invasive carcinoma. The cells are characteristically multinucleated, with inconspicuous cytoplasm that merges with the surrounding stroma. The nuclei vary from 2 to 15 per cell, tend to overlap, and are generally hyperchromatic. Mitoses are rare. These cells are randomly located in the interlobular stroma and rarely in the adipose tissue; occasionally, they are confined to the intralobular connective tissue (fig. 12-1) (94). Multinucleated stromal giant cells are seen in a variety of breast conditions such as fibroepithelial tumors (89), including fibroadenomas (6), and in 4.5 percent of non-neoplastic "ordinary" stroma of breasts removed for carcinoma (94).

The age of patients with multinucleated stromal giant cells varies according to the lesions in which the giant cells are found; patients are younger when the multinucleated giant cells are discovered in a fibroadenoma. The area showing giant cell changes can be limited to a microscopic field (94) or may affect the entire lesion (89). Most of these cells are randomly scattered and separated by abundant stroma, but in some cases, they are numerous and contiguous (89). The stroma is usually dense, but edematous changes are far from the exception. The diagnostic characteristic of the multinucleated giant cell reaction is the total lack of associated inflammatory changes.

Ultrastructurally, multinucleated stromal giant cells resemble fibroblasts (6,111). Immunohistochemically, they react with antivimentin and CD34 antibodies (89), and occasionally, desmin and smooth muscle actin, while cytokeratins and S-100 protein are absent.

A myoepithelial origin (82) for these cells is not tenable in view of the ultrastructural and immunohistochemical findings; a fibroblastic-histiocytic nature is more plausible (6,89). Multinucleated stromal giant cells are not confined to the breast stromal tissue since they are seen in a variety of organs, including the vagina and nasal mucosa (88). Identical cells are occasionally seen within the pseudovascular spaces in cases of pseudoangiomatous stromal hyperplasia whether or not associated with neurofibromatosis (5,17).

Multinucleated stromal giant cells are different from osteoclast-like giant cells of the type seen in sarcomatoid carcinoma (117). The latter, at variance with multinucleated giant cells, have prominent eosinophilic cytoplasm and ovoid nuclei that usually do not overlap, are not hyperchromatic, and display a centrally located nucleolus.

The recognition of multinucleated stromal giant cells is crucial as, due to nuclear hyperchromasia, the cells are easily visible at low-power microscopy and may simulate an invasive carcinoma (94). Another possible pitfall is failure to recognize these cells when they are

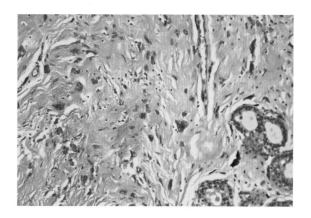

Figure 12-1

MULTINUCLEATED STROMAL CELLS

Multinucleated stromal cells are located in the interlobular stroma.

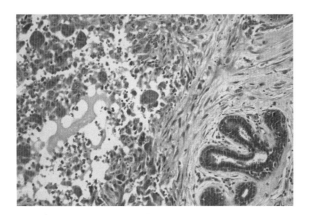

Figure 12-2

OSTEOCLAST-LIKE GIANT CELLS

Osteoclast-like giant cells intermingle with histiocytes, mononuclear cells, and red blood cells along the tract of needle-traumatized tissue.

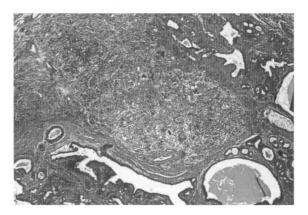

Figure 12-3

BENIGN FIBROEPITHELIAL LESION

The inflammatory changes are secondary to fine needle aspiration cytology (FNAC).

intermingled, as they are on rare occasion, with an invasive carcinoma, potentially upgrading the tumor. The same applies to fibroadenomas or benign cystosarcoma phyllodes tumors containing numerous giant cells that might result in their upgrading to a malignant neoplasm, as in the cases reported by Powell et al. (89).

Stromal Pseudomalignant Changes following Fine Needle Aspiration

The increasing use of fine needle aspiration cytology (FNAC) procedures in diagnostic breast pathology has led to the observation of numerous unexpected findings such as massive necrosis in a tumor (63), especially if oncocytic in nature, displacement of non-neoplastic epithelium into stroma and lymphatic spaces (121), and passive lymph node "benign" metastases (11). The most worrisome post-traumatic fine needle reaction is one similar to the postoperative spindle cell nodules described in the prostate (91). Reactive inflammatory cells along the needle tract can aggregate to form small nodules, 3.9 mm in average size (47). The reactive cells are ovoid to spindled, and have irregular nuclei and frequent mitoses. Of the 18 such lesions described by Gobbi et al. (47), 14 had "invasive" margins. The presence of hemosiderin and a lymphoplasmacytic infiltrate within the lesion help establish the reactive nature of the process. We feel that awareness of the existence of FNAC-generated traumatic changes, the histologic identification of the needle tract,

and the clinical information about the preceding fine needle procedures are vital for establishing the diagnosis of a reactive process.

Inflammatory giant cell reactions can also be a feature of FNAC-generated traumatic changes. One of the two cases reported by Marucci et al. (74) was composed of a microscopic nodule containing histiocytes intermingled with numerous osteoclast-like giant cells (fig. 12-2) and present within a benign fibroepithelial lesion of pseudoangiomatous stromal hyperplasia (PASH). The unexpected features led to a diagnosis of spindle cell carcinoma with osteoclast-like giant cells (117); this diagnosis resulted in unnecessary quadrantectomy with axillary lymph node dissection. The other case showed a microscopic nodule located within a fibroepithelial benign lesion. The nodule contained atypical multinucleated giant cells immersed in a dense lymphoid stroma. The pathologist in charge of the case had (fortunately) himself performed the FNAC on the patient and refused to sign out the diagnosis of malignant fibrohistiocytoma suggested by a reviewer, despite the atypicality of the giant cells (figs. 12-3, 12-4). No further treatment was given and the patient is alive and well 6 years after the FNAC procedure.

NODULAR FASCIITIS

Nodular fasciitis is a well-known pseudosarcomatous (probably reactive) myofibroblastic proliferation that can occur in the mammary region as well as at many other sites. It typically

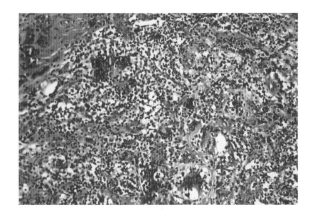

Figure 12-4

ATYPICAL MULTINUCLEATED GIANT CELLS

The cells are surrounded by a dense lymphoid reaction.

affects the subcutaneous tissue and rarely appears located within the breast parenchyma.

A brief history of tenderness is the most frequent symptom of nodular fasciitis. When the lesion is located deep in the parenchyma it appears as a small nodule, 4 cm (on average) in size, which can be clinically or radiologically mistaken for a malignant tumor (76).

As in nodular fasciitis at other sites, the reactive nodules are well circumscribed, with lymphoid inflammatory cells often present at the periphery. These lesions can be distinguished from myofibroblastomas (see below) by the constant lymphocytic infiltrate, multifocal red blood cell extravasation, and hypocellular central zone in late lesions. Fibromatosis has "infiltrative" borders while sarcomas and sarcomatoid carcinomas show atypical cells as well as irregular mitoses.

BENIGN STROMAL SPINDLE CELL TUMORS

Benign stromal spindle cell tumors (BSSCTs) are lesions composed of spindle cells that may show several lines of differentiation. Toker et al. (114) in 1981 described four cases designated as "benign spindle cell breast tumors." These lesions were composed of myofibroblasts, adipocytes, and smooth muscle cells. The authors suggested that the lesions belonged to a broad category of mesenchymal tumors capable of diverse lines of differentiation including fibroblasts, myofibroblasts, adipocytes, and smooth muscle cells. Two of these tumors had features of subsequently de-

scribed myofibroblastomas (119), one had features of benign spindle cell lipoma, and one probably showed some of the changes later described as pseudoangiomatous stromal hyperplasia (116).

All these lesions, to which we would add hemangiopericytomas/solitary fibrous tumors, share similar clinical characteristics (age of occurrence and benign course), the same macroscopic features (solid noncystic, well-circumscribed nodules), in most cases similar immunohistochemical findings (vimentin, CD34, bcl-2, CD10, CD99, smooth muscle actin, and desmin positivity) (68,69a), and in some cases the same cytogenetic profile (60,85). We share the view of Toker et al. (114) that these lesions originate from a common stromal stem cell and that the designation of benign stromal spindle cell tumors is the most appropriate for lesions that are not exclusive to the breast and can be seen in most sites in the body (68). The histologic variations depend on the predominant cell type present in each lesion, reflecting the features seen in the four types of myofibroblasts (V-vimentin; VA-vimentin and actin; VAD- vimentin, actin, and desmin; VADM- vimentin, actin, desmin, and myosin phenotypes) as codified by Schurch et al. (104).

BSSCT with Predominant Myofibroblastic Differentiation (Myofibroblastoma)

Definition. Wargotz et al. (119) in 1987 described 16 cases of a tumor composed predominantly of "cells having features of both fibroblasts and smooth muscle cells." The tumoral cells were regarded as myofibroblasts as they had, at the ultrastructure level, cytoplasmic stress fibers, cell junctions, and basal-like material that fulfilled the criteria used in the definition of these contractile cells by Schurch et al. (104). On these grounds, the name *myofibroblastoma* was generated.

Clinical Features. Myofibroblastomas occur over a wide age range (25 to 85 years) (76), with an average age of 63 years (119). Although originally reported to be more frequent in men, at present, they are believed to arise with equal frequency in both sexes (76). The lesion is unifocal and one case only of synchronous bilaterality has been described (52).

Clinically, myofibroblastoma appears as a mobile nodule not adherent to the skin and usually present for several months, with the

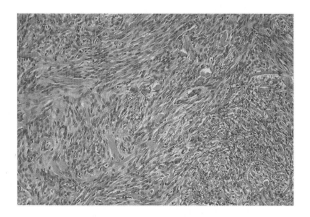

Figure 12-5

BENIGN STROMAL SPINDLE CELL TUMOR (BSSCT) WITH PREDOMINANT MYOFIBROBLASTIC DIFFERENTIATION

Numerous spindle cells are arranged in short fascicles.

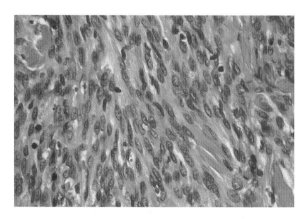

Figure 12-7

BSSCT WITH PREDOMINANT MYOFIBROBLASTIC DIFFERENTIATION

The spindle cells show elongated nuclei. The cells are intermingled with bands of hyalinized collagen.

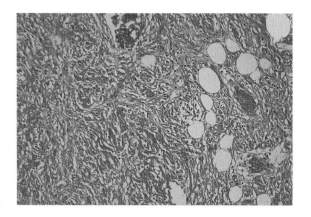

Figure 12-6

BSSCT WITH PREDOMINANT MYOFIBROBLASTIC DIFFERENTIATION

The proliferating spindle cells are loosely packed together. Numerous sclerohyaline short bundles and several adipocytes are visible.

exceptional case of a 66-year-old man in whom the lesion had been growing for 20 years (76). The neoplasm ranges in size from 1.0 to 4.0 cm, with a mean diameter of 2.3 cm (119), but may be massive considering the 10-cm tumor reported by Ali et al. (2) and those of 20 cm alluded to by McMenamin et al. (76).

Gross Findings. Myofibroblastomas display well-circumscribed margins. The cut surface shows a vague lobular appearance and a gray-pink color. The lesion is delimited by a pseudo-capsule and no glandular epithelium is visible

entrapped in the lesion. Rarely, the margins appear infiltrative.

Microscopic Findings. The cellularity of the lesion is variable. Some tumors contain numerous cells (fig. 12-5); others show a loose edematous (fig. 12-6), occasionally myxoid, stroma. In some cases, the cellularity varies from area to area within the same tumor. The proliferating cells are arranged in short fascicles and are spindle shaped and of similar size. The cytoplasm is eosinophilic. The nuclei are round to ovoid, and show an irregular nuclear membrane, dispersed chromatin, and distinct small nucleoli (fig. 12-7). Multinucleated floret-like giant cells are common. Mast cells are present in all cases. Mitoses are infrequent and necrotic areas are not seen.

The short cellular fascicles are separated by bands of hyalinized collagen, some of which are very thick. In rare cases, the cells appear epithelioid (93) and the nuclei are pleomorphic and irregular. Patients with these tumors, defined as *atypical myofibroblastomas* or *myxoid myofibroblastoma with atypical cells* (67a), do not have a significantly different prognosis than those with more conventional myofibroblastomas. Occasional cases containing foci of mature cartilage (36,61) or showing areas with smooth muscle cell differentiation (36,70a,113) have been reported.

Immunohistochemically, the proliferating cells feature the phenotypic profile of the VAD myofibroblasts as defined by Schurch et al. (104). They are immunoreactive with antivimentin,

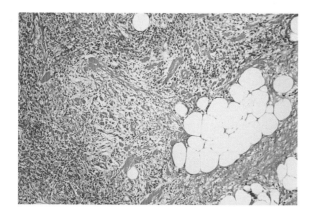

Figure 12-8

**BSSCT WITH PROMINENT
ADIPOCYTIC DIFFERENTIATION**

This tumor is composed of a proliferation of spindle cells containing numerous adipocytes. (Figs. 12-8 and 12-9 are from the same patient.)

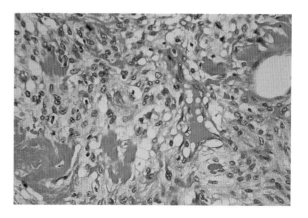

Figure 12-9

**BSSCT WITH PROMINENT
ADIPOCYTIC DIFFERENTIATION**

Several lipoblasts are adjacent to hyaline collagen bands.

CD34, smooth muscle actin, desmin, bcl-2, CD99, CD10, h caldesmon (69a,70a), and androgen receptor (AR) antibodies (62,70,70b, 76,80). This is a generalization, as some of these markers are not revealed (for instance, smooth muscle actin and h caldesmon) in otherwise typical cases. Pauwels et al. (85) have shown partial monosomy of 13q in two cases and partial monosomy of 16q in another.

Treatment and Prognosis. The lesion never recurs. Excision is the optimal treatment (93).

BSSCT with Predominant Adipocytic Component (Spindle Cell Lipoma)

Adipose tissue is frequently observed within myofibroblastomas (76). Seven of the nine cases reported by Hamele-Bena et al. (53) contained fat cells to a varying extent. Chan et al. (12) reported a case of spindle cell lipoma which they considered to be very similar to the tumors reported by Toker et al. (114). Toker et al. stated that their cases of spindle cell tumor contained spindle cell elements indistinguishable from those seen in spindle cell lipomas, a view also shared by McMenamin et al. (76) and by Rosen (93).

A case of benign spindle cell tumor with a prominent adipocytic component was reported by Magro et al. (69). We have seen a similar case also containing lipoblasts (figs. 12-8, 12-9). Magro et al. (69) agreed with Toker et al. (114) that myofibroblastomas and spindle cells tu-

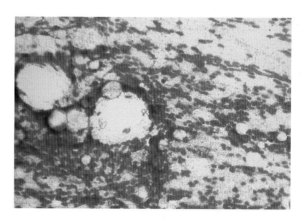

Figure 12-10

BSSCT WITH ADIPOCYTIC DIFFERENTIATION

FNAB shows numerous monotonous spindle cells and globoid mature adipocytes.

mors with a prominent adipocytic component belong to the same category of lesions and their features depend upon the predominate line of differentiation of a common precursor, whether myofibroblastic, fibroblastic, or adipocytic.

Cytologically, numerous spindle cells are apparent in spindle cell lipomas. These have evenly spaced, regular, elongated and ovoid nuclei (figs. 12-10–2-12). The immunohistochemical findings in both myofibroblastoma and spindle cell lipoma are nearly superimposable, as are the cytogenetic findings (85). Most of the available data point toward a link between these two lesions.

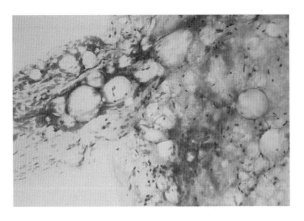

Figure 12-11

BSSCT WITH ADIPOCYTIC DIFFERENTIATION

Several globoid adipocytes intermingle with spindle cells.

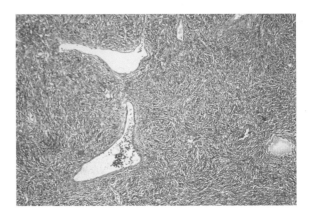

Figure 12-13

BSSCT WITH PREDOMINANT FIBROBLASTIC ELEMENTS

The vessels have an irregular angulated shape in this dense spindle cell proliferation.

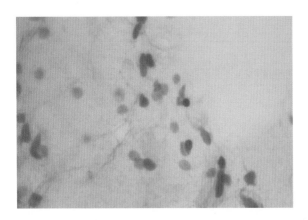

Figure 12-12

BSSCT WITH ADIPOCYTIC DIFFERENTIATION

FNAB shows spindle cells with ovoid bland nuclei.

BSSCT with Predominant Fibroblastic Elements (Solitary Fibrous Tumor, Hemangiopericytoma)

Solitary Fibrous Tumor. Damiani et al. (19) reported three solitary fibrous tumors (SFTs), which they considered to be identical to myofibroblastomas (fig. 12-13), a view suggested by Lee et al. (62). Two of these cases were studied immunohistochemically and smooth muscle actin was observed in one while desmin was present in both. Subsequently, Thomas et al. (113) stated that SFTs of the breast were closely related to myofibroblastomas but the latter were more committed toward myoid differentiation. Magro et al. (72) stated that SFT is a fibroblastic lesion,

while myofibroblastoma has to be regarded as a myofibroblastic tumor. This view was reached on the basis of immunohistochemical findings (SFTs are frequently actin and desmin negative; the opposite is true for myofibroblastomas) and on the pattern of growth (presence of a hemangiopericytoma-like vascular pattern in SFT and not in myofibroblastoma). The presence of a hemangiopericytoma vascular pattern was the most important criterion used to separate the two lesions by Nucci and Fletcher (83), who found that myofibroblastomas lack the hemangiopericytoma-like vascular pattern so often seen in SFTs.

We do not feel that these arguments are crucial enough to draw a sharp line between SFT and myofibroblastoma. The infrequent presence of desmin in SFT is probably not accurate since desmin is present in 6 out of 9 cases of SFT when the protein was investigated on fresh tissues as compared with only 3 positive cases out of 25 when formalin- fixed paraffin-embedded tissue was employed (54). The hemangiopericytoma-like pattern is not exclusive to SFT and has been reported in a case of myofibroblastoma of the breast (70). Finally, losses of 13q have been seen in SFTs of the pleura (60), similar to the findings in spindle cell lipomas (15) and myofibroblastomas. There are more similarities than differences between these tumors, with SFTs showing predominant fibroblastic differentiation and myofibroblastomas displaying a predominant myofibroblastic component.

Hemangiopericytoma. Fewer than 20 examples of hemangiopericytoma have been reported in the breast (111). This lesion affects a wide age range, with the peak at around 45 years (112). Hemangiopericytomas of the breast are well-circumscribed, pseudoencapsulated nodules. Histologically, the glandular breast structures appear pushed to the periphery of each tumor (93). They show uniformly the pattern classically reported in the morphologic descriptions of hemangiopericytomas of other sites. This pattern consists of cells arranged around small capillary-like vessels (fig. 12-14), which are often elongated to produce the classic "staghorn" features. The proliferating cells are usually spindle shaped and have round to ovoid nuclei. Mitoses are rare (112) and necrotic areas are absent. An adipocytic component may be present (40).

These lesions have been recently included in the spectrum of SFT as they share similar histologic and immunohistochemical features, including the rarity of actin-positive cells and intense staining with anti-CD34 antibodies. Ultrastructurally, clear-cut evidence of contractile elements is lacking in these tumors (83). However, the benign nature of hemangiopericytoma and the lack of recurrence in all cases reported in the breast (93,111) has led to the belief that excision of these tumors is curative (111).

Differential Diagnosis of BSSCT

There are several benign conditions simulating BSSCT. Spindle cell myoepitheliomas, as described by Toth (115), can be distinguished by the lack of collagen bundles among the proliferating cells as seen in myofibroblastomas and the immunohistochemical positivity for keratin that is not present in BSSCT (see chapter 11). Distinction from fibromatosis is addressed later.

Occasionally, sarcomatoid carcinomas have a hemangiopericytoma-like pattern (41). Usually these malignant tumors show irregular and frequent mitoses, irregular nuclei of the proliferating cells, and necrotic areas. Keratin, when positive, distinguishes a sarcomatoid carcinoma. Myofibrosarcomas share the same immunohistochemical profile as myofibroblastomas, but the epithelioid elements, necrotic areas, and frequent mitoses observed in the former (109) are not features of BSSCT. Spindle

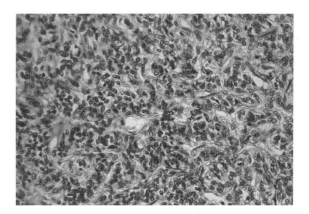

Figure 12-14

BSSCT WITH PREDOMINANT FIBROBLASTIC ELEMENTS

Small regular cells show a perivascular arrangement.

cell myoepithelial carcinomas have all the above malignant features and in addition stain for keratin (42). Spindle cell liposarcoma has never been described in the breast. They share with BSSCTs similar immunohistochemical features, but they have an invasive pattern, a small adipocytic component, and a lack of the collagen bundles that are features of BSSCTs (24).

PSEUDOANGIOMATOUS STROMAL HYPERPLASIA (PASH) AND THE PASH PHENOMENON

Definition. *Pseudoangiomatous stromal hyperplasia* (PASH) was originally described by Vuitch et al. (116) as a fibroepithelial nodule of the breast characterized by "mammary stromal proliferation with the formation of interanastomosing slits that simulate vascular spaces."

Clinical Features. The nodules appear mostly in premenopausal women although occasional cases are observed in women in the 6th decade of life (39). A solitary case of PASH was reported in a man (93). The classic clinical presentation is a nodular fibroadenoma-like lesion; exceptional cases measure 24 cm (39) or give the clinical impression of an inflammatory breast carcinoma (57). In most patients, PASH is a single nodular lesion, but sporadic multifocal and bilateral tumors have been reported (90).

Gross Findings. The nodules are well demarcated (fig. 12-15). Small cysts are a frequent finding (39).

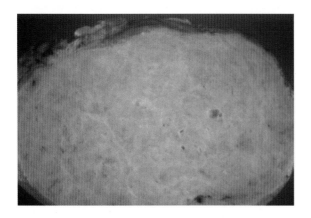

Figure 12-15

PSEUDOANGIOMATOUS STROMAL HYPERPLASIA (PASH)

A well-demarcated fibrous nodule with a uniform cut surface is typical of PASH. (Courtesy of Dr. H. Gobbi, Belo Horizonte, Brazil.)

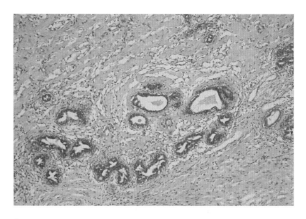

Figure 12-16

PSEUDOANGIOMATOUS STROMAL HYPERPLASIA

The fibroepithelial lesion contains a network of interanastomosing spaces in the interlobular and intralobular stroma.

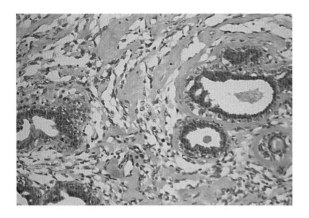

Figure 12-17

PSEUDOANGIOMATOUS STROMAL HYPERPLASIA

The spaces are empty, devoid of red blood cells.

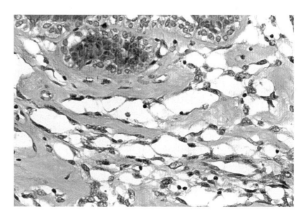

Figure 12-18

PSEUDOANGIOMATOUS STROMAL HYPERPLASIA

Single cells form delicate "bridges" between the walls of a space.

Microscopic Findings. PASH is recognizable at low-power microscopy because the nodule contains a network of interanastomosing, slit-like or elongated spaces that simulate a vascular proliferation; these spaces are present both in the intralobular and interlobular stroma (fig. 12-16). The spaces are generally empty, devoid of red blood cells, and their lumens vary from very thin slits to large elongated regular lacunae (fig. 12-17). They are lined by a discontinuous layer of flat cells having thin, elongated nuclei with pointed ends. Single cells frequently form delicate "bridges" between the walls of a space (fig. 12-18) (37). Adjacent spaces are separated

by dense collagen bands. Mitoses are extremely rare and necrotic areas are absent. The glandular epithelium may show bland hyperplasia and, rarely, apocrine differentiation.

The spaces are not artifacts secondary to the paraffin embedding process but true empty structures that are also observed in frozen tissues (5,39,116). We have seen cases of malignant lymphoma primary in the breast in which the neoplastic cells floated inside and propagated via the space network of PASH (fig. 12-19) (21). A similar case was depicted by Rosen (93).

There are variations to these classic features. In some areas PASH can show strap-like single

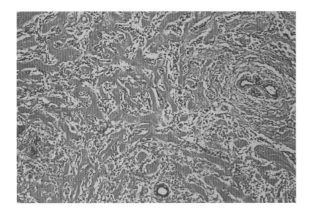

Figure 12-19

PSEUDOANGIOMATOUS STROMAL HYPERPLASIA

Large cell malignant lymphoma propagates via the space network of this PASH.

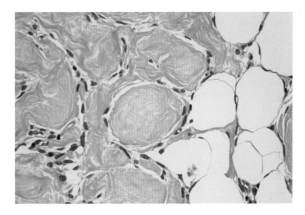

Figure 12-20

PSEUDOANGIOMATOUS STROMAL HYPERPLASIA

Strap-like cells dissect the collagenous stroma.

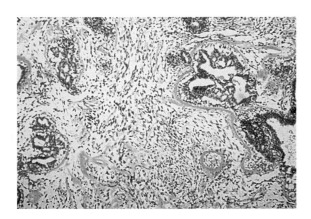

Figure 12-21

PSEUDOANGIOMATOUS STROMAL HYPERPLASIA

When the spaces are filled by proliferating fibroblasts, solid cellular areas are the result.

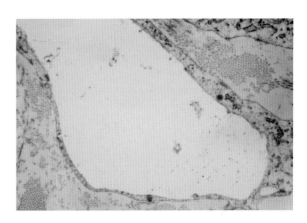

Figure 12-22

PSEUDOANGIOMATOUS STROMAL HYPERPLASIA

Thin cytoplasmic processes border the lumens and are in direct contact with the collagen. (Courtesy of Dr. G. Pasquinelli, Bologna, Italy.)

cells immersed in a dense collagenous stroma without lumen formation. These cells display the same features as the elements that line the spaces (fig. 12-20). Frequently, the cells that border the lumens acquire abundant cytoplasm and plump round to ovoid nuclei with one to two very small nucleoli. These cells can be numerous enough to fill the spaces and form small to large cellular solid nests (fig. 12-21).

Ultrastructurally, these cells display fibroblast characteristics (figs. 12-22, 12-23) (116).The immunohistochemical profile is identical to that seen in BSSCTs and includes immunoreactivity for vimentin, CD34 (figs. 12-24, 12-25), smooth muscle actin, desmin (39,90), and bcl-2.

Differential Diagnosis. PASH has to be distinguished from vascular lesions that include angioma and well-differentiated angiosarcoma (see below and chapter 13). As seen in Table 12-1, the main criteria useful in the differential diagnosis are a lack of red blood cells, the discontinuous layer of cells bordering the lumens, the elongated CD34-positive stromal cells, and the presence of the "bridge" cells, all features nearly exclusive to PASH.

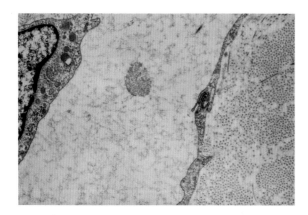

Figure 12-23

PSEUDOANGIOMATOUS STROMAL HYPERPLASIA

The cells have features of fibroblasts, are in direct contact with the collagen, and line a space that has amorphous granular content. (Courtesy of Dr. G. Pasquinelli, Bologna, Italy.)

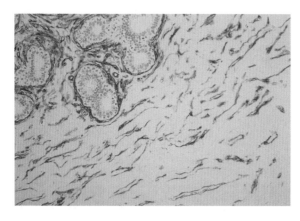

Figure 12-24

PSEUDOANGIOMATOUS STROMAL HYPERPLASIA

CD34 decorates cells lining the spaces as well as single spindle stromal cells and the intralobular stroma.

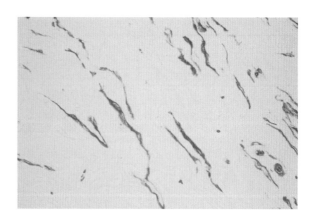

Figure 12-25

PSEUDOANGIOMATOUS STROMAL HYPERPLASIA

Single strap-like stromal cells are stained by CD34 antibody.

Table 12-1

DISTINGUISHING BETWEEN PSEUDOVASCULAR SPACES AND VASCULAR CHANNELS

	PASH[a]	Angioma/ Angiosarcoma
Elongated CD34+ single stromal cells	Present	Absent
Spaces	Slit or open, elongated, regular	Round to irregular
Bridging cells	Present	Absent
Red blood cells	Absent	Present
CD34	Positive	Positive
Desmin	Can be positive	Negative
CD31	Negative	Positive
Factor VIII	Negative	Positive
Basal lamina	Absent	Can be present

[a]PASH = pseudoangiomatous stromal hyperplasia.

Angiosarcomas are immunoreactive with anti-factor VIII and CD31 antibodies that are negative in PASH. Basal lamina is absent in PASH (39) while it can be a feature of angiosarcomas. Desmin is a feature of PASH and not of angiosarcomas.

PASH can also be confused with phyllodes tumor. The characteristic epithelial growth pattern of phyllodes tumor is never observed in PASH; mitoses, despite the cellularity, are rare in PASH.

Treatment and Prognosis. PASH is a benign lesion, but 6 cases in a series of 40 reported by Powell et al. (90) recurred ipsilaterally. In 3, the recurrences were multiple and 2 patients developed contralateral PASH. In 1 case, the lesions were so extensive as to require bilateral mastectomy. Complete excision of the lesion is required and follow-up is important in bilateral cases

The PASH Phenomenon. The term *PASH phenomenon* is reserved for those cases in which pseudoangiomatous stromal hyperplasia is an incidental microscopic finding and does not cause a clinical lump. This is a common phenomenon which has been demonstrated in up to 23 percent of 200 consecutive breast biopsies and mastectomies (57). PASH foci were multicentric in 60 percent of the cases and the age

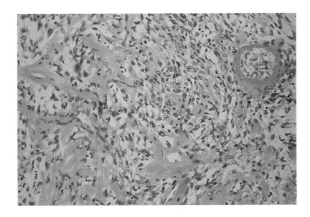

Figure 12-26

PSEUDOANGIOMATOUS STROMAL HYPERPLASIA

The nodular proliferation is reminiscent of a myofibroblastoma.

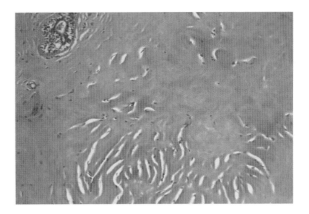

Figure 12-27

FIBROUS TUMOR

Sclerotic tissue with empty slits is reminiscent of the spaces seen in PASH. The bordering (myo)fibroblasts have probably disappeared.

incidence of these patients was 5 years younger than those in a series reported by Powell et al. (90). The PASH phenomenon was also observed in 47 percent of patients with gynecomastia (5). When multinucleated giant cells line the pseudovascular spaces in gynecomastia, the chances that the patient is affected by neurofibromatosis type 1 appear to be high (17).

PASH and BSSCT with Prominent Myofibroblastic Differentiation (Myofibroblastoma). The histologic and immunohistochemical profiles of the cells lining the spaces in PASH lesions parallel those of myofibroblastomas, as shown by Powell et al. (90). In addition, there are cases in which in some areas of PASH the stromal cells proliferate and form nodules identical to myofibroblastomas (fig. 12-26). These cases led Rosen (93) to state that PASH and myofibroblastoma are related conditions. A case of our own was characterized by a typical smooth muscle cell tumor that in the center showed areas reminiscent of PASH/BSSCT. This indicates that PASH cells can transform into smooth muscle cells in the same manner as myofibroblasts. The link between PASH and BSSCT had already been observed, among other findings, by Toker et al. (114), who reported that in one of their cases, a myofibroblastic proliferation with smooth muscle differentiation, was preceded 17 years earlier by a lesion showing a vascular pattern that was labeled as angiosarcoma. This was very likely a case of PASH, in view of the long clinical history.

PASH and Fibrous Tumor. Fibrous tumor is defined as a discrete nodule composed of collagenized mammary stroma and atrophic epithelium. It is the end point of various conditions including fibroadenomas as well as PASH. In the latter case, the sclerotic tissue shows the remnants of slits that are devoid of bordering myofibroblasts (fig. 12-27).

Histogenesis of PASH. It has been suggested that PASH is an exaggerated manifestation of the secretory phase of the menstrual cycle (90). This suggestion was made on the basis of the premenopausal appearance of most lesions and the nuclear immunohistochemical localization of progesterone receptors. Fisher et al. (39) did not find evidence of estrogen and progesterone receptors after a careful study of nine cases employing cytosolic and immunohistochemical methods. However, no fewer than five patients showing the PASH phenomenon were postmenopausal (57). Male patients with gynecomastia can show the PASH phenomenon. These data make implausible the theory of an exuberant response to progestins.

Fisher et al. (39) believe that PASH is hamartomatous in nature. This view is difficult to accept since some cases are bilateral, PASH phenomenon is multifocal, and some cases of PASH give rise to multiple recurrences. These data appear more consistent, as suggested by Rosen (93), with a neoplastic process.

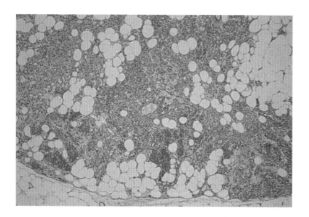

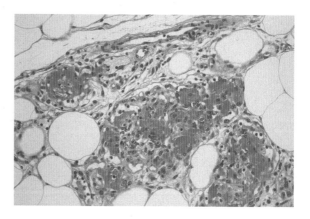

Figure 12-28

ANGIOLIPOMA

Adipose tissue intermingles with proliferating capillaries.

Figure 12-29

ANGIOLIPOMA

Microthrombi are present within the vascular lumens.

Fisher et al. (39) also suggested that the pseudovascular network might recapitulate the lymphatic labyrinth which constitutes the prelymphatic system through which the lymph flows before entering into well-formed lymphatic vessels. The labyrinth was also termed the missing lymphatic system by Hartveit (55) and appears to be a plausible normal counterpart to the existence of the genuine spaces that constitute PASH. More studies are needed for a better definition of the lymphatic labyrinth that probably has an important role in the dissemination of neoplastic conditions in the breast as suggested by the previously illustrated cases of malignant lymphoma in which the neoplastic cells float within spaces (fig. 12-19).

LIPOMAS

Definition. *Lipomas*, as might be expected, are the most frequent benign lesions in the male breast and the most common soft tissue tumor of the female breast (45). They are composed of mature fat, mostly located in the subcutaneous tissue (superficial lipomas) or deeply seated in the breast parenchyma or pectoral muscle.

Clinical Features. Lipomas are asymptomatic, mobile solitary nodules that develop in patients of all ages, with a peak around 47 years (50). Three percent of lipomas are bilateral and 10 percent appear as multiple nodules within the same breast (45). Eight of 292 patients with breast lipomas presented with lipomas in other parts of the body as well (50). Radiologically,

they appear as sharply defined, round to ovoid nodules with a radiolucent halo (4).

Gross Findings. All lipomas, including adenolipomas, show the same macroscopic features (38). These are so similar to normal fat as to require very close inspection to detect the thin pseudocapsule, but generally, they are yellower than the surrounding fatty tissue (50). Their average size is 2.5 cm but some exceed 10.0 cm (45).

Microscopic Findings. Histologically, all the features observed in lipomas of other organs are recapitulated in the breast. This also applies to immunohistochemical reactions which include S-100 protein and CD34 positivity (25,108). Lipomas vary from the classic form composed of mature fat as seen in the subcutis (4) to the lipoma variants represented by *angiolipoma* (figs. 12-28, 12-29) and *myolipoma* (111), *pleomorphic lipoma* (66), and *spindle cell-BSSCT-lipoma* (see above)(69).

Chondroid lipomas, defined by Enzinger and Weiss (33) as tumors formed by cartilage associated with white and brown fat, have never been reported in the breast. *Chondrolipomas* that contain only ordinary fat and cartilage are very rare (73), while most of the cases reported and seen by us contain glandular tissue in addition to fat and cartilage (43,79,93). Whether this glandular tissue represents preexisting entrapped epithelium or a "neoplastic" proliferation analogous to that of pleomorphic adenoma of salivary glands is open to question. All of the above-described lesions never recur if adequately excised.

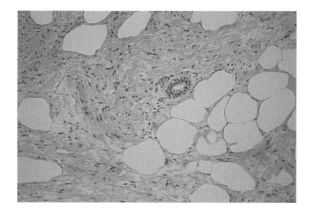

Figure 12-30

ADENOMYOLIPOMA

Smooth muscle cells intermingle with adipose tissue.

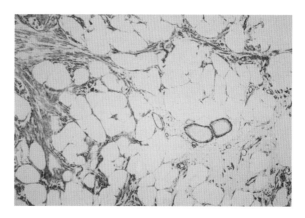

Figure 12-31

ADENOMYOLIPOMA

Smooth muscle cells stain with actin antibody. Actin is also evident in the myoepithelial cells that encircle the existing glands.

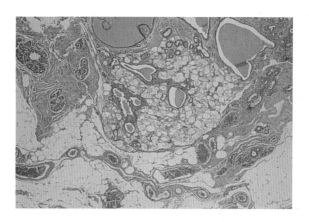

Figure 12-32

ADENOHIBERNOMA

Ducts in the center are surrounded by foamy cells. (Figs. 12-32 and 12-33 are from the same patient.)

Adenolipomas are mostly formed by "normal" lobules immersed in and in direct contact with adipose tissue (4,50,93,106). The epithelium does not show any proliferative changes, with the exception of a lobular carcinoma in situ reported by Mendiola et al. (77). Adenolipomas must be distinguished from fibroadenomas containing fat in the stroma and from cystosarcomas containing a liposarcomatous component. In adenolipomas, the glandular stromal relationship typical of fibroadenomas is not seen and the adipose tissue in fibroadenomas is separated from the epithelium by variable amounts of fibrous tissue (106). The liposarcomatous component of phyllodes tumors shows nuclear atypicalities that are not seen in adenolipomas.

There are cases of lipoma in which the smooth muscle cells outnumber the adipose tissue cells (figs. 12-30, 12-31). These cases have been variously named in the literature. "Muscular hamartoma" is the designation given to case 2 of the small series of Davies and Riddell (23) that presented as a 3.5-cm well-circumscribed nodule showing a prominence of smooth muscle cells and associated with glands and adipose tissue. Cases 1 and 3 of the series reported by Daroca et al. (22) were named "myoid hamartomas" for a lesion showing smooth muscle cells intermingled with mature adipose tissue and "entrapped" residual glands. The case of "muscular hamartoma" reported by Bussolati et al. (9) contained small cysts with apocrine epithelium in addition

to the other features. Some believe the smooth muscle component is of myoepithelial cell origin (27). The fact that smooth muscle cells and adipose tissue can be intermingled is not surprising since clonal chromosomal aberrations in lipomas and leiomyomas involve similar regions of chromosome 12 (78).

Hibernomas are rare in the breast (44). They occur mostly in the axillary tail (93). A case of *adenohibernoma* has been reported (figs. 12-32, 12-33) (20) and we have seen a case as well. Two *angiomyolipomas* (PECOMA) of the type seen in the renal region have been reported (16).

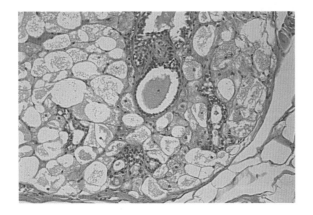

Figure 12-33

ADENOHIBERNOMA

The foam cells have the features of brown fat.

LEIOMYOMA

Leiomyomas are benign tumors containing only smooth muscle cells. In addition to myolipomas and adenomyomas, smooth muscle cells can be seen in the stroma of occasional fibroadenomas (34,48,67) and as limited areas in rare cases of fibroepithelial lesions designated as hamartomas (39,84).

Leiomyomas composed exclusively of smooth muscle cells are rare, and as with leiomyomas of other regions, can be superficial or deeply located in the breast parenchyma. The largest series reported by Jones et al. (59) consisted of 7 superficial and 11 deep leiomyomas. Four of the superficial cases were tumors of erector pili muscle and were located in the skin far from the nipple. Three cases were located in the nipple and were considered derived from the erector muscle. The average age of the patients was 43 years and in one case, occurring in a man, the skin contracted when touched.

Nipple leiomyomas range from 0.5 to 1.5 cm, and can cause contraction of the skin areola (50) and tenderness of the nipple. These tumors are formed by interlacing bundles of elongated cells with ovoid nuclei showing round ends and eosinophilic cytoplasm. The neoplastic proliferation blends with the surrounding stroma and entrapped preexisting ducts are usually observed. Irregular nuclei in the proliferating cells are not rare, but mitoses are not seen (81).

Leiomyomas located in the breast parenchyma are rare. With the exception of the Armed Forces Institute of Pathology (AFIP) series (59), sporadic

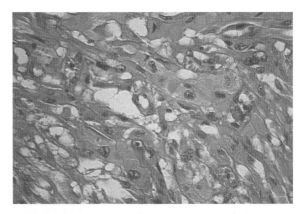

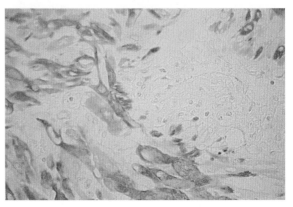

Figure 12-34

EPITHELIOID LEIOMYOMA

Top: The cells show abundant granular eosinophilic cytoplasm.
Bottom: Proliferating cells are positive with desmin antibody.

cases only have been reported (13,29). The tumors are well circumscribed, possess a thin fibrous pseudocapsule, and have a mean diameter of 1.4 cm with exceptional cases over 10 cm in greatest axis (13). Histologically, they show the features classically seen in leiomyomas of other sites and mitoses do not exceed 1 per 10 highpower fields (59). Immunohistochemically, the proliferating cells are positive for smooth muscle actin, vimentin, and desmin and stain, although weakly, with anti-CD34 antisera (67b,113). The parenchymal myoma reported by Roncaroli et al. (92) was formed by epithelioid smooth muscle cells with granular cytoplasm (fig. 12-34). The nuclei were round, with prominent nucleoli. No mitotic figures were seen. The granularity of the cytoplasm proved to be due to lysosomes and the patient was in good health 7 years after the excision of the nodule.

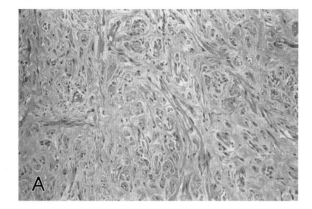

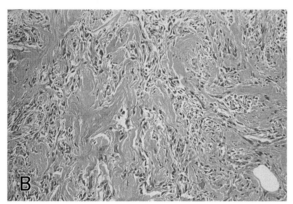

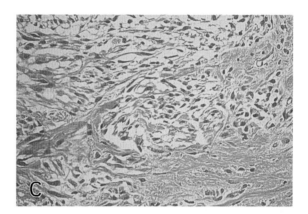

Figure 12-35

LEIOMYOMA

A: At the periphery of a tumor with circumscribed borders is a benign smooth muscle cell proliferation.

B: In the center of the lesion is a spindle cell proliferation. Hyaline collagen bands separate the cells.

C: Higher magnification of B shows the proliferating cells that are reminiscent of a BSSCT.

Two *adenomyomas*, formed exclusively of glands and smooth muscle cells, have been described (23,67b). Both cases were originally interpreted as hamartomas.

The origin of leiomyoma of the breast parenchyma has been a matter of debate for a long time. Hamperl (53) suggested an origin from myoepithelium, a dislodgement of mammillary muscle has been proposed (13), as well as an origin from vessel walls.

The fact that leiomyomas share with BSSCT many immunohistochemical features, that they share with lipomas similar cytogenetic changes, and that cases of BSSCT display areas of smooth muscle cells (113), indicate that leiomyomas originate from the same stromal precursor as BSSCT. In support of this was a case seen by the author that was characterized by a typical leiomyoma proliferation (fig. 12-35A). In the center of the nodule, encaseated by the smooth muscle cells, was a central core showing the typical features of BSSCT with a prominent myofibroblastic component (fig. 12-35B,C). This case is similar to the one reported by Thomas et al. (113).

FIBROMATOSIS

Definition. *Fibromatosis* is a clonal fibroblastic/myofibroblastic proliferation that tends to recur (76).

Clinical Features. Cases reported in the mammary region are included among extraabdominal deep fibromatoses (extraabdominal desmoids) that arise from the connective tissue of the pectoralis muscle or the overlying fascia. One case occurred as two independent lesions in the breast and the pectoralis muscle (71). Sporadic cases manifest after trauma or breast augmentation with implants (103). Cases occurring in families (122), associated with Gardner syndrome (51) or hereditary desmoid disease (31), have been described. Unlike abdominal desmoids, fibromatosis of the breast has not been associated with pregnancy and has been observed even in nulliparous women and in the male breast (111). Patients range in age from 13 to 80 years, but most patients are in the 3rd to 5th decades (76).

Primary mammary fibromatosis is a rare disease with an incidence of less than 0.2 percent of all primary lesions of the mammary gland (87).

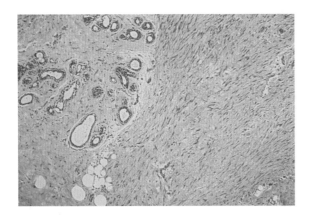

Figure 12-36

FIBROMATOSIS

The specialized stroma of the lobule is compressed but not invaded by the proliferating cells.

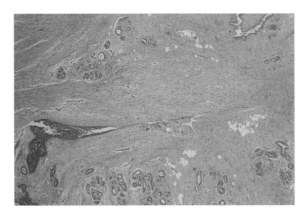

Figure 12-38

FIBROMATOSIS

The spindle cells are arranged in finger-like sweeping fascicles.

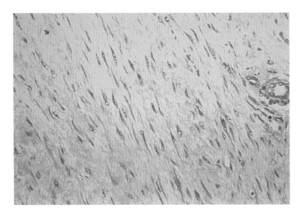

Figure 12-37

FIBROMATOSIS

Spindle cells of uniform appearance are separated by abundant collagen.

Bilaterality (mostly synchronous) is present in 6 percent of cases (93), but in most cases the lesion is unifocal. Lesions are palpated as mobile nodules when in the breast, while the mass is fixed to the chest wall in the musculoaponeurotic forms. Small lesions located in the breast parenchyma radiologically mimic invasive carcinomas (8,87,111). Skin dimpling can be observed when the lesion is superficially located (118). Tumor size varies from 0.7 to 10.0 cm (97,118), with a median size of 2.5 cm, which is notably smaller than other extraabdominal desmoid tumors (76).

Gross Findings. The gross features are those of an ill-defined firm nodule, but cases with a stellate appearance are not rare.

Microscopic Findings. FNAC is characterized by isolated spindle cells, small groups of cohesive benign elements, and scattered lymphocytes in a background of amorphous material (87). These features often lead to inconclusive diagnoses, one of which may be malignancy (8).

The histologic features of tumors of musculoaponeurotic origin are identical to those of any other site. Lesions primary in the breast show preexisting entrapped glandular epithelium, which usually is located at the periphery of the lesion. The epithelium consists mostly of atrophic ductules and lobules which preserve the original "specialized" stroma that is compressed, but not invaded by, the lesional cells (fig. 12-36). Tumor cells are elongated and spindle shaped, and of uniform appearance. They are immersed in and spaced from one another by abundant collagen (fig. 12-37) (33). The nuclei vary from round to elongated, and display one to three nucleoli. Mitoses and necrotic areas are absent. The presence of pleomorphic nuclei and multinucleated giant cells may suggest an incorrect diagnosis.

The spindle cells have pale cytoplasm and are arranged in finger-like sweeping fascicles (fig. 12-38). The amount of stromal collagen and consequently, the cellularity, can vary considerably. Many lesions display a central hyalinized zone with a scanty cellular component while the periphery shows greater cellularity with entrapped glands (zoning phenomenon). A myxoid fasciitis-like appearance is frequent (76).

Table 12-2

DISTINGUISHING FIBROMATOSIS, FIBROMATOSIS-LIKE METAPLASTIC MALIGNANT TUMOR, AND BSSCT[a]

	Zoning Phenomenon	Epithelium	Borders	Spindle Cells	Nuclei
Fibromatosis	Present	Entrapped	Pushing to invasive	Uniformly oriented, separated by abundant collagen	Ovoid, pale staining
Fibromatosis-like metaplastic malignant tumor	Absent	Part of the lesion	Invasive	Irregular with no orientation, unevenly spaced	Irregular, variable staining
BSSCT	Absent	Absent	Pushing	Uniformly oriented, in close contact, in nests	Ovoid

[a]BSSCT = benign stromal spindle cell tumors.

The proliferating cells stain for vimentin and smooth muscle actin. Some cells in each lesion stain for S-100 protein and desmin. CD34 is negative. The two cases reported by Pettinato et al. (86) showed cells with intracytoplasmic, spherical inclusion bodies that by light and ultrastructural microscopy and immunohistochemistry were indistinguishable from those seen in infantile digital fibromatosis and those observed in the "fibroepithelial tumor" of the breast described by Bittesini et al. (7). In 50 percent of cases, a lymphocytic infiltrate is observed at the periphery of the lesion (97).

Differential Diagnosis. Fibromatosis has to be distinguished from benign (nodular fasciitis and BSSCT) and malignant spindle cell tumors of which the most deceptive lesion is composed of bland looking spindle cell carcinomas such as those named "metaplastic breast tumors with a dominant fibromatosis-like phenotype" (46).

Nodular fasciitis is superficially located, has well-circumscribed borders, and does not contain elongated fascicles of spindle cells.

BSSCTs (Table 12-2) have neat circumscribed borders, absent epithelium in the lesion, cells that are in close contact with one another when arranged in nests, and cells not separated by collagen. CD34 is constantly found in the cells of BSSCT and not in those of fibromatosis.

Stringent criteria are critically important when differentiating fibromatosis and spindle cell fibromatosis-like sarcomatoid carcinoma. In the latter, no zoning phenomenon is observed (fig. 12-39, left) as the neoplastic spindle cells proliferate randomly. Specifically, epithelium is present irregularly throughout the lesion and not at the periphery, as seen in fibromatosis. In fibromatosis-like sarcomatoid carcinoma,

often there is proliferating epithelium that accompanies the tumor. If the epithelium does not show frank malignancy, it usually has the features of peripheral papilloma or minute well-differentiated clear cell adenomyoepithelioma (fig. 12-39, right) (110). The spindle cells of the sarcomatoid proliferation are irregularly spaced and oriented, cellularity is variable, and the nuclei have different shapes and sizes in different areas (fig. 12-40). Transition between the spindle cell component and the epithelial component within the lesion is a frequent finding (fig. 12-39, right), at variance with fibromatosis in which the epithelium appears entrapped. Keratin positive cells were present in 85 percent of fibromatosis-like metaplastic carcinomas (46); the cells of fibromatosis are keratin negative.

Prognosis. Recurrences are observed in up to 27 percent of cases. All of the recurrent cases had been inadequately excised (118). No histologic difference was observed between recurring and nonrecurring tumors. Most of the recurrences appear 3 to 5 years after excision (76).

BENIGN NERVE SHEATH TUMORS

Neurofibroma

Jones et al. (59) described 15 *neurofibromas* of the breast, the largest series reported. One case affected the skin overlying the breast, while the others were deep seated. Three patients had von Recklinghausen disease. The patients ranged in age from 17 to 77 years (mean, 38 years). Tumor size varied from 0.4 to 10.0 cm, with a median of 5.0 cm. All 11 patients who were followed for a mean period of 6.7 years were alive and well at the last contact.

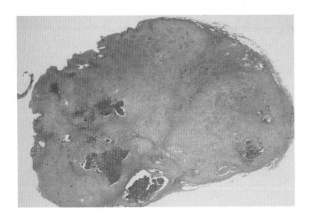
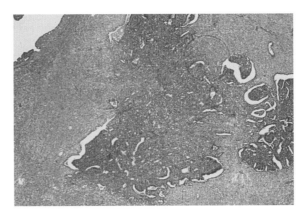

Figure 12-39

FIBROMATOSIS-LIKE SARCOMATOID CARCINOMA (METAPLASTIC BREAST TUMOR WITH A DOMINANT FIBROMATOSIS-LIKE PHENOTYPE)

Left: No zoning phenomenon is apparent. The papillary epithelium is visible throughout the lesion.
Right: The epithelium shows features of peripheral papilloma.

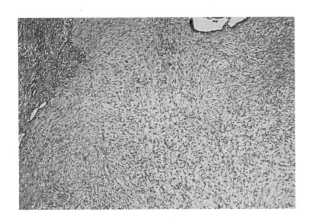
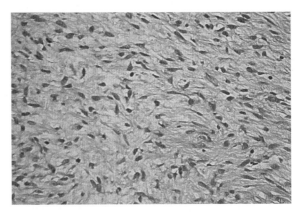

Figure 12-40

FIBROMATOSIS-LIKE SARCOMATOID CARCINOMA (METAPLASTIC BREAST TUMOR WITH A DOMINANT FIBROMATOSIS-LIKE PHENOTYPE)

The cellularity is variable. The nuclei vary in shape and size in different areas.

Pseudogynecomastia

Children with von Recklinghausen disease can have associated *pseudogynecomastia*. According to Lipper et al. (65), who collected six cases from the literature, pseudogynecomastia is a result of lipomatous infiltration associated with small subcutaneous neurofibromas of the mammary region. Pseudogynecomastia also occurred in the two patients with von Recklinghausen disease reported by Damiani et al. (17). In both cases, the typical features of PASH were present and in addition, multinucleated giant cells were observed within the empty spaces along the fibrous walls.

Perineurioma

A single case of *perineurioma* was reported by Carneiro et al. (10) in a 42-year-old woman. The 2-cm nodule contained monotonous spindle cells that were vimentin and epithelial membrane antigen positive while keratins, S-100 protein, and desmin were negative. Similar features were seen in a small series of perineuriomas from the AFIP (111).

Schwannoma

Schwannomas are rare in the breast. Only 15 cases are present in the files of AFIP, of which 9 were in men. Patients ranged in age 20 to 90 (mean, 30) years. Five of these cases were reported by Jones et al. (59). The nodules ranged from 0.6 to 4.0 cm in greatest dimension and all were well circumscribed. Differentiating schwannoma from BSSCT is usually not difficult although immunohistochemistry is not helpful. Cases of *ancient schwannoma* can lead to an erroneous diagnosis of malignancy. As in tumors of other sites, microcystic areas coupled with thick vessels, hemosiderin deposits, and total lack of mitoses balance the nuclear pleomorphism present in this type of schwannian proliferation.

Granular Cell Tumor

The first case of *granular cell tumor* (GCT) located in the breast was reported by Abrikossoff (1) in a 55-year-old diabetic woman. Numerous cases have been published since then describing this benign lesion that simulates an invasive carcinoma clinically (50), radiologically (18), macroscopically (26), cytologically (99), and at frozen section (18).

Microscopic examination is almost always the only reliable method for diagnosing these tumors (4). As with all other soft tissue sites, GCTs can arise from the skin as well as deep in the breast parenchyma. The deeply located tumors are rare, with only about 1 for every 1,000 malignancies; they constitute between 6 and 8 percent of all GCTs of the body (26). Ten percent of breast GCTs occur in men (93); the others usually affect middle-aged premenopausal women (26), although the age range varied from 17 to 73 years in one report (average, 40 years) (18).

The lesion is usually localized to the inner quadrants of the breast, and rarely, in the lower outer quadrant. This probably reflects the distribution of the supraclavicular nerve which does not contribute much to the lower outer quadrant (26).

Clinically, there is skin dimpling or nipple retraction in cases located in paraareolar region. In deeply located lesions, a firm nodule is the most frequent presentation, followed by a mass adherent to pectoralis fascia (50). GCTs are usually unifocal, but multifocality occasionally

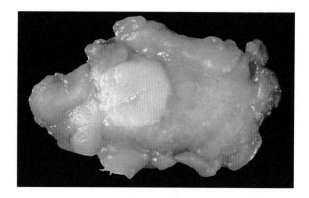

Figure 12-41

GRANULAR CELL TUMOR

The lesion has circumscribed borders. (Courtesy of Dr. F. Koerner, Boston, MA.)

occurs, most frequently in blacks. Some cases are discovered at mammography and invariably appear suspicious for malignancy (18). The clinical manifestations are usually of short duration (a few days to a few months) but in one patient, the lesion had been present for 14 years (18). The most frequent preoperative diagnoses are fibroadenoma and invasive carcinoma depending on the age of the patient.

The tumors were well circumscribed in 5 of the 12 cases reported by DeMay and Kay (26); the rest were ill defined. Three of the seven cases reported by Damiani et al. (18) showed circumscribed borders (fig. 12-41).

Histologically, GCTs are composed of sheets, nests, and rows of cells immersed in a fibrous stroma. The cells show abundant, granular and eosinophilic cytoplasm and round to ovoid nuclei (fig. 12-42), which occasionally display cytoplasmic pseudoinclusions. Nuclei vary from hyperchromatic to clear, with one to two nucleoli. Mitotic figures and necrotic areas are not observed. Well-formed nerve bundles are frequently seen, as well as entrapped mammary glands. The proliferating cells usually surround lobular structures, but it is not exceptional to see the "specialized" stroma of the lobules invaded. At the edge of some lesions isolated clusters of proliferating cells invade the adjacent adipose tissue.

The granules are periodic acid–Schiff (PAS) positive after diastase digestion and the cytoplasm stains with S-100 protein antiserum in 20 to 80 percent of the total neoplastic proliferations. The intensity of staining can be weak (fig.

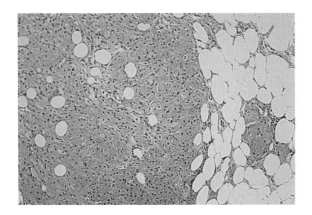

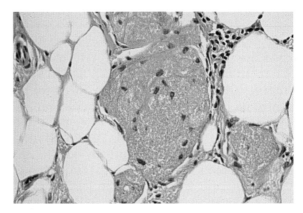

Figure 12-42

GRANULAR CELL TUMOR

The cells have abundant granular and eosinophilic cytoplasm and round nuclei.

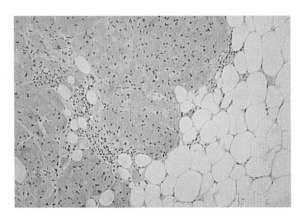

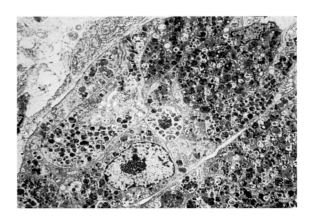

Figure 12-43

GRANULAR CELL TUMOR

S-100 protein is faintly positive.

Figure 12-44

GRANULAR CELL TUMOR

Many secondary lysosomes are seen in the cytoplasm. (Fig. 6 from Damiani S, Koerner FC, Dickersin GR, Cook MG, Eusebi V. Granular cell tumour of the breast. Virchows Arch A Pathol Anat Histopathol 1992;420:223.)

12-43). Vimentin stains the cytoplasmic borders of most of the cells that are negative for keratins, epithelial membrane antigen, gross cystic disease fluid protein (GCDFP)-15, myoglobin, steroid receptors, alpha-1-antitrypsin, lysozyme, and glial fibrillary acidic protein (GFAP) (18,58,120). Immunoreactivity with anticarcinoembryonic antigen (CEA) antibodies has been found by some authors (105), and denied by others (120); it seems that CEA positivity in GCTs is the result of a nonspecific cross reaction of some antibodies (75).

Ultrastructurally, the neoplastic cells are surrounded by basal lamina, but the most striking feature is that the cells are filled by myriads of secondary lysosomes (fig. 12-44) in the form of mem-

brane-bound vesicles. Some of these are empty, but most contain varying amounts of membranous, flocculent, electron-dense material (18).

The histogenesis of these lesions has led to a large number of hypotheses, more so than most of the lesions in human pathology. The general consensus is that the tumor arises from Schwann cells (3,107). This view is corroborated by the granular cell traumatic neuroma which supervenes in mammary scars after mastectomies (102) and which consists of the typical features of traumatic neuroma including granular, S-100 protein–positive cells, indistinguishable from those of GCT, intermingled with nerves.

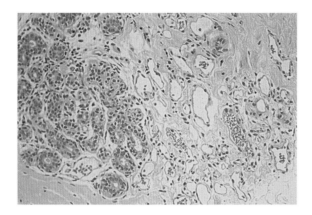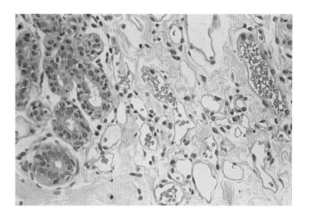

Figure 12-45

PERILOBULAR ANGIOMA

The lesion is the same size as an angioma. The vessels are delicate capillary-like spaces.

The most important entity in the differential diagnosis is myoblastomatoid (histiocytoid) invasive carcinoma. The latter can mimic GCT to a degree that no fewer than two cases of the series reported by Eusebi et al. (35) were originally diagnosed as GCT. Fortunately, keratins, which are lacking in GCT, are very useful in establishing the correct diagnosis of carcinoma.

Since only a single case of putative malignant GCT primary in the breast has been published (14), the initial surgical treatment should be conservative with tumor-free margins.

BENIGN VASCULAR LESIONS

Angiomas

Angioma, also called *hemangioma,* is a benign proliferation of endothelial cells that tends to be vasoformative. Angiomas of the breast region are identical to those of other areas and, accordingly, can arise in the skin, around the breast region (named *nonparenchymal hemangiomas* [96]), and within the breast tissue. In the latter location, angiomas are incidental microscopic findings in most cases while mammographic or palpable lesions are rare and need to be carefully distinguished from angiosarcoma (4,32).

Microscopic angiomas are minute cavernous angiomas that can be located anywhere in the breast stroma, including the specialized intralobular and periductal connective tissue. These minute lesions were generically named perilobular hemangioma (100) and were seen in 11 percent of cases in an accurate forensic

postmortem study of 210 patients (64). The lesions are usually bilateral and patient age ranges from 29 to 82 years, with a mean of 51.5.

Microscopically, angiomas are easily overlooked (4) since they are composed of small groups of delicate, mainly cavernous vascular spaces that usually occupy only one high-power field. There is little stroma between the endothelial channels, which are invested by smooth muscle actin-positive pericyte-like cells. Most of the lumens are filled with red blood cells. The lesions can be unifocal or multiple (fig. 12-45).

The unfortunate name of *atypical perilobular hemangioma* (93) has been given to some similar and clinically irrelevant lesions with hyperchromatic nuclei of the type seen in targetoid hemangiomas. We think that this term should be abandoned in order to avoid unnecessary caution as "it is unlikely that any one of these lesions would be mistaken for an angiosarcoma" (4).

Macroscopic angiomas are those rare lesions revealed either by mammography or clinically. Tavassoli (111) reported a series of 65 cavernous, 36 capillary, 2 epithelioid, and 8 arteriovenous hemangiomas, all of which were larger than 5 mm. An additional 85 were labeled by Tavassoli as not otherwise specified. These probably have to be grouped with the 18 lesions reported by Hoda et al. (56) that were named "hemangiomas with atypical histological features." Most of the latter lesions were atypical in the sense that they did not have the features of ordinary hemangiomas. In fact, Hoda et al. even included cases of sinusoidal cavernous hemangioma and spindle

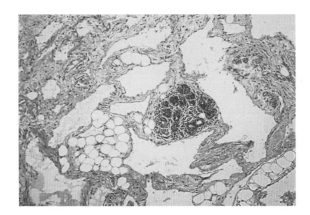 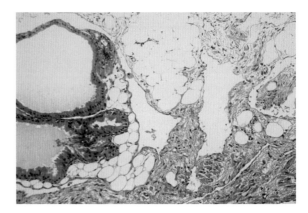

Figure 12-46

BENIGN LYMPHANGIOENDOTHELIOMA

Large and irregular empty spaces "dissect" the collagen and adipose tissue and surround single lobules.

cell hemangioma. Four venous hemangiomas were described by Rosen et al. (98).

Most clinically apparent angiomas are seen in female breasts, but occasional cases also appear in men (111). Their sizes range up to 3.5 cm. The patient age depends on the type of angioma: younger patients have capillary angiomas.

The best treatment for any form of macroscopic angioma is its complete excision with a view to accurate diagnosis. No patient with angioma has had local recurrence or metastasis with a follow-up period as long as 140 months and averaging 44 months (93). In children, the best treatment is still questionable since both surgery and radiotherapy may result in mammary hypoplasia (111).

Angiomatosis

To use Enzinger and Weiss' words, "Angiomatosis is a rare benign, but clinically extensive, vascular lesion of soft tissues, which almost invariably becomes symptomatic during childhood. Such lesions are histologically benign and affect a large segment of the body in a contiguous fashion" (33).

If the above definition of angiomatosis is adopted, then only one case described in the literature is consonant with it: case 2 of a series reported as angiomatosis of the breast by Rosen (95). All the other cases of putative angiomatosis have been reported in adult patients and most, if not all, can at present be categorized as benign lymphangioendothelioma (acquired progressive lymphangioma) (49).

Rosen's case 2 (95) was followed for 39 years from the age of 11 weeks when a "cavernous vascular tumor" extending from "beneath the right nipple upward...to the level of clavicle and outward...to the anterior vascular fold" was removed. The lesion recurred at ages 34 and 39 as nodules formed by vascular channels with flat endothelium with no atypia.

In all the other lesions reported as angiomatosis, patients ranged from 17 to 73 years, with a median of 40 (111). All lesions were described as large masses ranging from 9 to 20 cm but three cases seen by the authors did not exceed 3 cm in greatest dimension.

Benign lymphangioendothelioma (BLE) of soft tissues has the same age range, macroscopic size (49), and histologic findings as does so-called angiomatosis of the breast (93,111). Anastomosing, irregular empty spaces appear to "dissect" the stromal collagen and the adipose tissue. Rare vascular spaces may contain red blood cells. The endothelial cells are usually flat and no signs of atypia are evident (fig. 12-46). Lymphoid aggregates can be present around the vascular spaces.

Taking these histologic features into account, it is not surprising that there is a general worry about the difficulty of distinguishing BLE from well-differentiated angiosarcoma. Clinically, BLE is a longstanding, slow-growing lesion (49). Well-differentiated angiosarcoma is characterized by red blood cells within the vascular spaces while these are rare in BLE. Nuclear hyperchromatism in angiosarcoma is always present even if only to a minor degree; nuclear hyperchromatism is

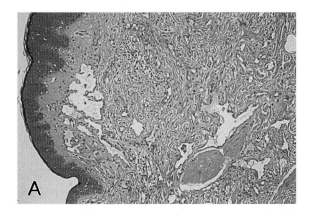

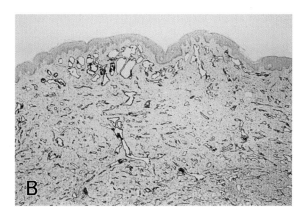

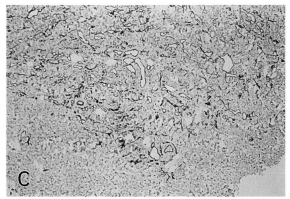

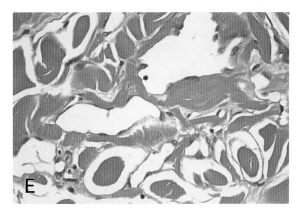

Figure 12-47

BENIGN LYMPHANGIOMATOUS PAPULES OF SKIN

A: Dilated vessels are present in the superficial dermis.
B: CD31 decorates the vessels, which are mostly parallel to the epidermis.
C: The wedge silhouette is shown using CD31 antibody.
D,E: The endothelium is flat and nuclei are regular.

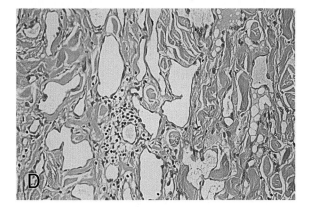

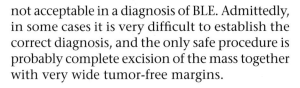

not acceptable in a diagnosis of BLE. Admittedly, in some cases it is very difficult to establish the correct diagnosis, and the only safe procedure is probably complete excision of the mass together with very wide tumor-free margins.

Benign Lymphangiomatous Papules of the Skin after Radiotherapy for Breast Carcinoma

Five cases of *benign lymphangiomatous papules of the skin* (BLAP) were reported by Diaz-Cascajo et al. (30); one lesion was named "acquired progressive lymphangioma of the skin follow-

ing radiotherapy for breast carcinoma" (101). However, the first description of this vascular change is credited to Fineberg and Rosen (38) who reported three skin lesions and one nodule in the breast, which they called "atypical vascular lesions after radiotherapy for breast carcinoma." All the lesions developed, on average, 3.1 years after radiotherapy for breast carcinoma. Most of the lesions were solitary to multiple, white-tan papules or transparent vesicles (30).

Histologically, BLAPs have specific characteristics that, together with the clinical features,

285

prevent an erroneous diagnosis of well-differentiated angiosarcoma. These characteristics include: 1) a wedge-shaped silhouette with the base on the epidermis; 2) markedly dilated vascular spaces in the upper part of the epidermis which result in the clinical appearance of vesicles; 3) empty vascular spaces of the type seen in BLE which are mostly parallel to the epidermis when superficially located; and 4) flat regular endothelium positive for CD31, with micropapillae (fig. 12-47).

Red blood cells are occasionally seen within the lumens, which contain proteinaceous material. Some lesions reach the subcutaneous tissue, as occurred in two of the cases of the series reported by Diaz-Cascajo et al. (30). In these two cases, the deeper vessels were described as smaller than the superficial ones.

BLAPs have to be distinguished from lesions with a deceptively benign appearance that resemble capillary hemangiomas but evolve into or represent cutaneous postradiation angiosarcoma (28). The clinical benign behavior of this condition is characterized by a lack of recurrence and metastasis, even in patients followed for more than 5 years (30,38).

REFERENCES

1. Abrikossoff AI. Weitere untersuchungen uber myoblastenmyome. Virchows Arch Pathol Anat Physiol Klin Med 1931;280:723-740.
2. Ali S, Teichberg S, DeRisi DC, Urmacherher C. Giant myofibroblastoma of the male breast. Am J Surg Pathol 1994;18:1170-1176.
3. Azzopardi JG. Histogenesis of the granular-cell myoblastoma. J Pathol Bacteriol 1956;71:85-94.
4. Azzopardi JG, Ahmed A, Millis RR. Problems in breast pathology. London: W.B. Saunders Company; 1979.
5. Badve S, Sloane JP. Pseudoangiomatous hyperplasia of male breast. Histopathology 1995;26:463-466.
6. Berean K, Tron VA, Churg A, Clement PB. Mammary fibroadenoma with multinucleated stromal giant cells. Am J Surg Pathol 1986;10:823-827.
7. Bittesini L, Dei Tos AP, Doglioni C, Della Libera D, Laurino L, Fletcher CD. Fibroepithelial tumor of the breast with digital-fibroma-like inclusions in the stromal component. Am J Surg Pathol 1994;18:296-301.
8. Bogomoletz WV, Boulenger E, Simatos A. Infiltrating fibromatosis of the breast. J Clin Path 1981;34:30-34.
9. Bussolati G, Ghiringhello B, Papotti M. Subareolar muscular hamartoma of the breast. Appl Pathol 1984;2:92-95.
10. Carneiro F, Brandao O, Correia AC, Sobrinho-Simoes M. The quarterly case. Spindle cell tumor of the breast. Ultrastruct Pathol 1989;13:593-599.
11. Carter BA, Jensen RA, Simpson JF, Page DL. Benign transport of breast epithelium into axillary lymph nodes after biopsy. Am J Clin Pathol 2000;113:259-265.
12. Chan KW, Ghadially FN, Algaratnam TT. Benign spindle cell tumour of the breast—a variant of spindle cell lipoma or fibroma of breast? Pathology 1984;16:331-337.
13. Craig JM. Leiomyoma of the female breast. Arch Pathol (Chic) 1947;44:314-317.
14. Crawford ES, DeBakey ME. Granular cell myoblastoma: two unusual cases. Cancer 1953;6:786-789.
15. Dal Cin P, Sciot R, De Smet L, Van Den Berghe H. Translocation 2;11 in a fibroma of tendon sheath. Histopathology 1998;32:433-435.
16. Damiani S, Chiodera P, Guaragni M, Eusebi V. Mammary angiomyolipoma. Virchows Arch 2002;440:551-552.
17. Damiani S, Eusebi V. Gynecomastia in type 1 neurofibromatosis with features of pseudoangiomatous stromal hyperplasia with giant cells. Report of two cases. Virchows Arch 2001;438:515-516.
18. Damiani S, Koerner FC, Dickersin GR, Cook MG, Eusebi V. Granular cell tumour of the breast. Virchows Arch A Pathol Anat Histopathol 1992;420:219-226.
19. Damiani S, Miettinen M, Peterse JL, Eusebi V. Solitary fibrous tumor (myofibroblastoma) of the breast. Virchows Arch 1994;425:89-92.
20. Damiani S, Panarelli M. Mammary adenohibernoma. Histopathology 1996;28:554-555.
21. Damiani S, Peterse JL, Eusebi V. Malignant neoplasms infiltrating "pseudoangiomatous" stromal hyperplasia of the breast: an unrecognized pathway of tumor spread. Histopathology 2002;41:208-215.
22. Daroca PJ, Reed RJ, Love GL, Kraus SD. Myoid hamartomas of the breast. Hum Pathol 1985;16:212-219.
23. Davies JD, Riddell RH. Muscular hamartomas of the breast. J Pathol 1973;111:209-211.

24. Dei Tos AP, Mentzel T, Newman PL, Fletcher CD. Spindle cell liposarcoma, a hitherto unrecognized variant of liposarcoma. Analysis of six cases. Am J Surg Pathol 1994;18:913-921.

25. Dei Tos AP, Wadden C, Fletcher CD. S-100 protein staining in liposarcoma. Its diagnostic utility in the hihg-grade myxoid (Rand cell) variant. Applied Immunohistochemistry 1996;4:95-101.

26. DeMay RM, Kay S. Granular cell tumor of the breast. Pathol Annu 1984;19:121-148.

27. Di Tommaso L, Pasquinelli G, Damiani S. Smooth muscle cell differentiation in mammary stromoepithelial lesions with evidence of a dual origin: stromal myofibroblasts and myoepithelial cells. Histopathology 2003;42:448-456.

28. Di Tommaso L, Rosai J. The capillary lobule: a deceptively benign feature of post-radiation angiosarcoma of the skin. Report of three cases. Am J Dermatopathol 2005;27:301-305.

29. Diaz-Arias AA, Hurt MA, Loy TS, Seeger RM, Bickel JT. Leiomyoma of the breast. Hum Pathol 1989;20:396-399.

30. Diaz-Cascajo C, Borghi S, Retzlaff H, Requena L, Metze D. Benign lymphangiomatous papules of the skin following radiotherapy: a report of five new cases and review of the literature. Histopathology 1999;35:319-327.

31. Eccles DM, van der Luijt R, Breukel C, et al. Hereditary desmoid disease due to a frameshift mutation at codon 1924 of the APC gene. Am J Hum Genet 1996;59:1193-1201.

32. Elston CW, Ellis IO. The breast, 3rd ed. Edinburgh: Churchill Livingstone; 1998.

33. Enzinger FM, Weiss SW. Soft tissue tumors, 3rd ed. St. Louis: Mosby; 1995.

34. Eusebi V, Cunsolo A, Fedeli F, Severi B, Scarani P. Benign smooth muscle cell metaplasia in breast. Tumori 1980;66:643-653.

35. Eusebi V, Foschini MP, Bussolati G, Rosen PP. Myoblastomatoid (histiocytoid) carcinoma of the breast. A type of apocrine carcinoma. Am J Clin Pathol 1995;19:553-562.

36. Fakunaga M, Ushigome S. Myofibroblastoma of breast with diverse differentiations. Arch Pathol Lab Med 1997;121:599-603.

37. Fechner RE, Mills SE. Breast pathology benign proliferations, atypias in situ carcinomas. Chicago: ASCP Press - American Society of Clinical Pathologists; 1990.

38. Fineberg S, Rosen PP. Cutaneous angiosarcoma and atypical vascular lesions of the skin and breast after radiation therapy for breast carcinoma. Am J Clin Pathol 1994;102:757-763.

39. Fisher CJ, Hanby AM, Robinson L, Millis RR. Mammary hamartoma—a review of 35 cases. Histopathology 1992;20:99-106.

40. Folpe AL, Devaney K, Weiss SW. Lipomatous hemangiopericytoma: a rare variant of hemangiopericytoma that may be confused with liposarcoma. Am J Surg Pathol 1999;23:1201-1207.

41. Foschini MP, Dina RE, Eusebi V. Sarcomatoid neoplasms of the breast: proposed definitions for biphasic and monophasic sarcomatoid mammary carcinomas. Semin Diagn Pathol 1993;10:128-136.

42. Foschini MP, Eusebi V. Carcinoma of the breast showing myoepithelial cell differentiation. A review of the literature. Virchows Arch 1998;432:303-310.

43. Fushimi H, Kotoh K, Nishihnara K, Fujinaka H, Takao T. Chondrolipoma of the breast: a case report with cytological and histological examination. Histopathology 1999;35:478-479.

44. Gardner-Thorpe D, Hirschowitz L, Maddox PR. Mammary hibernoma. Eur J Surg Oncol 2000;26:430.

45. Geschickter CF. Diseases of the breast. Diangois, pathology, treatment, 2nd ed. Philadelphia: J.B. Lippincott Company; 1945.

46. Gobbi H, Simpson JF, Borowsky A, Jensen RA, Page DL. Metaplastic breast tumors with a dominant fibromatosis-like phenotype have a high risk of local recurrence. Cancer 1999;85:2170-2182.

47. Gobbi H, Tse G, Page DL, Olson SJ, Jensen RA, Simpson JF. Reactive spindle cell nodules of the breast after core biopsy or fine-needle aspiration. Am J Clin Pathol 2000;113:288-294.

48. Goodman ZD, Taxy JB. Fibroadenomas of the breast with prominent smooth muscle. Am J Surg Pathol 1981;5:99-101.

49. Guillou L, Fletcher CD. Benign lymphangioendothelioma (acquired progressive lymphangioma): a lesion not to be confused with well-differentiated angiosarcoma and patch stage Kaposi's sarcoma. Clinicopathologic analysis of a series. Am J Surg Pathol 2000;24:1047-1057.

50. Haagensen C D: Diseases of the breast, 3rd ed. Philadelphia: W.B. Saunders; 1986.

51. Haggitt RC, Booth JL. Bilateral fibromatosis of the breast in Gardner's syndrome. Cancer 1970;25:161-166.

52. Hamele-Bena D, Cranor ML, Sciotto C, Erlandson R, Rosen PP. Uncommon presentation of mammary myofibroblastoma. Mod Pathol 1996;9:786-790.

53. Hamperl H. The myothelia (myoepithelial cells). Normal state; regressive changes; hyperplasia; tumors. Curr Top Pathol 1970;53:161-220.

54. Hanau CA, Miettinen M. Solitary fibrous tumor: histological and immunohistochemical spectrum of benign and malignant variants presenting at different sites. Hum Pathol 1995;26:440-449.

287

55. Hartveit E. Attenuated cells in breast stroma: the missing lymphatic system of the breast. Histopathology 1990;16:533-543.

56. Hoda SA, Cranor ML, Rosen PP. Hemangiomas of the breast with atypical histological features. Further analysis of histological subtypes confirming their benign character. Am J Surg Pathol 1992;16:553-560.

57. Ibrahim RE, Sciotto CG, Weidner N. Pseudoangiomatous hyperplasia of mammary stroma. Some observations regarding its clinicopathologic spectrum. Cancer 1989;63:1154-1160.

58. Ingram DL, Mossler JA, Snowhite J, Leight GS, McCarty KS Jr. Granular cell tumors of the breast. Steroid receptor analysis and localization of carcinoembryonic antigen, myoglobin, and S100 protein. Arch Pathol Lab Med 1984;108:897-901.

59. Jones MW, Norris HJ, Wargotz ES. Smooth muscle and nerve sheath tumors of the breast. A clinicopathologic study of 45 cases. Int J Surg Pathol 1994;2:85-92.

60. Krismann M, Adams H, Jaworska M, Muller KM, Johnen G. Patterns of chromosomal imbalances in benign solitary fibrous tumours of the pleura. Virchows Arch 2000;437:248-255.

61. Lazaro-Santander R, Garcia-Prats MD, Nieto S, et al. Myofibroblastoma of the breast with diverse histological features. Virchows Arch 1999;434:547-550.

62. Lee AH, Sworn MJ, Theaker JM, Fletcher CD. Myofibroblastoma of breast: an immunohistochemical study. Histopathology 1993;22:75-78.

63. Lee K, Chan JK, Ho LC. Histologic changes in the breast after fine-needle aspiration. Am J Surg Pathol 1994;18:1039-1047.

64. Lesueur GC, Brown RW, Bhathal PS. Incidence of perilobular hemangioma in the female breast. Arch Pathol Lab Med 1983;107:308-310.

65. Lipper S, Willson CF, Copeland KC. Pseudogynecomastia due to neurofibromatosis—a light microscopic and ultrastructural study. Hum Pathol 1981;12:755-759.

66. Lopez-Rios F, Alberti N, Perez-Barrios A, de Agustin PP. Aspiration biopsy of pleomorphic lipoma of the breast. A case report. Acta Cytol 2000;44:255-258.

67. Mackenzie DH. A fibro-adenoma of the breast with smooth muscle. J Pathol Bacteriol 1968;96:231-232.

67a. Magro G, Amico P, Gurrera A. Myxoid myofibroblastoma of the breast with atypical cells: a potential diagnostic pitfall. Virchows Arch 2007;450:483-485.

67b. Magro G, Bisceglia M. Muscular hamartoma of the breast. Case report and review of the literature. Pathol Res Pract 1998;194:349-355.

68. Magro G, Bisceglia M, Michal M, Eusebi V. Spindle cell lipoma-like tumor, solitary fibrous tumor and myofibroblastoma of the breast: a clinico-pathological analysis of 13 cases in favor of a unifyng histogenetic concept. Virchows Arch 2002;440:249-260.

69. Magro G, Bisceglia M, Pasquinelli G. Benign spindle cell tumor of the breast with prominent adipocytic component. Ann Diagn Pathol 1998;2:306-311.

69a. Magro G, Caltabiano R, Di Cataldo A, Puzzo L. CD10 is expressed by mammary myofibroblastoma and spindle cell lipoma of the soft tissue: an additional evidence of their histogenetic linking. Virchows Arch 2007;450:727-728.

70. Magro G, Fraggetta F, Torrisi A, Emmanuele C, Lanzafame S. Myofibroblastoma of the breast with hemangiopericytoma-like pattern and pleomorphic lipoma-like areas. Report of a case with diagnostic and histogenetic considerations. Pathol Res Pract 1999;195:257-262.

70a. Magro G, Gurrera A, Bisceglia M. H-caldesmon expression in myofibroblastoma of the breast: evidence supporting the distinction from leiomyoma. Histopathology 2003;42:233-238.

70b. Magro G, Lanzafame S. Sporadic subcutaneous angiomyolipoma with expression of estrogen and progesterone receptors. Virchows Arch 2007;450:123-125.

71. Magro G, Mesiti M. Breast and pectoralis musculo-aponeurotic fibromatosis: two independent lesions occurring in the same patient. A case report. Pathol Res Pract 1998;194:867-871.

72. Magro G, Sidoni A, Bisceglia M. Solitary fibrous tumor of the breast: distinction from myofibroblastoma. Histopathology 2000;37:189-191.

73. Marsh WL Jr, Lucas JG, Olsen J. Chondrolipoma of the breast. Arch Pathol Lab Med 1989;113:369-371.

74. Marucci G, Bondi A, Lorenzini P, Eusebi V. [Giant cell reaction in breast after fine-needle aspiration.] Pathologica 2001;93:15-19. [Italian.]

75. Matthews JB, Mason GI. Granular cell myoblastoma: an immunoperoxidase study using a variety of antisera to human carcinoembryonic antigen. Histopathology 1982;7:77-82.

76. McMenamin ME, Deschryver K, Fletcher CD. Fibrous lesions of the breast. A review. Int J Surg Pathol 2000;8:99-108.

77. Mendiola H, Henrik-Nielsen R, Dyreborg U, Blichert-Toft M, Al-Hariri JA. Lobular carcinoma in situ occuring in adenolipoma of the breast. Report of a case. Acta Radiol Diagn 1982;23:503-505.

78. Mentzel T, Fletcher CD. Lipomatous tumours of soft tissues: an update. Virchows Arch 1995;427:353-363.

79. Metcalf JS, Ellis B. Choristoma of the breast. Hum Pathol 1985;16:739-740.

80. Morgan MB, Pitha JV. Myofibroblastoma of the breast revisited: an etiologic association with androgens? Hum Pathol 1998;29:347-351.

81. Nascimento AG, Karas M, Rosen PP, Caron AG. Leiomyoma of the nipple. Am J Surg Pathol 1979;3:151-154.

82. Nielsen BB, Ladefoged C. Fibroadenoma of the female breast with multinucleated giant cells. Pathol Res Pract 1985;180:721-724.

83. Nucci MR, Fletcher CD. Myofibroblastoma of the breast: a distinctive benign stromal tumor. Pathology Case Reviews 1999;4:214-219.

84. Oberman HA. Hamartomas and hamartoma variants of the breast. Semin Diagn Pathol 1989;6:135-145.

85. Pauwels P, Sciot R, Croiset F, Rutten H, Van Den Berghe H, Dal Cin P. Myofibroblastoma of the breast: genetic link with spindle cell lipoma. J Pathol 2000;191:282-285.

86. Pettinato G, Manivel JC, Gould EW, Albores-Saavedra J. Inclusion body fibromatosis of the breast. Two cases with immunohistochemical and ultrastructural findings. Am J Clin Pathol 1994;101:714-718.

87. Pettinato G, Manivel JC, Petrella G, Jassim AD. Fine needle aspiration cytology, immunocytochemistry and electron microscopy of fibromatosis of the breast. Report of two cases. Acta Cytol 1991;35:403-408.

88. Pitt MA, Roberts IS, Agmabu DA, Eyden BP. The nature of atypical multinucleated stromal cells: a study of 37 cases from different sites. Histopathology 1993;23:137-145.

89. Powell CM, Cranor ML, Rosen PP. Multinucleated stromal giant cells in mammary fibroepithelial neoplasms. A study of 11 patients. Arch Pathol Lab Med 1994;118:912-916.

90. Powell CM, Cranor ML, Rosen PP. Pseudoangiomatous stromal hyperplasia (PASH). A mammary stromal tumor with myofibroblastic differentiation. Am J Surg Pathol 1995;19:270-277.

91. Proppe KH, Scully RE, Rosai J. Postoperative spindle cell nodules of genitourinary tract resembling sarcomas. A report of eight cases. Am J Surg Pathol 1984;8:101-108.

92. Roncaroli F, Rossi R, Severi B, Martinelli GN, Eusebi V. Epithelioid leiomyoma of the breast with granular cell change: a case report. Hum Pathol 1993;24:1260.

93. Rosen PP. Rosen's Breast pathology. Philadelphia: Lippincott-Raven; 1997.

94. Rosen PP. Multinucleated mammary stromal giant cells: a benign lesion that simulates invasive carcinoma. Cancer 1979;44:1305-1308.

95. Rosen PP. Vascular tumors of the breast. III. Angiomatosis. Am J Surg Pathol 1985;9:652-658.

96. Rosen PP. Vascular tumors of the breast. V. Nonparenchymal hemangiomas of mammary subcutaneous tissues. Am J Surg Pathol 1985;9:723-729.

97. Rosen PP, Ernsberger D. Mammary fibromatosis. A benign spindle-cell tumor with significant risk for local recurrence. Cancer 1989;63:1363-1369.

98. Rosen PP, Jozefczyk MA, Boram LH. Vascular tumors of the breast. IV. The venous hemangioma. Am J Surg Pathol 1985;9:659-665.

99. Rosen PP, Oberman HA. Tumors of the mammary gland. AFIP Atlas of Tumor Pathology, 3rd Series, Fascicle 7. Washington DC: American Registry of Pathology; 1993.

100. Rosen PP, Ridolfi RL. The perilobular hemangioma. A benign microscopic vascular lesion of the breast. Am J Clin Pathol 1976;68:21-23.

101. Rosso R, Gianelli U, Carnevali L. Acquired progressive lymphangioma of the skin following radiotherapy for breast carcinoma. J Cutan Pathol 1995;22:164-167.

102. Rosso R, Scelsi M, Carnevali L. Granular cell traumatic neuroma: a lesion occurring in mastectomy scars. Arch Pathol Lab Med 2000;124:709-711.

103. Schuh ME, Radford DM. Desmoid tumor of the breast following augmentation mammoplasty. Plast Reconstr Surg 1994;93:603-605.

104. Schurch W, Seemayer TA, Gabbiani G. The myofibroblast: a quarter century after its discovery. Am J Surg Pathol 1998;22:141-147.

105. Shousha S, Lyssiotis T. Granular cell myoblastoma: positive staining for carcinoembryonic antigen. J Clin Path 1979;32:219-224.

106. Sloane JP. Biopsy pathology of the breast. London: Chapman and Hall; 1985.

107. Sobel HJ, Marquet E, Schwarz R. Granular degeneration of appendiceal smooth muscle. Arch Pathol 1971;6:427-432.

108. Suster S, Nascimento AG, Miettinen M, Sickel JZ, Moran CA. Solitary fibrous tumors of soft tissue. Am J Surg Pathol 1995;19:1257-1266.

109. Taccagni G, Rovere E, Masullo M, Christensen L, Eyden B. Myofibrosarcoma of the breast: review of the literature on myofibroblastic tumors and criteria for defining myofibroblastic differentiation. Am J Surg Pathol 1997;21:489-496.

110. Tavassoli FA. Myoepithelial lesions of the breast. Myoepitheliosis, adenomyoepithelioma and myoepithelial carcinoma. Am J Surg Pathol 1991;15:554-568.

111. Tavassoli FA. Pathology of the breast, 2nd ed. Stamford, CT: Appleton-Lange/McGraw Hill; 1999.

112. Tavassoli FA, Weiss S. Hemangiopericytoma of the breast. Am J Surg Pathol 1981;5:745-752.

113. Thomas TM, Myint A, Mak CK, Chan JK. Mammary myofibroblastoma with leiomyomatous differentiation. Am J Clin Pathol 1997;107:52-55.

114. Toker C, Tang CK, Whitely JF, Berkheiser SW, Rachman R. Benign spindle cell breast tumor. Cancer 1981;48:1615-1622.

115. Toth J. Benign human mammary myoepithe-lioma. Virchows Arch A Pathol Anat Histol 1977;374:263-269.

116. Vuitch MF, Rosen PP, Erlandson RA. Pseudoan-giomatous hyperplasia of the mammary stroma. Hum Pathol 1986;17:185-191.

117. Wargotz ES, Deos PH, Norris HJ. Metaplastic car-cinomas of the breast. II. Spindle cell carcinoma. Hum Pathol 1989;20:732-740.

118. Wargotz ES, Norris HJ, Austin RM, Enzinger FM. Fibromatosis of the breast. A clinical and pathological study of 28 cases. Am J Surg Pathol 1987;11:38-45.

119. Wargotz ES, Weiss SW, Norris HJ. Myofibroblas-toma of the breast. Sixteen cases of a distinctive benign mesenchymal tumor. Am J Surg Pathol 1987;11:493-502.

120. Willen R, Willen H, Baldin G, Albrechtsson U. Granular cell tumour of the mammary gland simulating malignancy. A report of two cases with light microscopy, transmission electron mi-croscopy and immunohistochemical investiga-tion. Virchows Arch A Pathol Anat Histopathol 1984;403:391-400.

121. Youngson BJ, Cranor M, Rosen PP. Epithelial displacement in surgical breast specimens fol-lowing needling procedures. Am J Surg Pathol 1994;18:896-903.

122. Zayid I, Dihmis C. Familial multicentric fibro-matosis-desmoids. A report of three cases in a Jordanian family. Cancer 1969;24:786-795.

13 SARCOMAS

SARCOMAS

Sarcomas are the most problematic tumors of the breast. This is due to several factors, the most important of which is the rarity of the lesion. Most authors have accepted an incidence for sarcoma of 1 percent of all malignancies of the breast (2,69,88), but there are hints that these tumors are even rarer. During a 17-year period at a cancer institute, only 6 sarcomas were diagnosed among 5,382 malignancies of the breast (Dr. J. Lamovec, Ljubljana, personal communication, 2000).

An additional factor that causes confusion is the heterogeneity of the cases reported in the literature. In some series angiosarcomas are included as sarcomas (14,36), while in other series these tumors are not included but fibrosarcomas, liposarcomas, osteogenic sarcomas, and even rhabdomyosarcomas are (7,10,61). In some series malignant phyllodes tumors and "ordinary" sarcomas are analyzed together (14,89), while the former are excluded in other reports (7,10,61). Some series of sarcomas of the breast include even benign conditions such as hemangiopericytoma (10) and desmoid tumors (10,60) and semimalignant lesions such as dermatofibrosarcoma protuberans (10,60,61).

Numerous series reported before the immunohistochemical era may have included sarcomatoid carcinoma with sarcomas. The difficulty in recognizing a sarcomatous proliferation in the breast is that sarcomatoid breast carcinomas are relatively common and they may simulate any type of mesenchymal malignancy (26). Specifically, those neoplasms designated "monophasic sarcomatoid carcinomas" (26) are predominantly composed of spindle cells that closely mimic fibrosarcomas and can be distinguished only on the basis of immunohistochemistry and cytogenetics.

Most breast sarcomas are characterized by cells positive only for vimentin and occasionally for actin, while spindle cell (monophasic sarcomatoid) carcinomas show cells positive for cytokeratins in addition to vimentin (26). Along with positivity for cytokeratins (particularly high molecular weight cytokeratins), reactivity for smooth muscle actin (27) and losses at 17p and 17q (41) are seen if myoepithelial cell differentiation is present (Table 13-1). The proof that monophasic sarcomatoid carcinomas are morphologically similar to fibrosarcomas is shown by the remarkable case reported by Pitts et al. (65) of a cytokeratin-negative spindle cell putative sarcoma which led to an axillary metastasis with the features of carcinoma. This case indicates that spindle cell carcinomas can "lose" their cytokeratin reactivity and in such cases there are no diagnostic tools available to distinguish these lesions from spindle cell sarcomas. The impact of molecular pathology in diagnosing breast sarcomas is limited since tumors that occur in the breast do not have a known specific molecular pattern.

The possibility that biphasic sarcomatoid carcinomas are diagnosed as pure sarcoma as

		Smooth Muscle Actin	Low Weight Keratin	Cyto-keratin 14	CD34
	Vimentin				
MSCT[a]-fibroblast	present	absent	absent	absent	variable
MSCT-myofibroblast	present	present	absent	absent	present
Monophasic SC	present	variable	present	variable	absent
Myoepithelial cell carcinoma	present	present	variable	present	absent

Table 13-1

IMMUNOHISTOCHEMISTRY OF MALIGNANT STROMAL CELL TUMORS

[a]MSCT = malignant stromal cell tumor; SC = sarcomatoid carcinoma.

a consequence of sampling errors is more than plausible. In fact, there are cases of sarcomatoid carcinoma in which the epithelial component constitutes a minute part of an entire tumor that is predominantly composed of mesenchymal elements. A notable example of this phenomenon is a case that the authors have seen that was initially regarded as pure osteosarcoma. Three tiny nests of malignant epithelial cells appeared only in the deeper levels that were requested for immunohistochemical evaluation for keratin (20). Sampling errors also play a part in cases of malignant phyllodes tumors in which stromal overgrowth replaces the epithelial component; the epithelial component is then difficult to detect or entirely missed.

Distinguishing Sarcomas from Spindle Cell Carcinomas and Malignant Phyllodes Tumors. Sarcomas are difficult to differentiate from spindle cell carcinomas (squamous or myoepithelial). Pitts et al. (65) compared 20 sarcomas with an identical number of carcinomas showing mesenchymal metaplasia. No statistically significant differences were seen between the groups in terms of duration of symptoms, patient age, and tumor size. The 5-year disease-free survival rates were 36 percent for patients with sarcomas and 43 percent for those with sarcomatoid carcinomas; the overall 5-year survival rates were 64 percent versus 43 percent. Only the incidence of metastases was different between the two groups of patients: there were no axillary lymph node metastases among sarcoma patients while such metastases were present in no fewer than 25 percent of the patients with sarcomatoid carcinomas.

Studies have compared the biologic behavior of sarcoma and malignant phyllodes tumors. No statistical difference in death rate with long-term follow-up (minimum 15 years) was seen by Christensen et al. (14) between patients with spindle cell sarcomas and malignant phyllodes tumors (45 versus 38 percent, respectively). Terrier et al. (89) compared 16 patients with spindle cell sarcoma and 17 patients with malignant phyllodes tumor. They concluded that the clinical course and survival for the two groups were identical and local recurrence, metastasis, and death occurred within 30 months.

It seems, therefore, that all the effort we make to establish the correct diagnosis does not affect practical results. This is an argument strongly in favor of the many who like to be practical and lump the different conditions together, as for instance, Christensen et al. (14), who consider spindle cell sarcomas a "variety" of malignant phyllodes tumor with excessive stromal overgrowth. Nevertheless, given the rarity of sarcomas, knowledge of these tumors would benefit from more detailed studies. Analysis of a larger number of homogeneous lesions is required for a better understanding of these different entities. Therefore, a histogenetic classification is followed.

Clinical Features. Sarcomas of the breast have been described in patients ranging from 17 (14) to 89 years of age (65), with a mean of 45 to 50 years in most series. Mammary sarcomas vary considerably in size, from microscopic foci to 40 cm (36), but in most studies the mean size is between 3 and 4 cm (69). Gutman et al. (36) found that patients with lesions smaller than 5 cm have a significantly better prognosis irrespective of any other factors. In contrast, other studies found no correlation between size, survival (4), and metastatic spread (14,89).

Gross Findings. Breast sarcomas are unifocal; only rare bilateral cases have been reported. In some studies, sarcomas with macroscopically circumscribed borders confer a low risk of recurrence or death (4,14,60), while in other series the status of borders has no prognostic relevance (89). This is probably a reflection of tumor heterogeneity, especially in earlier reports.

Microscopic Findings. As in soft tissue sarcomas of other regions, the prognosis depends on the histologic type and grade of the tumor (68). Some authors use no grading system, implying that in sarcomas histology alone provides a reliable prognostic parameter (36). Several three-tiered grading systems were proposed by Tavassoli (88) and Terrier et al. (89), while Jones et al. (43) proposed a two-grade system. In the three-grade system, at 30 months, 89 percent of the patients with grade 1, 59 percent with grade 2, and 31 percent with grade 3 remained metastasis free (89). Whatever system is employed, as with sarcomas of other regions, the most powerful parameters for prognosis are the number of mitoses, the degree of nuclear atypia, and the extent of necrosis.

Patterns of Metastases. Sarcomas of the breast, at presentation, do not metastasize to axillary lymph nodes, and axillary lymph node metastases are seen only in the context of disseminated disease (36). Sarcomas of the breast metastasize to the lungs, liver, gastrointestinal tract, adrenal glands, brain, bone, pleura, and retroperitoneum (36,65,66).

Staging. As might be expected, there are no studies on large series of breast sarcomas. The TNM system was employed by Glenn et al. (31) in their six cases and it was found that patients with unresectable primary tumors and distant metastases had the worst prognosis (36). Whatever staging system is used, it is important to consider the breast as a superficial organ, located above the fascia.

Treatment and Prognosis. At present, the only therapeutic procedure that influences prognosis is the total removal of the tumor. No benefit is obtained by adjuvant chemotherapy or radiotherapy (31,36). Gutman et al. (36) stated that whatever surgical procedure is employed, the primary tumor has to be excised with adequate negative margins, and we would add to this statement that the more "adequate" the margins are, the better the chances of limiting recurrence. In keeping with this view, none of the five patients reported by Pollard et al. (66) who had radical mastectomies had tumor recurrence. On the contrary, wide local excision was associated with a 67 percent rate of local recurrence and simple mastectomy with a recurrence rate of 54 percent (36). Axillary dissection is not indicated.

NOMENCLATURE AND TYPES

Stromal sarcoma is a term introduced by Berg et al. (7) to designate 25 cases of malignant soft tissue tumors that "were of the breast proper rather than of the adjacent muscle, skin or axillary connective tissue...and did not show evidence of origin from a fibroadenoma or benign cystosarcoma phyllodes." By admission of the authors, the cases were heterogeneous and included fibrosarcomas, liposarcomas, and pleomorphic tumors with the features of myxoid "malignant fibrohistiocytoma." Berg et al. also stated that a "denser pattern" was analogous to interlobular stroma, and the "myxoid pattern" was analogous to intralobular stroma. In spite of the heterogeneity, the name stromal sarcoma gained credibility until Callery et al. (10) questioned the concept and adopted the name only for malignant lesions that originated from the "specialized" stroma of the breast.

Although the idea of recognizing a specific type of sarcoma derived from the specialized stroma seems intriguing, we feel that at present there are no specific diagnostic criteria to make this diagnosis, which might then impact the prognosis. We, therefore, think that for the moment sarcomas of the breast should be regarded and diagnosed in the same histogenetic way as soft part sarcomas of the rest of the body. Here sarcomas are grouped using the same criteria employed for benign soft tissue lesions described in chapter 12.

MALIGNANT STROMAL CELL TUMOR WITH PREDOMINANT FIBROBLASTIC DIFFERENTIATION

Definition. *Malignant stromal cell tumor with predominant fibroblastic differentiation* (MSCT-FI), also termed *fibrosarcoma* and *malignant fibrohistiocytoma*, is a tumor with a uniform fasciculated (herringbone) to storiform (cartwheel) histologic pattern consisting of spindle-shaped cells separated by interwoven collagen fibers (figs. 13-1, 13-2). Neoplastic cells are positive for vimentin only and lack any other marker including alpha-smooth muscle actin, desmin, S-100 protein, and keratins. Admittedly, this is a diagnosis of exclusion, as also suggested by Enzinger and Weiss (19) for fibrosarcoma and Fletcher (24) for malignant fibrous histiocytoma (MFH).

Most MSCTs-FI, especially in earlier reports (4,7,60), are mixed with other sarcomas of different types. The ultrastructural evidence of the fibroblastic nature of this type of breast tumor was provided by Tang et al. (87). The largest homogeneous series of MSCTs-FI consisted of 32 cases of fibrosarcoma-MFH reported by Jones et al. (43). These cases showed two patterns of growth: herringbone and storiform (16 cases each). The cell of origin was regarded, on the basis of ordinary histology and immunohistochemistry, as fibroblastic in nature. Taking into consideration mitoses and cellular atypia, the tumors were subdivided into low and high grades. Recurrences were seen only in 63 percent of patients with low-grade lesions, while recurrences (44 percent of the patients) in addition to metastases (25 percent) and deaths (31 percent) occurred in patients with

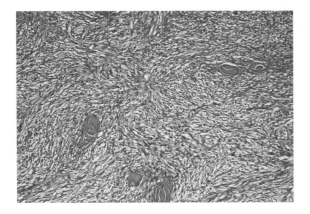

Figure 13-1

MALIGNANT STROMAL CELL TUMOR WITH FIBROBLASTIC DIFFERENTIATION (MSCT-FI)
Cartwheel pattern.

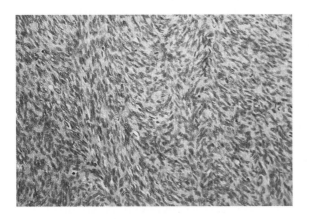

Figure 13-2

MSCT-FI

A herring-bone pattern is seen in this spindle cell tumor positive only for vimentin.

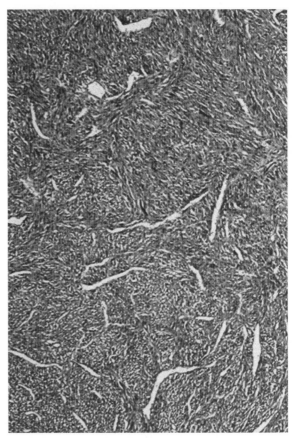

Figure 13-3

HIGH-GRADE MSCT-FI
The neoplastic cells are positive for vimentin only.

high-grade lesions (fig. 13-3). Low-grade lesions had more frequently a herringbone-fibrosarcoma pattern, but this was probably the result of selection of the cases, since most MFH-storiform tumors are high-grade sarcomas. All 20 tumors reported by Pitts et al. (65) had a MFH-storiform pattern. The overall survival rate was 64 percent. Five patients, including 4 who died, had distant metastases to the lungs (4 patients), liver (2), stomach (1), colon (1), and adrenal gland (1). The MFH-storiform pattern is probably more frequent than the herringbone-fibrosarcoma pattern as 21 cases reported by Terrier et al. (89) showed a MFH-storiform pattern while 6 were considered fibrosarcomas. The same ratio was evident in the series reported by Pollard et al. (66) in which 11 cases were MFH and 4 were fibrosarcomas.

Microscopic Findings. The neoplastic cells range from fusiform with little variation in size, little cytoplasm, and indistinct borders to cells that vary in size even in the same area and have abundant cytoplasm. Nuclei are round to ovoid and in high-grade lesions can be very irregular. Necrotic areas are more frequent in high-grade tumors (88). The average mitotic rate varies from 2 mitotic figures per 10 high-power fields in low-grade tumors to 12 per 10 high-power fields in high-grade lesions (43).

Immunohistochemically, the neoplastic cells are by definition immunoreactive to vimentin only. Myxoid areas are seen in both low-grade tumors (43), reminiscent of low-grade fibromyxoid sarcoma, as well as in high-grade lesions (66)

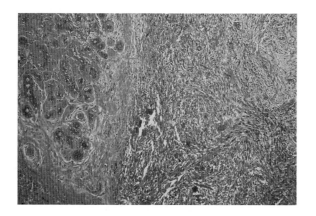

Figure 13-4

MSCT-FI WITH GIANT CELLS

The tumor is highly cellular and shows numerous giant cells. (Figs. 13-4 and 13-5 are from the same patient.)

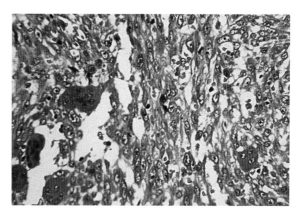

Figure 13-5

MSCT-FI WITH GIANT CELLS

Osteoclast-like reactive giant cells are intermingled with the neoplastic elements.

Table 13-2

DIFFERENTIATING MALIGNANT STROMAL CELL TUMOR, FIBROBLASTIC (MSCT-FI) AND SPINDLE CELL SARCOMATOID CARCINOMA (SC)

	MSCT-FI	SC
Herringbone pattern	frequent	very rare
Storiform pattern	frequent	frequent
Entrapped glands	unusual	frequent
Inflammatory reaction	unusual	frequent
Two cell types	not seen	frequent
Keratins	not present	by definition

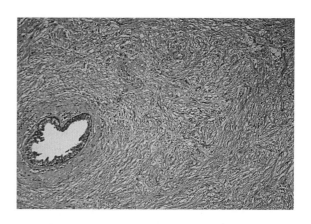

Figure 13-6

SPINDLE CELL SARCOMATOID CARCINOMA

Residual glands are entrapped within the neoplastic proliferation.

featuring myxoid MFH. Vimentin-rich sarcomas devoid of osteoid and with osteoclast-like reactive giant cells have been included in the spectrum of giant cell MFH (figs. 13-4, 13-5) (88). Probably five of the cases reported by Pollard et al. (66) that contained giant cells should be included in this group.

Differential Diagnosis. Distinguishing between MSCT-FI and spindle cell sarcomatoid carcinoma, as previously discussed, can be accomplished only with extensive sampling of the lesion as well as immunohistochemistry (Tables 13-1, 13-2). As a general rule, the herringbone pattern is the exception in spindle cell sarcomatoid carcinoma, which more frequently exhibits a storiform structure (20,26). Residual epithelial glands are more frequently entrapped within sarcomatoid carcinomas than in MSCT-FI, which tend to efface the breast tissue (fig. 13-6). Inflammatory mononuclear changes are frequent within sarcomatoid carcinomas but are rare in MSCT-FI. In sarcomatoid carcinoma showing a storiform pattern, two types of cells are frequently recognizable, with neoplastic cytokeratin-positive elements located in the center of the cartwheel, while the second type of cell, constituted by vimentin-positive (probably) reactive fibroblasts, is at the periphery (figs. 13-7, 13-8). In MSCT-FI, tumor cells tend to be more often of one type (Table 13-2).

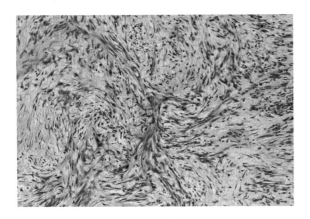

Figure 13-7

SPINDLE CELL SARCOMATOID CARCINOMA

Two types of cells are visible in this spindle cell proliferation. One has more eosinophilic cytoplasm.

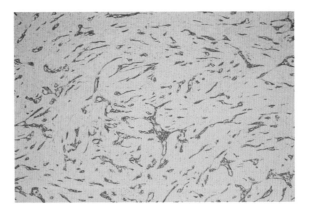

Figure 13-8

SPINDLE CELL SARCOMATOID CARCINOMA

The cells with eosinophilic cytoplasm are positive with high molecular weight keratin.

There are deceptive cases, like the one reported by Pitts et al. (65), in which the morphology (including immunohistochemistry) was inadequate for diagnosis since the neoplastic lesion was almost identical to a sarcoma. In years to come, advances in molecular pathology will help interpret these "gray zone" tumors. As a general rule, the more "nondescript" the "sarcoma" is and the more pleomorphic its cells, the greater the chance that one is dealing with a sarcomatoid carcinoma.

MALIGNANT STROMAL CELL TUMOR WITH PREDOMINANT MYOFIBROBLASTIC DIFFERENTIATION

Definition. *MSCT with predominant myofibroblastic differentiation (MSCT-MY),* also termed *malignant myofibroblastoma* and *myofibrosarcoma,* is a tumor with an irregular fascicular and/or storiform pattern consisting of a predominance of neoplastic cells showing immunohistochemical and/or ultrastructural evidence of myofibroblastic differentiation.

The accepted definition of a myofibroblast has been elaborated in chapter 12. Three MSCTs with predominant myofibroblastic proliferation of the breast have been reported (32,57,85) since Crocker and Murad (16) illustrated ultrastructurally a case of MSCT that they named "fibrosarcoma" but which was clearly composed of cells having the ultrastructural features of myofibroblasts. Five of the 32 tumors with fibrosarcoma/ MFH reported by Jones et al. (43) were positive

for actin, a finding that would qualify these tumors as myofibroblastic in nature. We have seen similar cases in our consultation files.

Despite the sporadic examples of this type of sarcoma reported to date in the breast, the incidence is probably underestimated (23). The current definition of a myofibroblast is strict and includes ultrastructural evidence of specific morphologic signs, of which fibronexus junctions constitute the highlight (74). To be strictly consistent with this definition, no tumor without ultrastructural study is acceptable as an MSCT with myofibroblastic differentiation. Despite this, we feel that tumors exist independent of any techniques and that some diagnoses should be accepted if other morphologic criteria (such as ordinary histology and actin positivity) point toward myofibroblastic differentiation.

Clinical Features. The age of the patients reported so far ranged from 51 to 72 years; one tumor occurred in a man (16). Tumor size varied from 2 to 5 cm. The tumor was described as well circumscribed in one case (85) and infiltrative in another. Two cases of our own were well circumscribed and two others were invasive.

Microscopic Findings. Histologically, as with sarcomas of other regions of the body showing myofibroblastic differentiation, there is a spectrum of appearances that varies from low-grade fasciitis-like lesions (fig. 13-9) to very cellular high-grade tumors with architecture resembling fibrosarcoma/MFH (fig. 13-10) (57). Several features are common to these lesions.

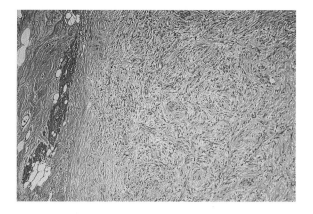

Figure 13-9

MSCT WITH MYOFIBROBLASTIC DIFFERENTIATION

The lesion has circumscribed borders and myxoid stroma.

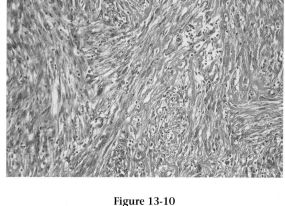

Figure 13-10

MSCT WITH MYOFIBROBLASTIC DIFFERENTIATION

This spindle cell tumor is highly cellular.

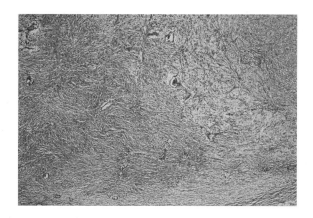

Figure 13-11

MSCT WITH MYOFIBROBLASTIC DIFFERENTIATION

The spindle cell solid pattern, reminiscent of myoid proliferation, is adjacent to a myxoid area.

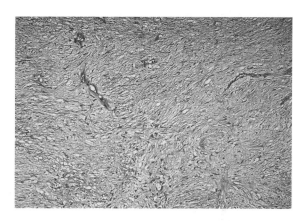

Figure 13-12

MSCT WITH MYOFIBROBLASTIC DIFFERENTIATION

Prominent myxoid features are seen.

The pattern varies from storiform to fascicular (figs. 13-11, 13-12). Neoplastic cells can be separated from each other by abundant stroma and myxoid areas may be seen (fig. 13-13). Broad collagenous hyaline bands may be present (fig. 13-14) (32,85). Spindle-shaped to stellate cells with moderately abundant eosinophilic to amphophilic cytoplasm may be seen (fig. 13-13). Globoid to spindle-shaped nuclei have tapered ends and prominent multiple nucleoli (fig. 13-15) (32).

Immunohistochemically, the neoplastic cells are diffusely vimentin and smooth muscle actin positive (fig. 13-16) while keratin is negative (85). Desmin can be positive in occasional cells in some lesions and CD34, bcl-2, and CD99 were strongly evident in two of our cases (fig. 13-17). The number of mitoses and pleomorphic nuclei vary according to the grade of the lesion.

Differential Diagnosis. Sarcomatoid monophasic carcinoma with myoepithelial cell differentiation (myoepithelial cell carcinoma) can easily be distinguished from MSCT since myoepithelial cells are positive for keratin antibodies, in addition to actin and p63. Squamous cell carcinoma with prominent myxoid stroma (28) resembles MSCT with a myofibroblastic component as the neoplastic cells are also stellate and float freely in stromal acidic mucopolysaccharides. Squamous

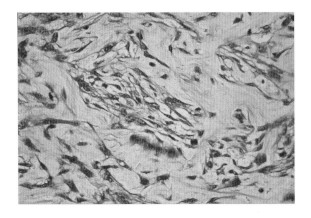

Figure 13-13

MSCT WITH MYOFIBROBLASTIC DIFFERENTIATION

Stellate to spindle cells are immersed in a myxoid stroma.

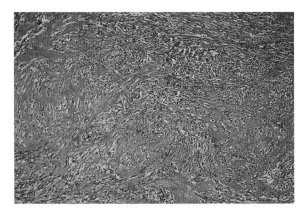

Figure 13-14

MSCT WITH MYOFIBROBLASTIC DIFFERENTIATION

The neoplastic cells are separated by broad collagenous bands.

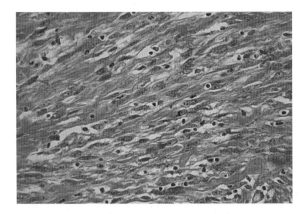

Figure 13-15

MSCT WITH MYOFIBROBLASTIC DIFFERENTIATION

The spindle cells have ovoid nuclei and prominent nucleoli.

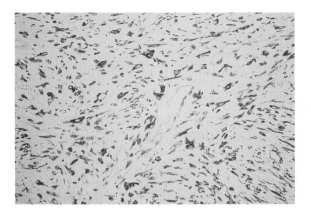

Figure 13-16

MSCT WITH MYOFIBROBLASTIC DIFFERENTIATION

Smooth muscle actin–positive cells have occasional stellate features.

pearls, when present, as well as keratin positivity, help distinguish squamous cell carcinoma.

Treatment and Prognosis. Myofibrosarcomas of the breast behave like those in other regions of the body: low-grade lesions tend to recur (52), while high-grade tumors may metastasize (57). The case reported by Taccagni et al. (85) was very cellular with myxoid areas, had 10 mitoses per 10 high-power fields, and showed areas of necrosis. It recurred 1 month after excision at the site of the surgical scar as a highly pleomorphic lesion and the patient died 11 months later with widespread lung metastases. Similar biologic behavior was reported by Montgomery et al. (57). The grade 2 sarcoma

recurred 5 months after local excision as a grade 3 tumor. The patient died 12 months later with multiple metastases to the lung, which surprisingly were described as less cellular and more "benign" looking than the primary.

As with other sarcomas of the breast, axillary lymph nodes are not involved. Excision alone, however, is not adequate for local control of the tumor.

LEIOMYOSARCOMA

Definition. *Leiomyosarcoma* in the breast is identical to leiomyosarcomas of other sites.

Clinical Features. This rare tumor has been reported mostly as single case reports and the

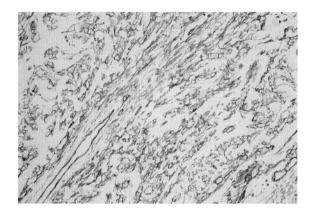

Figure 13-17

MSCT WITH MYOFIBROBLASTIC DIFFERENTIATION
The spindle cells are positive for CD34.

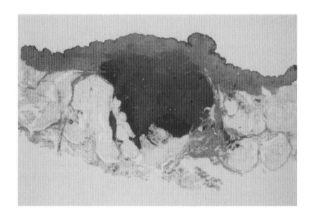

Figure 13-18

LEIOMYOSARCOMA

The tumor has circumscribed margins.

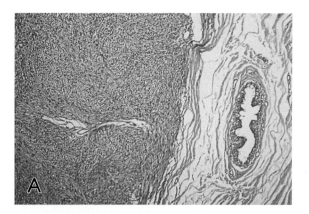

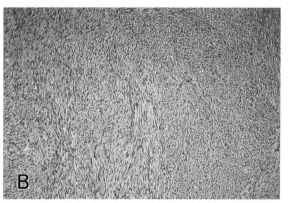

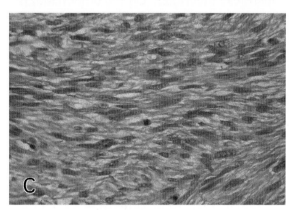

Figure 13-19

LEIOMYOSARCOMA

The cells are elongated (A) and have blunt-ended nuclei (B). The cytoplasm is eosinophilic and mitoses are present (C).

largest series from Armed Forces Institute of Pathology (AFIP) consists of only four cases (42). Patients are usually affected in the 5th decade (69), with an age range from 24 to 86 years. A longstanding lump is the most frequent clinical history and the tumor size at presentation varies from 1.0 to 9.0 cm, with a median of 5.6 cm (22). Nearly 50 percent of cases are located around the nipple areolar complex (69). Mammography suggests phyllodes tumor and macroscopy usually shows circumscribed margins (fig. 13-18).

Microscopic Findings. Histologically, there is a proliferation of smooth muscle cells, which include intersecting bundles of spindle to epithelioid elements with eosinophilic cytoplasm (fig. 13-19), occasionally intermingled with reactive osteoclast-like giant cells (22). The nuclei have a characteristic elongated, blunt-ended shape and pleomorphic cells can be numerous enough to be seen in fine needle aspiration cytology (FNAC) specimens (22).

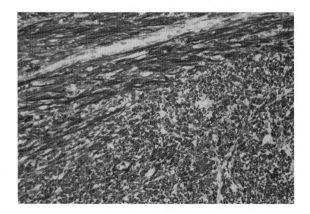

Figure 13-20

LEIOMYOSARCOMA

The neoplastic cells are intensely positive for smooth muscle actin.

Necrotic areas are occasionally present, but the mitotic count does not have the same prognostic impact as in uterine sarcomas. The leiomyosarcoma reported by Nielsen (59), which had 2 mitotic figures per 10 high-power fields, recurred three times and eventually killed the patient with widespread metastases. On the other hand, the patient with the tumor reported by Gonzales-Palacios (34), with 10 mitoses per high-power field, remained asymptomatic for 17 years. The size of the tumor does not correlate with prognosis.

Differential Diagnosis. The diagnosis is mainly based on the histologic findings and is enhanced by immunohistochemistry, as the neoplastic cells of leiomyosarcoma are vimentin, actin (fig. 13-20), and desmin positive. About 30 percent of leiomyosarcomas at all locations are positive for keratin (25). Fortunately, in the breast no such cases have been reported. If a tumor is keratin positive, differentiating it from spindle cell carcinoma with myoepithelial cell differentiation is difficult, if not impossible, since both tumors contain keratin, actin, and vimentin. It is not a coincidence that some authors have postulated a myoepithelial cell origin for leiomyosarcoma of the breast (11). P63 is at the moment the most appropriate marker to distinguish myoepithelial cell carcinoma from leiomyosarcoma.

Desmin positivity, when present in leiomyosarcoma, excludes myoepithelial cell differentiation since desmin is not present in myoepithelial cells. Cytogenetic studies are helpful because leiomyosarcomas and myoepithelial cell carcinomas have different karyotypic profiles which allow possible diagnostic distinction (41,48).

Treatment and Prognosis. From the cases published, it appears that mammary leiomyosarcomas are moderately aggressive neoplasms. Of the 10 cases recruited from the literature by Falconieri et al. (22), two patients died with widespread metastases (14 and 15 years after initial surgery) and two tumors recurred locally. It appears that mastectomy is the best treatment since only one recurrent lesion and one hepatic metastasis occurred in eight patients treated by mastectomy, while two patients whose tumors were excised locally had a recurrence, one of which caused the death of the patient. Two of the four tumors reported by Jones et al. (42) treated by excision, recurred. Complete excision of the tumor is the most important therapeutic procedure. Lumpectomy with generous free margins is adequate for small leiomyosarcomas, leaving mastectomy to the largest tumors. As with other sarcomas, leiomyosarcomas do not metastasize to the axillary lymph nodes.

LIPOSARCOMA

Definition. *Liposarcoma* is a malignant soft tissue tumor that contains lipoblasts as well as additional features.

Clinical Features. Despite the fact that the breast contains large quantities of adipose tissue and that lipomas are, in general, common lesions, liposarcoma is a very rare breast tumor (79). Ii et al. (39), in a survey of the literature, found 42 cases to which they added one of their own. They estimated that liposarcomas account for between 0.0001 and 0.03 percent of breast tumors. The incidence of liposarcoma among sarcomas of the breast varies from 6 percent (89) to 24 percent (66). Liposarcomas are particularly aggressive when they manifest during pregnancy (88).

Liposarcoma can arise de novo or, in about one quarter of the cases, within phyllodes tumors (79). One of the problems in assessing these tumors is determining whether they represent pure liposarcoma or a dominant liposarcoma overgrowth in a phyllodes tumor (2). They are virtually never seen in the context of sarcomatoid carcinomas (26).

The largest series from the AFIP (1) described 13 cases of pure liposarcoma (2 in men) and 7 cases of liposarcoma arising in phyllodes tumor. The patients ranged in age from 26 to 76 years (mean, 47 years), but case reports of younger patients are on record (39). The mean size for pure forms was 8 cm (range, 3 to 19 cm) while 11 cm was the mean size of lesions associated with phyllodes tumors (range, 4 to 23 cm). Liposarcomas are mostly unilateral, but rare bilateral cases have been reported (14).

Microscopic Findings. Microscopically, 5 of 13 tumors seen at the AFIP were classified as well-differentiated, 4 as myxoid liposarcoma, and 4 as pleomorphic liposarcoma (1). A predominance of myxoid cases (5 of 8) was found by Christensen et al. (14); the others were pleomorphic.

Differential Diagnosis. The lesion that most closely mimics well-differentiated liposarcoma is silicone granuloma. The latter contains numerous "lipoblast-like" cells showing microvacuoles in the cytoplasm. The diagnosis is based on finding silicone foreign body material and the conspicuous inflammatory changes that are part of the foreign body reaction. In addition, well-differentiated liposarcoma never has such numerous "lipoblasts" (25).

Treatment and Prognosis. From the AFIP series of 13 liposarcomas, 4 of the pure tumors recurred, of which 3 metastasized and 2 resulted in the death of the patient; only 1 of 7 phyllodes-related tumors recurred (1). Of 14 liposarcomas associated with phyllodes tumors reported by Powell and Rosen (67), 6 of which were high-grade pleomorphic tumors, only 1 recurred and no patient died of tumor. All recurrent tumors reported have been pleomorphic in type and all had invasive margins (1,67). Similar findings were reported by Pollard et al. (66), with three pleomorphic liposarcomas leading to the death of the patients. Of eight patients with liposarcoma reported by Christensen et al. (14), three died of tumor; these tumors were pleomorphic and had invasive margins, while no deaths were seen in the remaining five patients with myxoid liposarcoma with circumscribed margins.

Well-differentiated liposarcoma of the breast recapitulates the favorable clinical behavior of the analogous tumor of other sites. Considering that the breast can be regarded as a suprafascial organ, these nonrecurring tumors may be

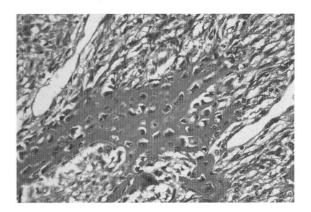

Figure 13-21

OSTEOSARCOMA

The osteoid in this spindle cell neoplastic tumor contains atypical osteoblasts.

termed *atypical lipomatous lesion* by analogy with such tumors in other sites in the body (53).

Complete excision with tumor-free margins is essential in all liposarcomas; mastectomy is not necessary provided excision margins are tumor free (79). Metastases, when they develop, usually occur within 3 years after diagnosis and involve sites like lungs and bone. Rare metastases are found within axillary lymph nodes, a finding that led Fred W. Stewart (82) to state that liposarcomas "... disregard the common textbook teaching about sarcoma in general and metastasize to axillary lymph nodes."

OSTEOSARCOMA

Definition. *Osteosarcoma* is a malignant soft tissue tumor containing malignant osteoid. It is not associated with biphasic tumors such as fibroadenoma, phyllodes tumor, and sarcomatoid carcinoma (fig. 13-21).

Extraskeletal osteosarcoma should be diagnosed as such only if multiple blocks of each tumor are examined because malignant osteoid can occupy 75 percent to nearly 100 percent of the whole neoplasm in phyllodes tumors (77). The same can be seen, although less frequently, in sarcomatoid carcinomas where carcinomatous cells may constitute a very small component of the whole tumor (20). This was clearly evident to F.W. Stewart (82) who stated that "the longer one searches, the less one is apt to find examples of the pure unadulterated mesenchymal tissue tumors of the breast."

Clinical Features. Mammary osteosarcomas constitute 12 percent of breast sarcomas (40). They affect patients between 27 and 89 years of age (mean, 64.2 years) (76). Most tumors are localized in the upper outer quadrant but some arise in the paraareolar region (58). The tumor is unifocal and, in 80 percent of cases (76), manifests clinically as a nodule that is often interpreted as a fibroadenoma at mammography.

Gross and Microscopic Findings. Osteosarcomas vary in size from 1.4 to 13.0 cm (mean, 4.6 cm). They are well circumscribed in about 60 percent of the cases (76), showing central cavitation in larger tumors (33). Most of the known histologic variants of osteosarcoma at other sites, including fibroblastic, osteoclast-rich, osteoblastic, chondroblastic (76), and even telangiectatic (58), have been reported in the breast.

Treatment and Prognosis. The prognosis of the patient depends on the size of the lesion, as patients with tumors smaller than 4.6 cm have a better survival rate (76). Patients with tumors in which cartilaginous or osseous tissue is a minor component appear to have a substantially better prognosis (2); also, those with the fibroblastic type have a better survival rate than those with other types (76). As a general rule, the more undifferentiated and mitotically active the tumor, the worse the survival. Exceptions do occur as even extremely well-differentiated tumors recur and metastasize (88).

Local recurrence and metastases are seen in 60 percent of patients, mostly within 2 years. Incomplete excision leads to recurrence within 2 to 4 months (40). Mastectomy, especially for larger infiltrative tumors, seems more beneficial than tumoral excision in terms of recurrence (76). Adjuvant chemotherapy has been reported to shrink the tumor (58). Metastases occur in the lungs in 80 percent of cases while axillary lymph nodes are spared. An overall 5-year survival rate of 38 percent and an estimated 10-year rate of 32 percent have been reported (76).

Osteosarcoma of the breast is a lethal tumor, and at present, all efforts to separate the pure form from those resulting from stromal overgrowth in phyllodes tumors or from the sarcomatous component of sarcomatous carcinoma are of limited practical value. All of these tumors are aggressive and incurable once they spread hematogenously. The size and probably the amount of neoplastic osteoid are the only two parameters that correlate with longer survival.

ANGIOSARCOMA

Angiosarcoma is a malignant tumor composed of neoplastic elements with the morphologic properties of normal endothelial cells. These tumors include lesions formerly termed hemangiosarcoma, hemangioblastoma, lymphangiosarcoma, and metastasizing hemangioma. The latter term was introduced by Borrmann (9) who described a histologically benign-looking neoplasm that recurred several times before the patient died of metastases 30 months later. *Lymphangiosarcomas* probably exist as a specific sarcoma of lymphatic endothelium, but at present, there are no reliable means of differentiating tumors derived from endothelia of hematic and lymphatic vessels including D2-40, the novel marker of lymphatic endothelia, which is present in about 50 percent of "ordinary angiosarcomas" (28a). Therefore, in keeping with Enzinger and Weiss (19), it is better at the moment to regard the term angiosarcoma as embracing malignant tumors of both hematic and lymphatic endothelia.

Most angiosarcomas of the breast region have distinct histologic features, but differ from a pathogenetic and clinical point of view. Accordingly, angiosarcoma is subdivided into: primary (de novo) forms of the breast parenchyma; secondary in the skin and soft tissues of the arm following ipsilateral radical mastectomy and subsequent lymphedema (Stewart Treves [S-T] syndrome); secondary in the skin and chest wall following radical mastectomy and local radiotherapy; and secondary in the skin, breast parenchyma, or both following conservative treatment and radiotherapy.

Angiosarcomas, as with other sarcomas of the breast, are rare: their incidence is about 0.05 percent of all primary malignancies of the organ (88). While the incidence of primary breast angiosarcoma has remained constant over the years, the incidence of secondary forms has been modified in the last two decades as a consequence of the introduction of more conservative therapeutic approaches. Halsted mastectomies, which underlined the prevalence of the S-T syndrome, have dramatically declined in recent years since most institutions have adopted more conservative surgical treatments including radiotherapy.

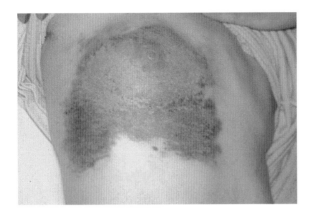

Figure 13-22

**ANGIOSARCOMA WITH
KASABACH-MERRITT SYNDROME**

Massive involvement of skin, breast, and pleura.

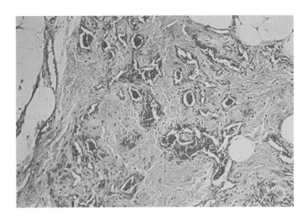

Figure 13-23

WELL-DIFFERENTIATED ANGIOSARCOMA

Dilated vascular channels are filled with red blood cells.

Accordingly, no new cases of S-T syndrome were reported in the population-based cancer registry for Los Angeles County after 1981, while six angiosarcomas of the breast that developed after conservative surgery with supplemental radiation therapy were diagnosed from the late 1980s onward (15).

Primary (De Novo) Angiosarcoma of Breast Parenchyma

Clinical Features. *Primary angiosarcoma of the breast parenchyma* affects mostly females; very rare cases have been reported in men (88). The 63 patients reported by Rosen et al. (70), one of the largest series reported from a single institution, ranged in age from 17 to 70 years (median, 38 years), with no prevalence of laterality (31 cases were located in the left breast).

Primary angiosarcomas are deeply located in the breast tissue (81). They have an insidious, painless, and rapid growth pattern that eventually manifests as a lump. Approximately 12 percent of patients present with diffuse enlargement of the breast (88). When the tumor involves the overlying skin, a bluish red discoloration may be seen. Bilateral synchronous and metachronous tumors have been reported (88). Three women were pregnant in the series reported by Rosen et al. (70).

Mammography is of little help in diagnosis since 33.0 and 37.5 percent of the angiosarcomas reported by Liberman et al. (45) and Wijnmaalen et al. (91), respectively, were mammographically undetectable. Sonography, on the contrary, although not specific, is far more sensitive than mammography for detecting angiosarcomas (73).

One patient with the Kasabach-Merritt syndrome had a well-differentiated angiosarcoma that recurred and led to death 8 years after the first appearance (51). There was widespread involvement of the skin (fig. 13-22) and the pleura.

Angiosarcoma of the male breast is extremely rare. No single case has been reported in the recent literature or has been seen by the authors.

Gross Findings. Angiosarcomas vary in size from 1 to 20 cm, with an average of 5.0 to 5.9 cm (69). They are ill-defined lesions, have a spongy appearance, and have a rim of vascular engorgement (19) that corresponds to a zone of well differentiation. Poorly differentiated tumors appear as ill-defined indurated fibrous lesions similar to other poorly differentiated sarcomas.

Microscopic Findings. Histologically, angiosarcomas vary depending on the degree of differentiation. Different areas of the same tumor may have different features, and consequently, these lesions have to be sampled extensively to include areas that constitute a minority of the tumor, such as poorly differentiated areas.

Two major systems have been proposed to grade angiosarcomas of the breast (18,54). Although similar, the one proposed (and here adopted) by Donnell et al. (18) has gained wide application as it was tested in 63 patients with adequate follow-up (70); the other system (54) was tested on only 15 cases.

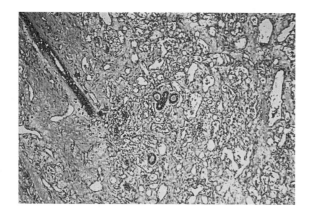

Figure 13-24

WELL-DIFFERENTIATED ANGIOSARCOMA

Interanastomosing vascular channels envelop preexisting glandular structures in a fashion simulating capillary angioma.

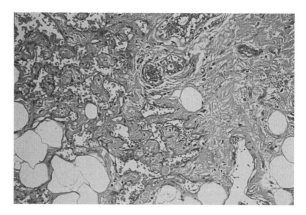

Figure 13-25

WELL-DIFFERENTIATED ANGIOSARCOMA

The vascular spaces are round to elongated and "dissect" the stroma. (Figs. 13-25 and 13-26 are from the same patient.)

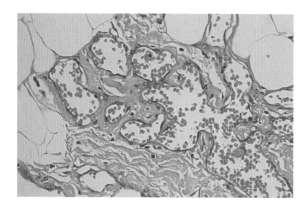

Figure 13-26

WELL-DIFFERENTIATED ANGIOSARCOMA

Hyperchromatic nuclei bulge into the lumens or lie along the wall of the vessel as thin hyperchromatic threads.

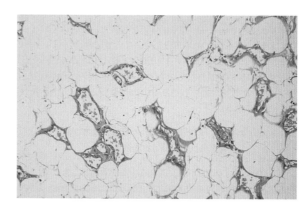

Figure 13-27

WELL-DIFFERENTIATED ANGIOSARCOMA

Innocent-appearing vessels dissect the adipose tissue at the periphery.

Grade 1 (well-differentiated) angiosarcoma shows interanastomosing vascular channels filled with red blood cells (figs. 13-23,13-24). The endothelial cells have hyperchromatic nuclei that bulge into the lumens or lie along the wall of the vessel as thin, elongated, hyperchromatic threads. The vascular spaces are round to ovoid or elongated with branches that anastomose with similar channels (figs. 13-25, 13-26). Ducts and lobules are often entrapped by the neoplastic proliferation but it is not unusual for channels to dissect the intralobular stroma. Lesions are often multifocal with normal non-neoplastic tissue between. Mitoses and necrotic areas are absent.

Even at a distance from the tumoral core, there is neoplastic involvement that is most evident in fatty tissue. In these peripheral areas, innocent-looking vessels dissect the adipose tissue and engulf single adipocytes (fig. 13-27). The neoplastic vessels have open lumens that tend to anastomose. The presence of anastomoses should alert the pathologist to the possibility of angiosarcoma and more tissue has to be obtained before conferring a definite diagnosis. The nuclei of the endothelial cells of these neoplastic vessels are prominent and hyperchromatic. No microthrombi are visible. This neoplastic invasion corresponds to the rim of engorgement seen

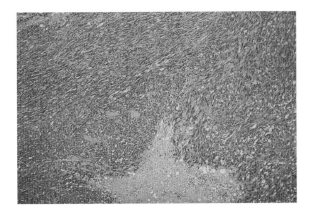

Figure 13-28

GRADE 3 ANGIOSARCOMA

There is a solid proliferation of spindle to polygonal cells with a necrotic area.

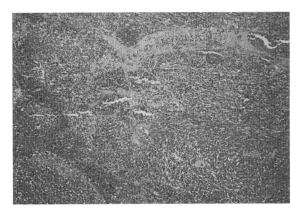

Figure 13-29

GRADE 3 ANGIOSARCOMA

Red blood cells are present within lacunae or cellular slits.

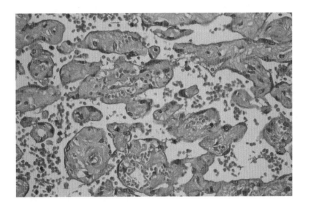

Figure 13-30

GRADE 2 ANGIOSARCOMA

Endothelial tufting and hyperchromatic nuclei are seen.

grossly and is diagnostically very deceptive. Probably these areas are the main cause of underdiagnosis in small biopsies and the reason why the malignant nature of the lesion was not recognized in the initial biopsy specimens in 37 percent of the cases (32/87) found in the literature by Chen et al. (13).

Grade 3 (poorly differentiated) angiosarcomas are easy to diagnose as such when the interanastomosing vascular channels are intermingled with solid or spindle cell areas that show necrotic foci and irregular mitoses (figs. 13-28, 13-29). These tumors are highly destructive as no residual entrapped preexisting tissue is visible. Invasiveness may be prominent and vessels and nerves can be enveloped by the neoplastic cells. A tumor qualifies as grade 3 angiosarcoma when more that 50 percent of the total neoplastic area is composed of solid and spindle cell components without evident vascular channels (69).

A tumor qualifies as grade 2 (intermediately differentiated) angiosarcoma when at least 75 percent of the bulk of the tumor is formed by the well-differentiated pattern seen in grade 1 tumors, but in addition, there are solid cellular foci scattered throughout the tumor. A feature that is also lacking in grade 1 tumors is endothelial tufting, which may be prominent in grade 2 lesions (fig. 13-30). In these endothelial vegetations mitoses are numerous.

When these tumors are subdivided in this fashion, no correlation is seen with size, but statistically significant correlations with age and survival are seen. Grade 1 angiosarcomas affect patients of an average of 43 years of age, while grades 2 and 3 angiosarcomas affect those of 34 and 29 years of age, respectively (18).

Immunohistochemical Findings. Factor VIII, CD34, and CD31 are the most widely used antibodies to characterize endothelial differentiation. We usually employ factor VIII and CD31 antibodies in combination since factor VIII, although the most specific of the three, is the least sensitive and does not stain poorly differentiated tumors and, in addition, highlights diffusion artifacts that on occasion cause substantial difficulties. CD31 is less specific than factor VIII, but it is more sensitive and does not show diffusion artifacts. The use of CD34 is

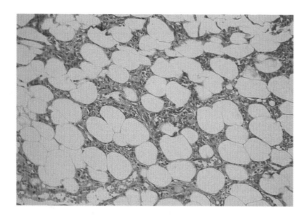

Figure 13-31

ANGIOSARCOMA

Spindle cells are present within adipocytes.

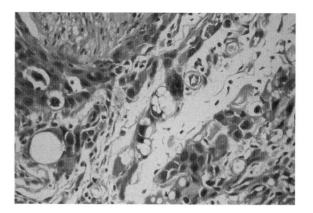

Figure 13-33

EPITHELIOID ANGIOSARCOMA

Multivacuolated cell simulates a lipoblast.

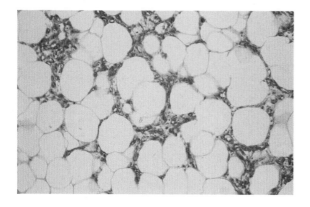

Figure 13-32

ANGIOSARCOMA

The spindle cells are positive for factor VIII.

avoided because benign and malignant spindle cell stromal tumors can be consistently positive with it. When stained with actin, well-differentiated angiosarcomas display a cuff of cells around the malignant endothelial cells (62).

Ultrastructural and Cytogenetic Findings. The ultrastructure of angiosarcoma of the breast has been well illustrated (88). It recapitulates the features seen in angiosarcomas of other regions. Although relevant to understanding the features of the cases illustrated, it has no diagnostic impact. In fact, Weibel-Palade bodies, which are the most specific electron microscopic marker of endothelial differentiation, are seldom observed in poorly differentiated angiosarcomas. One case studied cytogenetically showed multiple clonal rearrangements (30).

Differential Diagnosis. As pointed out by Rosen (69), there are well-differentiated angiosarcomas that closely simulate capillary angiomas. Fortunately, the former are larger in size and in the few cases we have seen, if adequately sampled, areas of typical grade 1 angiosarcoma sooner or later appear. Perilobular hemangiomas are of microscopic size, making Azzopardi's statement that "a benign angioma has never to date constituted a palpable or symptom producing breast tumor" still relevant (2), although such lesions exist, albeit rarely (see chapter 12).

Innocent-appearing endothelial spindle cells can be observed at the periphery of an angiosarcoma, insinuating among adipocytes. These cases simulate spindle cell lipomas and the correct diagnosis is established only with adequate sampling of the whole lesion as well as immunoreactivity with factor VIII and CD31 antibodies (figs. 13-31, 13-32).

Epithelioid neoplastic endothelial cells can simulate lipoblasts when their cytoplasm appears multivacuolated (fig. 13-33). Factor VIII and CD31 are extremely helpful in these cases (fig. 13-34). Epithelioid endothelial cells may have single cytoplasmic vacuoles that contain in the center one red blood cell (fig. 23-35). In these cases, neoplastic endothelial cells closely mimic invasive lobular carcinomas typically characterized by neoplastic elements that show intracytoplasmic lumens (Gad-Azzopardi phenomenon) (29). In these cases, the Alcian blue/periodic acid–Schiff (PAS) stain for mucins is far superior to the immunocytochemical stains for

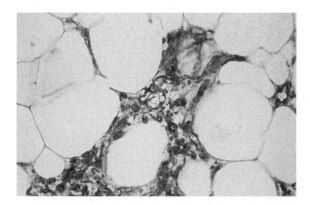

Figure 13-34

EPITHELIOID ANGIOSARCOMA

Factor VIII stains the lipoblast-looking cell.

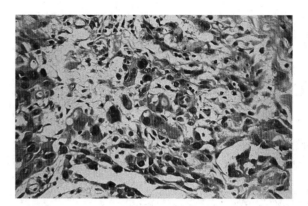

Figure 13-35

EPITHELIOID ANGIOSARCOMA

Intracytoplasmic lumens closely mimic those seen in cells of invasive lobular carcinoma.

keratins that are potentially present in epithelioid angiosarcomas. The only case of epithelioid angiosarcoma reported in the breast (46) was keratin negative and invasive carcinoma was the main concern.

The acantholytic variant of squamous cell carcinoma (ASCC) of the breast (21) mimics angiosarcoma so closely that the designation "pseudoangiosarcomatous carcinoma" has been applied to these lesions (3). Vascular-like spaces with intraluminal papillations and vascular-like channels that dissect collagen, similar to those seen in angiosarcoma, are the morphologic constituents of ASCC. The diagnosis resides in finding squamous cell nests in ASCC, a feature lacking in angiosarcoma (Table 13-3). The lumens of the vessel channels of ASCC contain eosinophilic amorphous material and are devoid of red blood cells. In some instances, neoplastic cells are seen floating in this material. These cells are round, with intense eosinophilic cytoplasm. Factor VIII, CD31, and CD34 are negative in ASCC, while high molecular weight keratins are consistently positive (21).

Poorly differentiated angiosarcomas can mimic malignant spindle cell fibroblastic tumors as well as metastatic malignant melanomas when no vascular channels are present. When solid areas constitute the only component of the tumor, the correct diagnosis is only established with immunohistochemistry. Metastatic malignant melanomas are closely mimicked when hemosiderin pigment is abundant within the cytoplasm of the neoplastic cells (fig. 13-36). In these cases, in addition to

Table 13-3
DIFFERENTIATION OF ANGIOSARCOMA AND ACANTHOLYTIC SQUAMOUS CELL CARCINOMA (ASCC)

	Angio-sarcoma	ASCC
Luminal red blood cells	present	absent
Intraluminal neoplastic cells	absent	present
Squamous nests	absent	present
Cytokeratins	+/−	+
Factor VIII	+	−
CD31	+	−
CD34	+	−

immunohistochemistry, the Perl stain for iron is helpful for excluding melanin.

Treatment and Prognosis. If well-differentiated (grade 1) angiosarcomas are excluded, this breast tumor is very lethal. Azzopardi (2) stated that "angiosarcoma is perhaps the most devastatingly deadly of all malignant breast tumors." Enzinger and Weiss (19) were of the same opinion as they stated that "of the approximately 50 cases [of angiosarcoma] reported in the literature, about 90 percent of the patients have died of the disease, usually within 2 years of diagnosis." The careful review of the world literature by Chen et al. (13) showed that 77 percent of the 87 patients reported had died of the disease, with mean survival time of 22 months. Twenty-eight patients (38 percent) survived 3

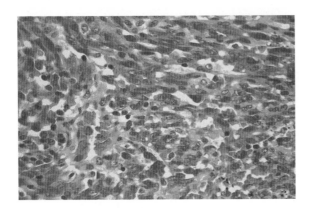

Figure 13-36

GRADE 3 ANGIOSARCOMA

The solid proliferation of spindle cells and the hemosiderin pigment mimic a metastatic malignant melanoma.

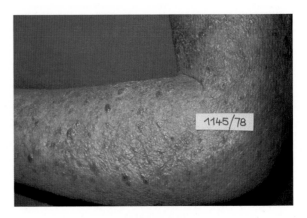

Figure 13-37

STEWART-TREVES SYNDROME

The edematous brawny arm has the slightly raised, purplish red macular lesions of the Stewart-Treves syndrome (S-T syndrome). (Courtesy of Dr. J. Lamovec, Ljubljana, Slovenia.)

years and 13.6 percent were disease free at 3 years. Eight patients (9 percent) survived longer than 5 years, five of whom were disease free.

When angiosarcomas are subdivided by grade, both grading systems highlight the relative malignancy of well-differentiated forms. The estimated survival probability for patients with grade 1 tumors is 91 percent at 5 years and 81 percent at 10 years. For patients with grade 3 tumors, the survival probability is 31 percent at 2 years and 14 percent at 5 and 10 years. Patients with grade 2 lesions have a survival rate of 68 percent at 5 and 10 years. Recurrence-free survival at 5 years was 76 percent for those with grade 1, 70 percent for those with grade 2, and 15 percent for those with grade 3 angiosarcomas (70). Exceptions do occur as some cases of well-differentiated angiosarcoma are rapidly lethal (88) and a 29-year-old woman with a grade 3 tumor survived 18 years with no evidence of disease (70).

The original impression that the small size of the tumor and the short duration of symptoms were significantly correlated with a better prognosis (81) has not been confirmed by Rosen (69). Metastases are mainly to lung, skin, bone, and liver. Rarely, axillary lymph nodes show metastases at presentation while the contralateral breast shows metastatic deposits in 21 percent of cases (13). The grade can vary between the primary tumor and its metastases (88).

Radiation therapy is ineffective. Chemotherapy is of little help. Twenty-nine patients treated with chemotherapy at recurrence showed 4 complete and 10 partial responses (48 percent) (74a). Radical mastectomy appears to be superior to simple mastectomy for control of local recurrence, but not metastases (81).

Angiosarcoma of the Skin of the Arm after Radical Mastectomy followed by Lymphedema (Stewart-Treves Syndrome)

Stewart and Treves in 1949 (83) provided a lucid description of a condition that since has been referred to as the S-T syndrome. They reported six patients who had undergone mastectomy for breast cancer and had developed an "immediate postmastectomy edema" in the ipsilateral arm. Five of the six patients had been irradiated in the breast area and the axilla. The edema had started in the arm and extended to the forearm and finally to the dorsum of the hands and digits. The edema was described as brawny, and after an interval of 6 to 24 years (average, 12.6 years), "a purplish-red, subdermal, slightly raised, macular lesion appeared" (fig. 13-37). To this masterly description can only be added that the macule spreads superficially, while in the center a nodule develops. Small papules or little nodules can also manifest around the main nodular lesion (44). The nodule eventually undergoes a bullous change. The bulla ruptures and ulcerations appear. Deeply located nodules are also observed (83).

The age of the patients in the Stewart and Treves series (83) varied from 37 to 60 years, while 64 years was the mean patient age in a larger series (92). In a review of the literature by Schafler et al. (72), two thirds of tumoral lesions arose on the medial aspect of the upper arm and the remainder at the elbow or in the forearm.

The skin tumors were interpreted histologically as angiosarcomas by Stewart and Treves (83), although their case 5 was associated (in addition to the previous breast carcinoma) with a squamous cell carcinoma of the skin of the ipsilateral hand. The angiosarcomatous differentiation, most frequently of high-grade malignancy, has been conclusively proven with ultrastructural analysis and immunohistochemistry in most cases studied. The skin lesions have the same ultrastructural and immunohistochemical features as do the de novo angiosarcomas, including Weibel-Palade bodies and factor VIII and CD31 immunoreactivity (35,44,55,78).

Since the original description by Stewart and Treves (83), the syndrome has been enlarged to include angiosarcomas arising in edematous limbs not associated with breast carcinoma. Of the 400 cases recruited from the literature by Bisceglia et al. (8), at least 40 cases arose in limbs (mainly leg) that were edematous as a consequence of various non-neoplastic causes including congenital lymphedema and even filariasis. Other malignant processes can be superimposed on edematous arms, like the case of malignant melanoma reported by Sarkany (71) or the two cases of large cell malignant lymphoma reported by d'Amore et al. (17). MacKenzie (47) and Schafler et al. (72) reported two cases of postmastectomy lymphedema with supervening malignancy consisting of metastatic carcinoma. To emphasize the possibility of carcinomatous metastases to the edematous limbs, the term *S-T pseudosyndrome* was proposed (75).

Considering the many different conditions that can cause S-T syndrome, it may be more appropriate to define it in a more liberal way as a high-grade malignant neoplasm, represented mostly by angiosarcomas (8), that arises in longstanding edematous limbs. The edema in 90 percent of cases is preceded by radical mastectomy for breast carcinoma (8) and develops within 12 months after mastectomy. Nearly 65 percent of these patients have also had irradia-

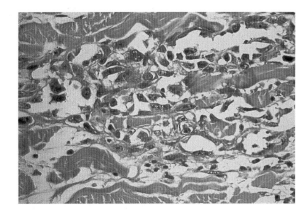

Figure 13-38

STEWART-TREVES SYNDROME

Grade 3 angiosarcoma is in the center of an elevated lesion.

tion of the chest wall and axilla (69). The interval between mastectomy and tumor appearance varies considerably from 1 to 49 years (69), but in the majority of cases, tumor becomes evident about 10 years following mastectomy (80,92).

Histologically, the lesion in most cases is an angiosarcoma, as previously mentioned. There is a topographic distribution of the tumor, with a central nodular core showing a grade 3 angiosarcoma (fig. 13-38), while the peripheral, flat, superficially spreading lesion shows a well-differentiated malignant vascular proliferation (fig. 13-39). This pattern is similar to that seen in de novo angiosarcomas, which also are characterized by the central part of the tumor containing definite angiosarcoma, surrounded by well-differentiated vascular channels (44). The latter can be very deceptive and easily misdiagnosed, resulting in an ambiguous diagnosis of lymphangiomatosis (92).

The early malignant changes have been illustrated by Bisceglia et al. (8) as superficial lymphangiectasia and dermal proliferation of thin-walled dissecting vessels, with only slight focal endothelial atypia (fig. 13-40). These subtle early neoplastic changes are similar to those of lymphangioma circumscriptum, and in such cases, a diagnosis of "atypical vascular proliferation" seems reasonable, reserving the diagnosis of angiosarcoma for cases having more definitive features (68).

Whatever type of malignancy is superimposed on the edema, with the exception of lymphoma, S-T syndrome is a lethal disease with

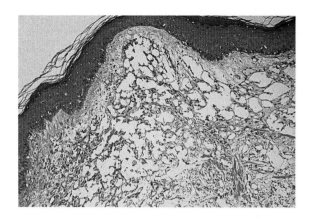

Figure 13-39

STEWART-TREVES SYNDROME

Differentiated features are seen at the periphery of a lesion.

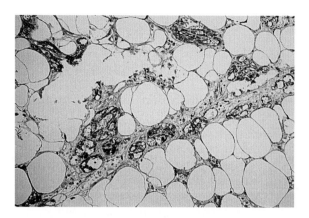

Figure 13-40

STEWART-TREVES SYNDROME

Deep small vessels are positive for CD31. (Courtesy of Dr. M. Bisceglia, Monterotondo, Italy.)

a median survival period of 19 months (92). The lung is the most frequent site of metastasis. In one study, 11 patients with S-T syndrome survived for more than 5 years, of whom 7 were treated by amputation, 2 by wide excision, 1 by radiation therapy, and 1 with intraarterially administered radioactive yttrium (92).

Tertiary Neoplasms Associated with S-T Syndrome

Tertiary neoplasms, i.e., the development first of a breast carcinoma, followed by angiosarcoma in the edematous arm, and finally the development of a new independent neoplasm, have been reported in about 10 percent of patients with S-T syndrome (72). This has led some to postulate the presence of a circulating carcinogen.

The main cause of S-T syndrome is the edema of the arm, which is present in all cases. Radiotherapy has been administered in only 65 percent of these patients, and in addition, the tumors develop in the arms that are not usually included in the irradiation field. This led Haagensen (37), who claimed that his patients infrequently developed edema of the arm after mastectomy, to state that he had never seen a case of S-T syndrome. This is also the reason why, as discussed earlier, most cases of S-T syndrome were reported in the literature before 1980, the year in which the Halsted mastectomy was abandoned in most centers in favor of more conservative surgical procedures that do not cause edema of the arm.

Angiosarcoma Postradiotherapy

Angiosarcomas can manifest after radiotherapy in two separate settings. First, they can occur in the chest wall when radiotherapy is administered after mastectomy for invasive breast carcinoma. Twenty such cases were found in a literature review in 1995 (63). The latency period for the development of these angiosarcomas was 30 to 156 months (mean, 70 months). Patient age was more advanced than that of patients with de novo angiosarcomas and ranged from 61 to 78 years (64). In these cases, the neoplastic endothelial proliferation is by definition confined to the skin (12).

The second setting is in the breast after conservative radiotherapy for breast carcinoma. Fifty-two cases were reported as of 1997, with the first case described in 1987 (49). The angiosarcomas involved only the skin in more than half the cases, while exclusive breast parenchymal involvement was seen in 4 cases. In the remaining cases, the breast parenchyma and the skin were involved simultaneously. Nine of 18,115 patients with breast carcinomas treated conservatively developed angiosarcomas. This represents 5 cases of angiosarcoma per 10,000 patients, which is the same prevalence of de novo angiosarcoma occurring in healthy breasts. The same view was shared by Virtanen et al. (90a) who found an increased risk of angiosarcoma among cancer patients not strictly related to radiation therapy. Patients with this type of angiosarcoma range from 46 to 95 years (mean, 68.5 years). The latency period ranges from 6 to 150 months, with a median of 63 months. Discoloration of the skin or a breast lump is the predominant clinical finding. Mammography is often silent (91). FNAC is frequently negative with sporadic exceptions in which atypical spindle cells are seen (84). Most cases (81 percent) are multifocal and most patients harbor grade 2 to 3 tumors. This is the main reason why the median time until recurrence is 7.5 months regardless of treatment and the median survival period is 15.5 months, with only 1 patient out of 9 alive without progressive disease at 32 months after salvage surgery for recurrence of angiosarcoma (49). Radiation and chemotherapy are ineffective (88).

As discussed in chapter 12, benign lymphangiomatous papules of the skin (BLAP) that occur after radiotherapy have to be distinguished from well-differentiated postradiation angiosarcoma.

MISCELLANEOUS SARCOMAS

Pure extraskeletal chondrosarcomas have been reported occasionally (6,88). They have myxochondroid features and when high grade, they can be aggressive, as in the case reported by Beltaos and Banerjee (6) that killed the patient within 9 months of diagnosis. Chondroid tissue is present in most sarcomas as well as within phyllodes tumors and in sarcomatoid carcinomas. Histologic sampling and immunohistochemistry are very helpful in establishing the diagnosis. Keratin stains do not stain cartilage but cartilage may be positive for S-100 protein and epithelial membrane antigen; the latter can lead to an incorrect diagnosis.

Rhabdomyosarcomas primary in the breast are more common in association with phyllodes tumors (5) or with sarcomatoid carcinomas (26) than in their pure form. Barnes and Pietruszka (5) found 25 cases in the literature. All were of pleomorphic type, appearing in adult females with an age range of 34 to 84 years (mean, 50.7 years). They behaved as high-grade tumors since 8 recurred and 4 patients died shortly after the diagnosis. Of the four primary rhabdomyosarcomas reported by Tavassoli (88), two patients died of disease within 12 months. Metastatic rhabdomyosarcomas to the breast are usually of alveolar type and affect children or young adults. Of the seven cases re-

ported by Howarth et al. (38), no patient survived longer than 24 months from the diagnosis. The primary site is usually the limbs, but cases in the perineum have been reported.

Alveolar rhabdomyosarcoma may mimic invasive lobular carcinoma with an alveolar pattern (50), especially since some of these tumors metastasize to the breast and the axillary lymph nodes at the same time. The young age of patients affected by rhabdomyosarcoma militates against invasive lobular carcinoma. Immunohistochemistry is helpful, since desmin, skeletal muscle actin, and myogenin are all positive in rhabdomyosarcomas. Keratin stains can be deceptive since rhabdomyosarcomas as well as carcinomas can be positive (56).

Malignant peripheral nerve sheath tumors were included in a larger series of soft tissue tumors of the breast and, consequently, it is difficult to assess their behavior (42,66). They were all high-grade lesions. At least one case was associated with von Recklinghausen disease and one case presented as focal rhabdomyoblastic differentiation consistent with malignant triton tumor.

A *clear cell sarcoma* that caused the death of the patient has been reported (66). There are two cases of *alveolar soft part sarcoma* reported (93).

POSTRADIATION SARCOMAS

In addition to angiosarcomas, rare cases of sarcoma arising after radiotherapy have been reported. The criteria for diagnosing a *postradiation sarcoma* should follow the guidelines proposed by Enzinger and Weiss (19): the initial lesion treated must be histologically different from the subsequent tumor; the sarcoma must arise within the radiation field; and a period of latency has to be demonstrated.

In a review of the literature by Pendlebury et al. (63), 81 postradiation sarcomas were found, of which 51 arose from the underlying bone and 30 from the soft tissues. The most frequent tumors were osteosarcomas (24 cases), followed by fibrosarcomas (16 cases) and angiosarcomas (14 cases). The median latent period was 11 years for bone sarcomas, followed by 8 years for soft tissue tumors, and 5.5 years for sarcomas arising in breast tissue after conservative treatment. The cumulative incidence varied from 0.05 percent at 5 years to 0.2 percent at 10 years (86,90).

REFERENCES

1. Austin RM, Dupree WB. Liposarcoma of the breast: a clinicopathologic study of 20 cases. Hum Pathol 1986;17:906-913.
2. Azzopardi JG. Problems in breast pathology. London: W.B. Saunders Company; 1979.
3. Banerjee SS, Eyden BP, Wells S, McWilliam LJ, Harris M. Pseudoangiosarcomatous carcinoma: a clinicopathological study of seven cases. Histopathology 1992;21:13-23.
4. Barnes L, Pietruszka M. Sarcomas of the breast: a clinicopathologic analysis of ten cases. Cancer 1977;40:1577-1585.
5. Barnes L, Pietruszka M. Rhabdomyosarcoma arising within a cystosarcoma phyllodes. Case report and review of the literature. Am J Surg Pathol 1978;2:423-429.
6. Beltaos E, Banerjee TK. Chondrosarcoma of the breast. Report of two cases. Am J Clin Pathol 1979;71:345-349.
7. Berg JW, DeCrosse JJ, Fracchia AA, Farrow J. Stromal sarcomas of the breast. A unified approach to connective tissue sarcomas other than cystosarcoma phyllodes. Cancer 1962;15:418-424.
8. Bisceglia M, Attino V, D'Addetta C, Murgo R, Fletcher CD. [Early-stage Stewart-Treves syndrome: report of two cases and review of the literature.] Pathologica 1996;88:483-490. [Italian.]
9. Borrmann R. Metastasenbildung bei histologisch gutartigen geschwülsten (fall von metastasierendem angiom). Beitr Pathol Anat 1906;40:372-392.
10. Callery CD, Rosen PP, Kinne DW. Sarcoma of the breast. A study of 32 patients with reappraisal of classification and therapy. Ann Surg 1985;201:527-532.
11. Cameron HM, Hamperl H, Warambo W. Leiomyosarcoma of the breast originating from myothelium (myoepithelium). J Pathol 1974;114:89-92.
12. Cancellieri A, Eusebi V, Mambelli V, Ricotti G, Gardini G, Pasquinelli G. Well-differentiated angiosarcoma of the skin following radiotherapy. Report of two cases. Path Res Pract 1991;187:301-306.
13. Chen KT, Kirkegaard DD, Bocian JJ. Angiosarcoma of the breast. Cancer 1980;46:368-371.
14. Christensen L, Schiodt T, Blichert-Toft M, Hansen JP, Hansen OH. Sarcomas of the breast: a clinicopathological study of 67 patients with long term follow-up. Eur J Surg Oncol 1988;14:241-247.
15. Cozen W, Bernstein L, Wang F, Press MF, Mack TM. The risk of angiosarcoma following primary breast cancer. Br J Cancer 1999;81:532-536.
16. Crocker DJ, Murad TM. Ultrastructure of fibrosarcoma in a male breast. Cancer 1969;23:891-899.
17. D'Amore ES, Wick MR, Geisinger KR, Frizzera G. Primary malignant lymphoma arising in postmastectomy lymphedema. Another facet of the Stewart-Treves syndrome. Am J Surg Pathol 1990;14:456-463.
18. Donnell RM, Rosen PP, Lieberman PH, et al. Angiosarcoma and other vascular tumors of the breast. Am J Surg Pathol 1981;5:629-642.
19. Enzinger FM, Weiss SW. Soft tissue tumors. St. Louis: Mosby; 1995.
20. Eusebi V, Cattani MG, Ceccarelli C, Lamovec J. Sarcomatoid carcinomas of the breast: an immunocytochemical study of 14 cases. Recent Progress Surg Pathol 1989;9:83-99.
21. Eusebi V, Lamovec J, Cattani MG, Fedeli F, Millis RR. Acantholytic variant of squamous-cell carcinoma of the breast. Am J Surg Pathol 1986;10:855-861.
22. Falconieri G, Della Libera D, Zanconati F, Bittesini L. Leiomyosarcoma of the female breast: report of two new cases and a review of the literature. Am J Clin Pathol 1997;108:19-25.
23. Fisher C. Myofibrosarcoma. Virchows Arch 2004;445:215-223.
24. Fletcher CD. Pleomorphic malignant fibrous histiocytoma: fact or fiction? A critical reappraisal based on 159 tumors diagnosed as pleomorphic sarcoma. Am J Surg Pathol 1992;16:213-228.
25. Fletcher CD. Soft tissue tumors. In: Fletcher CD, ed. Diagnostic histopathology of tumors, 2nd ed. London: Churchill Livingstone; 2000:1473-1540.
26. Foschini MP, Dina R, Eusebi V. Sarcomatoid neoplasms of the breast: proposed definitions for biphasic and monophasic sarcomatoid mammary carcinomas. Semin Diagn Pathol 1993;10:128-136.
27. Foschini MP, Eusebi V. Carcinomas of the breast showing myoepithelial cell differentiation. A review of the literature. Virchows Arch 1998;432:303-310.
28. Foschini MP, Fulcheri E, Baracchini P, Ceccarelli C, Betts CM, Eusebi V. Squamous cell carcinoma with prominent myxoid stroma. Hum Pathol 1990;21:859-865.
28a. Fukunaga M. Expression of D2-40 in lymphatic endothelium of normal tissue and in vascular tumours. Histopathology 2005;46:396-402.
29. Gad A, Azzopardi JG. Lobular carcinoma of the breast: a special variant of mucin-secreting carcinoma. J Clin Pathol 1975;28:711-716.
30. Gil-Benso R, Lopez-Gines C, Soriano P, Almenar S, Vazquez C, Llombart-Bosch A. Cytogenetic study of angiosarcoma of the breast. Genes Chromosomes Cancer 1994;10:210-212.

31. Glenn J, Kinsella T, Glatsein E, et al. A randomized, prospective trial of adjuvant chemotherapy in adults with soft tissue sarcomas of the head and neck, breast, and trunk. Cancer 1985;55:1206-1214.

32. Gocht A, Bosmuller HC, Bassler R, et al. Breast tumors with myofibroblastic differentiation: clinico-pathological observations in myofibroblastoma and myofibrosarcoma. Pathol Res Pract 1999;195:1-10.

33. Going JJ, Lumsden AB, Anderson TJ. A classical osteogenic sarcoma of the breast: histology, immunohistochemistry and ultrastructure. Histopathology 1986;10:631-641.

34. Gonzalez-Palacios F. Leiomyosarcoma of the female breast. Am J Clin Pathol 1998;109:650-651.

35. Govoni E, Pileri S, Bazzocchi F, Severi B, Martinelli G. Postmastectomy angiosarcoma: ultrastructural study of a case. Tumori 1981;67:79-86.

36. Gutman H, Pollok RE, Ross MI, et al. Sarcoma of the breast: implications for extent of therapy. The M.D. Anderson experience. Surgery 1994;116:505-509.

37. Haagensen CD. Diseases of the breast, 3rd ed. Philadelphia: W.B. Saunders; 1986.

38. Howarth CB, Caces JN, Pratt CB. Breast metastases in children with rhabdomyosarcoma. Cancer 1980;46:2520-2524.

39. Ii K, Hizawa K, Okazaki K, Morimoto T, Uyama Y. Liposarcoma of the breast—fine structural and histochemical study of a case and review of 42 cases in the literature. Tokushima J Exp Med 1980;27:45-56.

40. Jernstrom P, Lindberg AL, Meland ON. Osteogenic sarcoma of the mammary gland. Am J Clin Pathol 1963;40:521-526.

41. Jones C, Foschini MP, Chaggar R, et al. Comparative genomic hybridization analysis of myoepithelial carcinoma of the breast. Lab Invest 2000;80:831-836.

42. Jones MW, Norris HJ, Wargotz ES. Smooth muscle and nerve sheath tumors of the breast. A clinicopatholgic study of 45 cases. Int J Surg Pathol 1994;2:85-92.

43. Jones MW, Norris HJ, Wargotz ES, Weiss SW. Fibrosarcoma-malignant fibrous histiocytoma of the breast. Am J Surg Pathol 1992;16:667-674.

44. Kindblom LG, Stenman G, Angervall L. Morphological and cytogenetic studies of angiosarcoma in Stewart-Treves syndrome. Virchows Arch A Pathol Anat Histopathol 1991;419:439-445.

45. Liberman L, Dershaw DD, Kaufman RJ, Rosen PP. Angiosarcoma of the breast. Radiology 1992;183:649-654.

46. Macias-Martinez V, Murrieta-TIburcio L, Molina-Cardenas H, Dominguez-Malagon H. Epithelioid angiosarcoma of the breast. Clinicopathological, immunohistochemical, and ultrastructural study of a case. Am J Surg Pathol 1997;21:599-604.

47. Mackenzie DH. Lymphangiosarcoma arising in chronic congenital and idiopathic lymphoedema. J Clin Path 1971;24:524-529.

48. Mandahl N, Fletcher CD, Dal Cin P, et al. Comparative cytogenetic study of spindle cell and pleomorphic leiomyosarcomas of soft tissues: a report from the CHAMP Study Group. Cancer Genet Cytogenet 2000;116:66-73.

49. Marchal C, Weber B, de Lafontan B, et al. Nine breast angiosarcomas after conservative treatment for breast carcinoma: a survey from French comprehensive cancer centers. Int J Radiat Oncol Biol Phys 1999;44:113-119.

50. Martinez V, Azzopardi JG. Invasive lobular carcinoma of the breast: incidence and variants. Histopathology 1979;3:467-488.

51. Mazzocchi A, Foschini MP, Marconi F, Eusebi V. Kasabach-Merritt syndrome associated to angiosarcoma of the breast. A case report and review of the literature. Tumori 1993;79:137-140.

52. Mentzel T, Dry S, Katenkamp D, Fletcher CD. Low-grade myofibroblastic sarcoma: analysis of 18 cases in the spectrum of myofibroblastic tumors. Am J Surg Pathol 1998;22:1228-1238.

53. Mentzel T, Fletcher CD. Lipomatous tumours of soft tissues: an update. Virchows Arch 1995;427:353-363.

54. Merino MJ, Carter D, Berman M. Angiosarcoma of the breast. Am J Surg Pathol 1983;7:53-60.

55. Miettinen M, Lehto VP, Virtanen I. Postmastectomy angiosarcoma (Stewart-Treves syndrome). Light-microscopic, immunohistological, and ultrastructural characteristics of two cases. Am J Surg Pathol 1983;7:329-339.

56. Miettinen M, Rapola J. Immunohistochemical spectrum of rhabdomyosarcoma and rhabdomyosarcoma-like tumors. Expression of cytokeratin and the 68-kD neurofilament protein. Am J Surg Pathol 1989;13:120-132.

57. Montgomery E, Goldblum JR, Fisher C. Myofibrosarcoma: a clinicopathologic study. Am J Surg Pathol 2001;25:219-228.

58. Mufarrij AA, Feiner HD. Breast sarcoma with giant cells and osteoid. A case report and review of the literature. Am J Surg Pathol 1987;11:225-230.

59. Nielsen BB. Leiomyosarcoma of the breast with late dissemination. Virchows Arch A Pathol Anat Histopathol 1984;403:241-245.

60. Norris HJ, Taylor HB. Sarcomas and related mesenchymal tumors of the breast. Cancer 1968;22:21-28.

61. Oberman HA. Sarcomas of the breast. Cancer 1965;18:1233-1243.

62. Parham DM, Fisher C. Angiosarcomas of the breast developing post radiotherapy. Histopathology 1997;31:189-195.

63. Pendlebury SC, Bilous M, Langlands AO. Sarcomas following radiation therapy for breast cancer: a report of three cases and a review of the literature. Int J Radiat Oncol Biol Phys 1995;31:405-410.

64. Peters GN, Wolff M. Adenoid cystic carcinoma of the breast. Report of 11 new cases: review of the literature and discussion of biological behavior. Cancer 1983;52:680-686.

65. Pitts WC, Rojas VA, Gaffey MJ, et al. Carcinomas with metaplasia and sarcomas of the breast. Am J Clin Pathol 1991;95:623-632.

66. Pollard SG, Marks PV, Temple LN, Thompson HH. Breast sarcoma. A clinicopathologic review of 25 cases. Cancer 1990;66:941-944.

67. Powell CM, Rosen PP. Adipose differentiation in cystosarcoma phyllodes. A study of 14 cases. Am J Surg Pathol 1994;18:720-727.

68. Rosai J. Soft tissues. In: Rosai J, ed. Ackerman's surgical pathology. St. Louis: Mosby; 1996:2021-2134.

69. Rosen PP. Rosen's breast pathology. Philadephia: Lippincott-Raven; 1997.

70. Rosen PP, Kimmel M, Ernsberger D. Mammary angiosarcoma. The prognostic significance of tumor differentiation. Cancer 1988;62:2145-2151.

71. Sarkany I. Malignant melanomas in lymphoedematous arm following radical mastectomy for breast carcinoma (an extension of the syndrome of Stewart and Treves). Proc Soc Med 1972;65:253-254.

72. Schafler K, McKenzie CG, Salm R. Postmastectomy lymphangiosarcoma: a reappraisal of the concept, a critical review and report of an illustrative case. Histopathology 1979;3:131-152.

73. Schnarkowski P, Kessler M, Arnholdt H, Helmberger T. Angiosarcoma of the breast: mammographic, sonographic, and pathological findings. Eur J Radiol 1997;24:54-56.

74. Schurch W, Seemayer TA, Gabbiani G. The myofibroblast: a quarter century after discovery. Am J Surg Pathol 1998;22:141-147.

74a. Sher T, Hennessy BT, Valero V, et al. Primary angiosarcomas of the breast. Cancer 2007;110:173-178.

75. Sigal M, Grossin M, Bilet S, Basset F, Belaich S. [Stewart-Treves pseudo-syndrome caused by cutaneolymphatic metastases of contralateral breast carcinoma.] Ann Dermatol Venereol 1987;114:677-683. [French.]

76. Silver SA, Tavassoli FA. Primary osteogenic sarcoma of the breast: a clinicopathologic analysis of 50 cases. Am J Surg Pathol 1998;22:925-933.

77. Silver SA, Tavassoli FA. Osteosarcomatous differentiation in phyllodes tumors. Am J Surg Pathol 1999;23:815-821.

78. Silverberg SG, Kay S, Koss LG. Postmastectomy lymphangiosarcoma: ultrastructural observations. Cancer 1971;27:100-108.

79. Sloane JP. Biopsy pathology of the breast. London: Chapman and Hall; 1985.

80. Sordillo PP, Chapman R, Hajdu SI, Magill GB, Golbey RB. Lymphangiosarcoma. Cancer 1981;48:1674-1679.

81. Steingaszner LC, Enzinger FM, Taylor HB. Hemangiosarcoma of the breast. Cancer 1965;18:352-361.

82. Stewart FW. Tumors of the breast. Washington, DC: AFIP; 1950.

83. Stewart FW, Treves N. Lymphangiosarcoma in postmastectomy lymphedema. A report of six cases in elephantiasis chirurgica. Cancer 1948;1:64-81.

84. Stokkel MP, Peterse HL. Angiosarcoma of the breast after lumpectomy and radiation therapy for adenocarcinoma. Cancer 1992;69:2965-2968.

85. Taccagni G, Rovere E, Masullo M, Christensen L, Eyden B. Myofibrosarcoma of the breast: review of the literature on myofibroblastic tumors and criteria for defining myofibroblastic differentiation. Am J Surg Pathol 1997;21:489-496.

86. Taghian A, de Vathaire F, Terrier P, et al. Long-term risk of sarcoma following radiation treatment for breast cancer. Int J Radiat Oncol Biol Phys 1991;21:361-367.

87. Tang PH, Petrelli M, Robechek PJ. Stromal sarcoma of the breast. A light and electron microscopic study. Cancer 1979;43:209-217.

88. Tavassoli FA. Pathology of the breast, 2nd ed. Stamford, CT: Appleton-Lange/McGraw Hill; 1999.

89. Terrier PH, Terrier-Lacombe MJ, Mouriesse H, Friedman S, Spielman M, Contesso G. Primary breast sarcoma: a review of 33 cases with immunohistochemistry and prognostic factors. Breast Cancer Res Treat 1989;13:39-48.

90. Tountas AA, Fornasier V, Harwood AR, Leung PM. Postirradiation sarcoma of bone: a perspective. Cancer 1979;43:182-187.

90a. Virtanen A, Pukkala E, Auvinen A. Angiosarcoma after radiotherapy: a cohort study of 332,163 Finnish cancer patients. Br J Cancer 2007;97:115-117.

91. Wijnmaalen A, Van Ooijen B, Van Geel BN, Henzen-Logmans SC, Treurniet-Donker AD. Angiosarcoma of the breast following lumpectomy, axillary lymph node dissection, and radiotherapy for primary breast cancer: three case reports and a review of the literature. Int J Radiat Oncol Biol Phys 1994;26:135-139.

92. Woodward AH, Ivins JC, Soule EH. Lymphangiosarcoma arising in chronic lymphedematous extremities. Cancer 1972;30:562-572.

93. Wu J, Brinker DA, Haas M, Montgomery EA, Argani P. Primary alveolar soft part sarcoma (ASPS) of the breast: report of a deceptive case with xantomatous features confirmed by TFE3 immunohistochemistry and electron microscopy. Int J Surg Pathol 2005;13:81-85.

14 BIPHASIC TUMORS

Characterized by a simultaneous proliferation of both epithelial and mesenchymal elements, biphasic tumors of the breast constitute a distinctive group of lesions. The major tumors in this category are fibroadenoma and phyllodes tumor; carcinosarcomas and periductal stromal sarcomas are far less frequently observed variants. Various combinations of benign and malignant alterations within either the mesenchymal or the epithelial component occur.

FIBROADENOMA

Definition. *Fibroadenoma* is characterized by the proliferation of a generally hypocellular, exuberant stroma around relatively sparse epithelial-/myoepithelial-lined spaces. The dominant and most conspicuous abnormality is the stromal proliferation. In the juvenile variant, the stroma is actually hypercellular.

General Features. Fibroadenoma is the third most common mammary lesion following fibrocystic changes (FCC) and carcinoma; it is the most common lesion among women younger than 25 years of age (15,16). Cheatle (15,16) found fibroadenomas in 25 percent of normal breasts at postmortem examination. Frantz (29) found fibroadenomas in 9 percent of 225 postmortem examinations; one third of the fibroadenomas were microscopic lesions not detected on gross examination.

Fibroadenomas originate in the terminal duct lobular unit (TDLU) (82); this has been confirmed with three-dimensional reconstruction of serially sectioned lesions (20). Four stages in the development of a fibroadenoma have been defined (69). The initial processes of epithelial and stromal proliferation in multiple lobules either occur spontaneously or are precipitated by hormonal alterations (hyperestrogenic states). Next, a gradual confluence of the hyperplastic lobules develops, followed by the eventual formation of fibroadenomatous nodules. Finally, the fibroadenomatous nodules coalesce to form the fibroadenoma.

It is common to find fibroadenomatous hyperplasia around fully developed fibroadenomas. This is one reason why excision of a fibroadenoma is followed sometimes by the development of one or more new tumors. Also, some women appear to have a predisposition for the development of multiple fibroadenomas.

Clinical Features. Fibroadenoma generally presents as a painless, solitary, well-circumscribed and freely movable mass. Multiple fibroadenomas develop either synchronously or metachronously in one or both breasts in a quarter of the women with fibroadenomas and do so more frequently among black patients (23,30,67). The average age of women with fibroadenoma ranges from 20 to 33 years (15,16,21, 31,37,41). Generally, around 2 to 3 cm in size, some (particularly the juvenile variant) may assume massive proportions (*giant fibroadenoma*), replacing most of the mammary tissue.

It is believed that fibroadenomas develop as a result of unopposed estrogenic influences (32). Its frequent occurrence during the reproductive age and its lower prevalence in an involuted form (small, sclerotic, hyalinized) in postmenopausal women who are not on hormone replacement therapy support the role of hormones in the development and maintenance of fibroadenomas. Fibroadenomas do occur in postmenopausal women (41), and with the increasing use of postmenopausal hormone replacement therapy, it should not be surprising to find fibroadenomas without hyalinization in postmenopausal women. Given the origin of fibroadenoma in the TDLU and the absence of this structure in the normal male mammary duct system, this lesion is rarely observed in the male breast. When it does develop in the male breast, it is generally in the setting of estrogenic or estrogen-mimicking influences that have induced the development of TDLUs (2). A variety of drugs may induce estrogen-like effects (62).

Myxoid mammary fibroadenomas have been observed in some patients with Carney syndrome,

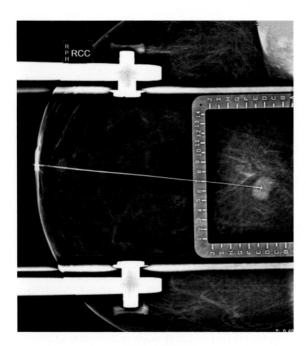

Figure 14-1

FIBROADENOMA

Mammographically, fibroadenoma presents as a well-delineated nodular density.

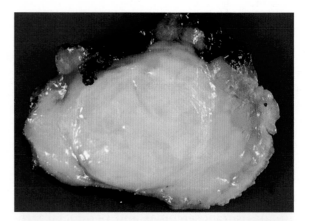

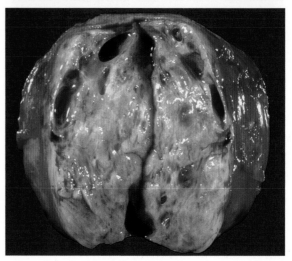

Figure 14-2

FIBROADENOMA

Top: Fibroadenomas are typically solid and well delineated.

Bottom: The bulging cut surface contains blue-domed cysts; these correspond to the fibrocystic changes within the tumor.

a complex of cardiac and cutaneous myxomas, spotty pigmentation, and endocrine overactivity (11,12,17). Inquiry about other components of this complex is prudent when a patient presents with myxoid fibroadenoma.

Recent studies have suggested that fibroadenomas constitute a minor risk factor of about 1.6 to 2.17 times for the subsequent development of invasive breast carcinoma compared to women without fibroadenomas (14,21,45,47,52,58). This is especially true when the fibroadenomas contain epithelial proliferations or sclerosing adenosis (21). In an Australian study, daily vitamin C intake and duration of cigarette smoking were both shown to have an inverse association with risk of fibroadenoma; the use of oral contraceptives prior to age 20 years increased the risk, while the number of full-term pregnancies decreased the risk (84).

Mammographically, fibroadenoma typically presents as a well-circumscribed, often lobulated density (fig. 14-1), occasionally with a radiolucent halo. Calcifications may be present in hyalinized tumors. Fibroadenomas are among lesions that can simulate malignancy on magnetic resonance imaging (MRI). The MRI appearance of fibroadenomas is variable depending on the degree of stromal cellularity. MRI cannot readily distinguish between these lesions and malignant tumors on the basis of signal intensity and enhancement (39,40); the lobulations and "internal septations" commonly observed in fibroadenomas provide a more reliable basis for distinction (39,40,42).

Gross Findings. Well-circumscribed and oval to round, the typical fibroadenoma has a bulging cut surface that is uniformly solid, fleshy, and gray-white; small slit-like spaces and small cysts are sometimes observed (fig. 14-2).

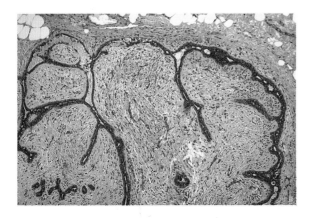

Figure 14-3

FIBROADENOMA

In this intracanalicular variant, duct lumens are compressed by the proliferating stroma.

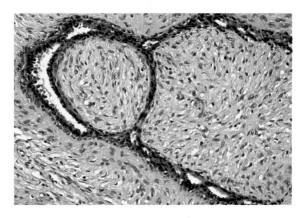

Figure 14-4

FIBROADENOMA

Epithelial and myoepithelial cell layers line the slit-like ductal spaces.

Fibroadenomas occurring during adolescence may have a more fleshy consistency due to a more cellular stromal component while those with myxoid stromal change display a gelatinous appearance. Hyalinized fibroadenomas have a rock-hard consistency. Often appearing encapsulated, fibroadenoma is generally 2 to 3 cm in size but may become massive (over 10 cm) (8,35,70).

Microscopic Findings. Fibroadenoma consists of a combined proliferation of epithelial and mesenchymal elements. The stroma proliferates around tubular (pericanalicular) or compressed cleft-like (intracanalicular) ducts. With the intracanalicular pattern (fig. 14-3), the stroma exhibits radial growth with deposition of reticulin fibers perpendicular to the epithelial elements, highlighted with silver stains. One pattern often dominates. Focal intracanalicular growth is seen in many juvenile fibroadenomas in which the pericanalicular pattern dominates. The intracanalicular pattern is frequently present in pure form, however, and rarely exhibits areas of pericanalicular growth.

The ducts, whether compressed (in the intracanalicular variant) or tubular (in the pericanalicular variant), are lined by two cell layers: a luminal epithelial cell layer and an underlying layer of myoepithelial cells (fig. 14-4). The margins of the lesion are generally pushing, with a well-developed capsule around some tumors; focal marginal irregularities are seen in rare cases. Rarely, an otherwise typical fibroadenoma displays fo-

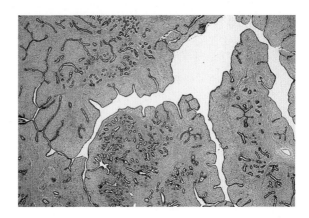

Figure 14-5

FIBROADENOMA PHYLLODES

Leaf-like processes (phyllodes structures) occasionally develop in an otherwise classic fibroadenoma.

cal leaf-like processes (phyllodes arrangement) protruding into dilated ductal spaces or cysts (fig. 14-5); the term *fibroadenoma phyllodes* is appropriate for this lesion. The stroma in the phyllodes areas is the same as in the more typical adjacent fibroadenomatous areas.

The epithelial and stromal components of fibroadenoma may undergo a variety of age related, metaplastic, and proliferative changes. The epithelium becomes attenuated and atrophic in elderly women. Apocrine epithelial differentiation is relatively common, present in 11 to 35 percent of fibroadenomas (3,5,7). Squamous metaplasia has also been observed (76), with lower frequency, and neuroendocrine

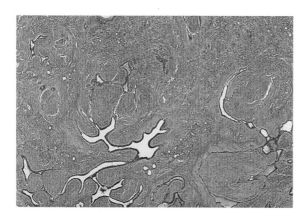
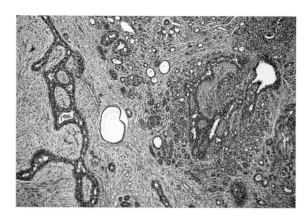

Figure 14-6

FIBROADENOMA

Sclerosing adenosis may involve a fibroadenoma either diffusely or focally.

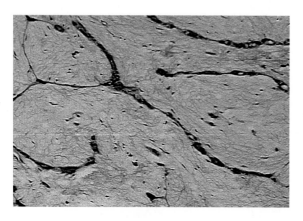

Figure 14-7

FIBROADENOMA

Myxoid stromal change is evident.

type differentiation may develop (5,22a). In a small proportion of fibroadenomas, fibrocystic changes and a variety of proliferative and atypical changes develop in the epithelial component (49,60). In some lesions, abundant sclerosing adenosis may be confused with invasive carcinoma (fig. 14-6). The persistent myoepithelial cell layer and a concentrically oriented collagen or basement membrane around other tubules identify the lesion as benign.

Prominence or hyperplasia of the myoepithelial cells may result in an unusually myoid appearance. This myoid transformation of the myoepithelial cells should not be confused with smooth muscle metaplasia of the stromal component.

Abundant hyalinization and diffuse myxoid change are among the more common alterations in the stroma (fig. 14-7) (50); calcification is observed in hyalinized lesions. Fibroadenomas with myxoid stroma occurring in women younger than 40 years of age appear to be associated with the development of multiple recurrences (81). Extensive hyalinization is observed more frequently, but not exclusively, in fibroadenomas removed from breasts of elderly postmenopausal women. Less commonly, atypical and bizarre multinucleated giant cells are identified focally or diffusely in the stroma (7,63,73,75); they are benign and have no prognostic significance (see chapter 12, Benign Stromal Lesions). Occasionally, adipose tissue (72) as well as chondroid and osseous metaplasia are seen (78,83). Among the more infrequent stromal alterations is smooth muscle metaplasia (36,55,81).

Rarely, a sarcoma may develop in a fibroadenoma; these can be quite aggressive and have been distinguished from a phyllodes tumor by the absence of leaf-like processes in the biphasic areas of the lesion. Thorough sampling is required in such cases to exclude the possibility of a phyllodes tumor. It is unlikely that the behavior of this lesion would differ significantly from a similar tumor with phyllodes architecture, however.

Spontaneous infarction is rare (significantly less than 1 percent of cases) and occurs most often during pregnancy and lactation (18,38). Thrombosed vessels may be seen in the areas of infarction. Hemorrhagic infarction of fibroadenoma may occur following fine needle aspiration

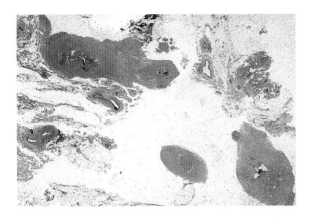

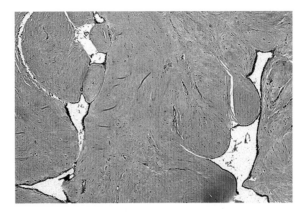

Figure 14-8

FIBROADENOMA

Several tissue fragments obtained by core biopsy show abundant hyalinized stroma around compressed ducts.

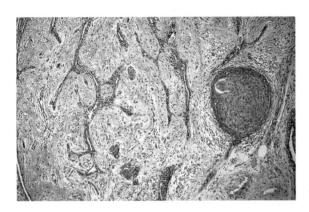

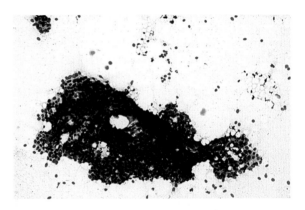

Figure 14-9

FIBROADENOMA

Squamous metaplasia forms around a core biopsy site. A lymphoplasmacytic infiltrate surrounds the immediate vicinity of the prior core biopsy site.

Figure 14-10

FIBROADENOMA

Fine needle aspiration specimen shows fenestrated sheets of evenly spaced, multilayered, polygonal epithelial cells. A few myoepithelial cells appear as bipolar naked nuclei in the background. (Courtesy of Dr. Philip Branton, Fairfax, VA.)

cytology (FNAC) (57). Oral contraceptive steroids may induce epithelial prominence and/or proliferation (9,35), but no epithelial atypia.

Core Biopsy. Fibroadenomas are easily recognizable on core biopsies (fig. 14-8). The classic biphasic pattern often is evident, even in small samples. Squamous metaplasia at the site of the core biopsy (fig. 14-9) or other needle instrumentation is observed with increasing frequency.

Cytologic Findings. The typical FNAC smears appear far more cellular than would be anticipated from a fibroadenoma. A pattern of fenestrated sheets of evenly spaced, polygonal or multilayered epithelial cells in branching formations (antler horn clusters), with myoepithelial cells adherent to the clusters or loose in the background and often appearing as bipolar naked nuclei, is characteristic (fig. 14-10). Fragments of acellular stroma may be present. The epithelial elements may display various degrees of atypia. Misinterpretation of the findings as carcinoma occurs on rare occasions (6). Carcinomas are also rarely misdiagnosed as fibroadenoma (54). The simultaneous presence of numerous multilayered fragments of proliferating glandular epithelium and numerous bare nuclei can significantly improve the predictive value of the aspiration cytology (56).

Immunohistochemical and Ultrastructural Findings. The stromal cells of fibroadenoma immunoreact for smooth muscle-specific actin in most tumors (34), particularly those with a cellular stroma and those composed of myofibroblastic cells (77); the immunoreaction is weak in tumors with either a myxoid or sclerotic stroma (68). Lesions that display smooth muscle metaplasia of the stromal cells are immunoreactive for desmin as well. The stromal cells in fibroadenomas are mostly CD34-positive fibroblasts/myofibroblasts; factor XIIIa-positive dendritic histiocytes comprise 5 to 20 percent of the stromal cells (77). The epithelial cells in fibroadenoma have the same immunoprofile observed in epithelial cells elsewhere in the breast: immunoreactivity with kermix (AE1/AE3), CAM5.2, cytokeratin (CK)7, and epithelial membrane antigen (EMA). Similarly, the myoepithelial cells are immunoreactive with all the myoepithelial cell markers (smooth muscle actin, calponin, caldesmon, p63, and others). The epithelial cells in fibroadenomas show variable immunoreactivity with estrogen receptor (ER) (33,59), but are more frequently positive for progesterone receptor (PR) (74). ER and PR expression may vary during different phases of the menstrual cycle (48). Immunoexpression of Caveolin-1 has been assessed in the epithelial cells of 167 fibroadenomas (53); no significant expression was noted.

At the ultrastructural level, fibroblasts and myofibroblasts constitute the main cells in the stroma, while a luminal layer of epithelial cells overlying an interrupted myoepithelial cell layer is separated from the stroma by a distinct basement membrane (1,13,26). The multinucleated stromal giant cells appear to be multinucleated fibroblasts. A fibroblastic/myofibroblastic nature is favored for the stromal cells (43).

Molecular Findings. A polyclonal cell population has been identified in both the epithelial and the stromal components of fibroadenoma; in contrast, the stromal elements in phyllodes tumor display monoclonality, while the epithelial cells are polyclonal (64,65). Progression of rare monoclonal fibroadenomas to phyllodes tumors has been reported (66). This would imply that clonality could be a useful tool in distinguishing the two tumors and possibly predicting the future course of fibroadenoma.

A cytogenetic abnormality has been identified in 20 to 30 percent of fibroadenomas (10, 27,80). Chromosomal aberrations have also been seen in some cases (10,26,79,80), with an identical aberration identified in three fibroadenomas from the same patient (10). Two types of translocation [t(4;12)(q27; q15)] and t(6;14) have been noted in fibroadenomas (79,136). Using the fluorescence in situ hybridization (FISH) technique, a translocation [t(4;12)(q27;q15)] as the sole cytogenetic abnormality was found in a single fibroadenoma; the breakpoint region was narrowed to a 230-kb fragment belonging to the *HMGI-C* gene that maps an area recently designated as the multiple aberration region (MAR) (79). Another translocation, t(6;14), was noted in a fibroadenoma by another group (136).

Differential Diagnosis. The major lesion in the differential diagnosis of fibroadenoma is a phyllodes tumor. Characterized by the formation of leaf-like processes that project into cystic spaces and a densely cellular stroma, phyllodes tumor is easily distinguished from fibroadenoma in most cases. Borderline lesions with only minimal and localized stromal cellularity pose a major diagnostic problem. The term *cellular fibroadenoma* is used when the lesion lacks well-formed leaf-like processes and the stroma is minimally cellular. When the stroma is hypocellular or of the degree of cellularity expected in typical fibroadenomas, but the lesion contains well-formed leaf-like processes, the term *fibroadenoma phyllodes* is used (see fig. 14-5). In the case of a borderline lesion, the designation of fibroadenoma is favored when the patient is younger than 20 years. In core biopsies, stromal cellularity, stromal overgrowth, tissue fragmentation, and stromal adipose tissue favor a phyllodes tumor in borderline cases (51).

Another lesion in the differential diagnosis, albeit less frequently, is tubular adenoma. A tubular adenoma lacks the abundant stroma typical of fibroadenoma. Sometimes, fibroadenomas have a minor component of tubular adenoma, or vice versa; in such cases, the diagnosis is based on the dominant component, with a comment regarding the other element. The designation of a combined tubular-fibroadenoma is suitable for lesions in which both components are conspicuous, with the minor component comprising at least 10 percent of the

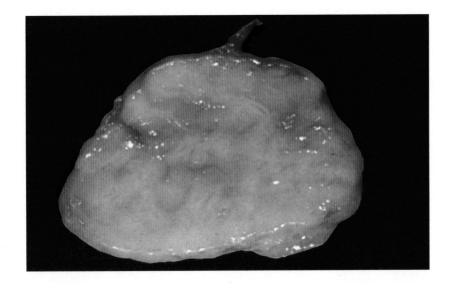

Figure 14-11

JUVENILE FIBROADENOMA
The cut surface is yellow-tan.

lesion; often, however, the two components are nearly equally represented.

Other lesions to consider in the differential include hamartoma and adenosis tumor. Adipose tissue is a more abundant component of hamartoma and the epithelial elements are in the form of normal or mildly altered ducts and lobules irregularly dispersed in a fibroadipose stroma lacking the organized epithelial stromal relationship of fibroadenomas. Adenosis tumor is composed of an aggregation of variably expanded lobules without either hyperplastic stroma or the epithelial stromal-relationship typical of fibroadenoma (see chapter 2).

Treatment. Most fibroadenomas can be removed without any complications or recurrences. A small number are associated with significant fibroadenomatous hyperplasia around the main tumor mass; these may lead to the development of additional lesions that are generally interpreted as recurrences because of their proximity to the previous lesion. Rarely, fibroadenomatous hyperplasia involves the entire breast.

Juvenile Fibroadenoma

The most common mammary lesion in the adolescent female (23,67), *juvenile fibroadenoma* is characterized by rapid growth, massive size, stretching of the overlying skin, and dilatation of superficial veins (in less than 10 percent of patients) (44,61). The cut surface is often yellow-tan (fig. 14-11) and has a softer consistency than adult type fibroadenoma. Often characterized by a pericanalicular growth pattern (fig. 14-12),

the stroma is more cellular than in the adult type and may occasionally appear hypercellular either focally or diffusely (4,22,25,81). When the rare intracanalicular stromal proliferation, myxoid degeneration, and metaplastic changes occur, they are mostly focal.

Even in the hypercellular juvenile fibroadenoma, mitotic activity is in the range of 2 to 3 per 10 high-power fields and rarely exceeds 4 to 5 per high-power field, noted focally in the lesion. On rare occasions, focal areas of marginal irregularity are present (fig. 14-12). In lesions with borderline features, it is important to ascertain complete excision and recommend follow-up for 2 to 3 years.

Gynecomastoid hyperplasia (a low-risk ductal intraepithelial neoplasia), characterized by the formation of irregular epithelial tufts overlying a stratified epithelium, similar to that seen in gynecomastia (fig. 14-12C), is often associated with juvenile fibroadenoma. Other patterns of hyperplasia also occur, although less frequently. The presence of atypical intraductal hyperplasia or ductal carcinoma in situ (DCIS)/ductal intraepithelial neoplasia 1 (DIN1) should be interpreted conservatively. Assessment of the surrounding breast tissue excised along with the fibroadenoma to rule out similar changes within the breast proper is recommended. When such changes are focal and confined to the fibroadenoma, follow-up of the patient in the form of annual examination of the breasts by palpation is advised.

Juvenile fibroadenoma should be distinguished from juvenile hypertrophy and

Figure 14-12

JUVENILE FIBROADENOMA

A: This juvenile fibroadenoma is characterized by pericanalicular growth of stroma around small tubular ducts.

B: The stroma is often slightly more cellular than in the adult variant.

C: Epithelial proliferation within juvenile fibroadenomas often assumes a gynecomastoid pattern. This degree of epithelial proliferation is common, and it is not essential to include its presence in the diagnosis although it could be included in the microscopic description.

D,E: This tumor from a 19-year-old showed increased stromal cellularity and, while nearly entirely encapsulated, had focal marginal irregularity (E). Complete excision of the tumor and follow-up of the patient are advised for lesions with borderline features in adolescent females.

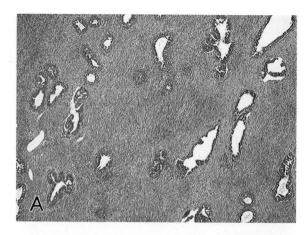

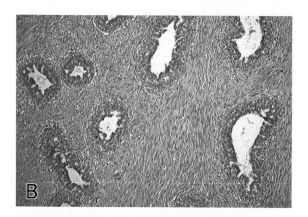

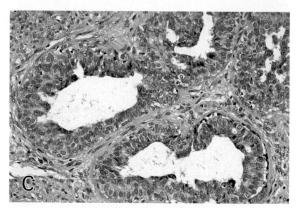

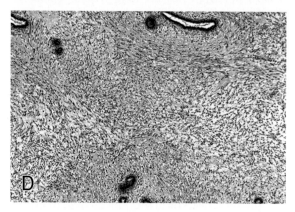

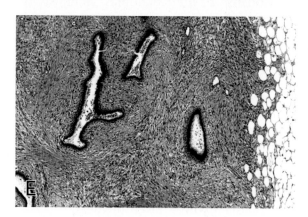

phyllodes tumor. A diffuse enlargement of the entire breast with a dense, sclerotic stroma and generally without a discrete, palpable mass characterizes juvenile hypertrophy. Phyllodes tumor has a more cellular stroma with a cambium layer and leaf-like processes, only rarely displays a prominent pericanalicular growth pattern, and occurs in an older age group. When leaf-like processes rarely and focally develop within an otherwise classic juvenile fibroadenoma, the term *juvenile fibroadenoma phyllodes* would be appropriate.

Intraepithelial and Invasive Epithelial Neoplasms Arising in a Fibroadenoma

Fibroadenomas harbor intraepithelial and/or invasive neoplasia (ductal or lobular type) in less than 0.5 percent of cases (4a,5,19,22a,28,39,58a). More than half of the nearly 270 carcinomas reported have been completely confined to

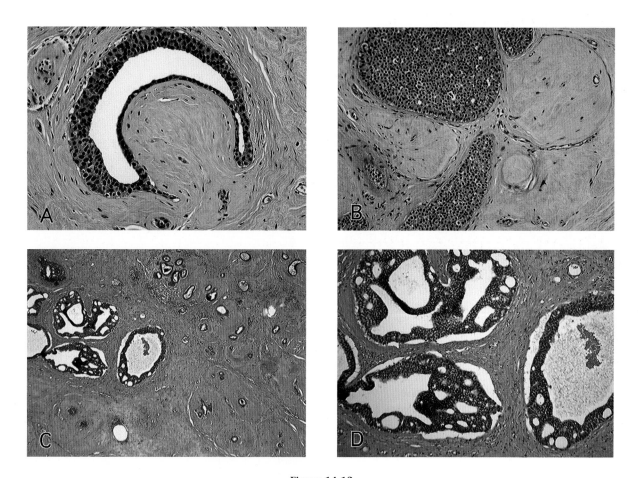

Figure 14-13

EPITHELIAL NEOPLASMS IN FIBROADENOMA

A: Flat epithelial atypia (flat ductal intraepithelial neoplasia [DIN]1).
B: Ductal carcinoma in situ, grade 1, solid type (DCIS/DIN1, solid type).
C,D: Ductal carcinoma in situ, grade 1, cribriform type (DIN1, cribriform type).

the fibroadenoma (4a,5,20,22a,39,58a,71,81). Because of the presence of similar lesions in the adjacent breast tissue in a significant proportion of the women, reexcision of tissue around the fibroadenoma is advised (20). The epithelium lining the ducts may show various forms of epithelial proliferation (all grades of DIN) (fig. 14-13); follow-up is required when focal atypia is present (60). The presence of DCIS/DIN1-3 requires reexcision if the fibroadenoma had been shelled out to exclude the possible presence of similar changes in the surrounding breast tissue.

Epithelial neoplasia in fibroadenoma consists of lobular intraepithelial neoplasia (LIN) (about 50 percent of cases) (fig.14-14), DCIS (nearly 25 percent of cases), and invasive carcinoma (the remainder) (fig. 14-15). Since LIN within fibroadenoma

is believed to have the same behavior as when it is present within the breast proper (20), its treatment should follow the current management principles for LIN (20). An invasive carcinoma arising in a fibroadenoma may lead to death, however (71), and should be managed as an invasive mammary carcinoma.

PHYLLODES TUMOR

Definition. *Phyllodes tumor* is a proliferation of hypercellular, spindled mesenchymal cells around benign epithelial/myoepithelial-lined spaces. The spaces are distended by leaf-like protrusions of stromal elements covered by epithelial/myoepithelial cell layers. In some cases, a soft tissue sarcoma develops and may become dominant in the lesion.

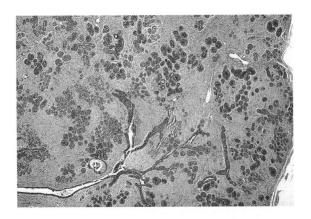

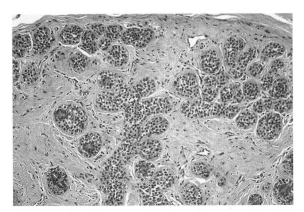

Figure 14-14

LOBULAR INTRAEPITHELIAL NEOPLASIA

This is the most common neoplastic alteration in a fibroadenoma.

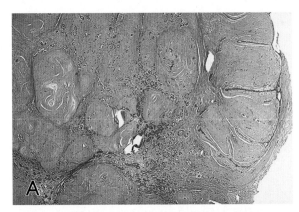

Figure 14-15

FIBROADENOMA WITH INVASIVE CARCINOMA

A: A hyalinized fibroadenoma has an area of increased cellularity.

B,C: An invasive tubulolobular carcinoma is confined to the fibroadenoma.

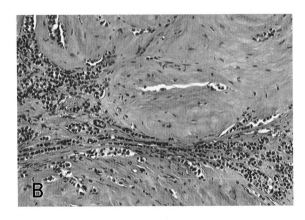

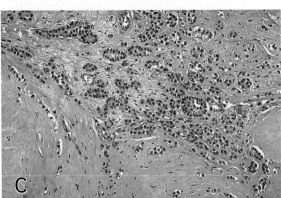

General Features. The origin of this tumor appears to be in the TDLU, similar to fibroadenomas. Described by Johannes Mueller in 1838 (147), it was initially designated as cystosarcoma phyllodes, "sarcoma" for the fleshy nature of the lesion and "phyllodes" for the leaf-like processes. This designation, widely used until recently, has been replaced by the term "phyllodes tumor" because of the very low frequency of aggressive behavior and the current malignant connotation of the term "sarcoma." The introduction of the term phyllodes tumor has been embraced by most pathologists; in 2003, the World Health Organization (WHO) continued to support the term phyllodes tumor in its classification of breast tumors (183).

Clinical Features. Accounting for less than 1 percent of all breast tumors (89,127,135,186), phyllodes tumor is rarely encountered in the general practice of pathology. While it is observed in a wide age range, it occurs most frequently among women 45 to 49 years of age (114,151). Rare cases have been reported in the male breast (2,159). Women with phyllodes tumors are about 15 to 20 years older than those with fibroadenoma; those with aggressive phyllodes tumors are even older, by approximately 7 years, compared to all patients with phyllodes tumors (151). Interestingly, rapid growth of malignant phyllodes tumor has been noted during pregnancy (150). Generally presenting as a unilateral mass, rare bilateral tumors have been reported (152,165).

Because of the increasing use of radiotherapy in the management of breast carcinomas and the report of a phyllodes tumor manifesting 15 years following radiation therapy for a presumable breast carcinoma (133), documentation of any phyllodes tumors and sarcomas following radiation therapy to the anterior chest wall is necessary.

The vast majority (over 85 percent) of patients with phyllodes tumors are white, 8 percent are black, and 5 percent are of other racial extractions (121,151). Asians and Latin American patients with phyllodes tumor in Los Angeles county were significantly younger than other patients with phyllodes tumor in the same county (92).

The clinical presentation is that of a painless, lobulated and freely movable breast mass. Preoperative diagnosis is difficult; rapid growth and large size are useful clues (113,150). A history of rapid growth resulting in changes in the overlying skin, nipple retraction, and associated pain, suggest an aggressive phyllodes tumor, but identical changes have been observed in benign tumors (166). Large tumors, whether benign or malignant, may cause stretching and ulceration of the overlying skin and distension of the superficial veins. Bilaterality is rare, but may occur either simultaneously or within months to years of the initial lesion (135,151,152,165,186).

Axillary lymph node enlargement, observed in 17 percent of cases (151), is generally due to reactive changes. Actual lymph node involvement occurs rarely by contiguous growth (145).

Mammographically, phyllodes tumor presents as a well-circumscribed and occasionally lobulated density (105). Sonographically, a well-defined solid, hypoechoic mass is characteristic (98,138). Delayed magnetic resonance imaging (MRI) may have a potential for separating low-grade from malignant phyllodes tumors (156). Larger studies are needed to confirm these mammographic and sonographic findings. A multi-lobulated appearance is characteristic of benign phyllodes tumor on dynamic MRI (155).

The development of phyllodes tumor in a background of fibroadenoma (172) has raised the possibility that a similar stimulus may initiate the development of both lesions.

Gross Findings. Phyllodes tumors have a median size of around 6 cm, but may be quite small or over 20 cm in diameter (91,127,151,178,186). The typical phyllodes tumor is solitary, well circumscribed, and solid, with cystic areas; fleshy leaf-like processes protrude into cystic spaces (fig. 14-16, left). Some lesions are predominantly to exclusively solid on cut surface (fig. 14-16, right), or contain barely visible cysts. The bulging cut surface is gray-white or yellow. Focal hemorrhage and/or necrosis is apparent in some of the larger tumors.

Microscopic Findings. Composed of a benign epithelial component and a cellular, spindle cell stroma, phyllodes tumor is characterized by the formation of leaf-like processes protruding into cystic spaces (fig. 14-17). The cellular, hyperplastic stroma of phyllodes tumor is in sharp contrast to the hypocellular appearance of fibroadenoma. The degree of cellularity, atypia, and mitotic activity varies significantly in different lesions and in different areas within the same lesion, sometimes with more intense hypercelullarity in the subepithelial zone (cambium layer) (figs. 14-18, 14-19). This cellularity and the presence of the leaf-like processes are the most helpful features distinguishing phyllodes tumor from fibroadenoma. Leaf-like processes qualify the lesion as a phyllodes tumor only if there is increased stromal cellularity.

The benign epithelium lining the ducts and slit-like spaces or covering the leaf-like processes consists of two cell layers: epithelial cells along the luminal aspect and myoepithe-

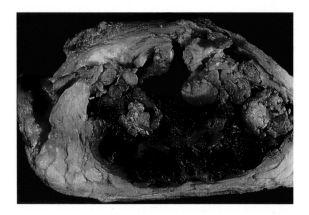
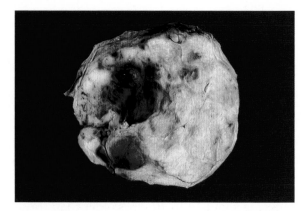

Figure 14-16

PHYLLODES TUMOR

Variable in its gross appearance, phyllodes tumor is more often characterized by large, fleshy, broad papillae projecting into complex cystic spaces (left), or it may appear rather solid (right) with only a suggestion of compressed cystic spaces at the periphery.

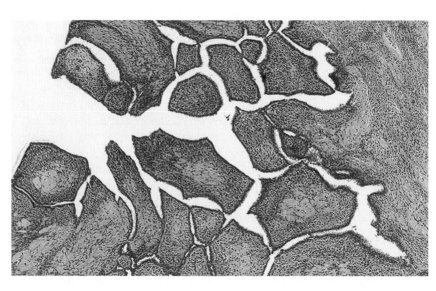

Figure 14-17

PHYLLODES TUMOR

The typical leaf-like processes and a moderately cellular stroma are seen.

lial cells beneath them. The stromal cells are spindle shaped and either fibroblastic or myofibroblastic (96). A variety of mesenchymal metaplasias may develop within the stroma. These include benign and malignant osseous (fig. 14-20A), chondroid, adipose (fig. 14-20B,C), rhabdomyoblastic, and smooth muscle differentiation (125,150,156a,159,161,162,176,177). A rarely observed alteration is characterized by actin-positive aggregates of myofibrils or digital fibroma-like inclusions (94,120,175). A multinucleated floret type stromal giant cell is present in some cases. Hemangiopericytoma and malignant fibrous histiocytoma also develop in phyllodes tumors (143,159).

More than one type of differentiation can be seen within the sarcomatous component. The sarcomatous component may develop significant overgrowth with minimal residual biphasic elements, recognizable only focally after exhaustive sampling. It is, therefore, important to thoroughly evaluate all mammary sarcomas to exclude sarcomatous overgrowth in a phyllodes tumor. The sarcomatous component should be classified according to its differentiation whenever possible; in a significant proportion of cases, the sarcomatous component defies classification as a distinct soft tissue sarcoma.

Assessment of the tumor margin is important. It is generally the sarcomatous component that

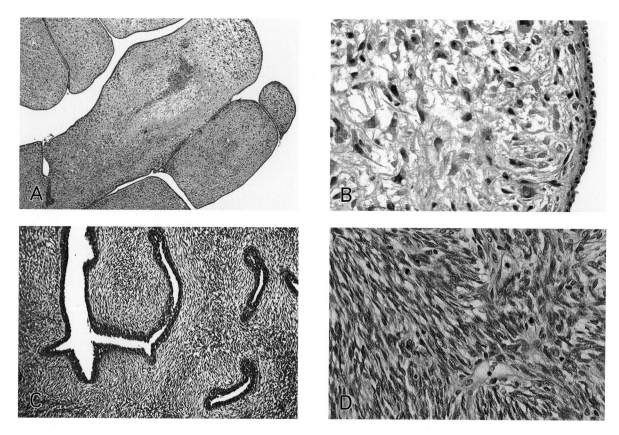

Figure 14-18

PHYLLODES TUMOR

The leaf-like processes (A) and stromal cells without significant atypia (B) are seen. This phyllodes tumor has a hypercellular stroma (C), but lacks nuclear pleomorphism (D).

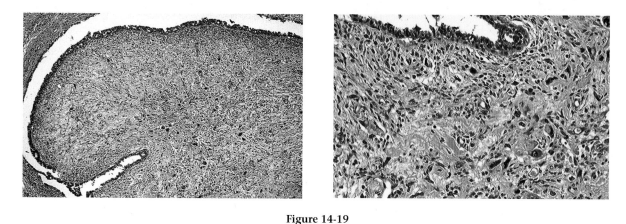

Figure 14-19

PHYLLODES TUMOR

The stromal atypia is significant and the mitotic figures are readily identifiable.

is at the margin and it may display either a pushing (fig. 14-21) or an infiltrating (fig. 14-22) growth pattern.

The most common alterations in the epithelial element of phyllodes tumor are focal apocrine change or squamous metaplasia (fig. 14-23)

Figure 14-20

PHYLLODES TUMOR

Phyllodes tumor may contain a variety of sarcomas including osteosarcoma (A) and liposarcoma (B,C).

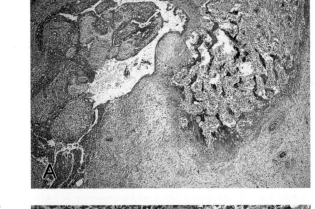

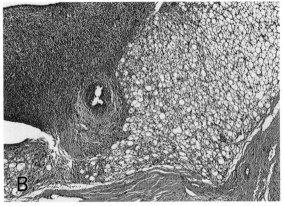

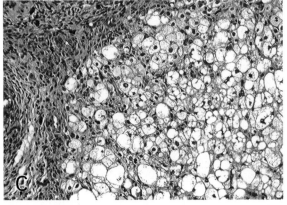

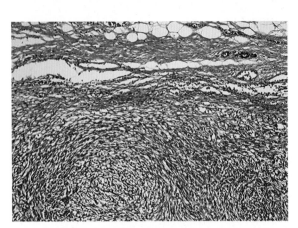

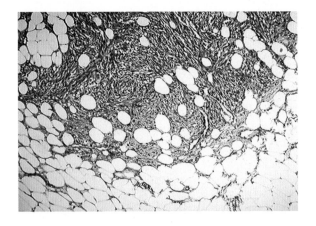

Figure 14-21

PHYLLODES TUMOR

This tumor has a pushing growth margin

Figure 14-22

PHYLLODES TUMOR

The infiltrating margin requires excision with a margin of uninvolved breast tissue to minimize the chance of local recurrence.

(131,151), areas of adenosis, and cystic changes. All grades of in situ (intraepithelial) and invasive carcinomas of both lobular and ductal types, including squamous carcinoma, occur in phyllodes tumor, but they are uncommon (invasive carcinoma oc-

curs in 2 percent of cases) (89a,104a,115a,116a, 117a, 129a,134a,151,156a,168a,186).

Cytologic Findings. A combination of epithelial cell clusters, naked nuclei, atypical cells, and

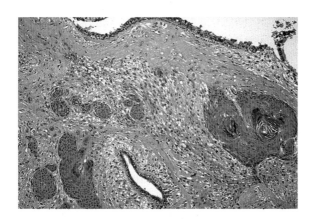

Figure 14-23

PHYLLODES TUMOR

Spontaneous squamous metaplasia is far more common in phyllodes tumors than fibroadenomas. With increasing use of needle core biopsies, however, squamous metaplasia along the needle track is observed more frequently in fibroadenomas.

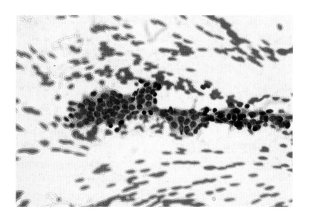

Figure 14-24

PHYLLODES TUMOR

The cytology of some phyllodes tumors is indistinguishable from that of a fibroadenoma and consists of multilayered sheaths of epithelial cells. (Courtesy of Dr. Parvin Ganjei, Miami, FL.)

myxoid changes in a background of mitotically active bipolar stromal cells raises the possibility of a biphasic tumor (fig. 14-24) (173,174). The cytologic features of low-grade phyllodes tumor can be indistinguishable from those of a fibroadenoma. Misinterpretation of phyllodes tumor as a carcinoma may result when there is a paucity of stromal cells in the background (107). The stromal cells of phyllodes tumor may have cytoplasm in contrast to the naked nuclei of stromal cells that form the background in aspirates of fibroadenoma.

Immunohistochemical Findings. Positive immunoreactions for vimentin and actin have been noted in the stromal cells of phyllodes tumor in over two thirds of cases; focal positivity for desmin is present in a quarter of the cases (88). The stromal cells are negative for epithelial markers (CAM5.2, EMA, CK7, and AE1/AE3) and S-100 protein. The stromal cells express p53 when there is significant atypia, but rarely in low-grade lesions (128,173). Immunoexpression of p53 has been associated with known negative prognostic factors, but is not a useful determinant of tumor recurrence or long-term survival (110,181). Both CD117 (181) and CD10 (184,191) expression have been noted in the stromal cells of phyllodes tumors. The findings have been variable and more data are needed to determine their utility in either the diagnosis or management of these tumors.

Significant differences have been noted in the stromal proliferative activity of different grades of phyllodes tumor using MIB-1, which reacts with Ki-67 (187) and appears to correlate with the histologic grade (130).

Hormone Receptors. Expression of estrogen and progesterone receptors (ER, PR) has been assessed in a small number of cases and the findings are variable (31,59,164), suggesting that neither estrogen nor progesterone plays a major role in the histogenesis of phyllodes tumor. In one study, immunoreactivity only with PR, but not ER, was noted in the stromal cells (164). ER-beta expression has been noted in the stromal cells of phyllodes tumors and its expression correlates with the expression of smooth muscle markers in the stromal cells (170).

Ultrastructural Findings. The stromal cells in a majority of phyllodes tumors are fibroblastic-myofibroblastic in nature (185). When specific types of soft tissue sarcoma develop, smooth muscle (123), rhabdomyoblastic, and other differentiation may be noted at the ultrastructural level.

Molecular Findings. While some have suggested that polyclonality of the epithelial component and monoclonality of the stromal elements imply that the stroma is the only neoplastic component, other studies of phyllodes tumors have supported a clonal origin (65,66,93). Allelic imbalance on chromosomes 3p and 1q occurs in both the stroma and the epithelial components, sometimes as independent genetic events, supporting the neoplastic nature of both elements (171). Allelic imbalance at one or more markers on 3p has been noted in 24 percent of phyllodes tumors; allelic imbalance on chromosome 1q has been noted in 30 percent (171). Another group looked for deletions in chromosome 3p at the *FHIT* and *hMLH1* loci in eight tumors (four benign, four malignant). No loss of heterozygosity was found in any of these tumors (129).

Gains on chromosome 1q were noted as one of the more common alterations among low-grade phyllodes tumors (160). Structural alteration of 10q was the second most common change (160). Lae et al. (132) found that benign phyllodes tumors have none or only a few chromosomal alterations, while malignant phyllodes tumors have numerous chromosomal changes, in particular 1q gain and 13q loss. Using single nucleotide polymorphism (SNP) array analysis, frequent and sometimes extensive loss of heterozygosity (LOH) has been noted in phyllodes tumors, but rarely in fibroadenomas. Furthermore, primary and recurrent phyllodes tumors share common regions of LOH, supporting their kinship (189). A germline mutation has been reported in codon 162 of the *TP53* gene in two simultaneous phyllodes tumors; this mutation results in the replacement of isoleucine by asparagine (96).

Cytometric and fluorescent in situ hybridization (FISH) analysis performed on two samples taken 4 weeks apart revealed loss of chromosome 21 in both samples and the presence of two different chromosome 1 derivatives; the first sample had a dic(1;10)(q10;q24) and the second had an i(1)(q10) alteration (93). Using short-term cultures, cytogenetic evaluation of five benign phyllodes tumors showed interstitial deletions of the short arm of chromosome 3, del(3)(p12p14) and del(3)(p21p23), as the only aberrations in two cases (106). The only malignant tumor evaluated had a near-triploid stemline, indicating that karyotyping complexity is a marker of malignancy in phyllodes tumor (106). Cytogenetic polyclonality was observed in three benign tumors.

Differential Diagnosis. When sarcomatous overgrowth is pronounced, a pure sarcoma becomes an important entity in the differential diagnosis (see chapter 13). In such cases, adequate sampling of the tumor (one tissue section per each centimeter of maximum tumor diameter) is necessary to identify or to rule out the presence of epithelial elements. Furthermore, since the recurrence of some phyllodes tumors may be in the form of a pure sarcoma, the availability of a thorough history concerning any previous biopsies is essential.

The distinction from cellular fibroadenoma is made predominantly on the basis of absent phyllodes structures (see Differential Diagnosis, Fibroadenoma). In core biopsies, the presence of abundant squamous metaplasia in a borderline biphasic tumor (fig. 14-23) favors a phyllodes tumor if the patient has not had prior instrumentation of the tumor.

Factors Affecting Prognosis. It is currently recognized that phyllodes tumors have an aggressive potential; this is generally in the form of local recurrences, sometimes with progression to a more aggressive morphologic appearance and far less frequently in the form of metastases. It is, however, extremely difficult to predict reliably the behavior of a phyllodes tumor on the basis of its histologic features. Rare histologically benign tumors have metastasized (85), while many histologically malignant tumors do not even recur. A fairly good estimate of the behavior of a phyllodes tumor can be made by evaluating several pathologic features including tumor size, contour, stromal cell atypia, mitotic activity (118,151), and sarcomatous overgrowth (190).

Based on a composite evaluation of the number of mitotic figures, the degree of atypia, and the tumor contour, numerous investigators have proposed subdividing phyllodes tumors into benign, intermediate (borderline), and malignant groups (101–103,146,166,188). The criteria proposed by various investigators differ primarily in the number of mitotic figures allowed for each subgroup and the weight of stromal cellularity and atypia as factors influencing the subdivision (101,116,159). In some studies, the borderline category behaves more like the benign variant, with mainly local recurrences, sometimes with increased frequency. Other investigators (169) have found no difference between borderline and malignant tumors in terms of local recurrence or distant metastases. In our opinion, a three-tiered subdivision does not separate clinically distinct categories. Although the addition of a morphologically intermediate category may appear useful, the criteria advanced so far seem more helpful in creating an arbitrary histologic separation than in providing clinically predictive values.

Stromal overgrowth is another factor of prognostic significance; this feature has been quantified only recently (118,190). Defined as an overgrowth of the stromal component to the point that epithelial elements are absent in at least one low-power field (40X magnification), stromal overgrowth was found in 6 of 7 tumors that caused patient death in a review of 26 phyllodes tumors by Ward and Evans (190). While it is agreed that stromal overgrowth is a significant prognostic variable, the threshold should be raised significantly to refer only to neoplasms that display a predominance of sarcoma on multiple sections in which residual phyllodes tumor elements are barely identifiable. In our unpublished experience, this higher threshold is a better predictor of aggressive behavior.

A classic study from Armed Forces Institute of Pathology (AFIP) (151) concluded that no single histologic feature could predict reliably the behavior of a phyllodes tumor; a combination of tumor size, type of margin, degree of atypia, and amount of mitotic activity was helpful as a guide in predicting the behavior of these lesions, but not in an absolute way. None of the 15 tumors that proved fatal was smaller than 4 cm, but recurrences did develop in 11 percent of those cases smaller than 4 cm. More than a third (38 percent) of tumors with infiltrating margins recurred and 35 percent of the patients died of their infiltrating tumor. Of tumors with "pushing" margins, 15 percent recurred and the tumor was lethal in only 3 percent of patients. Of the 15 tumors that proved fatal, 5 (33 percent) had 3+ stromal atypia (scale of 1 to 3), whereas of the 30 lesions with 1+ stromal atypia, 27 percent recurred and 7 percent proved fatal. Tumors with 5 or more mitotic figures per 10 high-power fields accounted for 11 of the 15 deaths. Of tumors with 0 to 2 mitotic figures per 10 high-power fields, 17 percent recurred, and 18 percent of tumors with only 3 to 4 mitotic figures proved fatal, despite radical mastectomy in one case.

Because of the difficulty in predicting the behavior of phyllodes tumors and because local recurrences develop even in histologically benign tumors, it is preferable, although not mandatory, to use the term low-grade rather than benign phyllodes tumor. Most phyllodes tumors have a potential for local recurrence, but are very unlikely to metastasize. The term "high-grade or malignant" is used to designate a tumor with the potential for distant metastasis that is characterized by invasive or pushing margins, moderate to severe atypia (2+ to 3+), and at least 3 and often more mitotic figures per 10 high-power fields; sarcomatous overgrowth also would qualify a phyllodes tumor as high grade. Of course, if a specific sarcoma is identified, then it is included in the diagnosis; for example, liposarcoma arising in a phyllodes tumor. Lesions are designated as low grade if they have a pushing growth margin, mild (1+) to moderate (2+) atypia, and fewer than 3 mitotic figures per 10 high-power fields; these tumors also have a potential for local recurrence, but are very unlikely to metastasize. Tumors with intermediate features may be simply designated phyllodes tumor without further qualification; local recurrence is the main concern for these lesions. In essence, this is also a three-tier system, but avoids the use of term "benign" for any phyllodes tumor.

The presence of tumor at the resection margin is a major determinant of local recurrence. It should be noted in the assessment of these lesions (100,109a,146).

While in several studies, aneuploidy or high S-phase has been associated with aggressive behavior (108,109,148,157), the value of ploidy and S-phase as prognostic factors is controversial. El-Naggar and associates (108) performed flow cytometric DNA and cell cycle analyses on 30 phyllodes tumors to determine the potential prognostic utility of these procedures. Multivariate regression analysis of their results showed that DNA content is a significant predictor of the patient's clinical outcome. Neither DNA content nor S-phase fraction correlated with outcome in many other studies, however (116,126,134).

There is no immunohistochemical marker that can predict the behavior of a phyllodes tumor. Both the Ki-67 labeling index and p53 have been studied as possible markers predictive of recurrence. The Ki-67 labeling index cannot reliably predict recurrences (129), although there is a good correlation between conventional assessment of mitotic activity of phyllodes tumor and

MIB-1 indices (129,130) (MIB-1 is a monoclonal antibody directed against cell proliferation-associated Ki-67 antigen; the MIB-1 index expresses the percentage of MIB-1–positive proliferating stromal cells). Likewise, increased p53 expression has been noted among higher-grade phyllodes tumors, but not in lower-grade tumors or fibroadenomas. Also, a distinctive pattern of p53 immunostaining at areas of periepithelial stromal condensation and atypia is observed among high-grade phyllodes tumors (144). Nonetheless, p53 immunoexpression does not reliably predict the behavior of phyllodes tumors (129). Expression of p53 is associated with known negative prognostic factors (stromal overgrowth, nuclear pleomorphism, increased mitotic count among stromal cells, an infiltrative tumor margin, and high nuclear grade among stromal cells), but is not a useful determinant of tumor recurrence or long-term survival (110).

Recurrence and Metastases. Recurrences have been reported in 7 to 70 percent of patients with phyllodes tumors. The wide range is due to the variable proportion of aggressive lesions in different studies (91,103,104,111,117, 134,135,142,146,151,153,159,169,179,192). In general, approximately 30 percent of phyllodes tumors recur, a majority doing so within 2 years of diagnosis (90,151); they may recur several times. Recurrences generally retain the histologic features of the original neoplasm, but may develop a more aggressive phenotype (95,100,117,124,129,148). Some have suggested that the presence of a positive resection margin (incomplete excision) most closely correlates with recurrence (148). Metastases, usually preceded by local recurrences, develop in about 15 percent of patients. Rarely, extension of recurrent tumor to vital organs causes fatality in the absence of distant metastasis (159).

Metastases through the bloodstream occur in less than 10 percent of patients. A majority of the tumors metastasize to the lungs (66 percent) (180); the skeleton is involved in 28 percent, the heart in 9.4 percent (141), and the liver in 5.6 percent (168) of cases with metastases. Metastases to almost all organ sites have been reported, including intraneural and central nervous system (116,182), adrenal gland, pancreas, spleen, omentum, stomach, larynx, cervical and paraaortic lymph nodes, pleura, subpleura, gum, scalp, vulva, and even the sole of the foot (182). Lymph node metastases are generally absent (139) but have been described in less than 2 percent of cases (151,178). With rare exceptions, the metastatic tumors are devoid of epithelial elements.

Treatment and Prognosis. While the large size of even a low-grade phyllodes tumor or highly infiltrative margins around a relatively smaller tumor may necessitate a simple mastectomy, and all types of mastectomy have been used in the past (97,151), the current treatment of choice is wide local excision to achieve complete excision of the tumor (91, 112,142,151,169), preferably with a rim of uninvolved breast tissue, particularly in cases of high-grade or highly infiltrative tumors. The frequent presence of a lobulated margin has made wide local excision preferable to prevent local recurrences even for those tumors lacking an infiltrative growth pattern (139). Given the rarity of axillary lymph node metastases by phyllodes tumor, axillary node dissection is not necessary. Simple mastectomy is reserved for massive tumors, lesions with highly infiltrating margins, those with aggressive histologic features that would defy total excision with a clear margin by a lesser procedure (183,192), and for local recurrences of borderline and malignant lesions (116,169). Based on Surveillance, Epidemiolgy, and End Results data, women undergoing wide local excision have similar or improved cause-specific survival rates compared to those who have had mastectomy on both univariate and multivariate analyses; the role of radiotherapy is uncertain (140).

While pulmonary metastases may be resectable (111), surgical management for metastatic disease has proven discouraging. Combination chemotherapy (cisplatin and etoposide or ifosfamide and doxorubicin), with or without radiation therapy, has been reported to be effective in the management of symptomatic metastases (99,119). The efficacy of these therapeutic approaches has not been established, however. Cure and survival over 10 years are rare after metastasis since currently available therapies are not particularly effective for metastastic phyllodes tumor.

Patients with phyllodes tumor have an overall survival rate of 90 percent (116). The 5-year survival rate drops to about 65 percent for those

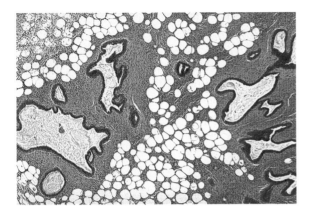

Figure 14-25

PERIDUCTAL STROMAL SARCOMA

A proliferation of stromal cells with an infiltrating pattern forms around a cluster of ducts with open lumens.

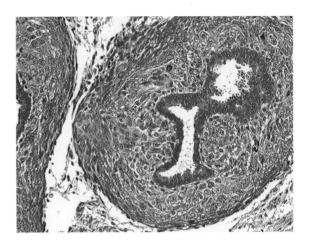

Figure 14-26

PERIDUCTAL STROMAL SARCOMA

Periductal stromal sarcoma displays a proliferation of highly atypical and mitotically active stromal cells around otherwise normal-appearing ducts.

with high-grade tumors (148,166). Among cases accumulated from 1988 to 2003 in the California Cancer Registry, the relative cumulative survival rate of patients with malignant phyllodes tumor was 87.4 percent (115b).

For practical purposes, phyllodes tumors can be divided into two groups, those with a potential for local recurrence (benign/low-grade and intermediate-grade lesions) and high-grade lesions that have the potential for metastasis (high-grade lesions). Most phyllodes tumors are low grade. In a majority of cases, the potential for recurrence is not realized and there are no reliable methods for consistent and accurate prediction of recurrences or metastases. The presence of any specific soft tissue sarcoma in a phyllodes tumor should be noted in the diagnosis (e.g., rhabdomyosarcoma arising in a phyllodes tumor).

Phyllodes Tumor in Children and Men

Given the origin of phyllodes tumor in lobules, its rarity in children and men is not surprising. In a series of the 94 patients, only 3 were younger than 20 years (151). The number of affected children is low in other reports as well (86,87,115,122, 137,159,163,182). Complete excision is crucial in the management of these tumors. Infiltrative tumor margins and positive resection margins are associated with an increased likelihood of recurrence (163).

While total excision of the lesion is the goal in the management of phyllodes tumor in children and men, special care should be taken to avoid damaging uninvolved developing breast tissue in children and adolescent females. Follow-up of the patient is necessary for those whose neoplasms display morphologically aggressive features. Special attention should be paid to distinguishing juvenile fibroadenoma from phyllodes tumor in children. It should be noted that the potential for either recurrence or metastasis is not realized in the vast majority of phyllodes tumors and we lack the ability to accurately predict which tumor will recur or metastasize.

Phyllodes tumors are particularly rare in men. None or only single cases are reported in some series (2,149,158,167).

PERIDUCTAL STROMAL TUMORS

Characterized by a cellular, sarcomatous, spindle cell proliferation around rounded or slightly irregular tubules, often with open lumens, *periductal stromal sarcoma* (PSS) lacks the leaf-like processes of typical phyllodes tumor (figs. 14-25, 14-26). PSS invariably and irregularly dissects the adjacent breast tissue, but may have a partially delineated margin. Mitotic activity is in the range of 3 to 5 per 10 high-power fields; atypia is often minimal. PSS may reflect the malignant counterpart of the pericanalicular growth pattern of fibroadenoma. In contrast to pericanalicular fibroadenoma, which occurs more often in adolescent girls, PSS rarely occurs in women younger than 40 years of age. The term *cellular periductal stromal tumor* has been applied to conventional phyllodes tumors by some pathologists (153,154).

PSS generally behaves as a low-grade sarcoma that sometimes progresses or assumes the mor-phology of typical phyllodes tumor when it recurs (193). A benign counterpart (*periductal stromal hyperplasia*) is characterized by a peri-ductal proliferation of stromal cells without significant atypia or mitotic activity.

REFERENCES

Fibroadenoma

1. Ahmed A. Atlas of the ultrastructure of human breast diseases. Edinburgh: Churchill Living-stone; 1978:58-64.
2. Ansah-Boateng Y, Tavassoli FA. Fibroadenoma and cystosarcoma phyllodes of the male breast. Mod Pathol 1992;5:114-116.
3. Archer F, Omar M. Pink cell (oncocytic) metaplasia in a fibroadenoma of the breast: electron micro-scopic observations. J Pathol 1969;119-124.
4. Ashikari R, Farrow JH, O'Hara J. Fibroadenomas in the breast of juveniles. Surg Gynecol Obstet 1971;132:259-262.
4a. Austin WE, Fidler HK. Carcinoma developing in fibroadenoma of the breast. Am J Clin Pathol 1953;23:688-690.
5. Azzopardi JG. Problems in breast pathology. In: Bennington JL, ed. Major problems in pathology, Vol. 11. Philadelphia: WB Saunders; 1979.
6. Benoit JL, Kara R, McGregor SE, Duggan MA. Fibroadenoma of the breast: diagnostic pitfalls of the fine-needle aspiration. Diagn Cytopathol 1992;8:643-648.
7. Berean K, Tron VA, Churg A, Clement PB. Mam-mary fibroadenoma with multinucleated stromal giant cells. Am J Surg Pathol 1986;10:823-827.
8. Block GE, Zlatnik PA. Giant fibroadenomata of the breast in a prepubertal girl. A case report with observations of hormonal influences. Arch Surg 1960;80:665-669.
9. Brown JM. Histological modification of fibroade-noma of the breast associated with oral hormonal contraceptives. Med J Aust 1970;1:276-277.
10. Calabrese G, Di Virgilio C, Cianchetti E, et al. Chro-mosome abnormalities in breast fibroadenoma. Genes Chromosome Cancer 1991;3:202-204.
11. Carney JA, Gordon H, Carpenter PC, Shenoy BV, Go VL. The complex of myxomas, spotty pig-mentation, and endocrine overactivity. Medicine 1985;64:270-283.
12. Carney JA, Toorkey BC. Myxoid fibroadenoma and allied conditions (myxomatosis) of the breast. A heritable disorder with special associa-tions including cardiac and cutaneous myxomas. Am J Surg Pathol 1991;15:713-721.
13. Carstens PH. Ultrastructure of human fibroad-enoma. Arch Pathol 1974;98:23-32.
14. Carter CL, Corle DK, Micozzi MS, Schatzkin A, Taylor PR. A prospective study of the de-velopment of breast cancer in 16,692 women with benign breast disease. Am J Epidemiol 1988;128:467-477.
15. Cheatle GL. Hyperplasia of epithelial and con-nective tissues in the breast: Its relation to fibro-adenoma and other pathologic conditions. Br J Surg 1923;10:436-455.
16. Cheatle GL, Cutler M. Tumours of the breast. Their pathology, symptoms, diagnosis and treat-ment. London: Arnold & Co; 1931:455-475.
17. Courcoutsakis NA, Chow CK, Shawker TH, Car-ney JA, Stratakis CA. Syndrome of spotty skin pigmentation, myxomas, endocrine overactivity, and schwannomas (Carney complex): breast im-aging findings. Radiology 1997;205:221-227.
18. Delarue J, Redon H. Les Infarctus des fibroad-enomes mammaires. Problem clinique et patho-genique. Sem Hop 1949;25:2991-2996.
19. Demetrakopoulos NJ. Three-dimensional recon-struction of a human mammary fibroadenoma. Q Bull Northwestern Univ Med Sch 1958;32:221–228.
20. Diaz NM, Palmer JO, McDivitt RW. Carcinoma arising within fibroadenomas of the breast. A clinicopathologic study of 105 patients. Am J Clin Pathol 1991;95:614-622.
21. Dupont WD, Page DL, Parl FF, et al. Long-term risk of breast cancer in women with fibroad-enoma, N Engl J Med 1994;331:10–15.
22. Duray PH, Holahan K, Merino M, et al. Ado-lescent cellular fibroadenomas: a clinical and pathologic study. Abstracts, annual meeting of IAP. Lab Invest 1984;50:17A.
22a. Eusebi V, Azzopardi JG. Lobular endocrine neo-plasia in fibroadenoma of the breast. Histopa-thology 1980;4:413-428.

23. Farrow JH, Ashikari H. Breast lesions in young girls. Surg Clin North Am 1969;49:261-269.

24. Fechner RE. Fibroadenomas in patients receiving oral contraceptives: a clinical and pathologic study. Am J Clin Pathol 1970;53:857-864.

25. Fekete P, Petrek J, Majmudar B, Someren A, Sandberg W. Fibroadenomas with stromal cellularity. A clinicopathologic study of 21 patients. Arch Pathol Lab Med 1987;111:427-432.

26. Fisher ER. Ultrastructure of human breast and its disorders. Am J Clin Pathol 1976;66:291-375.

27. Fletcher JA, Pinkus GS, Weidner N, Morton CC. Lineage-restricted clonality in biphasic solid tumors. Am J Pathol 1991;138:1199-1207.

28. Fondo EY, Rosen PP, Fracchia AA, et al. The problem of carcinoma developing in a fibroadenoma. Recent experience at Memorial Hospital. Cancer 1979;43:563-567.

29. Frantz VK, Pickren JW, Melcher GW, Auchincloss H Jr. Incidence of chronic cystic disease in so-called "normal breast." A study based on 225 postmortem examinations. Cancer 1951;4:762-783.

30. Funderburk WW, Rosero E, Leffall LD. Breast lesions in blacks. Surg Gynecol Obstet 1972;135:58-60.

31. Geschickter CF. Diseases of the breast. Diagnosis, pathology, treatment. 2nd ed. Philadelphia: JB Lippincott; 1945:291-324.

32. Geschickter CF, Lewis D, Hartman CG. Tumors of the breast related to the oestrin hormone. Am J Cancer 1934;21:828-859.

33. Giani C, D'Amore E, Delarue JC, et al. Estrogen and progesterone receptors in benign breast tumors and lesions: relationship with histological and cytological features. Int J Cancer 1986;37:7-10.

34. Gibert MA, Noel P, Faucon M, Pavans de Ceccatty M. Comparative immunohistochemical localization of fibronectin and actin in human breast tumor cells in vivo and in vitro. Virchows Arch B Cell Pathol Incl Mol Pathol 1982;40:99-112.

35. Goldenberg VE, Wiegenstein L, Mottet NK. Florid breast fibroadenomas in patients taking hormonal oral contraceptives. Am J Clin Pathol 1968;49:52-59.

36. Goodman ZD, Taxy JB. Fibroadenomas of the breast with prominent smooth muscle. Am J Surg Pathol 1981;5:99–101.

37. Haagensen CD. Diseases of the breast, 3rd ed. Philadelphia: WB Saunders Co; 1986:267-283.

38. Hasson J, Pope CH. Mammary infarcts associated with pregnancy presenting as breast tumors. Surgery 1961;49:313-316.

39. Heywang SH, Wolf A, Pruss E, Hilbertz T, Eirmann W, Permanetter W. MR imaging of the breast with Gd-DTPA use and limitation. Radiology 1989;171:95-103.

40. Hochman MG, Orel SG, Powell CM, Schnall MD, Reynolds CA, White LN. Fibroadenomas: MR imaging appearances with radiologic-histopathologic correlation. Radiology 1997;204:123-129.

41. Hunter TB, Roberts CC, Hunt KR, Fajardo LL. Occurrence of fibroadenomas in postmenopausal women referred for breast biopsy. J Am Geriatr Soc 1996;44:61-64.

42. Iglesias A, Arias M, Santiago P, Rodriguez M, Manas J, Saborido C. Benign breast lesions that simulate malignancy: magnetic resonance imaging with radiologic-pathologic correlation. Curr Probl Diagn Pathol 2007;36:66-82.

43. Jao W, Vazquez LT, Keh PC, et al. Myoepithelial differentiation and basal lamina deposition in fibroadenoma and adenosis of the breast. J Pathol 1978;126:107-112.

44. Jordal K, Sorensen B. Giant fibroadenoma of the breast. Report of two cases, one treated with mammoplasty. Acta Chir Scand 1961;122:147-151.

45. Kodlin D, Winger EE, Morgestern NL, Chen U. Chronic mastopathy and breast cancer. A follow-up study. Cancer 1977;39:2603-2607.

46. Koerner FC, O'Connell JX. Fibroadenoma: morphological observations and a theory of pathogenesis. Pathol Annu 1994;29:1-19.

47. Krieger N, Hiatt RA. Risk of breast cancer after benign breast diseases. Variation by histologic type, degree of atypia, age at biopsy, and length of follow-up. Am J Epidemiol 1992;136:619-631.

48. Kutten F, Fournier S, Durand JC, Mauvais-Jarvis P. Estradiol and progesterone receptors in human breast fibroadenomas. J Clin Endocrinol Metab 1981;52:1225-1229.

49. Lacombe MJ, Llombart-Bosch A, Lecluse Y, Bertin F, Contesso G. [Fibroadenoma of the breast with atypical clear-cell epithelial hyperplasia.] Ann Pathol 1986;1:37-44. [French.]

50. Lefer LG. Fibroadenoma of the breast with prominent mucinous stromal component. Arch Pathol Lab Med 1982;106:649-650.

51. Lee AH, Hodi Z, Ellis IO, Elston CW. Histological features useful in the distinction of phyllodes tumour and fibroadenoma on needle core biopsy of the breast. Histopathology 2007;51:336-44.

52. Levi F, Randimbison L, Te VC, La Vecchia C. Incidence of breast cancer in women with fibroadenoma. Int J Cancer1994;57:681-683.

53. Liedke C, Kersting C, Burger H, Kiesel L, Wulfing P. Caveolin-1 expression in benign and malignant lesions of the breast. World J Surg Oncol 2007;5:110-118.

54. Lopez-Ferrer P, Jimenez-Heffernan JA, Vicandi B, Ortega L, Viguen JM. Fine needle aspiration cytology of breast fibroadenoma. A cytohistologic correlation study of 405 cases. Acta Cytol 1999;43:579-586.

55. MacKenzie DH. A fibro-adenoma of the breast with smooth muscle. J Pathol Bacteriol 1968;96: 231-232.

56. Malberger E, Yerushalmi R, Tamir A, Keren R. Diagnosis of fibroadenoma in breast fine needle aspirates devoid of typical stroma. Acta Cytol 1997;41:1483-1488.

57. McCutcheon JM, Lipa M. Infarction of a fibroadenoma of breast following fine needle aspiration. Cytopathology 1993;4:247-250.

58. McDivitt RW, Stephens JA, Lee NC, Wingo PA, Rubin GL, Gersell D. Histologic types of benign breast disease and the risk of breast cancer. Cancer 1992;69:1408-1414.

58a. McDivitt RW, Stewart FW, Farrow JH. Breast carcinoma arising in solitary fibro-adenomas. Surg Gynecol Obstet 1967;125:572-576.

59. Mechtersheimer G, Kruger KH, Born IA, Moller P. Antigenic profile of mammary fibroadenoma and cystosarcoma phyllodes. A study using antibodies to estrogen and progesterone receptors and to a panel of cell surface molecules. Pathol Res Pract 1990;186:427-438.

60. Mies C, Rosen PP. Juvenile fibroadenoma with atypical epithelial hyperplasia. Am J Surg Pathol 1987;11:184-190.

61. Nambiar R, Kutty MK. Giant fibroadenoma (cystosarcoma phyllodes) in adolescent female—a clinicopathological study. Br J Surg 1974;61:113-117.

62. Nielsen BB. Fibroadenomatoid hyperplasia of the male breast. Am J Surg Pathol 1990;14:774-777.

63. Nielsen BB, Ladefoged C. Fibroadenoma of the female breast with multinucleated giant cells. Pathol Res Pract 1985;180:721-724.

64. Noguchi S, Aihara T, Motomura K, et al. Demonstration of polyclonal origin of giant fibroadenoma of the breast. Virchows Arch 1995;427:343-347.

65. Noguchi S, Motomura K, Inaji H, Imaoki S, Koyama H. Clonal analysis of fibroadenoma and phyllodes tumor of the breast. Cancer Res 1993;53:4071-4074.

66. Noguchi S, Yokouchi H, Aihara T, et al. Progression of fibroadenoma to phyllodes tumor demonstrated by clonal analysis. Cancer 1995;76:1779-1785.

67. Oberman HA. Breast lesions in the adolescent female. Pathol Annu 1979;14:175-201.

68. Ohtani H, Sasano N. Stromal cells of the fibroadenoma of the breast. An immunohistochemical and ultrastructural study. Virchows Arch A Pathol Anat Histopathol 1984;404:7-16.

69. Orcel L, Douvin D. Contribution a l'etude histogenetique des fibroadenomes mammaries. Ann Anat Pathol 1973;18:255-276.

70. Owens FM, Adams WE. Giant intracanalicular fibroadenoma of the breast. Arch Surg 1941;43:588-598.

71. Ozzello L, Gump FE. The management of patients with carcinomas in fibroadenomatous tumors of the breast. Surg Gynecol Obstet 1985;160:99-104.

72. Pike AM, Oberman HA. Juvenile (cellular) adenofibromas. A clinicopathologic study. Am J Surg Pathol 1985;9:730-736.

73. Powell CM, Cranor ML, Rosen PP. Multinucleated stromal giant cells in mammary fibroepithelial neoplasms. A study of 11 patients. Arch Pathol Lab Med 1994;118:912-916.

74. Rao BR, Meyer JS, Fry CG. Most cystosarcoma phyllodes and fibroadenomas have progesterone receptors but lack estrogen receptor: stromal localization of progesterone receptor. Cancer 1981;47:2016-2921.

75. Rosen PP. Multinucleated mammary stromal giant cells: a benign lesion that stimulates invasive carcinoma. Cancer 1979;44:1305-1308.

76. Salm R. Epidermoid metaplasia in mammary fibroadenoma with formation of keratin cysts. J Pathol Bacteriol 1957;74:221-222.

77. Silverman JS, Tamsen A. Mammary fibroadenoma and some phyllodes tumour stroma are composed of CD34+ fibroblasts and factor XIIIa+ dendrophages. Histopathology 1996;29:411-419.

78. Spagnolo DV, Shilkin KB. Breast neoplasms containing bone and cartilage. Virchows Arch A Pathol Anat Histopathol 1983;400:287-295.

79. Staats B, Bonk U, Wanschura S, et al. A fibroadenoma with a t(4;12) (q27;q15) affecting the HMG1-C gene, a member of the high motility group pattern gene family. Breast Cancer Res Treat 1996;38:299-303.

80. Stephenson CF, Davis RI, Moore GE, Sandberg AA. Cytogenetic and fluorescence in situ hybridization analysis of breast fibroadenomas. Cancer Genet Cytogenet 1992;63:32-36.

81. Tavassoli FA. Pathology of the breast, 2nd ed. Stamford, CT: Appleton-Lange.McGraw Hill; 1999.

82. Wellings SR, Jensen HM, Marcum RG. An atlas of subgross pathology of the human breast with special reference to possible precancerous lesions. J Natl Cancer Inst 1975;55:231-273.

83. Willis RA. Pathology of tumors, 4th ed. London: Butterworths; 1967:215-216.

84. Yu H, Rohan TE, Cook MG, Howe GR, Miller AB. Risk factors for fibroadenoma: a case-control study in Australia. Am J Epidemiol 1992;135:247-258.

Phyllodes Tumor

85. Ackerman LV, Taylor HB. Seminar on lesions of the breast. In: Proceedings of the American Society of Clinical Pathologists. Chicago: American Society of Clinical Pathology; 1956.

86. Adami HO, Hakelius L, Rimsten A, Willen R. Malignant locally recurrent cystosarcoma phyllodes in an adolescent female. Acta Chir Scand 1984;150:93-100.

87. Amerson JR. Cystosarcoma phyllodes in adolescent females. A report of seven patients. Ann Surg 1970;171:849-858.

88. Aranda FI, Laforga JB, Lopez JI. Phyllodes tumor of the breast. An immunohistochemical study of 28 cases with special attention to the role of myofibroblasts. Pathol Res Pract 1994;190:474-481.

89. Ariel L. Skeletal metastases in cystosarcoma phyllodes. A case report and review. Arch Surg 1961;82:275-280.

89a. Azzopardi JG. Problems in breast pathology, Vol 11. In: Major problems in pathology. Philadelphia: Saunders; 1979:354-355.

90. Barth RJ Jr. Histologic features predict local recurrence after breast conserving therapy of phyllodes tumors. Breast Cancer Res Treat 1999;57:291-295.

91. Bartoli C, Zurrida SM, Clemente C. Phyllodes tumor in male patients with bilateral gynecomastia induced by oestrogen therapy for prostatic carcinoma. Eur J Surg Oncol 1991;17:215-217.

92. Bernstein L, Deapen D, Ross RK. The descriptive epidemiology of malignant cystosarcoma phyllodes tumors of the breast. Cancer 1993;71:3020-3024.

93. Birdsall SH, Summersgill BM, Egan M, Fentiman IS, Gusterson BA, Shipley JM. Additional copies of 1q in sequential samples from a phyllodes tumor of the breast. Cancer Genet Cytogenet 1995;83:111-114.

94. Bittesini L, Dei Tos AP, Doglioni C, Della Libera D, Laurino L, Fletcher CD. Fibroepithelial tumor of the breast with digital fibroma-like inclusions in the stromal component. Case report with immunocytochemical analysis. Am J Surg Pathol 1994;18:296-301.

95. Blichert-Toft M, Hansen JP, Hansen OH, Schiodt T. Clinical course of cystosarcoma phyllodes related to histologic appearance. Surg Gynecol Obstet 1975;140:929-932.

96. Bot FJ, Sleddens HF, Dinjens WN. Molecular assessment of clonality leads to the identification of a new germ line TP53 mutation associated with malignant cystosarcoma phyllodes and soft tissue sarcoma. Diagn Mol Pathol 1998;7:295-301.

97. Buchanan EB. Cystosarcoma phyllodes and its surgical management. Am Surg 1995;61:350-355.

98. Buchberger W, Strasser K, Heim K, Muller E, Schrocksnadel H. Phylloides tumor: findings on mammography, sonography, and aspiration cytology in 10 cases. AJR Am J Roentgenol 1991;157:715-719.

99. Burton GV, Hart LL, Leight GS Jr, Iglehart JD, McCarty KS Jr, Cox EB. Cystosarcoma phyllodes. Effective therapy with cisplatin and etoposide chemotherapy. Cancer 1989;63:2088-2092.

100. Cheng SP, Chang YC, Liu TP, Lee JJ, Tzen CY, Liu CL. Phyllodes tumor of the breast: the challenge persists. World J Surg 2006;30:1414-1421.

101. Chowdhury C, Chattopadhyay TK, Pramanik M, Sarathy VV, Verma K. Cystosarcoma phyllodes—A clinicopathologic analysis of 32 cases. Indian J Cancer 1984;21:23-30.

102. Christensen L, Schiodt T, Blichert-Toft M. Sarcomatoid tumours of the breast in Denmark from 1977 to 1987. A clinicopathological and immunohistochemical study of 100 cases. Eur J Cancer 1993;29A:1824-1831.

103. Ciatto S, Bonardi R, Cataliotti L, Cardona G. Phyllodes tumor of the breast: a multicenter series of 59 cases. Eur J Surg Oncol 1992;18:545-549.

104. Cohn-Cedermark G, Rutqvist LE, Rosendahl T, Rosendahl I, Silversward C. Prognostic factors in cystosarcoma phyllodes. A clinicopathologic study of 77 patients. Cancer 1991;68:2017-2022.

104a. Cornog JL, Mobini J, Steiger E, et al. Squamous carcinoma of the breast. Am J Clin Pathol 1971;55:410-417.

105. Czum JM, Sanders LM, Titus JM, Kalisher L. Breast imaging of the day. Benign phyllodes tumor. Radiographic 1997;17:548-551.

106. Dietrich CU, Pandis N, Rizou H, et al. Cytogenetic findings in phyllodes tumors of the breast. Karyotypic complexity differentiates between malignant and benign tumors. Hum Pathol 1997;28:1379-1382.

107. Dusenbery D, Frable WJ. Fine needle aspiration cytology of phyllodes tumor. Potential diagnostic pitfalls. Acta Cytol 1992;36:215-221.

108. El-Naggar AK, Mackay B, Sneige N, Batsakis JG. Stromal neoplasms of the breast: a comparative flow cytometric study. J Surg Oncol 1990;44:151-156.

109. El-Naggar AK, Ro JY, McLemore D, Garnsy L. DNA content and proliferative activity of cystosarcoma phyllodes of the breast. Potential prognostic significance. Am J Clin Pathol 1990;93:980-985.

109a. Esposito NN, Mohan D, Brufsky A, Lin Y, Kapali M, Dabbs DJ. Phyllodes tumor: a clinicopathologic and immunohistochemical study of 30 cases. Arch Pathol Lab Med 2006;130:1516-1521.

110. Feakins RM, Mulcahy HE, Nickols CD, Wells CA. P53 expression in phyllodes tumours is associated with histological features of malignancy but does not predict outcome. Histopathology 1999;35:162-169.

111. Fernandez BB, Hernandez FJ, Spindler W. Metastatic cystosarcoma phyllodes: a light and electron microscopic study. Cancer 1976;37:1737-1746.

112. Fou A, Schnabel FR, Hamela-Bena D, et al. Long-term outcomes of malignant phyllodes tumors patients: an institutional experience. Am J Surg 2006;192:492-495.

113. Foxcroft LM, Evans EB, Porter AJ. Difficulties in the pre-operative diagnosis of phyllodes tumours of the breast: a study of 84 cases. Breast 2007;16:27-37.

114. Geisler DP, Boyle MJ, Malnar KF, et al. Phyllodes tumors of the breast: a review of 32 cases. Am J Surg 2000;66:360-366.

115. Gibbs BF, Roe RD, Thomas DF. Malignant cystosarcoma phyllodes in a pre-pubertal female. Ann Surg 1968;167:229-231.

115a. Gilks B, Tavassoli FA. Coexistence of intracytoplasmic lumens and membrane bound vesicles in an invasive carcinoma arising in a cystosarcoma phyllodes. Ultrastruct Pathol 1988;12:631-642.

115b. Grabowski J, Salztein SL, Sadler GR, Blair SL. Malignant phyllodes tumors: a review of 752 cases. Am Surg 2007;73:967-969.

116. Grimes M. Cystosarcoma phyllodes of the breast: histological features, flow cytometric analysis, and clinical correlations. Mod Pathol 1992;5:232-239.

116a. Grove A, Kristensen LD. Intraductal carcinoma within a phyllodes tumor of the breast: a case report. Tumori 1986;72:187-190.

117. Hajdu SI, Espinosa MH, Robbins GF. Recurrent cystosarcoma phyllodes: a clinicopathologic study of 32 cases. Cancer 1976;38:1402-1406.

117a. Harris M, Persaud V. Carcinosarcoma of the breast. J Pathol 1974;112:99-105.

118. Hawkins RE, Schofield JB, Fisher C, Wiltshaw E, McKinna JA. The clinical and histologic criteria that predict metastases from cystosarcoma phyllodes. Cancer 1992;69:141-147.

119. Hawkins RE, Schofield JB, Wiltshaw E, Fisher C, McKinna JA. Ifosfamide is an active drug for chemotherapy of metastatic cystosarcoma phyllodes. Cancer 1992;69:2271-2275.

120. Hiroaka N, Mukai M, Hosoda Y, Hata J. Phyllodes tumor of the breast containing the intracytoplasmic inclusion bodies identical with infantile digital fibromatosis. Am J Surg Pathol 1994;18:506-511.

121. Holthouse DJ, Smith PA, Naunton-Morgan R, Minchin D. Cystosarcoma phyllodes: the Western Australian experience. Aust N Z J Surg 1999;69:635-638.

122. Hoover HC, Trestioreanu A, Ketcham AS. Metastatic cystosarcoma phyllodes in an adolescent girl: an unusully malignant tumor. Ann Surg 1975;181:279-282.

123. Horie A. Fine structure of cystosarcoma phyllodes with reference to smooth muscle tumors. Acta Pathol Jpn 1981;31:1015-1028.

124. Inoshita S. Phyllodes tumor (cystosarcoma phyllodes) of the breast. A clinicopathologic study of 45 cases. Acta Pathol Jpn 1988;38:21-33.

125. Kay S. Light and electron microscopic studies of a malignant cystosarcoma phyllodes featuring stromal cartilage and bone. Am J Clin Pathol 1971;55:770-776.

126. Keelan PA, Myers JL, Wold LE, Katzmann JA, Gibney DJ. Phyllodes tumor: clinicopathologic review of 60 patients and flow cytometric analysis in 30 patients. Hum Pathol 1992;23:1048-1054.

127. Kessinger A, Foley JF, Lemon HM, Miller DM. Metastatic cystosarcoma phyllodes: a case report and review of the literature. J Surg Oncol 1972;4:131-147.

128. Kim CJ, Kim WH. Patterns of p53 expression in phyllodes tumors of the breast—an immunohistochemical study. J Korean Med Sci 1993;8:325-328.

129. Kleer CG, Giordano TJ, Braun T, Oberman HA. Pathologic, immunohistochemical and molecular features of benign and malignant phyllodes tumors of the breast. Mod Pathol 2001;14:185-190.

129a. Knudsen PJ, Ostegaard J. Cystosarcoma phyllodes with lobular and ductal carcinoma in situ. Arch Pathol Lab Med 1987;111:873-875.

130. Kocava L, Skalova A, Fakan F, Rousarova M. Phyllodes tumour of the breast: immunohistochemical study of 37 tumours using MIB1 antibody. Pathol Res Pract 1998;194:97-104.

131. Kube MJ, Greenberg ML. Cytology of a benign phyllodes tumor with keratin cyst formation: a spectrum of diagnostic pitfalls. Cytopathology 1995;6:121-125.

132. Lae M, Vincent-Salomon A, Savignoni A, et al. Phyllodes tumors of the breast segregate in two groups according to genetic criteria. Mod Pathol 2007;20:435-444.

133. Lamovec J, Us-Krasovec M. Malignant phyllodes tumor following irradiation of the breast. Pathol Res Pract 1985;180:727-732.

134. Layfield LJ, Hart J, Neuwirt H, Bohman R, Trumbull WE, Guiliano AE. Relation between DNA ploidy and the clinical behavior of phyllodes tumors. Cancer 1989;64:1486-1489.

134a. Leong AS, Meredith DJ. Tubular carcinoma developing within a recurring cystosarcoma phyllodes of the breast. Cancer 1980;46:1863-1967.

135. Lester J, Stout AP. Cystosarcoma phyllodes. Cancer 1954;7:335-353.

136. Leuschner E, Meyer-Bolte K, Caselitz J, Bartnitzke S, Bullerdiek J. Fibroadenoma of the breast showing a translocation (6;14), a ring chromosome and two markers involving parts of chromosome 11. Cancer Genet Cytogenet 1994;76:145-147.

137. Leveque J, Meunier B, Wattier E, Burtin F, Grall JY, Kerisit J. Malignant cystosarcoma phyllodes of the breast in adolescent females. Eur J Obstet Gynecol Reprod Biol 1994;18:197-203.

138. Liberman L, Bonaccio E, Hamele-Bene D, Abramson AF, Cohen MA, Deershaw DD. Benign and malignant phyllodes tumors: mammographic and sonographic findings. Radiology 1996;198:121-124.

139. Mangi AA, Smith BL, Gadd MA, Tanabe KK, Oh J, Souba WW. Surgical management of phyllodes tumors. Arch Surg 1999;134:487-492.

140. Macdonald QK, Lee CM, Tward JD, Chappel CD, Gaffney DK. Malignant phyllodes tumor of the female breast. Association of primary therapy with cause-specific survival from the Surveillance, Epidemiology, and End Results (SEER) Program. Cancer 2006;107:2127-2133.

141. McCullough K, Lynch JM. Metastatic sarcoma of the heart from cystosarcoma phyllodes of the breast. Md Med J 1960;9:66-68.

142. McGregor GI, Knowling MA, Este FA. Sarcoma and cystosarcoma phyllodes tumors of the breast—a retrospective review of 58 cases. Am J Surg 1994;167:477-480.

143. Mentzel T, Kosmehl H, Katenkamp D. Metastasizing phyllodes tumour with malignant fibrous histiocytoma-like areas. Histopathology 1991;19:557-560.

144. Millar EK, Beretov J, Marr P, et al. Malignant phyllodes tumours of the breast display increased stromal p53 protein expression. Histopathology 1999;34:491-496.

145. Minkowitz S, Zeichner M, Di Maio V, Nicastri AD. Cystosarcoma phyllodes: a unique case with multiple unilateral lesions and ipsilateral axillary metastasis. J Pathol Bacteriol 1986;96:514-517.

146. Moffat CJ, Pinder SE, Dixon AR, Elston CW, Blamey RW, Ellis IO. Phyllodes tumours of the breast: a clinicopathologic review of thirty-two cases. Histopathology 1995;27:205-218.

147. Mueller J. Ueber den feinern Bau und die Formen der krankhaften Geschwuelste. Berlin: G. Reimer; 1838:56.

148. Murad TM, Hines JR, Beal J, Bauer K. Histopathological and clinical correlations of cystosarcoma phyllodes. Arch Pathol Lab Med 1988;112:752-756.

149. Nielsen VT, Andreasen C. Phyllodes tumor of the male breast. Histopathology 1987;11:761-762.

150. Nejc D, Pasz-Walczak G, Piekarski J, et al. Astonishingly rapid growth of malignant cystosarcoma phyllodes tumor in a pregnant woman—a case report. Int J Gynecol Cancer 2007 [Epub ahead of print].

151. Norris HJ, Taylor HB. Relationship of histologic features to behavior of cystosarcoma phyllodes. Analysis of ninety-four cases. Cancer 1967;20:2090-2099.

152. Notley RG, Griffiths HJ. Bilateral malignant cystosarcoma phyllodes. Br J Surg 1965;52:360-362.

153. Oberman HA. Cystosarcoma phyllodes. A clinicopathologic study of hypercellular periductal stromal tumors of the breast. Cancer 1965;18:697-710.

154. Oberman HA, Nosanchuk JS, Finger JE. Periductal stromal tumors of the breast with adipose metaplasia. Arch Surg 1969;98:384-387.

155. Ogawa Y, Nishioka A, Tsuboi N, et al. Dynamic MR appearance of benign phyllodes tumor of the breast in a 20-year-old woman. Radiat Med 1997;15:247-250.

156. Ohta H, Yamamoto S, Ukikusa M, Awane H, Shintaku M, Irie K. Tc-99 sestamibi and Tc-99m HMDP uptake in a malignant phyllodes tumor of the breast. Clin Nucl Med 1997;22:553-554.

156a. Padmanabhan V, Dahlstrom JE, Chong G, Bennett G. Phyllodes tumor with lobular carcinoma in situ and liposarcomatous stroma. Pathology 1997;29:224-226.

157. Palko MJ, Wang SE, Shackney SE, Cottington EM, Levitt SB, Hartsock RJ. Flow cytometric S fraction as a predictor of clinical outcome in cystosarcoma phyllodes. Arch Pathol Lab Med 1990;114:949-952.

158. Pantoja E, Llobet RE, Lopez E. Gigantic cystosarcoma phyllodes in a man with gynecomastia. Arch Surg 1976;111:611.

159. Pietruszka M, Barnes L. Cystosarcoma phyllodes: a clinicopathologic analysis of 42 cases. Cancer 1978;41:1974-1983.

160. Polito P, Cin PD, Pauwels P, et al. An important subgroup of phyllodes tumors of the breast is characterized by rearrangements of chromosomes 1q and 10q. Oncol Rep 1998;5:1099-1102.

161. Powell CM, Rosen PP. Adipose differentiation in cystosarcoma phyllodes. A study of 14 cases. Am J Surg Pathol 1994;18:720-727.

162. Qizilbash AH. Cystosarcoma phyllodes with liposarcomatous stroma. Am J Clin Pathol 1976;65:321-327.

163. Rajan PB, Cranor ML, Rosen P. Cystosarcoma phyllodes in adolescent girls and young women. A study of 45 patients. Am J Surg Pathol 1998;22:64-69.

164. Rao BR, Meyer JS, Fry G. Most cystosarcoma phyllodes and fibroadenomas have progesterone receptors but lack estrogen receptor: stromal localization of progesterone receptors. Cancer 1981;47:2016-2021.

165. Reich T, Solomon C. Bilateral cystosarcoma phyllodes, malignant variant, with a 14-year follow-up: case report. Ann Surg 1958;147:39-43.

166. Reinfuss M, Mitus J, Duda K, et al. The treatment and prognosis of patients with phyllodes tumor of the breast: an analysis of 170 cases. Cancer 1996;77:910-916.

167. Reingold IM, Ascher GS. Cystosarcoma phyllodes in a man with gynecomastia. Am J Clin Pathol 1970;53:852-856.

168. Riepl M, Strnad V. [Radiochemotherapy in the liver metastases of cystosarcoma phyllodes.] Strahlenther Onkol 1994;170:668-672. [German.]

168a. Ross ED. Malignancy occurring in cystosarcoma phyllodes. Am J Surg 1954;88:243-247.

169. Salvadori B, Cosumano F, Del Bo R, et al. Surgical treatment of phyllodes tumors of the breast. Cancer 1989;63:2532-2536.

170. Sapino A, Bosco M, Cassoni P, et al. Estrogen receptor-beta is expressed in stromal cells of fibroadenoma and phyllodes tumors of the breast. Mod Pathol 2006;19:599-606.

171. Sawyer EJ, Hanby AM, Ellis P, et al. Molecular analysis of phyllodes tumors reveals distinct changes in the epithelial and stromal components. Am J Pathol 2000;156:1093-198.

172. Seijo L, Sidhy J, Mizrachy B, Shfir M, Tartter P, Bleiweiss IJ. Malignant phyllodes tumor of the breast. A report of four cases with associated fibroadenomata. Int J Surg Pathol 1995;3:17-22.

173. Shabalova IP, Chemeris GJ, Ermilova VD, Rodionova LM, Pavlikova NA, Syrjanen KJ. Phyllodes tumour: cytologic and histologic presentation of 22 cases, and immunohistochemical demonstration of p53. Cytopathology 1997;8:177-187.

174. Shabb NS. Phyllodes tumor. Fine needle aspiration cytology of eight cases. Acta Cytol 1997;41:321-326.

175. Shin SJ, Rosen PP. Bilateral presentation of fibroadenoma with digital fibroma-like inclusions in the male breast. Arch Pathol Lab Med 2007;131:1126-1129.

176. Silver S, Tavassoli FA. Osteosarcomatous differentiation in phyllodes tumors. Am J Surg Pathol 1999;23:815-821.

177. Smith BH, Taylor HB. The occurrence of bone and cartilage in mammary tumors. Am J Clin Pathol 1969;51:610-618.

178. Staren ED, Lynch G, Boyle C, Witt TR, Bines SD. Malignant cystosarcoma phyllodes. Am Surg 1994;60:583-585.

179. Stebbing JF, Nash AG. Diagnosis and management of phyllodes tumour of the breast: experience of 33 cases at a specialist center. Ann R Coll Surg Engl 1995;77:181-184.

180. Takahashi M, Murata K, Mori M, et al. Giant metastatic cystosarcoma phyllodes to the lung: CT and MR findings. Radiat Med 1992;10:210-213.

181. Tan PH. 2005 Galloway Memorial Lecture: Breast phyllodes tumours—morphology and beyond. Ann Acad Med Singapore 2005;34:671-677.

181. Tavassoli FA. Pathology of the breast, 2nd ed. Stamford, CT: Appleton & Lange/McGraw Hill; 1999.

183. Tavassoli FA, Devilee P. WHO classification of tumors. Tumors of the breast and female genital organs. Lyon: IARC; 2003:100-103.

184. Tsa WC, Jin JS, Yu JC, Sheu LF. CD10, actin, and vimentin expression in breast phyllodes tumors correlates with the grades of WHO grading system. Int J Surg Pathol 2006;14:922-936.

185. Toker C. Cystosarcoma phyllodes: an ultrastructural study. Cancer 1968;21:1171-1179.

186. Treves N. A study of cystosarcoma phyllodes. Ann N Y Acad Sci 1964;114:922-936.

187. Umekita Y, Yoshida H. Immunohistochemical study of MIB1 expression in phyllodes tumor and fibroadenoma. Pathol Int 1999;49:807-810.

188. Uribe A, Bravo G, Uribe A, Blada R, Capetillo M, Villarroel T. [Phyllodes tumor: diagnosis and treatment.] Rev Chir Obstet Ginecol 1995;60:17-22. [Spanish.]

189. Wang ZC, Buraimoh A, Iglehart JD, Richardson AL. Genome-wide analysis for loss of heterozygosity in primary and recurrent phyllodes tumor and fibroadenoma of the breast using single nucleotide polymorphism arrays. Br Cancer Res Treat 2006;97:301-309.

190. Ward RM, Evans HL. Cystosarcoma phyllodes. A clinicopathologic study of 26 cases. Cancer 1986;58:2282–2289.

191. Zamecnik M, Kinkor Z, Chlumska A. CD10+ stromal cells in fibroadenomas and phyllodes tumors of the breast. Virchows Arch 2006;448:871-872.

192. Zurrida S, Bartoli C, Galimberti V, et al. Which therapy for unexpected phyllodes tumour of the breast? Eur J Cancer 1992;28:654-657.

Periductal Stromal Tumors

193. Burga A, Tavassoli FA. Periductal stromal tumor: a rare lesion with low-grade sarcomatous behavior. Am J Surg Pathol 2003;27:343-348.

15 DISEASES OF THE NIPPLE

NIPPLE ADENOMA

Definition. *Nipple adenoma* is a benign epithelial proliferation localized within and/or around the collecting ducts. Synonyms include *nipple duct adenoma, papillary adenoma, erosive adenomatosis, florid papillomatosis*, and *papillomatosis of the nipple*. The large number of synonyms is attributable to the several morphologic lesions (some of which overlap) that are included in this condition.

Jones (27) reported the first five cases of nipple adenoma in 1955. This account was followed by larger series, including 65 cases reported by Perzin and Lattes (48) and 29 cases by Taylor and Robertson (66). A full clinicopathologic delineation is found in the series of 49 cases of "florid papillomatosis of the nipple" reported by Rosen and Caicco (54). These authors described a spectrum of lesions that they divided into two types of benign proliferative lesion. The most frequent type was described in 20 patients who had either *sclerosing adenosis* in its classic form (3 patients) or, more commonly, sclerosing adenosis complicated by pseudoinvasive features (17 patients). This type is also called *sclerosing papillomatosis* (54) and *infiltrative epitheliosis* (2). The second type, seen in 12 patients, was *epithelial hyperplasia of the collecting ducts*, also known as *papillomatosis* (54) and *epitheliosis* (2). A combination of epithelial hyperplasia and sclerosing adenosis constituted a third "mixed" type (seen in 17 patients). In addition to these types, an intraductal papilloma located deep to the adenoma was seen in 12 cases in the series of Perzin and Lattes.

The term nipple adenoma was used for the first time by Handley and Thackray in 1962 (23). It was subsequently adopted by Azzopardi et al. (2) as a practical compromise because, to use the words of Fechner and Mills (16), "it is simple, accurate and generic."

Clinical Features. Nipple adenomas are rare: only 38 cases in a total of 305,000 surgical specimens were reported by Perzin and Lattes (47).

The age ranges from 20 to 87 years (average, 43 years) (66). Cases outside this age range are anecdoctal, as was a case of a nipple adenoma present at birth (54). Less than 5 percent affect male patients (54). The duration of symptoms is extremely variable, from a month to 15 years (65), although 14 lesions in the series reported by Perzin and Lattes were incidental findings. Presenting symptoms in 51 patients from the same series were sanguineous and serous discharge in 33 patients, erosion of the nipple in 17, and a nodule in 10. A clinical impression of Paget's disease is frequent.

Sclerosing Adenosis Type of Nipple Adenoma. In this lesion, proliferating glands sprout from the collecting ducts, as was demonstrated by Perzin and Lattes (48) in three nipple adenomas in which serial sections were obtained. If the nipple is examined in perpendicular sections, the proliferating glands are seen along and around the ducts. If the nipple is cut across, then the proliferating glands show a concentric arrangement (fig. 15-1).

The glandular proliferation is usually located in the center of the nipple, within the superficial dermis; there is no contact with the malpighian

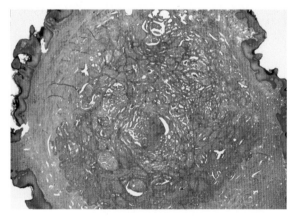

Figure 15-1

NIPPLE ADENOMA, SCLEROSING ADENOSIS TYPE
The proliferating glands have a concentric arrangement.

341

layers of the epidermis. The proliferating glands may compress the ducts, which undergo cystic dilatation. As a consequence, this type of lesion manifests clinically as a discrete nodule (fig. 15-2).

If the epidermis undergoes hyperkeratosis, the nipple is described as scaly. Rarely, the adenosis expands and results in atrophy and subsequent erosion of the epidermis. Redness, inflammation, and ulceration of the nipple are rare in this type of nipple adenoma (54).

The lesion has an edematous stroma, and its proliferating glands are composed of two-layered tubules (fig. 15-3). The luminal cells are positive for cytokeratin (CK) 7 and epithelial membrane antigen (EMA), and the basal myo-epithelial cells are positive for alpha smooth muscle actin, calponin, CK14, and S-100 protein (fig. 15-4). Apocrine differentiation of the luminal cells is rarely observed, and microcalcifications are surprisingly absent in all types of nipple adenoma.

When the pseudoinfiltrative pattern (synonym: sclerosing papillomatosis, infiltrative epitheliosis) complicates the lesion and is prominent, then an invasive carcinoma is closely simulated (fig. 15-5). This explains why this type of adenoma is the most prominent type in cases seen in consultation (54).

The pseudoinvasive changes can manifest either in the center or at the periphery of the lesion and constitute only a part of and not the entire lesion. The proliferating epithelium streams into the stroma, which reacts variably by either showing loose myxoid features or large collagenous bands similar to the keloids or elastosis that on occasion is present to a severe degree (2). The "infiltrative" epithelium appears as irregular tubules, elongated strands, or even strongly eosinophilic isolated cells.

Distinction from an invasive carcinoma depends on several factors. First, the recognition that the infiltrating area of nipple adenoma is

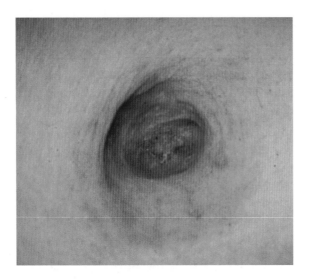

Figure 15-2

NIPPLE ADENOMA, SCLEROSING ADENOSIS TYPE

The adenoma results in a clinical nodule.

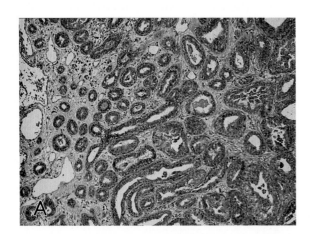
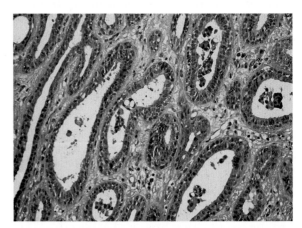

Figure 15-3

NIPPLE ADENOMA, SCLEROSING ADENOSIS TYPE

Left: The proliferating glands have edematous stroma.
Right: Two cell layers line the glands.

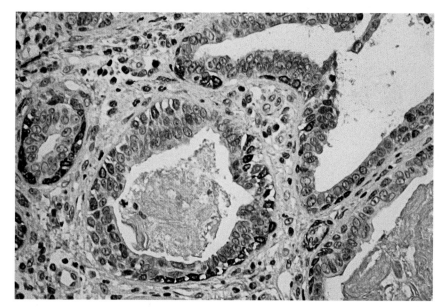

Figure 15-4

**NIPPLE ADENOMA,
SCLEROSING ADENOSIS TYPE**

The basal layer is composed of actin-rich myoepithelial elements.

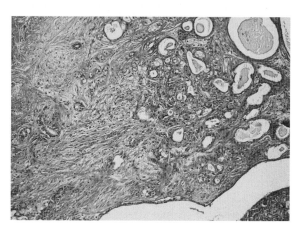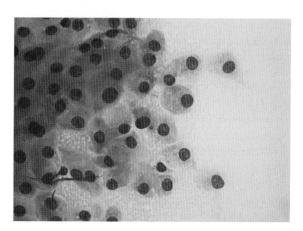

Figure 15-5

NIPPLE ADENOMA, SCLEROSING ADENOSIS TYPE

Left: The glands are distorted, have a pseudoinfiltrative pattern of growth, and occasionally show an apocrine epithelium.

Right: The apocrine epithelium, as seen in a fine needle aspiration cytology (FNAC) specimen, is composed of globoid, granular cells with round nuclei.

only part of the entire lesion, which is formed by regular, benign-looking, two-layered glands; second, that myoepithelial cells are easily identified (especially with immunohistochemistry) encircling the infiltrating epithelium; and third, the lack of anaplasia and hyperchromatism in the proliferating cells. The worrisome features relate more to the architecture rather than to the cytologic profile.

A lesion similar to sclerosing type nipple adenoma is subareolar sclerosing duct hyperplasia

(52). The only difference between the two is the deeper location of the latter.

Epithelial Hyperplasia (Papillomatosis, Epitheliosis) Type of Nipple Adenoma. This lesion is composed of the same florid benign epithelial hyperplasia ordinarily seen in other parts of the mammary duct system (see chapter 2). The epithelial proliferation is mainly located within the collecting ducts, of which several are simultaneously affected (fig. 15-6). It usually stops at the squamous-columnar junction where

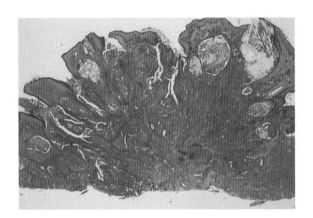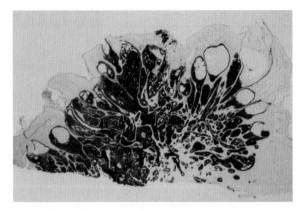

Figure 15-6

NIPPLE ADENOMA, EPITHELIAL HYPERPLASIA TYPE

Left: The nipple is transected perpendicularly. Several collecting ducts are filled by benign proliferating epithelial cells.
Right: The epithelial cells are highlighted by anticytokeratin 7 antibody.

the keratin plug of the galactophore ostium lies (fig. 15-7A). In some cases, the epithelium proliferates in a polypoid fashion causing noticeable enlargement of the collecting ducts as well as of the galactophore ostia. The keratin of the ostium unplugs and the epithelial proliferation is exposed to the exterior in a fashion reminiscent of an ectropion in the uterine cervix (fig. 15-7B–E). These cases are often clinically reported to have an ulcer and to be suspicious of Paget's disease. The hyperplastic epithelial proliferation can be so exuberant (fig. 15-8) as to give the impression of a wart (66). If trauma ensues or there is superimposed infection, a true ulcer with granulation tissue may develop (fig. 15-9).

The epithelial hyperplasia has to be distinguished from an in situ carcinoma. This can be done by applying the criteria described in chapter 2. There are two major pitfalls that have to be taken into account to avoid a diagnosis of malignancy. First, the solid exuberant intraductal proliferation frequently undergoes "comedo type" necrosis (fig. 15-10). Also, a proliferation of clear (Toker) cells (see chapter 1) is frequently observed in the epidermis bordering the ostium and overlying the adenoma. This phenomenon is mostly evident if CK7 or CAM5.2 antibodies are used (73), but Toker cells are also apparent in specimens stained with hematoxylin and eosin (H&E) (39). The Toker cell hyperplasia can be so exuberant (fig. 15-11) that Paget's disease is closely simulated, especially when an ectropion-like proliferation is present. Toker cells appear regular and are usually suprabasally

located, while Paget cells have irregular nuclei and can be found scattered through all malpighian layers. Toker cells are only positive with CK7 and CAM5.2 (35,39), while Paget cells are also EMA and c-erbB-2 positive (Table 15-1).

Nipple Adenoma and Malignancy. A review of the literature revealed 24 nipple adenomas associated with carcinoma (18 percent of total cases) (54). Nine subsequent cases were reported by Santini et al. (59) and by Jones and Tavassoli (29). The carcinomas are most frequently concurrent and are located at a distance from the nipple adenoma. The percentage of carcinomas independent of nipple adenoma varies from 1 to 5 percent. Fisher et al. (17) found 12 nipple adenomas (1.2 percent) in 967 mastectomies for breast carcinoma. Concurrent carcinomas may be located in the contralateral breast (50).

Carcinomas can supervene in the same area after the excision of a nipple adenoma (50). One patient developed an in situ carcinoma 10 years after the removal of a nipple adenoma (50). Invasive carcinoma appeared in two patients 3 and 17 years excision of a nipple adenoma. The latter developed lung metastases.

Carcinoma can develop in the areola, at a distance from a nipple adenoma. One such case was reported by Jones and Tavassoli (29), who also described two invasive carcinomas in close contact with a nipple adenoma. In situ or invasive carcinomas arising within a nipple adenoma have been reported in about 10 patients (29).

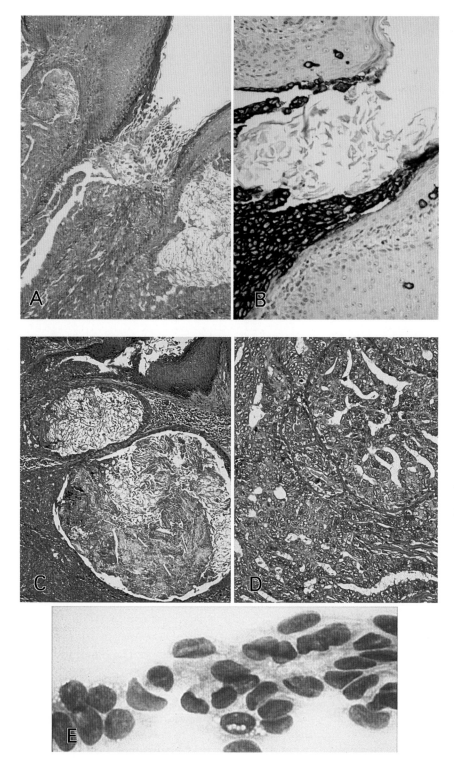

Figure 15-7

NIPPLE ADENOMA, EPITHELIAL HYPERPLASIA TYPE

A: The benign epithelium proliferates in a polypoid fashion within the terminal duct, stopping below the keratin plug at the squamous-ductal junction.

B: The ostium of this terminal duct appears enlarged and the proliferating glandular epithelium is exposed to the exterior. Dendritic Toker cells are within the epidermis (CK7).

C: Two cystic glandular dilatations are present within the benign proliferating epithelium.

D: Florid epitheliosis (epithelial hyperplasia) shows the characteristic irregular spaces. The epithelial proliferation is formed by at least two cell types.

E: FNAC of this lesion shows spindle to polygonal elements with regular nuclei. (Courtesy of Dr. R. van Pel, Amsterdam, the Netherlands.)

Treatment. Total removal of the lesion is the best treatment of nipple adenoma since occasional cases have recurred after partial excision. Radical excision requires the removal of the nipple. Patients and surgeons (as well as the authors) are reluctant to accept the aesthetically unpleasant results of tylectomy, and often "a wait and see" approach is adopted as recurrences are

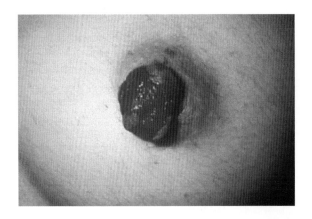

Figure 15-8

NIPPLE ADENOMA, EPITHELIAL HYPERPLASIA TYPE

Cases with exuberant epithelial hyperplasia appear clinically as wart-like lesions.

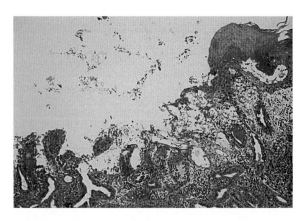

Figure 15-9

NIPPLE ADENOMA, EPITHELIAL HYPERPLASIA TYPE

This ectropion of the glandular epithelium has undergone erosion with superimposed inflammatory changes.

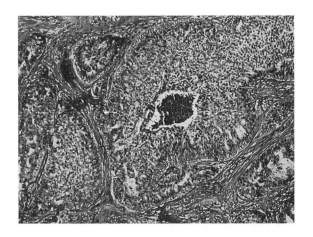

Figure 15-10

NIPPLE ADENOMA, EPITHELIAL HYPERPLASIA TYPE

Comedo necrosis is apparent within the proliferating benign epithelium.

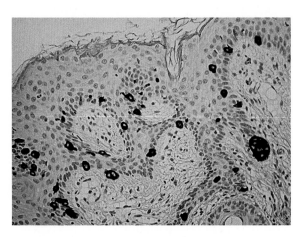

Figure 15-11

NIPPLE ADENOMA, TOKER CELL HYPERPLASIA

The epidermis shows Toker cell hyperplasia. The Toker cells are highlighted by CK7, are dendritic, and are suprabasally located. These cells were negative for c-erbB-2.

rare even in partially removed lesions. Several mastectomies have been performed in the past for nipple adenomas; in most cases, this was the result of an erroneous diagnosis of invasive carcinoma.

SYRINGOMATOUS TUMOR

Definition. *Syringomatous tumor* (SyT) is a nonmetastasizing, recurring, and locally invasive tumor of the nipple/areolar region that shows sweat duct differentiation histologically. Synonyms include *syringomatous adenoma of the nipple* and *infiltrating syringomatous adenoma of the nipple.*

This lesion of the nipple region was probably illustrated for the first time by Handley and Thackray (23), but it was fully described by Rosen in 1983 (53) who reported five cases, one of which was in a male patient. It was named syringomatous adenoma as it was composed of a proliferation of glands similar to sweat ducts, had bland cytology, and had no evidence of metastasis. Infiltrating syringomatous adenoma was the term adopted by Jones et al. (28) because the proliferating glands were seen invading nerves and muscle fibers of the nipple and the lesion recurred in 5 out of 11 patients (45 percent).

Table 15-1

DIFFERENTIAL DIAGNOSIS OF PAGET CARCINOMA AND SIMILAR LESIONS

	PC[a]	Bowen	CCDy	DNS	PMC	TCHy
Basal involvement	Possible	Constant	No	Constant	Constant	Very rare
Inflammatory band-like dermal reaction	Constant	Possible	No	Possible	No	No
Dendritic cells	Yes	No	No	Yes	Yes	Yes
Cytoplasmic melanin	Possible	Possible	Possible	Yes	No	Possible
CK7	Positive	Negative	Negative	Negative	Positive	Positive
CK20	Negative	Negative	Negative	Negative	Positive	Negative
EMA	Positive	May be positive	Negative	Negative	Negative	Rare positivity
S-100 protein	May be positive	Negative	Negative	Positive	Negative	Negative
HMB45	Negative	Negative	Negative	Positive	Negative	Negative
c-erbB-2	Positive	Negative	Negative	Negative	Negative	Negative

[a]PC: Paget carcinoma; Bowen: intraepidermal squamous cell carcinoma; CCDy: clear cell dyskeratosis; DNS: dysplastic nevus/in situ malignant melanoma; PMC: Merkel cell carcinoma with intraepidermal spread; TCHy: Toker cell hyperplasia; CK = cytokeratin; EMA = epithelial membrane antigen.

These features, not totally consistent with a benign process, led Ward et al. (72) to adopt the noncommittal term of syringomatous tumor that we feel is the most appropriate term at the present time. Ward et al. also stated that SyT belongs to a large family of neoplasms showing locally invasive growth (including perineural and smooth muscle invasion), bland cytology, and resemblance to syringoid structures.

SyTs, in addition to the nipple, have a predilection for the skin of the face, and are variously named microcystic adnexal carcinoma, sclerosing sweat duct carcinoma, malignant syringoma, sweat gland carcinoma with syringomatous features, and syringoid carcinoma (58). They also have a predilection for the breast parenchyma and in this site are named low- grade adenosquamous carcinoma (54) and syringomatous squamous tumor (64). For SyTs in the minor salivary glands, terms include syringomatous tumor (26) and syringomatous adenocarcinoma (6).

Clinical Features. SyT is a rare lesion that is mostly seen in consultation files or in slide seminars. Of the five cases reported by Rosen (52), four were derived from the author's consultation files and the fifth was a conference case. In spite of its rarity, the lesion has acquired extensive coverage in major textbooks. This is because the lesion needs to be distinguished from low-grade adenosquamous carcinoma (LASC) which is its analogue in the breast parenchyma, a histologically identical, potentially metastasizing lesion (70), as well as from tubular carcinoma. Also, it is pictorially characteristic.

Patient age range varies from 11 to 67 years, with an average of 40 years (28). SyT is described as a firm discrete mass, 1 to 3 cm, situated in the nipple and subareolar regions. The duration of the lesion prior to biopsy ranges from 3 months to several years (28).

Gross Findings. SyT is a firm, ill-defined nodule.

Microscopic Findings. Microscopically, the lesion consists of nests, branching cords, glandular structures, and small cysts containing well-developed lamellar keratin (fig. 15-12). The proliferating epithelium dissects the collagenous stroma of the nipple, encircles the lactiferous ducts (fig. 15-13), invades the smooth muscle of the nipple (fig. 15-14), and occasionally is seen in perineural spaces (28,72). The margin of invasion of these lesions is difficult to assess because neoplastic nests or branching glands can be present at a great distance from the bulk of the tumor, separated by normal tissue. The epidermis is often acanthotic and overlies keratin cysts located in the upper dermis.

The branching glands and cords are occasionally so tortuous as to resemble Chinese ideograms. The glands show small lumens in

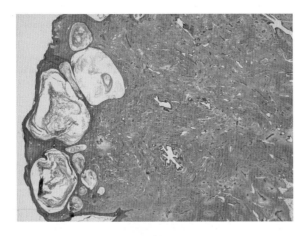

Figure 15-12

SYRINGOMATOUS TUMOR

Subepidermal keratinous cysts are numerous and the irregularly scattered syringoid glands are easily spotted since they are surrounded by edematous stroma.

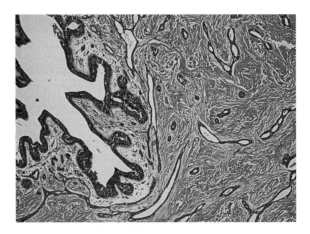

Figure 15-13

SYRINGOMATOUS TUMOR

The proliferating glands "dissect" the stroma of the nipple and surround the ducts.

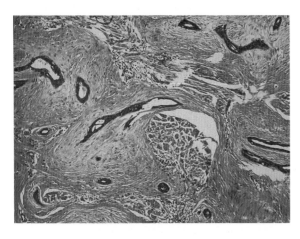

Figure 15-14

SYRINGOMATOUS TUMOR

The glands, surrounded by edematous stroma, invade the muscular tissue of the nipple.

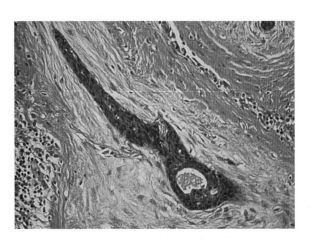

Figure 15-15

SYRINGOMATOUS TUMOR

Squamoid differentiation is readily seen in this gland, which has a lumen at one pole and a pointed end at the other.

which granular eosinophilic material is present. This material is periodic acid–Schiff (PAS) positive in the center and weakly alcianophilic at the periphery. Some lumens are very small and appear to contain nuclear debris. The branching structures occasionally show a feature unique to this tumor: squamous cords that have a pointed end and at the opposite end, a glandular lumen, resembling a needle (fig. 15-15). The glands are haphazardly intermingled with the nests and solid cords.

Cytologic Findings. Cytologically, most of the proliferating elements appear to be bland squamous cells with scant eosinophilic cytoplasm and regular round nuclei. The cells lining the lumens are cuboidal or flat and their cytoplasm, on occasion, resembles a cuticle. Frequently, the glandular structures display two rows of cells (inner luminal and outer cuboidal basal cells). The nature of the latter type of cell has not been defined (49). In the author's experience, the results of staining with smooth muscle actin antibody showed that evidence of myoepithelial cell differentiation in these basal cells is poor. There are numerous actin-positive flat cells that invest the glands in a fashion resembling myofibroblasts but most of the neoplastic structures do not contain myoepithelial actin-positive cells (fig. 15-16). Myofibroblasts are a source of major confusion in the interpretation of myoepithelial cells; ultrastructure is the only technique that can confidently demonstrate myoepithelial cells. Unfortunately, the only two cases of SyT studied ultrastructurally led to inconclusive results (28).

Mitoses are rare and necrotic areas are absent. The stroma is composed of sclerotic collagen, but areas of myxoid stroma containing spindle cells are frequent. This type of stroma forms cuffs around individual cell aggregates and is very helpful in the identification of tumor foci at low-power microscopy, a finding emphasized by Ward et al. (72).

Histogenesis. An origin from ducts of apoeccrine sweat glands of the nipple/areolar complex is highly probable. These ducts are not surrounded by myoepithelial cells. In addition, SyT is often located at the interphase between the nipple and the areola where apoeccrine glands are frequent.

Differential Diagnosis. The differential diagnosis of SyT includes low-grade adenosquamous carcinoma (LASC) of the breast parenchyma (55) and tubular carcinoma (Table 15-2). LASC is very similar to SyT, but subtle differences are present. LASCs are macroscopically larger, ranging from 0.6 to 8.6 cm (mean, 2.8 cm) (70) while SyTs range from 1 to 3 cm (mean, 1.6 cm). Twelve out of 32 cases of LASC reported by Van Hoeven et al. (70) were associated with intraductal "papillary tumors," of which 3 cases were adenomyoepithe-liomas. Three cases reported by Foschini et al. (19) were also associated with an adenomyoepithelioma. Five cases of LASC associated with complex sclerosing lesions were reported by Denley et al. (12). On the contrary, no associated epithelial proliferating changes have been associated with SyTs. Myoepithelial cells are constituents of LASC, as demonstrated by immunohistochemical (18) and ultrastructural (70) techniques, while these cells are variable in SyT (fig. 15-16). The stroma of LASC frequently contains mature lymphocytes, a finding uncommon in SyT. Differentiating these two similar lesions is important since some SyTs may invade the breast parenchyma (72) while LASCs, which are potentially metastasizing tumors, can invade the areola (55).

Tubular carcinoma rarely involves the nipple (fig. 15-17). If nipple invasion occurs, it closely mimics SyT. Tubular carcinoma is frequently associated with an in situ malignancy, a finding not seen in SyT. The tubules in tubular carcinoma

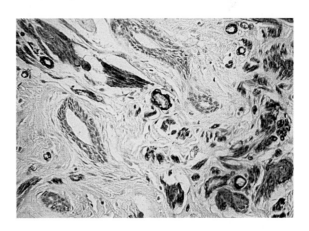

Figure 15-16

SYRINGOMATOUS TUMOR

No actin-positive myoepithelial elements are visible.

	Table 15- 2						
	FEATURES OF SYRINGOMATOUS TUMOR (SYT), LOW-GRADE ADENOSQUAMOUS CARCINOMA (LASC), AND TUBULAR CARCINOMA (TC)						
	Epithelial Proliferation	Squamous Differentiation	EMA[a]	Luminal Snouts	Myoepithelial Cells	Stromal Lymphocytes	Elastosis
SyT	No	Yes	+/–	No	+/–	No	No
LASC	Papillary Tumors	Yes	+/–	No	Yes	Yes	No
TC	DCIS	No	Yes	Yes	No	No	Yes

[a]EMA = epithelial membrane antigen; DCIS = ductal carcinoma in situ.

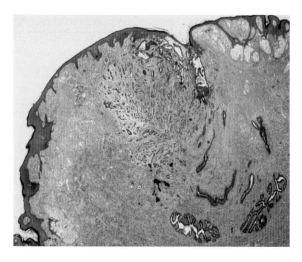

Figure 15-17

TUBULAR CARCINOMA IN THE NIPLE

The nipple is involved by a minute tubular carcinoma.

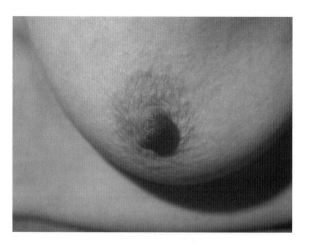

Figure 15-18

PAGET'S CARCINOMA

The nipple is eroded.

are lined by a single layer of epithelial cells. Squamous differentiation and squamous cysts are not a feature of tubular carcinoma, while they are a regular finding in SyT. Prominent "secretory snouts" are seen at the luminal pole of the neoplastic glands in over 50 percent of tubular carcinomas (15), but are absent in the cells lining the glandular lumens of SyT, which often have a cuticle-like luminal edge. Finally, periductal and perivenous elastosis (4) are features of tubular carcinoma but not SyT.

Treatment and Prognosis. Five of 9 lesions reported by Jones et al. (28) recurred but no metastases developed. Recurrences were seen at the site of excision in all five patients. The time of recurrence ranged from 1.5 months to 4.0 years and one patient had three recurrences in 4 years. SyTs are slow-growing tumors with a duration as long as 22 years (53). The best treatment is excision of the lesion with generous margins since these tumors invade insidiously at a long distance from their center.

PAGET'S CARCINOMA

Definition. *Paget's carcinoma* (PC) is an intraepidermal carcinoma of the nipple-areolar region with glandular cell differentiation. *Paget's disease* is another term for this lesion.

Clinical Features. PC represents 1.0 to 3.2 percent of all breast carcinomas (1,43). It is usually a unilateral process and affects women

between 28 and 82 years of age (average, 54 years) (1). PC is also seen in about 12 percent of male patients with invasive breast carcinomas (44). It has been found in cases of supernumerary nipple (38), ectopic breast tissue (30), and congenital absence of ducts (47).

Redness and roughness as well as erosion of the nipple epithelium (fig. 15-18) were the signs reported by Haagensen (22), who believed that the latter reflected progression of the disease. The lesion appears first in the nipple, subsequently spreads to the areola, and eventually may involve the surrounding skin. An eczematoid lesion of the areola not involving the nipple is almost invariably a dermatitis (22). On the contrary, "eczema," crust, or ulceration of the nipple is a presenting symptom in 34 to 76 percent of patients affected by PC (32,47), followed by discharge or bleeding of the nipple in 26 percent (46). Persistent eczematoid lesions of the nipple and areola were the main complaints of the patients reported by Ashikari et al. (1). The edge of the eczematoid reaction is slightly raised, has irregular borders, and is sharply demarcated from the surrounding skin (58). Some cases appear pigmented and simulate a malignant melanoma (fig. 15-19), as in the remarkable case in a male breast reported by Stretch et al. (63).

The mean duration of symptoms prior to presentation is 6.5 months (25) but a delay of up to 11 years has been reported (22). Since the diagnosis of PC is missed clinically in 33 percent of

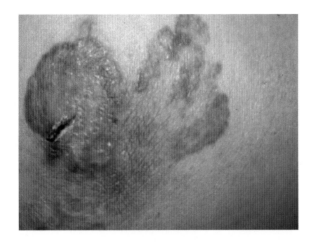

Figure 15-19

PAGET'S CARCINOMA

The nipple is ulcerated and the intraepidermal growth expands radially beyond the areola in an irregular fashion. It is so pigmented as to simulate a melanoma.

cases, all erosions and dermatitis-like lesions that involve the nipple epithelium should be regarded as highly suspicious for malignancy (22).

About 50 percent of patients with PC have, in addition to the clinical changes in the nipple, a palpable breast mass. Such cases were more numerous in earlier reports; 61 percent of the patients of Nance et al. had a palpable mass (43). In more recent series, the incidence of cases in which a palpable mass is detected is about 40 percent (61).

Subclinical PC, defined as microscopic involvement of the nipple without any clinical evidence of the disease, is discovered incidentally after a mastectomy for invasive carcinoma. Its incidence is difficult to assess as studies centered on establishing the incidence of subclinical PC in a large series of breast carcinomas are lacking. Subclinical PC was present in 12 of 80 PCs (15 percent) reported by Kollmorgen et al. (32). The highest incidence recorded (29 percent) is that of Sheen-Chen et al. (61).

The sensitivity of mammography in detecting the presence of an underlying carcinoma is remarkably high in cases of PC associated with a breast lump (97 percent) (25). In cases without clinical evidence of a breast mass, the mammogram is read as normal in a majority of cases (62 to 70 percent). Mammograms were reported as normal in a series of 44 patients without a clinical lump (71). Most of the patients with PC who do not have a palpable tumor have an underlying in situ duct carcinoma (DCIS)/ductal intraepithelial neoplasia grade 3 (DIN3). Therefore, it seems that the low sensitivity of mammography in these cases is more than coincidental and probably reflects the true insensitivity of mammography in diagnosing DCIS/DIN.

Microscopic Findings. The recognition of PC would be easier if wedge or punch biopsies were not so often used as routine diagnostic procedures. These result in an underestimation of the neoplastic process as a consequence of the small quantity of tissue sampled.

At low-power magnification, some noteworthy features are seen. The epidermis appears to be of normal thickness and is rarely acanthotic, and features of pseudoepitheliomatous hyperplasia are exceptional. Hyperkeratosis with parakeratosis is observed in longstanding processes. The neoplastic cells are located within the epidermis and, as will be described shortly, are "easily" distinguished from the normal keratinocytes with which they intermingle.

In the upper part of the dermis, a band-like inflammatory infiltrate is constantly present, very similar to the one that accompanies regressing pigmented lesions. It is composed mainly of lymphocytes with rare plasma cells and is observed below the areas where the neoplastic cells are located (fig. 15-20). It usually disappears abruptly where the neoplastic cells are no longer visible within the epidermis.

Histologic Variants. Three histologic types of PC are recognized.

Classic PC. The classic variant shows neoplastic cells that are individually dispersed among non-neoplastic keratinocytes or are clumped in small nests within the epidermis (fig. 15-21). The neoplastic cells are located anywhere within the malpighian layer although a suprabasal location is the most frequent. They have abundant, weakly eosinophilic cytoplasm that contrasts with the intense eosinophilia of the keratinocytes (fig. 15-22).

Mucosubstances are present within the cytoplasm of the neoplastic cells in about 38 percent of cases (71). A clear halo often encircles these elements, which appear detached from the adjacent keratinocytes (fig. 15-23). The halo is an artifact since it disappears when the tissue is fixed for electron microscopy (57). Melanin granules are easily seen within the cytoplasm and are a frequent feature (fig. 15-24). The

transfer of melanin pigment from melanocytes to carcinomatous cells has been recognized for a long time in the breast (3,40) and this phenomenon is responsible for those heavily pigmented carcinomas that closely simulate malignant melanomas (63).

The nuclei of classic PC cells are round to ovoid, frequently pleomorphic, and often display prominent nucleoli. Mitoses are infrequently seen.

The neoplastic cells may extend to sebaceous glands or can be observed along the basal layer

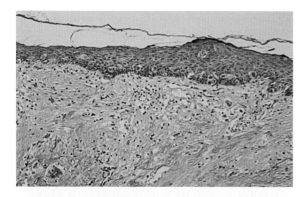

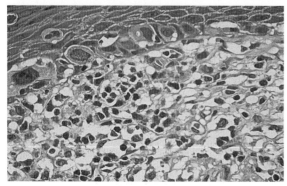

Figure 15-20

PAGET'S CARCINOMA

The band-like inflammatory infiltrate (top) is mostly composed of mature lymphocytes (bottom).

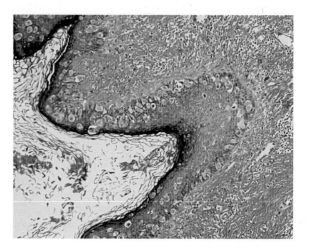

Figure 15-21

CLASSIC PAGET'S CARCINOMA

The neoplastic cells are individually dispersed among non-neoplastic keratinocytes or are clustered in small nests.

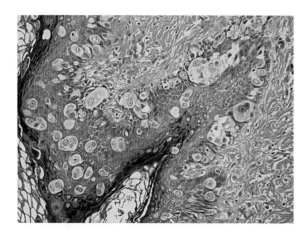

Figure 15-22

CLASSIC PAGET'S CARCINOMA

The neoplastic cells display faintly stained, abundant cytoplasm.

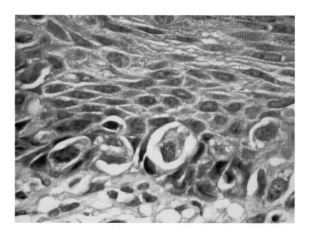

Figure 15-23

CLASSIC PAGET'S CARCINOMA

An artifactual clear halo surrounds the neoplastic cells.

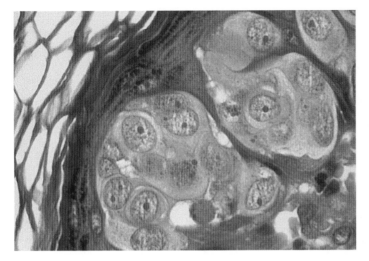

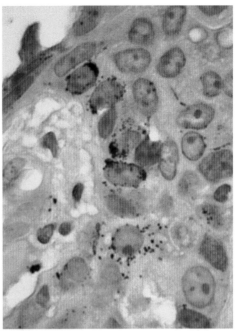

Figure 15-24

CLASSIC PAGET'S CARCINOMA

Above: Coarse melanin granules are visible within the cytoplasm.
Right: The granules are stained by the Masson-Fontana stain.

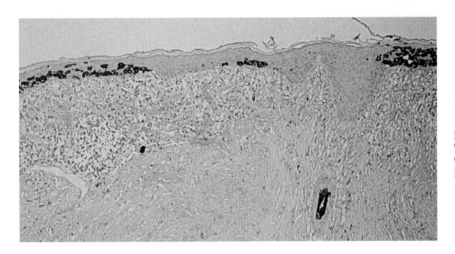

Figure 15-25

CLASSIC PAGET'S CARCINOMA

Apparent multifocality is present in this lesion stained for CK7. This is probably the result of an artifact consequent to the plane of sectioning.

of the epidermoid cysts occasionally present in the dermis. The spread of the neoplastic cells can be continuous but cases showing areas of neoplastic clumping separated by normal epidermis occur. This is probably artifactual as a result of the two-dimensional plane of section and not to a genuine multifocality (fig. 15-25).

Bowenoid PC. This is an infrequent histologic subtype of PC. Some of these cases were included in a small series of six patients showing "anaplastic" PC (48). Bowenoid PC is characterized by intraepidermal atypical cells that involve half to the full thickness of the epidermis in a continuous fashion, without the intermingled non-neoplastic keratinocytes seen in classic PC (fig. 15-26). Their nuclei are irregular and pleomorphic but mitoses are rare. The neoplastic cells may involve the basal layer, and when this occurs, the distinction from an in situ epidermoid carcinoma is difficult (see below). The immunocytochemical profile of the neoplastic cells is identical to that of classic PC cells, however, only they are not dendritic (fig. 15-27) (see Immunohistochemical Findings).

Pemphigus-Like PC. Pemphigus-like PC is also a rare variant of PC, and was probably included in the series of anaplastic PCs (49) as a lesion that presented "cleft-like acantholysis." These

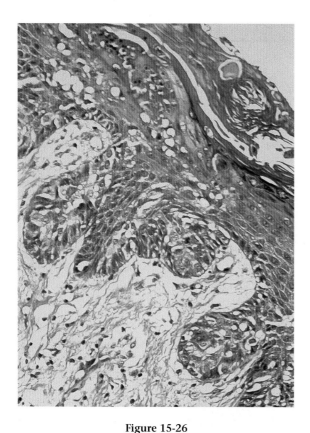

Figure 15-26

BOWENOID PAGET'S CARCINOMA

The neoplastic cells are present in half of the thickness of the epidermis and grow in a continuous fashion.

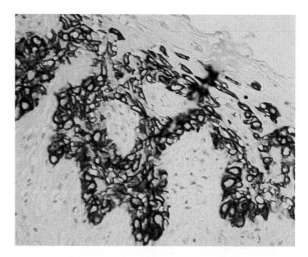

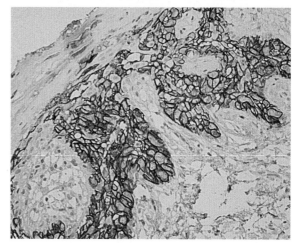

Figure 15-27

BOWENOID PAGET'S CARCINOMA

The neoplastic cells stain for CK7 (top) and c-erbB-2 (bottom). These cells do not show any dendritic projections.

cases are characterized by hyperplasia of the epidermis where the neoplastic cells grow in a continuous fashion, specifically the lowest layers of the epidermis, including the basal layer (fig. 15-28). The cells are not cohesive and cleft-like spaces parallel to the epidermis feature intraepidermal bulla. The neoplastic cells may encircle the dermal papillae that appear "sequestered" by neoplastic cells (fig. 15-29). The upper layers of the epidermis may detach and result in nipple erosion. The floor of the erosion is composed of "denuded" dermal papillae, which on occasion are bordered by residual, basally located neoplastic cells (fig. 15-30). As a consequence, as pointed out by Rosen (50), if a wedge biopsy is obtained from the center of a nipple erosion, the neoplastic condition can go undetected. The immunohistochemical profile of the neoplastic cells is identical to that of ordinary PC but no cytoplasmic dendritic projections are seen (see Immunohistochemical Findings).

Immunohistochemical Findings. Abundant data exist in the literature on the immunohistochemical features of PC. Some studies are mostly directed to the diagnosis, others more concerned with the histogenesis of PC. One of the first pivotal studies demonstrated casein within the cytoplasm of PC cells (7), which was the first evidence that PC cells were different than keratinocytes, which are devoid of the substance.

Virtually all PC cells are positive for CK7 (35,39) and CAM 5.2 (24). The cytoplasm of the vast majority of neoplastic cells stains intensely for both markers. The cell profile varies from globoid to polygonal, but some cells show dendritic cytoplasmic projections that insinuate

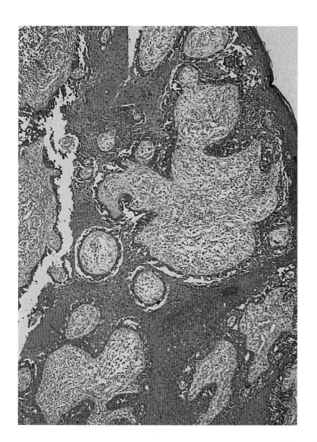

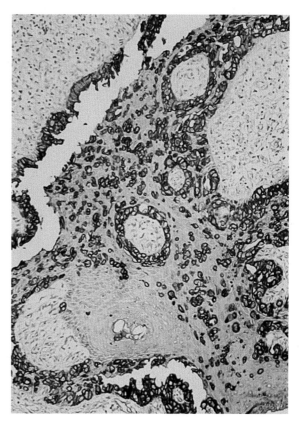

Figure 15-28

PEMPHIGUS-LIKE PAGET'S CARCINOMA

Left: The neoplastic cells grow in a continuous fashion along the lower layers of the epidermis.
Right: The cells are not cohesive and this results in the formation of an intraepidermal bulla.

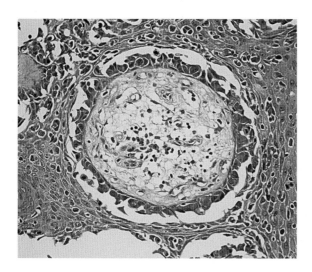

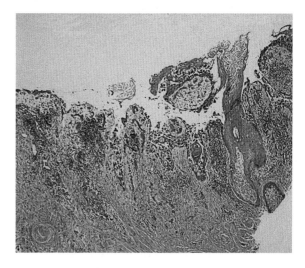

Figure 15-29

PEMPHIGUS-LIKE PAGET'S CARCINOMA

A "sequestered" dermal papilla.

Figure 15-30

PEMPHIGUS-LIKE PAGET'S CARCINOMA

Erosion of the epidermis with "denuded" dermal papillae.

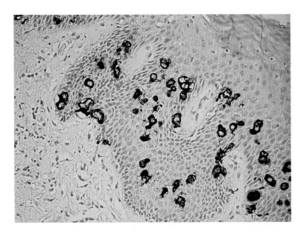

Figure 15-31

PAGET'S CARCINOMA

CK7 stains the neoplastic cells, which have evident dendritic projections.

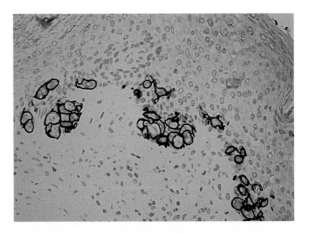

Figure 15-32

PAGET'S CARCINOMA

The cell membranes of the neoplastic cells are positive for c-erbB-2. The positivity can be traced along the dendritic processes.

among non-neoplastic keratinocytes (fig. 15-31). The dendritic appearance of PC cells has never been mentioned in the literature but is self-evident from the illustrations of various papers in which PC cells stained for low-weight keratins. The dendritic nature of PC cells was emphasized in only two of four cases studied by Marucci et al. (39), who interpreted this phenomenon as a sign of cell motility. In this respect PC cells are similar to Toker cells, which also show dendritic cytoplasmic processes.

Lammie et al. (34) were the first to demonstrate c-erbB-2 in 91 percent of PC cells. With the currently available monoclonal antibodies, virtually 100 percent of cases of PC show positive staining of the majority of neoplastic cells (24,39). The cell membrane stains intensely and positivity can be traced along the dendritic processes (fig. 15-32).

Positivity for carcinoembryonic antigen (CEA) varies from 62.5 to 100 percent of the cases studied (45). The same range of positivity is seen for EMA (38 to 100 percent) (24,45). Gross cystic disease fluid protein (GCDFP)-15 is present in about 50 percent of cases (45) while p53 is overexpressed in 43 percent (21). In the latter study, cyclin D was expressed in all cases, Ki-67 in 86 percent, and estrogen and progesterone receptors in only 29 percent of the cases. The immunohistochemical profile of PC cells is identical to that of the associated underlying carcinoma when present.

Ultrastructural Findings. Sagebiel (57) performed the first ultrastructural study on four cases of PC. He gave a very lucid description to which little can be added. PC cells are identified within the epidermis since their cytoplasm appears less dense than the adjacent epidermal cells. Microvilli are seen along the plasma membrane of some cells, a finding confirmed by Azzopardi et al. (2). Rare intracytoplasmic lumens are bordered by microvilli. The plasma membranes of contiguous PC cells are joined by desmosomes, which are also seen between a neoplastic cell and an adjacent keratinizing epidermal cell. Desmosomes are never as numerous along the PC cell membrane as in the normal epidermal cells. Intimate hemidesmosomal attachments with the basal lamina of the epidermis were seen by Lagios et al. (3) while their existence was denied by Ordonez et al. (45), who also stated that the underlying breast carcinomas appeared ultrastructurally identical to the PC cells.

Histogenesis. The histogenesis of PC remains poorly understood. The view that PC cells represent altered melanocytes (46) is no longer tenable since the overwhelming demonstration that PC cells have an adenocarcinomatous nature.

There is evidence that these cells are "foreign" elements to the epidermis caused by epidermotropic migration of cancer cells from a carcinoma of lactiferous ducts. This is suggested by the high frequency and intimate connection between PC and underlying DCIS/DIN; the fact that cells from PC and DCIS/DIN are identical, even in terms of immunohistochemistry; the dendritic nature of PC cells, which suggests motility of these cells; and the suggestion, and demonstration in vitro, that epidermal keratinocytes secrete the motility factor heregulin-alpha and that PC cells express heregulin receptors of which c-erbB-2 is a member. Therefore, the binding of heregulin to the receptor complex in PC results in chemotactic migration of the neoplastic cells into the nipple epidermis (60).

Despite these facts, there are several data difficult to reconcile to an exclusively epidermotropic view. There are cases, albeit rare, with exclusive involvement of the skin with no underlying DCIS/DIN. This includes the remarkable case of PC of the areola in a patient with congenital absence of the nipple (47).

There are also cases in which the carcinoma is located far away from the nipple with no apparent connection to it (47). These data have led Marucci et al. (39) to propose that these specific cases are the result of malignant transformation of Toker cells, a view also suggested by Toker himself (67). The case of mammary PC confined to the areola and associated with multifocal Toker cell hyperplasia (69) is consonant with this view as is the case of PC of a supernumerary nipple that was difficult to distinguish from Toker cell hyperplasia (11). Also, at the edge of typical PC, it is common to see CK7-positive and c-erbB-2-negative cells consistent with Toker cells, which share with PC a dendritic structure.

Morandi et al. (41) have shown that 2 of 10 PCs with underlying carcinoma had clonal diversities between the intraepidermal and the ductal carcinoma cells, while the other 8 cases displayed cells of similar clonality. The clonal difference was interpreted as the result of neoplastic transformation of preexisting intraepidermal non-neoplastic cells. Consequently, the underlying tumors were regarded as coincidental neoplastic lesions (collision tumors). From a molecular point of view, both histogenetic theories described above are possible and supplement each other.

In the pemphigus-like and bowenoid types of PC, there is nearly constant involvement of the basal layer and the continuous growth of neoplastic cells which is difficult to explain on

the basis of epidermotropic spread or a neoplastic transformation of Toker cells. These cases, as proposed by Mai (36), have features similar to those seen in extramammary PC where a multipotential epidermal stem cell with the capacity for divergent differentiation is the accepted histogenesis.

PC and Underlying Duct Carcinoma. Most PCs of the breast are associated with an underlying duct carcinoma. Cases in which there is involvement of the skin alone are rare. Their incidence varies from 0 to 26 percent according to different authors (8,32,61). This incidence depends on selection criteria and on the extent of sampling of nipple and paraareolar tissue. Probably the most realistic figure is the one reported by Ashikari et al. (1) who found 6 (5.3 percent) of 209 cases of PC confined to the skin of the nipple only.

DCIS/DIN is the most frequent lesion associated with PC in patients without a clinical lump. The incidence of DCIS/DIN ranges from 65 to 95 percent (1,8,61). In patients who present with a mass, the incidence is much lower, ranging from 0 to 9 percent (8,61). When a clinical lump is present, the predominant lesion is an invasive duct carcinoma (91 to 100 percent of cases) (8,61).

The extent of DCIS/DIN is highly variable in different reports. The discrepancies again depend on the criteria of selection and, to a greater extent, on sampling accuracy. The 12 cases of DCIS/DIN (44 percent of the cases of PC) reported by Sheen-Chen et al. (61) were limited to the subareolar area. In another study, 2 of 32 PCs showed DCIS/DIN confined exclusively to the large ducts immediately beneath the nipple (8). In a three-dimensional study of mastectomies for PC, Mai et al. (37) found 5 (26 percent) lesions only extending up to 1.5 cm from the nipple while the remaining cases extended far beyond this. The DCIS/DIN was very extensive in 25 (70 percent) patients and in 8 there was also multicentric invasive carcinoma (8). From these reports, it seems likely that in about 30 percent of cases, the DCIS/DIN is localized to the paraareolar tissue only.

The vast majority of DCIS/DIN lesions related to PC are of poorly differentiated type and show the same immunohistochemical reactions as seen in PC cells. Calcifications are seen in up to 60 percent of cases (8) and probably this is one of the reasons for the low sensitivity

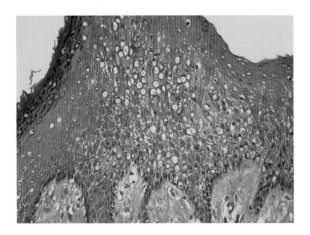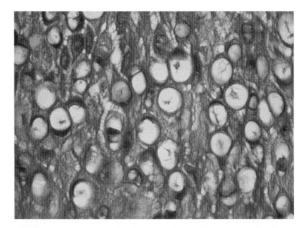

Figure 15-33

PAGETOID DYSKERATOSIS

Left: Numerous signet ring cells are present in most of the epidermal layers.

Right: The nuclei are located at one pole of the cell. The vacuoles contain eosinophilic debris, probably remnants of cytoplasm.

of mammography in detecting PC without a clinical lump.

In most cases, the underlying invasive carcinoma is of high-grade ductal type. Invasive lobular carcinomas are exceedingly rare in PC and sporadic cases of medullary and papillary invasive carcinomas have been reported (1). The size of the invasive tumor averages 4.4 cm (9). Invasive carcinoma is often found in a subareolar location, but in 45 percent of cases it is in the upper outer quadrant (8).

Secondary PC is the term given to metastatic or primary invasive carcinomas that grow beneath the skin which can be cancerized by single neoplastic cells over a small area (42). This type of skin cancerization is not necessarily localized to the nipple, but can be seen anywhere in the breast skin (as well as outside the breast).

Differential Diagnosis. A number of conditions can simulate PC histologically (Table 15-1). Bowenoid squamous cell carcinoma in situ characteristically appears on sun-exposed skin, although it can affect areas not exposed to the sun (31). This condition, together with the more classic intraepidermal (Bowen) carcinoma, can be difficult to distinguish from PC. Architecture and cytology can be unhelpful and the correct diagnosis depends upon immunohistochemistry. PCs are positive for CK7, CAM5.2, and c-erbB-2, while these markers are not seen in epidermoid in situ carcinomas. E-cadherin is expressed by

all types of PC as well as in situ squamous carcinoma, however.

Dysplastic nevi/in situ malignant melanomas are frequently located around the areola in patients with the familial dysplastic nevus syndrome (14). Clinically, PC can be very similar to an in situ malignant melanoma and histologically PC cells can contain melanin. Therefore, a confident diagnosis is obtained in difficult cases only with immunohistochemistry: dysplastic nevi/malignant melanoma in situ do not stain for keratins while they are positive for HMB45, all features distinguishing them from PC. S-100 protein can be deceptive, as occasional PC cells are positive. Fortunately, solitary melanomas of the nipple/areolar complex are rare.

Pagetoid dyskeratosis is frequently localized in the nipple-areolar complex (see chapter 1). The dyskeratotic cells are located suprabasally and extend to the stratum corneum. The cytoplasm of dyskeratotic cells varies from pale to clear and their nuclei are pyknotic and centrally to peripherally located. In some cases, signet ring cells are numerous since the nuclei are crescentic and are pushed to the periphery of the cell by a large vacuole with a remnant of the cytoplasm in the center (fig. 15-33). These cells are devoid of mucosubstances and do not stain for CK7, EMA, c-erbB-2, CEA, and human papilloma virus (68). Merkel cell carcinoma with pagetoid intraepidermal spread has characteristic nuclear features and is positive for CK20 as cytoplasmic paranuclear dots, a feature constantly absent in PC.

One of the most difficult entities to distinguish from PC is Toker cell hyperplasia. This distinction is such a problem that Decaussin et al. (11) honestly admitted that they were unable to establish whether the intraepidermal cell proliferation was PC or Toker cell hyperplasia. It is also quite likely that the intraepidermal, single cell proliferations above some adenomas of the nipple and interpreted as PC (51) are in fact examples of Toker cell hyperplasia (73). Toker cells are difficult to recognize in the context of the epidermis with routine H&E staining and lack nuclear signs of atypicality (see chapter 1). On the contrary, PC cells are characterized as "easily" visible cells located within the epidermis and the nuclei have an irregular profile and prominent nucleoli. The most reliable criterion is the immunocytochemical constant lack of c-erbB-2 and p53 in Toker cells; p53 is overexpressed in about 40 percent and c-erbB-2 in virtually all PC cells.

Prognosis and Treatment. Axillary lymph nodes metastases, as expected, are directly related to the presence of a clinical lump. When a palpable mass is present (and consequently, an invasive carcinoma), the percentage of lymph node metastases varies from 50 to 65 percent (1,61). The nodal metastatic rate drops to 13 to 21 percent when there is no clinical evidence of a mass (1,32).

The prognosis of patients with PC is determined by the type of the underlying carcinoma and the treatment chosen. Radical mastectomy has been proposed by most authors as the standard therapy (8). Of 63 patients with DCIS/DIN localized beneath the nipple, cure with mastectomy was 100 percent (1). The same result was obtained in 14 patients with PC and DCIS/DIN reported by Chaudary et al. (8), with the exception of 2 patients who died of breast cancer probably as the result of an invasive carcinoma missed on histopathologic examination .

After mastectomy, the overall survival rate of patients who did not have a palpable mass is 87 percent at 10 years while the survival rate of patients with a palpable mass is only 40 percent at 10 years (1). Patients who have no palpable mass and negative nodes have a 10-year survival rate of 94.5 percent, while those with positive nodes in the lower axilla have a survival rate of

75 percent. Patients with a palpable mass, with and without positive nodes, have survival rates of 38 and 68 percent, respectively, at 10 years (1). A significant difference in 5-year overall survival rate (94 versus 19 percent) was seen between patients without and with a palpable mass in another series (61). Paone and Baker (47) found that the 10-year survival rates of patients with PC and a palpable breast mass were similar to those of patients with infiltrating duct carcinoma; positive axillary nodes were the most important prognostic factor, with a 10-year survival rate of 9.9 percent for those patients.

Excision alone is a conservative option occasionally proposed in selected patients. Five patients without palpable tumors, axillary adenopathy, and suspicious mammographic lesions were treated by total excision of the affected nipple-areolar complex (33). One patient only had a recurrence as PC of the residual areolar skin. All the other patients were well over a period ranging from 15 to 36 months (average, 36 months). Dixon et al. (13) reported on 10 cases with similar criteria of selection. At a median follow-up period of 56 months, 4 local recurrences were detected, of which 2 were invasive duct carcinomas with nodal metastases.

Radiotherapy alone was the treatment in 17 selected patients studied by Fourquet et al. (20). The patients were followed for 15 to 276 months (median, 90 months). The overall 7-year actuarial survival rate was 93 percent. No patients died of breast disease and no axillary metastases occurred. Three patients had recurrent PC in the irradiated breast that was treated by mastectomy. No residual tumor was found. Similar results were obtained by Stockdale et al. (62) in 19 selected patients. Sixteen patients remained free of disease after a median of 5 years (range, 11 months to 13 years). Three patients noticed an invasive carcinoma after 3 to 6 years. A mastectomy was performed and no patient treated (initially) with radiotherapy died of breast carcinoma.

Cone excision and radiotherapy were used in a prospective series of 61 carefully selected patients with PC who were followed until death (median, 6.4 years; maximum, 12.5 years) (5). All patients had histologically proven PC with or without (7 percent of cases with exclusive involvement of the skin) underlying grade 3 DCIS/DIN3, which was not permitted to extend more that 5 cm from the nipple. In addition, the tissue had to be excised with histologically confirmed tumor-free margins, defined as DCIS that had not transected the inked margins. Four patients had a recurrence (5-year recurrence rate 5.2 percent), 1 with DCIS/DIN3 and 3 with invasive disease. One of the latter patients died of disseminated breast carcinoma.

There is a wide range of opinions on the treatment for PC which, especially for cases with underlying DCIS/DIN3, recapitulates the options proposed for DCIS alone. Mastectomy offers the best treatment for DCIS/DIN, but the histologic assessment of tumor-free margins of a cone biopsy, followed by radiotherapy, appears to be a reasonable alternative.

MISCELLANEOUS LESIONS OF THE NIPPLE

The skin of the nipple-areolar complex can harbor any lesion that arises in the epidermis, in the adnexa, and in the connective tissues that compose the dermis. Most of the skin lesions are more frequent in men, which probably reflects the greater sun exposure of the male nipple (56).

About 15 cases of basal cell carcinoma have been reported in the nipple, one of which metastasized to the axillary lymph nodes (65). Nodular hidroadenomas, eccrine spiroadenomas, sebaceous adenomas, and sweat duct carcinomas have all been described or illustrated (53). Leiomyomas, leiomyosarcomas, and vascu-

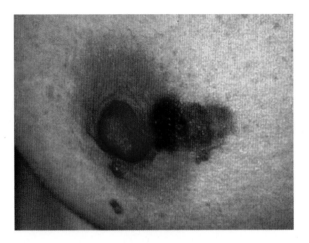

Figure 15-34

MELANOMA OF THE NIPPLE

Paraareolar superficially spreading malignant melanoma in a dysplastic nevus syndrome.

lar tumors have been discussed in the chapters related to soft tissue lesions.

Nevi and melanomas are also, albeit rarely, seen in and around the nipple areolar complex. In the dysplastic nevus syndrome, pigmented lesions are found in this location (fig. 15-34). Pigmented lesions have to be carefully distinguished from PC. CK7 and c-erbB-2 positivity in PC and HMB45 positivity in melanoma cells are vital for establishing the correct diagnosis.

REFERENCES

1. Ashikari R, Park K, Huvos AG, Urban JA. Paget's disease of the breast. Cancer 1970;26:680-685.
2. Azzopardi JG, Ahmed A, Millis RR. Problems in breast pathology. London: W.B. Saunders Company; 1979.
3. Azzopardi JG, Eusebi V. Melanocyte colonization and pigmentation of breast carcinoma. Histopathology 1977;1:21-30.
4. Azzopardi JG, Laurini RN. Elastosis in breast cancer. Cancer 1974;33:174-183.
5. Bijker N, Rutgers EJ, Duchateau L, Peterse JL, Julien JP, Cataliotti L: The EORTC Breast Cancer Cooperative Group. Breast-conserving therapy for Paget disease of the nipple: a prospective European Organization for Research and Treatment of Cancer study of 61 patients. Cancer 2001;91:472-477.
6. Bondi R, Urso C. Syringomatous adenocarcinoma of minor salivary glands. Tumori 1990;76:286-289.
7. Bussolati G, Pich A. Mammary and extramammary Paget's disease. An immunocytochemical study. Am J Pathol 1975;80:117-128.
8. Chaudary MA, Millis RR, Lane EB, Miller NA. Paget's disease of the nipple: a ten year review including clinical, pathological, and immunohistochemical findings. Breast Cancer Res Treat 1986;8:139-146.
9. Coyne JD, Dervan PA, Barr L, Baildam AD. Mixed apocrine/endocrine ductal carcinoma in situ of the breast coexistent with lobular carcinoma in situ. J Clin Path 2001;54:70-73.

10. Cruz DJ. Sweat gland carcinomas: a comprehensive review. Semin Diagn Pathol 1987;4:38-74.

11. Decaussin M, Laville M, Mathevet P, Frappart L. Paget's disease versus Toker cell hyperplasia in a supernumerary nipple. Virchows Arch 1998;432:289-291.

12. Denley H, Pinder SE, Tan PH, et al. Metaplastic carcinoma of the breast arising within a complex sclerosing lesion: a report of five cases. Histopathology 2000;36:203-209.

13. Dixon AR, Galea MH, Ellis IO, Elston CW, Blamey RW. Paget's disease of the nipple. Br J Surg 1991;78:722-723.

14. Elder DE, Greene MH, Bondi EE, Clark WH. Acquired melanocytic nevi and melanoma: the dysplastic nevus syndrome. In: Ackerman AB, ed. Pathology of malignant melanoma. New York: Masson Publishing USA; 1981:185-216.

15. Eusebi V, Betts CM, Bussolati G. Tubular carcinoma: a variant of secretory breast carcinoma. Histopathology 1979;3:407-419.

16. Fechner RE, Mills SE. Breast pathology benign proliferations, atypias in situ carcinomas. Chicago: ASCP Press - American Society of Clinical Pathologists; 1990.

17. Fisher ER, Gregorio R, Redmond C, Vellios F, Sommers SC, Fisher B. Pathologic findings from the national surgical adjuvant breast project (protocol no. 4). I. Observations concerning the multicentricity of mammary cancer. Cancer 1975;35:247-254.

18. Foschini MP, Eusebi V. Carcinomas of the breast showing myoepithelial cell differentiation. Virchows Arch 1998;432:303-310.

19. Foschini MP, Pizzicannella G, Peterse JL, Eusebi V. Adenomyoepithelioma of the breast associated with low-grade adenosquamous and sarcomatoid carcinomas. Virchows Arch 1995;427:243-250.

20. Fourquet A, Campana F, Vielh P, Schlienger P, Jullien D, Vilcoq JR. Paget's disease of the nipple without detectable breast tumor: conservative management with radiation therapy. Ital J Radiat Oncol Biol Phys 1987;13:1463-1465.

21. Fu W, Lobocki CA, Silberberg BK, Chelladurai M, Young SC. Molecular markers in Paget disease of the breast. J Surg Oncol 2001;77:171-178.

22. Haagensen CD. Diseases of the breast, 3rd ed. Philadelphia: W.B. Saunders; 1986.

23. Handley RS, Thackray AC. Adenoma of nipple. Br J Cancer 1962;16:187-194.

24. Hitchcoch A, Topham S, Bell J, Gullick W, Elston CW, Ellis IO. Routine diagnosis of mammary Paget's disease. A modern approach. Am J Surg Pathol 1992;16:58-61.

25. Jamali FR, Ricci A Jr, Deckers PJ. Paget's disease of the nipple-areola complex. Surg Clin North Am 1996;76:365-381.

26. Johnston CA, Toker C. Syringomatous tumors of minor salivary gland origin. Hum Pathol 1982;13:182-184.

27. Jones DB. Florid papillomatosis of the nipple ducts. Cancer 1955;8:315-319.

28. Jones MW, Norris HJ, Snyder RC. Infiltrating syringomatous adenoma of the nipple. A clinical and pathological study of 11 cases. Am J Surg Pathol 1989;13:197-201.

29. Jones MW, Tavassoli FA. Coexistence of nipple duct adenoma and breast carcinoma: a clinicopathologic study of five cases and review of the literature. Mod Pathol 1995;8:633-636.

30. Kao GF, Graham JH, Helwig EB. Paget's disease of the ectopic breast with an underlying intraductal carcinoma: report of a case. J Cutan Pathol 1986;13:59-66.

31. Kohler S, Rouse RV, Smoller BR. The differential diagnosis of pagetoid cells in the epidermis. Mod Pathol 1998;11:79-92.

32. Kollmorgen DR, Varanasi J, Edge SB, Carson WE 3rd. Paget's disease of the breast: a 33-year experience. J Am Coll Surg 1998;187:171-177.

33. Lagios MD, Westdahl PR, Rose MR, Concannon S. Paget's disease of the nipple. Alternative management in cases without or with minimal extent of underlying breast carcinoma. Cancer 1984;54:545-551.

34. Lammie GA, Barnes DM, Millis RR, Gullick WJ. An immunohistochemical study of the presence of c-erbB-2 protein in Paget's disease of the nipple. Histopathology 1989;15:505-514.

35. Lundquist K, Kohler S, Rouse RV. Intraepidermal cytokeratin 7 expression is not restricted to Paget cells but is also seen in Toker cells and Merkel cells. Am J Surg Pathol 1999;23:212-219.

36. Mai KT. Morphological evidence for field effect as a mechanism for tumour spread in mammary Paget's disease. Histopathology 1999;35:567-576.

37. Mai KT, Yazdi HM, Perkins DG. Mammary Paget's disease: evidence of diverse origin of the disease with a subgroup of Paget's disease developing from the superficial portion of lactiferous duct and a discontinuous pattern of tumor spread. Pathol Int 1999;49:956-961.

38. Martin VG, Pellettiere EV, Miller AW. Paget's disease in an adolescent arising in a supernumerary nipple. J Cutan Pathol 1994;21:283-286.

39. Marucci G, Betts CM, Golouh R, Peterse JL, Foschini MP, Eusebi V. Toker cells are probably precursors of Paget cell carcinoma: a morphological and ultrastructural description. Virchows Arch 2002;441:117-123.

40. Masson PT. Tumeurs humaines. Histologie. Diagnostics et techniques, 2nd ed. Paris: Librairie Maloine; 1968.

41. Morandi L, Pession A, Marucci GL, et al. Intraepidermal cells of Paget's carcinoma of the breast can be genetically different from those of the underlying carcinoma. Hum Pathol 2003;34:1321-1330.

42. Muir R. Further observations on Paget's disease of the nipple. J Pathol Bacteriol 1939;49:299-312.

43. Nance FC, DeLoach DH, Welsh RA, Becker WF. Paget's disease of the breast. Ann Surg 1970;171:864-874.

44. Norris HJ, Taylor HB. Carcinoma of the male breast. Cancer 1969;23:1428-1435.

45. Ordonez NG, Awalt H, Mackay B. Mammary and extramammary Paget'ts disease. An immunocytochemical and ultrastructural study. Cancer 1987;59:1173-1183.

46. Orr JW, Parish DJ. The nature of the nipple changes in Paget's disease. J Path Bact 1962;84:201-206.

47. Paone JF, Baker RR. Pathogenesis and treatment of Paget's disease of the breast. Cancer 1981;48:825-829.

48. Perzin KH, Lattes R. Papillary adenoma of the nipple (florid papillomatosis, adenoma, adenomatosis). A clinicopathologic study. Cancer 1972;29:996-1009.

49. Rayne SC, Santa Cruz DJ. Anaplastic Paget's disease. Am J Surg Pathol 1992;16:1085-1091.

50. Rosen PP. Rosen's breast pathology. Philadelphia: Lippincott-Raven; 1997.

51. Rosen PP. Rosen's breast pathology, 2nd ed. Philadelphia: Lippincott Williams & Wilkins; 2001.

52. Rosen PP. Subareolar sclerosing duct hyperplasia of the breast. Cancer 1987;59:1927-1930.

53. Rosen PP. Syringomatous adenoma of the nipple. Am J Surg Pathol 1983;7:739-745.

54. Rosen PP, Caicco JA. Florid papillomatosis of the nipple. A study of 51 patients, including nine with mammary carcinoma. Am J Surg Pathol 1986;10:87-101.

55. Rosen PP, Ernsberger D. Low-grade adenosquamous carcinoma. A variant of metaplastic mammary carcinoma. Am J Surg Pathol 1987;11:351-358.

56. Rosen PP, Oberman HA. Tumors of the mammary gland. AFIP Atlas of Tumor Pathology, 3rd Series, Fascicle 7. Washington DC: American Registry of Pathology; 1993.

57. Sagebiel RW. Ultrastructural observations on epidermal cells in Paget's disease of the breast. Am J Pathol 1969;57:49-64.

58. Sakorafas GH, Blanchard K, Sarr MG, Farley DR. Paget's disease of the breast. Cancer Treat Rev 2001;27:9-18.

59. Santini D, Taffurelli M, Gelli MC, et al. Adenoma of the nipple. A clinico-pathological study and its relation with carcinoma. Breast Dis 1990;3:153-163.

60. Schelfhout VR, Coene ED, Delaey B, Thys S, Page DL, De Potter CR. Pathogenesis of Paget's disease: epidermal heregulin-alpha motility factor, and the HER receptor family. J Natl Cancer Inst 2000;92:622-628.

61. Sheen-Chen SM, Chen HS, Chen WJ, Eng HL, Sheen CW, Chou FF. Paget disease of the breast-an easily overlooked disease? J Surg Oncol 2001;76:261-265.

62. Stockdale AD, Brierley JD, White WF, Folkes A, Rostom AY. Radiotherapy for Paget's disease of the nipple: a conservative alternative. Lancet 1989;2:664-666.

63. Stretch JR, Denton KJ, Millard PR, Horak E. Paget's disease of the male breast clinically and histopathologically mimicking melanoma. Histopathology 1991;19:470-472.

64. Suster S, Moran CA, Hurt MA. Syringomatous squamous tumors of the breast. Cancer 1991;67:2350-2355.

65. Tavassoli FA. Pathology of the breast, 2nd ed. Stamford, CT: Appleton & Lange/McGraw Hill; 1999.

66. Taylor HB, Robertson AG. Adenomas of the nipple. Cancer 1965;18:995-1002.

67. Toker C. Clear cells of the nipple epidermis. Cancer 1970;25:601-610.

68. Val-Bernal JF, Pinto J, Garijo MF, Gomez MS. Pagetoid dyskeratosis of the cervix: an incidental histologic finding in uterine prolapse. Am J Surg Pathol 2000;24:1518-1523.

69. Van der Putte SC, Toonstra J, Hennipman A. Mammary Paget's disease confined to the areola and associated with multifocal Toker cell hyperplasia. Am J Dermatopathol 1995;5:487-493.

70. Van Hoeven KH, Drudis T, Cranor ML, Erlandson RA, Rosen PP. Low-grade adenosquamous carcinoma of the breast. A clinicopathologic study of 32 cases with ultrastructural analysis. Am J Surg Pathol 1993;17:248-258.

71. Vielh P, Validire P, Kheirallah S, Campana F, Fourquet A, Di Bonito L. Paget's disease of the nipple without clinically and radiologically detectable breast tumor. Histochemical and immunohistochemical study of 44 cases. Pathol Res Pract 1993;189:150-155.

72. Ward BE, Cooper PH, Subramony C. Syringomatous tumor of the nipple. Am J Clin Pathol 1989;92:692-696.

73. Zeng Z, Melamed J, Symmans PJ, et al. Benign proliferative nipple duct lesions frequently contain CAM 5.2 and anti-cytokeratin 7 immunoreactive cells in the overlying epidermis. Am J Surg Pathol 1999;23:1349-1355.

16 LYMPHOID AND HEMATOPOIETIC LESIONS

LYMPHOMAS

Definition. *Lymphomas* involving the breast are divided into three groups: primary breast lymphomas, secondary disseminated lymphomas, and recurrent lymphomas. Primary breast lymphomas (PBL) are diagnosed only when the lesion is confined to the breast, without involvement of ipsilateral lymph nodes and clinically enlarged axillary lymph nodes; lymph node involvement is incidentally discovered on microscopic study (4). Secondary disseminated lymphomas with breast involvement are accompanied by distant disease upon full staging. Patients have recurrent lymphoma if the tumor recurs in the breast (10).

Clinical Features. Lymphomas (either primary or secondary) are rare tumors. They represent less than 1 percent of all non-Hodgkin lymphomas, about 1.7 percent of all extranodal non-Hodgkin lymphomas (10), and 0.13 percent of all breast malignancies (14). Lymphomas are almost exclusive to females, who range in age from 16 to over 80 years.

Twenty percent of PBLs are bilateral (14). When the bilaterality is synchronous (13 percent of cases), it usually manifests in young women with onset during puberty, pregnancy, or lactation. It spreads widely, involving the central nervous system, ovaries, and gastrointestinal tract, and rarely to the lymph nodes (32). Several of the bilateral cases are Burkitt lymphomas of endemic or sporadic type (9,23,31). Both breasts enlarge very fast, in a matter of weeks, simulating an inflammatory carcinoma.

Synchronous bilaterality can also manifest in women above 45 years of age and in this case the lymphoma has more indolent behavior (4). It is not surprising that there is a statistically significant longer survival period in the older group (41.3 months) than the younger group (9.1 months) (19). The fast growth of Burkitt lymphoma in pregnant and lactating patients is probably due to the reported presence of prolactin receptors in Burkitt lymphoma cells (9).

Bilaterality is asynchronous in 7 percent of cases. A contralateral non-Hodgkin lymphoma can occur up to 10 years after the first lesion (14). These cases are seen in patients older than 45 years of age and they are usually small cell indolent tumors (19).

Unilateral PBL is seen in about 80 percent of cases (14), and affects mostly women in their sixties (14,20). The presentation is similar to that of a unilateral carcinoma. Most are of the diffuse large B-cell lymphoma type (see below). Prognosis is variable and depends on the histologic type and clinical stage of the tumor (see below).

In about 90 percent of cases, the diagnosis of lymphoma is made after the histologic evaluation of a palpable mass. Screening mammography identifies only 1 out of 32 PBLs, indicating a very low sensitivity of this diagnostic method for breast lymphomas (10). This is partly due to the absence of microcalcifications in lymphomas.

Frozen sections are a major source of erroneous diagnoses; in one series, evaluation of frozen sections led to the diagnosis of medullary/lobular carcinoma in 34 percent of the cases. Fine needle aspiration cytology (FNAC), in contrast, results in an accurate diagnosis of lymphoma in 70 percent of cases (19).

Gross Findings. PBLs and secondary lymphomas appear as well-circumscribed tumors, varying in size from 1.5 to 20.0 cm in greatest dimension (7). The cut surface is white-gray, with necrotic areas, similar to the macroscopic appearance of ordinary invasive carcinoma. Elastotic streaks are lacking (fig. 16-1). Some lymphomas show an ill-defined area of growth that can occupy an entire quadrant (fig. 16-2). In occasional cases, especially those manifesting bilaterally, multiple nodules are seen, which, according to one investigator, "resembled a bag of marbles" (31).

Microscopic Findings. With occasional exceptions, lymphomas of the breast are of B-cell lineage (3,4,10). Most are classifiable as diffuse large B cell lymphomas.

Fifty to 80 percent of lymphomas are composed of intermediate- and high-grade components in both the primary and secondary lesions (1,4,14,18a). Cases reported in the past as reticulum cell sarcoma, lymphosarcoma, and histiocytic lymphoma would now be included in this group.

In about 20 percent of cases, the B-cell lymphomas are of variable subtypes that include Burkitt lymphoma, extranodal marginal zone B-cell lymphoma of mucosa associated lymphoid tissue (MALT lymphoma), and follicular lymphoma. Less frequently, mantle cell lymphoma, lymphoblastic lymphoma (B and T cell), and T-cell lymphomas of various subtypes have been reported (2).

Diffuse Large B-Cell Lymphomas. These lymphomas can be infiltrative, but their margin of invasion is usually circumscribed (fig. 16-3). The preexisting breast tissue is effaced, but remnants of ducts and lobules are occasionally seen. Areas of necrosis are abundant and the bulk of the tumor is composed of neoplastic cells without evident stroma. Rarely, the stroma is sclerohyaline type and shows keloid-like features when the neoplastic cells diffusely permeate Hartveit channels (fig. 16-4) (8). Vessels at the periphery of the tumor are frequently invaded.

Diffuse large B-cell lymphomas histologically closely simulate an invasive carcinoma (fig. 16-5), especially the single file pattern of invasion typical of invasive lobular carcinomas (fig. 16-6). Invasion of preexisting glandular epithelium, reminiscent of pagetoid spread, is a frequent feature (fig. 16-7). When the neoplastic cells fill the ductal lumens, a poorly differentiated ductal carcinoma in situ (grade 3 DCIS/ductal intraepithelial neoplasia [DIN]3) is closely simulated (29). The rare signet ring cell lymphoma can also lead to the erroneous diagnosis of invasive carcinoma (fig. 16-8). In frozen section specimens, medullary carcinoma is a common source of error.

Cytokeratin (CK)7 is positive in carcinomas while CAM5.2, CK8, and CK18 are less reliable for diagnostic purposes since they are also present in

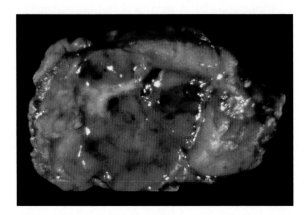

Figure 16-1

LYMPHOMA

The neoplastic (lymphoma) nodule has circumscribed margins, no sclerotic center, and no streaks of elastosis. (Courtesy of D. J. Lamovec, Ljubljana).

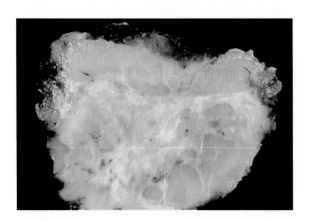
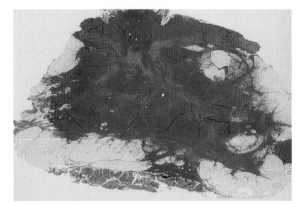

Figure 16-2

LYMPHOMA

Left: The lymphoma is infiltrative, occupies an entire quadrant, and reaches the skin (evident in the upper right corner).
Right: The skin, present in the upper part, is invaded by the same lymphoma, as is the pectoral muscle that is seen in the lower part.

diffuse large B-cell lymphomas (13,21). The latter are immunoreactive for CD20, CD79a, and CD45RB, while CD3 and CD45R0 are negative. CD30 is negative with rare exceptions (1).

Burkitt Lymphomas. The tumors in the breast have morphologic features similar to those seen in other organs. The tumor is locally as destructive as diffuse large B-cell lymphoma and shares the features that simulate an invasive carcinoma. Immunohistochemically, Burkitt lymphoma expresses B cell-associated antigens (CD19, CD20, and CD22) as well as CD10, bcl-6, and membrane immunoglobulin (Ig)M with light chain restriction. Bcl-2, CD5, CD23, and terminal deoxynucleotidyltransferase (TdT) are not expressed. Epstein-Barr virus (EBV) genomes can be demonstrated in nearly all endemic cases and less frequently in sporadic cases (9).

Extranodal Marginal Zone B-Cell Lymphoma of Mucosa-Associated Lymphoid Tissue (MALT Lymphoma). The occurrence of MALT lymphoma in the breast was first mentioned by Lamovec and Jancar (20). The data on the frequency of these lymphomas vary substantially from none (5) to 44 percent of primary breast lymphomas (25).

According to the World Health Organization (WHO), the incidence of MALT lymphomas of the breast is regarded as rare and accepted as 4 percent of all MALT lymphomas (18).

It is important to correctly diagnose MALT lymphomas because they are indolent lymphomas and they frequently disseminate from

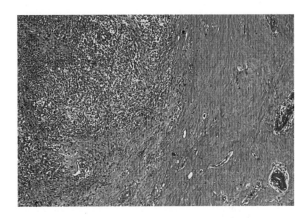

Figure 16-3

DIFFUSE LARGE B-CELL LYMPHOMA

The invasive edge of the lesion is well circumscribed.

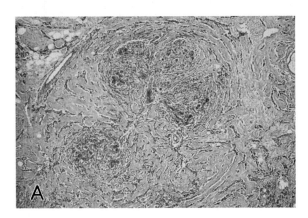

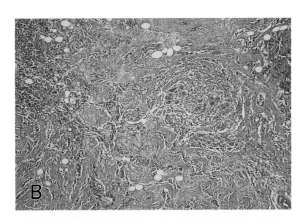

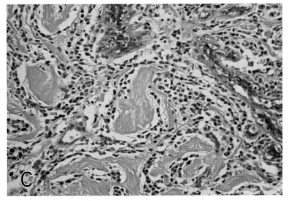

Figure 16-4

DIFFUSE LARGE B-CELL LYMPHOMA

A,B: The neoplastic cells have a plexiform architecture due to invasion of preexisting channels (Hartveit prelymphatic channels).

C: The neoplastic cells float within the prelymphatic space.

365

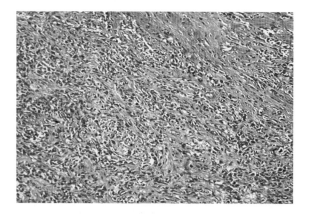

Figure 16-5

DIFFUSE LARGE B-CELL LYMPHOMA

The neoplastic lymphoid cells invade in cords and sheets and simulate an invasive carcinoma.

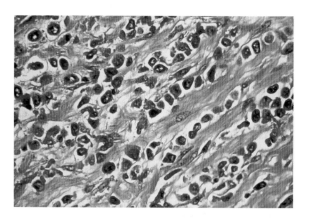

Figure 16-6

DIFFUSE LARGE B-CELL LYMPHOMA

A single file pattern of cells is seen in this large cell lymphoma showing plasmacytoid differentiation.

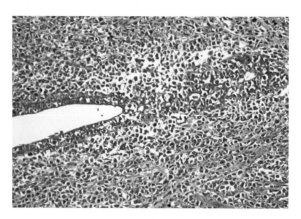

Figure 16-7

LYMPHOEPITHELIAL COMPLEX

The neoplastic cells of this diffuse large B-cell lymphoma have extended into a duct and simulate pagetoid spread.

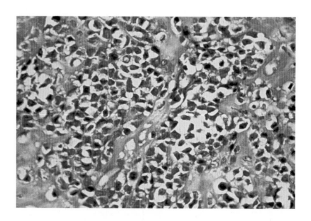

Figure 16-8

DIFFUSE LARGE B-CELL LYMPHOMA

Some cells have clear cytoplasm. The nucleus is dislodged at the periphery. A signet ring cell carcinoma is simulated.

the original site to another MALT area before nodal dissemination. Of three cases reported by Lamovec and Jancar (20), there was subsequent involvement of larynx, epimesopharynx, and contralateral breast. These are the tumors that may show bilateral nonsynchronous involvement.

Histologically, MALT lymphomas are composed of morphologically heterogeneous small B cells: marginal zone cells, cells that resemble monocytoid elements, small lymphocytes, and scattered immunoblasts. Monotypic plasma cells are frequently seen. Occasionally, the latter are so numerous that the distinction from an extraosseous plasmacytoma is difficult (16).

A lymphoepithelial lesion composed of monocytoid neoplastic cells and infiltrating glandular epithelium is rarely seen (20) and is not exclusive to MALT lymphomas. Similarly rare is lymphocytic lobulitis (lymphocytic mastopathy) accompanying the neoplasm. The high incidence (10 out of 11 cases) seen in one series (3) is probably the result of some selection bias.

Immunohistochemically, MALT lymphoma cells are CD20, CD79a, and bcl-2 positive. IgM is frequently expressed and shows light chain restriction. CD5, CD10, and CD23 are negative.

The translocation t(11;18)(q21;q21), found in many cases of MALT lymphoma, has never been demonstrated in the breast. The same is true of trisomy 3.

Treatment and Prognosis. The prognosis of patients with breast lymphomas varies in different studies but in large series from single institutions the overall survival rate at 5 years is 40 to 50 percent (14,23). The 5-year survival rate and the probability of freedom from progression at 5 years are, respectively, 61percent and 50 percent for patients with stage 1 tumors and 27 percent and 26 percent for those with stage 2 disease (14). As with other extranodal lymphomas, the survival rate appears most closely related to histology and stage of disease (7,32).

Wiseman and Liao (34) proposed a surgical approach (mastectomy) for breast lymphoma. Mastectomy is avoided today (18a,29a). Most patients generally benefit from chemotherapy and radiotherapy appropriate for the histologic grade of the tumor (10).

EXTRAOSSEOUS PLASMACYTOMA

Extraosseous plasmacytoma of the breast is a neoplasm confined to the breast without evidence of plasma cell myeloma on bone marrow examination or by radiography. Anemia, hypercalcemia, or renal failure are not present.

If this definition is applied, only five cases have been reported in the breast (29). Secondary involvement of the breast in cases of plasma cell myeloma is more frequent.

Plasmacytoma has to be distinguished from MALT lymphoma with numerous monotypic plasma cells and from benign reactive plasma cell infiltrates. Polyclonal kappa and lambda light chain expression indicates a reactive process that contrasts with the monoclonal pattern of plasmacytoma. Radiotherapy is the current treatment.

PSEUDOLYMPHOMA

Pseudolymphoma of the breast, like similar lesions of other organs, is an ill-defined, reactive lymphoid process. As outlined by Lin et al. (22), the lymphoid proliferation has sharp borders, and is composed of a polymorphic inflammatory infiltrate with mature lymphocytes and histiocytes. Germinal centers are often present and no destruction of the glandular epithelium is evident. A previous history of trauma is reported in most cases. Kappa and light chain immunoglobulins invariably char-

acterize the lymphocytes (12). Tumoral excision is curative.

PRIMARY HODGKIN LYMPHOMA

Primary Hodgkin lymphoma is exceptional in the breast. The breast is usually involved in stage IV Hodgkin lymphoma.

MYELOID SARCOMA

Myeloid sarcoma of the breast is a rare tumor that is composed of myeloblasts or immature myeloid cells. Myeloid sarcoma can occur concurrently with acute or chronic myeloid leukemia or with other myeloproliferative disorders, it can be the initial manifestation of relapse in a patient with acute myeloid leukemia in remission, or a single tumor mass may precede myeloid leukemia (26,27,29,32). This last occurrence is mostly seen in consultation centers as the lesion is easily misinterpreted as a large cell lymphoma or anaplastic carcinoma.

The 10 patients seen at the Armed Forces Institute of Pathology (AFIP) were 21 to 56 years of age. As a general rule, when a malignant tumor of the breast superficially resembles a large cell lymphoma but lacks B- and T-cell markers, then a myeloid sarcoma has to be considered. Immunohistochemical positivity for lysozyme, CD68, myeloperoxidase, CD117, CD34, and chloracetate esterase is very useful in the recognition of these lesions.

EXTRAMEDULLARY MYELOID METAPLASIA

Extramedullary myeloid metaplasia, also known as *extramedullary hematopoiesis*, occasionally manifests in the breast. The breast lesions are preceded by chronic idiopathic myelofibrosis (myelosclerosis), which in one case was diagnosed 16 years earlier (6). The lesion presents invariably as a palpable breast nodule that measured up to 8 cm in one report (6) and was associated with an enlarged lymph node in another (24) so as to simulate metastatic carcinoma. In one remarkable case, myeloid metaplasia was seen intermingled with a tubular carcinoma (30).

Histologically, there is dense intralobular fibrosis in which mononuclear and binuclear cells with granular cytoplasm are intermingled with abnormal megakaryocytes. The same pleomorphic infiltrate is seen in the specialized stroma

Figure 16-9

MYELOID METAPLASIA

A: The stroma of the breast, lobular and extralobular, is invaded by a mononuclear and pleomorphic cellular proliferation.

B: Large pleomorphic "atypical" megakaryocytes are seen.

C: Plump lobulation of the nuclei of megakaryocytes is surrounded by precursors of granulocytes.

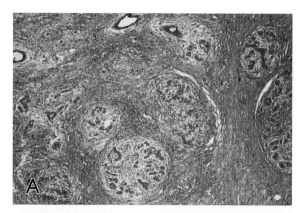

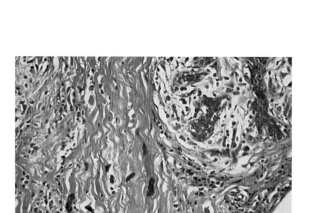

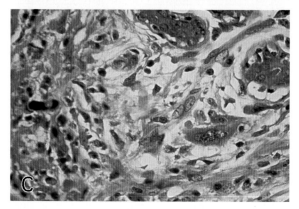

of the lobules. The megakaryocytes have an abnormal nuclear to cytoplasmic ratio, irregular chromatin, hyperchromatic nuclei, and plump lobulation of some nuclei (fig. 16-9).

As pointed out by Martinelli et al. (24), myeloid sarcomas do not exhibit the mixed proliferation of elements belonging to the granulocytic, erythroid, and megakaryocytic series as is seen in myeloid metaplasia. Pleomorphic invasive lobular carcinomas closely mimic extramedullary myeloid metaplasia. Immunohistochemistry is useful in the differential diagnosis. Keratins are positive in carcinomas and factor VIII is positive in megakaryocytes.

FOLLICULAR DENDRITIC CELL SARCOMA

Follicular dendritic cell sarcoma developing as a primary tumor in the breast is very rare. The two reported cases were in women of 41 and 40 years of age, with respective tumor size of 2.5 and 4.3 cm (11,28). Both patients were free of tumor at their last contact after surgery, which was 3 years in one case and 19 months in the other. The histology of this tumor is remarkably

similar to that seen in lymphoepithelial-like carcinomas (LEC) of Schmincke type.

The neoplastic cells are spindle to polygonal with eosinophilic cytoplasm. The nuclei are round to ovoid and have small nucleoli. Numerous small lymphocytes are intermingled with these cells (fig. 16-10). The case reported by Fisher et al. (11) showed a prominent myxoid stroma, while in the case reported by Pruneri et al. (28), the myxoid stroma was visible only in one small area. Cells were CD21 positive, as in all follicular dendritic cell sarcomas, but some elements were keratin positive (28). CD21 is the only marker useful in distinguishing dendritic cell sarcoma from LEC. An interdigitating dendritic cell tumor located in the breast involved a cervical lymph node (33).

EXTRANODAL ROSAI-DORFMAN DISEASE

Rosai-Dorfman disease occasionally involves the breast. Patients range in age from 15 to 84 years (15,17). Of the seven cases reported by Green et al. (15), four patients had the disease confined to the breast, one had involvement of the breast and

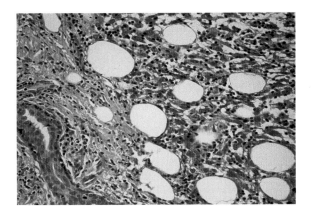 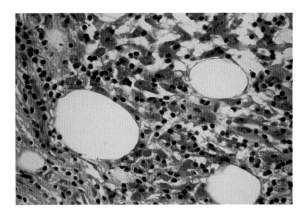

Figure 16-10

FOLLICULAR DENDRITIC CELL SARCOMA

Left: "Epithelioid" cells surround breast glands. (Courtesy of Dr. C. Fisher, London, England.)
Right: The neoplastic cells have abundant eosinophilic cytoplasm and are intermingled with numerous mature lymphocytes.

ispsilateral axillary lymph nodes, and two had bilateral involvement and systemic disease. The lesions were well circumscribed and all patients were treated with excisional surgery.

Histologically, the lesions are multinodular. The pale S-100 protein–positive histiocytes are located in the stroma, including the specialized stroma of the lobules.

Rosai-Dorfman disease has to be distinguished from idiopathic granulomatous mastitis. Apart from the different clinical and morphologic features, the inflammatory histiocytes in the latter are S-100 protein negative.

REFERENCES

1. Abbondanzo SL, Seidman JD, Lefkowitz M, Tavassoli FA, Krishnan J. Primary diffuse large B-cell lymphoma of the breast. Pathol Res Pract 1996;192:37-43.
2. Anania G, Baccarani U, Risaliti A, et al. Primary non-Hodgkin's T-cell lymphoma of the breast. Eur J Surg 1997;163:633-635.
3. Aozasa K, Ohsawa M, Saeki K, Horiuchi K, Kawano K, Taguchi T. Malignant lymphoma of the breast. Immunologic type and association with lymphocytic mastopathy. Am J Clin Pathol 1992;97:699-704.
4. Arber DA, Simpson JF, Weiss LM, Rappaport H. Non-Hodgkin's lymphoma involving the breast. Am J Surg Pathol 1994;18:288-295.
5. Bobrow LG, Richards MA, Happerfield LC, et al. Breast lymphomas: a clinicopathologic review. Hum Pathol 1993;24:274-278.
6. Brooks JJ, Krugman DT, Damjanov I. Myeloid metaplasia presenting as a breast mass. Am J Surg Pathol 1980;4:281-285.
7. Cohen PL, Brooks JJ. Lymphomas of the breast. A clinicopathological and immunohistochemical study of primary and secondary cases. Cancer 1991;67:1359-1369.
8. Damiani S, Peterse JL, Eusebi V. Malignant neoplasms infiltrating "pseudoangiomatous" stromal hyperplasia of the breast: an unrecognized pathway of tumor spread. Histopathology 2002;41:208-215.
9. Diebold J, Jaffe ES, Raphael M, Warnke RA. Burkitt lymphoma. In: Jaffe ES, Harris NL, Stein H, Vardiman JW, eds. World Health Organization Classification of Tumours. Pathology and genetics of tumours of haematopoietic and lymphoid tissues. Lyon: IARC Press; 2001:181-184.

10. Domchek SM, Hecht JL, Fleming MD, Pinkus GS, Canellos GP. Lymphomas of the breast. Primary and secondary involvement. Cancer 2002;94:6-13.

11. Fisher C, Magnusson B, Hardarson S, Smith ME. Myxoid variant of follicular dendritic cell sarcoma arising in the breast. Ann Diagn Pathol 1999;3:92-98.

12. Fisher ER, Palekar AS, Paulson JD, Golinger R. Pseudolymphoma of breast. Cancer 1979;44:258-263.

13. Frierson HF, Bellafiore FJ, Gaffey MJ, McCary WS, Innes DJ Jr, Williams ME. Cytokeratin in anaplastic large cell lymphoma. Mod Pathol 1994;7:317-321.

14. Giardini R, Piccolo C, Rilke F. Primary non-Hodgkin's lymphomas of the female breast. Cancer 1992;69:725-735.

15. Green I, Dorfman RF, Rosai J. Breast involvement by extranodal Rosai-Dorfman disease: report of seven cases. Am J Surg Pathol 1997;21:664-668.

16. Grogan TM, Van Camp B, Kyle RA, Muller-Hermelink HK, Harris NL. Plasma cell neoplasms. In: Jaffe ES, Harris NL, Stein H, Vardiman JW, eds. World Health Organization Classification of Tumours. Pathology and genetics of tumours of haemotopoietic and lymphoid tissues. Lyon: IARC Press; 2001:142-156.

17. Hammond LA, Keh C, Rowlands DC. Rosai-Dorfman disease in the breast. Histopathology 1996;29:582-584.

18. Isaacson PG, Muller-Hermelink HK, Piris MA, et al. Extranodal marginal zone B-cell lymphoma of mucosa-associated lymphoid tissue (MALT lymphoma). In: Jaffe ES, Harris NL, Stein H, Vardiman JW, eds. World Health Organization Classification of tumours. Pathology and genetics of tumours of haematopoietic and lymphoid tissues. Lyon: IARC Press; 2001:157-160.

18a. Jennings WC, Baker RS, Murray SS, et al. Primary breast lymphoma: the role of mastectomy and the importance of lymph node status. Ann Surg 2007;245:784-789.

19. Jeon HJ, Akagi T, Hoshida Y, et al. Primary non-Hodgkin malignant lymphoma of the breast. An immunohistochemical study of seven patients and literature review of 152 patients with breast lymphoma in Japan. Cancer 1992;70:2451-2459.

20. Lamovec J, Jancar J. Primary malignant lymphoma of the breast. Lymphoma of the mucosa-associated lymphoid tissue. Cancer 1987;60:3033-3041.

21. Lasota J, Hyjek E, Ko CH, Blonski J, Miettinen M. Cytokeratin-positive large cell lymphomas of B-cell lineage. A study of five phenotypically unusual cases verified by polymerase chain reaction. Am J Surg Pathol 1996;20:346-354.

22. Lin JJ, Farha GJ, Taylor RJ. Pseudolymphoma of the breast. I. In a study of 8,654 consecutive tylectomies and mastectomies. Cancer 1980;45:973-978.

23. Mambo NC, Burke JS, Butler J. Primary malignant lymphomas of the breast. Cancer 1977;39:2033-2040.

24. Martinelli G, Santini D, Bazzocchi F, Pileri S, Casanova S. Myeloid metaplasia of the breast. A lesion which clinically mimics carcinoma. Virchows Arch A Pathol Anat Histopathol 1983;401:203-207.

25. Mattia AR, Ferry JA, Harris NL. Breast lymphoma. A B-cell spectrum including the low-grade B-cell lymphoma of mucosa-associated lymphoid tissue. Am J Surg Pathol 1993;17:574-587.

26. Meis JM, Butler JJ, Osborne BM, Manning JT. Granulocytic sarcoma in nonleukemic patients. Cancer 1986;58:2697-2709.

27. Neiman RS, Barcos M, Berard C, et al. Granulocytic sarcoma. Cancer 1981;48:1426-1437.

28. Pruneri G, Masullo M, Renne G, et al. Follicular dendritic cell sarcoma of the breast. Virchows Arch 2002;441:202-204.

29. Rosen PP. Rosen's breast pathology, 2nd ed. Philadelphia: Lippincott Williams & Wilkins; 2001.

29a. Ryan G, Martinelli G, Kuper-Hommel M, et al. Primary diffuse large B-cell lymphoma of the breast: prognostic factors and outcome of a study by the International Extranodal Lymphoma Study Group. Ann Oncol 2008;19:233-241.

30. Setsu Y, Oka K, Naoi Y, et al. Breast carcinoma with myeloid metaplasia—a case report. Pathol Res Pract 1997;193:219-222.

31. Shepherd JJ, Wright DH. Burkitt's tumour presenting as bilateral swelling of the breast in women of child-bearing age. Br J Surg 1967;54:776-780.

32. Sloane JP, Trott PA, Lakhani SR, eds. Biopsy pathology of the breast. London: Arnold; 2001.

33. Uluoglu O, Akyurek N, Uner A, Coskun U, Ozdemir A, Gokcora N. Interdigitating dendritic cell tumor with breast and cervical lymph-node involvement: a case report and review of the literature. Virchows Arch 2005;446:546-554.

34. Wiseman C, Liao KT. Primary lymphoma of the breast. Cancer 1972;29:1705-1712.

17 MALE BREAST LESIONS

Mammary tumors, benign or malignant, are uncommon in men, except for gynecomastia. Most lesions in the male breast are of ductal origin since the normal male breast is devoid of fully developed terminal duct lobular units (TDLUs), the structure that is the source of the vast majority of mammary lesions in females. Even under conditions of relative or absolute hyperestrogenism, including the influence of estrogen-mimetic drugs, TDLUs rarely develop in the male breast. Once they do develop, however, a variety of lesions may originate within these structures (e.g., fibroadenoma, lobular neoplasia).

GYNECOMASTIA

Definition. *Gynecomastia* is a non-neoplastic enlargement of the male breast characterized by a proliferation of epithelial and mesenchymal elements.

General Features. Gynecomastia is characterized by a nodular or diffuse enlargement of the breast. Normal palpable breast tissue is so prevalent among men that it has been suggested that it should be distinguished from clinically significant gynecomastia (8). Gynecomastia is most often bilateral (synchronous or asynchronous); unilateral gynecomastia favors the left breast (5). The frequency of gynecomastia peaks during periods of relative hyperestrogenism and hormonal fluctuations: the neonatal period, adolescence, and the male climacteric. The newborn male often displays gynecomastia due to in utero exposure to maternal estrogenic hormones (8); with the termination of estrogenic stimulation, the changes revert within a few weeks. Bilateral gynecomastia is also observed among up to 40 percent of adolescent males, generally due to hormonal surges during this period (28). It may also occur in the prepubertal (4,21) and adult (26,37) male.

Gynecomastia appears to be more common than generally realized (27). It was found in 55 percent of 100 consecutive male autopsies (2). About 7 percent of these patients had severely atypical intraductal proliferations of either the atypical ductal hyperplasia (ADH)/cribriform ductal carcinoma in situ (DCIS)/ductal intraepithelial neoplasia (DIN) 1 types, or rarely, the lobular type (2). In a study of 306 adult males (17 to 58 years of age), 36 percent had palpable breast tissue; the prevalence of gynecomastia increased with advancing age to a peak of 57 percent among those over 44 years of age (27). A prevalence of palpable gynecomastia of 32 percent was noted among 100 male veterans (9).

A variety of conditions are associated with or predispose to the development of gynecomastia. A regular feature of Klinefelter syndrome, gynecomastia also develops in association with a variety of systemic diseases including cirrhosis of the liver, hypogonadism, chronic renal disease, chronic pulmonary disease, hormonally active (human chorionic gonadotropin [HCG]-producing) tumors, and hyperthyroidism (1,6,7,22,39). Estrogens and androgens (endogenous or exogenous), as well as a variety of drugs including digitalis (23), cimetidine, marijuana, spironolactone (24), cyclic antidepressants, Levothyroxin, finasteride used for prostatic hyperplasia (1,16,23), and tricyclic antidepressants (1,22) can cause gynecomastia. Unilateral gynecomastia has been reported among men seropositive for human immunodeficiency virus (HIV) who had prolonged exposure to protease inhibitors (13), but the contribution of liver disease, long-term use of marijuana, and other medications known to induce gynecomastia cannot be excluded. Interestingly, in a cohort of 446 men who had surgery for gynecomastia of all causes, a significantly increased risk for testicular cancer and squamous cell carcinoma of the skin was noted (30). There is no definitive evidence, however, that gynecomastia is associated with an increased risk for the subsequent development of invasive breast carcinoma.

Clinical Features. Breast enlargement and a palpable mass are the major clinical presentations of gynecomastia (fig. 17-1), occasionally

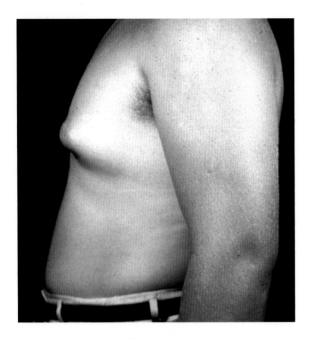

Figure 17-1

GYNECOMASTIA

A middle-aged man presents with idiopathic breast enlargement.

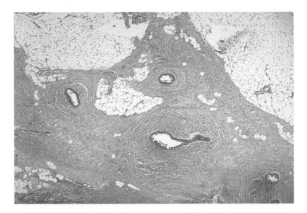

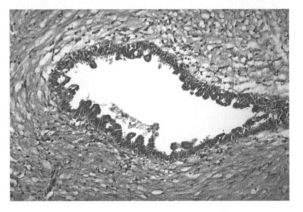

Figure 17-2

GYNECOMASTIA, PROLIFERATIVE PHASE

Top: The periductal stromal proliferation is pronounced.
Bottom: Epithelial proliferation is evident in the ducts.

accompanied by pain and/or tenderness. When bilateral, the breasts are diffusely enlarged, whereas a palpable discrete mass is more characteristic of unilateral lesions. Rarely, the mass may exceed 10 cm, however, it is more frequently about 3 to 4 cm in maximum diameter. The palpable mass is most frequently subareolar and may occasionally result in expansion of the nipple-areolar complex, but nipple discharge or retraction is uncommon.

Mammographically, gynecomastia is generally characterized by a subareolar density displaying either a dendritic configuration with prominent radial extensions into the surrounding mammary tissue when long standing (6 months or more) and reflecting the fibrous phase of the disease, or as a triangular nodule lacking extensions into the adjacent tissue when of shorter duration, reflecting the florid phase of the disease (9a,35). In a study of 206 men between 12 and 82 years of age, the mammographic patterns of gynecomastia were designated as nodular (34 percent), dendritic (35 percent), and diffuse (31 percent) (18). Invasive carcinomas that develop in the setting of gynecomastia can be detected mammographically.

Using high frequency (10-13 MHz) ultrasound examinations, it is possible to accurately diagnose gynecomastia and differentiate florid from fibrous gynecomastia (10).

Gross Findings. Whether discrete or ill-defined, gynecomastia tissue is characteristically gray-white, rubbery, and firm. This is in contrast to the fatty appearance of lipomastia.

Microscopic Findings. Microscopically, the appearance depends on the duration of the lesion (25). Gynecomastia has an active proliferative phase and ends in an inactive fibrous phase (1). The initial florid phase typically shows various degrees of intraductal proliferation (fig. 17-2), periductal stromal edema, increased vascularity, and lymphocytic infiltrates. Cytologic atypia was seen in a 53-year-old man with finasteride-induced gynecomastia (38) as well as in gynecomastia associated with flutamide therapy for prostatic carcinoma (32). In a study

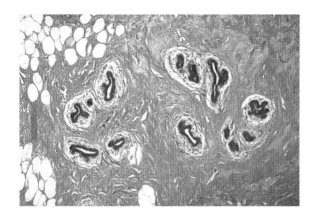

Figure 17-3

GYNECOMASTIA, FIBROUS PHASE

Mild periductal edema, collagenous background stroma, and no epithelial proliferations are seen.

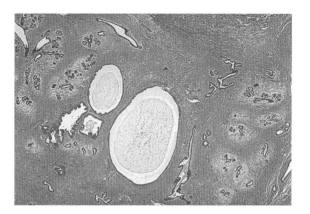

Figure 17-4

GYNECOMASTIA

Lobular development and cystic change are associated with spironolactone therapy. (Fig. 16-4 from Tavasolli FA. Pathology of the breast, 2nd ed. Stamford, CT: Appleton & Lange/McGraw Hill, 1999:836.)

of 83 patients with gynecomastia, ADH/cribriform DCIS (DIN1) was present in 6.5 percent (1). Squamous metaplasia may develop in florid gynecomastia and may become extensive (15). Apocrine change occurs in about 3 percent of cases detectable by aspiration cytology (19). The florid phase generally lasts about 6 months and is followed by a gradual transition to the fibrous phase; the period of transition is referred to as the intermediate phase.

In the fibrous phase, the epithelial proliferation is diminished, the periductal stromal edema subsides, and the stroma becomes more collagenous and less vascular (fig. 17-3). Apocrine metaplasia and pseudoangiomatous stromal hyperplasia occur in either the florid or fibrous phases.

Rarely, lobular development occurs secondary to a variety of endogenous and exogenous influences. The formation of lobules (fig. 17-4) is not necessarily related to the administration of exogenous estrogenic hormones, however (1,21,34). Interestingly, gynecomastia-like lesions have been described in women ranging from 33 to 60 years of age (35,36).

Cytologic Findings. The typical characteristics of gynecomastia, recognizable on aspiration cytology, confirm the clinical impression of gynecomastia and distinguish it from carcinoma (19,20,33). The aspirate is generally highly cellular, with cohesive sheets of round to cuboidal epithelial cells admixed with the naked nuclei of myoepithelial cells. The epithelial cell membranes are mostly ill-defined, while the nuclei are round to oval with finely granular chromatin; nuclear atypia is rare, but may occur (20).

Immunohistochemical Findings. The epithelial cells in the proliferating ducts of gynecomastia are estrogen receptor (ER) positive by immunohistochemistry in nearly 90 percent of cases (3). Immunoreactivity for progesterone (11,17) and androgen receptors (PR, AR) (31) has also been reported. In 28 percent of patients with gynecomastia, ductal epithelial cells (normal and hyperplastic) react with prostate-specific antigen (PSA), causing diagnostic problems and confusion with metastatic carcinoma from the prostate (14). The cells in gynecomastia show no immunoreaction for antiprostatic acid phosphatase (PsAP), however, and this feature could be helpful in difficult cases (14).

Molecular Findings. Few examples of gynecomastia have been analyzed at the molecular level. Comparative genomic hybridization (CGH) of two cases demonstrated overexpression of 8q in both (29). In one case, del(1)(q41) was detected by both cytogenetics and CGH. The other case had gain of 1p34.3, 11p14-q12, and 17p11.2-qter, but loss of 1q41-qter and 4q33-qter. Neither patient had Klinefelter syndrome or a family history of breast cancer and neither had received any therapy prior to specimen collection (29).

Cytogenetic studies are limited, but those available have shown a deletion of 12p and monosomies of chromosomes 9, 17, 19, and 20 (12).

Treatment. In most cases, gynecomastia requires no therapy other than removal of the inciting factor. Regression of gynecomastia secondary to hyperthyroidism (6) and alcoholic liver disease may occur once the underlying condition has been treated (7). Treatment is indicated only when there is sufficient pain, embarrassment, or emotional discomfort to interfere with the patient's life style. Management options include both surgical and medical intervention.

Before initiating medical therapy, it is important to keep in mind that 1) the high rate of spontaneous regression of gynecomastia makes it difficult to judge the efficacy of any therapy and 2) medical treatment is most effective during the proliferative phase of the disease. In the absence of concern for primary or metastatic carcinoma, surgery is attempted only if a trial of medical therapy (e.g., tamoxifen, danazol) is unsuccessful.

OTHER BENIGN MAMMARY LESIONS AND ALTERATIONS

In addition to gynecomastia, a wide variety of benign lesions, including papillomas (42,44, 48,49), juvenile papillomatosis (47,50), nipple duct adenomas (52), duct ectasia (43,51), sclerosing adenosis, and fibrocystic changes (41,45), occurs in the male breast. The criteria for diagnosis are similar to those in the female counterpart.

Among benign mesenchymal tumors, myofibroblastomas were initially thought to occur more commonly in the male breast (40) but subsequent reports have shown equal frequency in male and female breast (see chapter 12). Rare examples of adenomyoepithelioma (46) and benign mesenchymoma have also been reported in the male breast.

CARCINOMA OF THE MALE BREAST

General Features. Carcinoma of the male breast is rare, accounting for less than 1 percent of all breast carcinomas and fewer than 0.1 percent of deaths from cancer among men (141,182). In 2008, an estimated 1,990 new cases were diagnosed in the United States, with 450 deaths due to breast cancer among men (128). Mortality from breast cancer among men in the 1990s was about 2/million men both in the United States and the European Union

compared to a figure of 3/million men a decade earlier (136). Most countries report an annual incidence of less than 1/100,000 men (175), which has remained stable over a four-decade period (136). There is a linear increase in incidence with increasing age (145,147,182,189). Curiously, 6 percent of all breast carcinomas diagnosed in Tanzania occur in men (175). A higher proportion of male breast carcinoma has been noted in west and central African countries as well as among blacks in the United States (54,185,193). There is a lower incidence among Japanese males (147).

Pathogenesis. Factors associated with increased male breast cancer risk appear related to hormonal alterations, in particular, to estrogen and androgen imbalance, as well as a family history of breast cancer in female and male first-degree relatives (70,86,120,134,166,175). Klinefelter syndrome (47, XXY karyotype, small testis, azospermia, gynecomastia) is an important risk factor (64,86,98,122,127,134,175,180). About 4 to 20 percent of men with breast carcinoma have Klinefelter syndrome compared to a frequency of only 0.1 percent in the general population (126,175,193,203); men with Klinefelter syndrome have up to a 50-fold increased risk for breast carcinoma (126). An elevated risk has also been noted among males with prolactinoma (113), undescended testis, orchiectomy, orchitis, testicular injury, and infertility (193,198,210). Obesity and diabetes mellitus may be associated with some increased risk, most probably through hormonal influences (125,175,210). A high incidence of breast carcinoma has been noted in Egypt where the liver infection bilharziasis is endemic; this has been attributed to altered estrogen metabolism secondary to the liver disease (96). The development of breast carcinoma in transsexuals on prolonged oral estrogen therapy has been cited as strong supportive evidence for the role of a hormonal influence on the development of male breast carcinoma (103,160,194). Radiation exposure (95,206,210); exposure to electromagnetic fields among electricians, telephone wire workers (90,142), and railway engine drivers (68); and testicular heat exposure among workers in blast furnaces, steel works, and rolling mills (74,140,167) are among suggested risk factors. The suggestion that there is an increased risk associated with a higher socioeconomic status (86,175) is controversial (135,198). Dietary factors do not seem to play a major role in breast cancer among men (166). A higher risk has also been reported among never married and Jewish men (141,175,198). While 10 to 17 percent of patients report trauma to the affected breast prior to tumor manifestation, it is believed that trauma simply serves to increase awareness of the region.

The odds ratio for developing breast carcinoma among men with a positive family history of breast cancer in a female relative is 3.98; this increases with young age and increasing number of affected first-degree relatives (193). While epidemiologic studies have not demonstrated a higher frequency of breast carcinoma in men with prostatic carcinoma (144), prolonged estrogen therapy may be a cause of breast carcinoma in this population (69,181,213). Since prostatic carcinoma has a predilection for metastases to the breast, confirmation of a second primary carcinoma in the breast is important. Rare synchronous prostate/breast carcinomas have been reported (195).

A causal relationship between gynecomastia and carcinoma has not been proven. Gynecomastia has been reported to be associated with male breast carcinomas in 40 percent of patients by some (119,179), while others have noted gynecomastia in only about 3 percent of males with breast carcinoma (75). Among healthy men, 35 percent (8) have clinical gynecomastia and 40 percent (37) have histologic gynecomastia, indicating that the frequency of gynecomastia is not substantially higher among those with breast carcinoma (37).

Genetic Predisposition. The presence of certain germline mutations in the *BRCA1* and *BRCA2* genes confers a very high risk of developing breast cancer (94,196,199). The estimated cumulative risk of breast carcinoma for male *BRCA1* mutation carriers at age 70 years is 1.2 percent, and for *BRCA2* mutation carriers, 6.8 percent (194a); both the relative and cumulative risks are higher for *BRCA2* mutation carriers than for *BRCA1* mutation carriers. Immunohistochemical assessment of BRCA1 protein showed diminished expression in all male breast cancers (26 cases) compared to normal epithelium; marked loss was associated with increased cell proliferation (192). After evaluation of 22 families with at least one case of male breast carcinoma for

linkage to *BRCA1* on chromosome 17q, Stratton et al. (190) concluded that genes other than *BRCA1* confer an increased risk of male breast cancer. Among families with one or more male breast carcinomas, 76 percent are attributable to the presence of *BRCA2* mutation (101).

First identified by Wooster (218), who also described multiple cases of male breast carcinoma with linkage to this area, the *BRCA2* gene was localized to 13q12-13. Among breast cancer families with even one affected male, the likelihood of carrying a *BRCA2* mutation is 60 to 76 percent (101). Of 111 families with *BRCA2* mutations, men accounted for 11 percent of those with breast carcinoma compared to only 1 percent in the general population (151). In Iceland, 40 percent of male breast carcinomas are attributable to a single cancer-predisposing *BRCA2* mutation (999del5) (199), but other populations have a lower mutation frequency of 4 to 33 percent (78,102,114). Of 18 Hungarian men with breast cancer who had a family history of breast carcinoma, 6 (33 percent) carried a truncating mutation of the *BRCA2* gene (84). It is important to fully investigate all new patients with breast carcinoma to rule out hereditary *BRCA*-related disease (94).

Other heritable mutations observed among men with breast carcinoma include the androgen receptor (*AR*) gene (138,217), CYP17 polymorphism, Cowden syndrome, *CHEK2* (209), and the mismatch repair (MMR) genes associated with the hereditary familial nonpolyposis coli carcinoma (HNPCC) or Lynch syndrome (62,70). Germline mutations in the *AR* gene have been suggested as possible predisposing factors for male breast carcinoma (139,217). The *AR* gene is located at Xq11-q12, codes for a 917-amino acid transcription factor, and plays a critical role in mediating androgenic effects on cells. It has highly polymorphic polyglutamine (CAG) and polyglycine (GGC) tracts in the coding area of the first exon. It has been suggested that long CAG repeats increase the risk for breast cancer in women, probably by decreasing the capacity of the receptor to activate transcription (106). The presence of somatic mutations of the *AR* gene is not required, however, for the development of male breast carcinoma (122).

There is not a lot of information about molecular events related to the development and progression of sporadic male breast carcinoma. While the frequency of genetic aberrations has been lower in men, somatic genetic changes similar to those associated with sporadic breast carcinoma in women have been noted using comparative genomic hybridization, loss of heterozygosity (LOH), and cytogenetic analysis (173,201,211,213,220). Among the chromosomes, those most frequently amplified are 1q, 8q21-22, 17q12qter (*BRCA1* and *ERB-B2* genes are also located on chromosome 17q), 16p, and 20q13, while losses have affected mostly chromosomes 13q13-22, 6q14-23, 8p21-pter, and 9q (201); these are basically the regions showing loss in female breast carcinomas. LOH has been noted on chromosomes 8p22 (71), 11q13 (more common among carcinomas with lymph node metastases) (71), and 13q (this chromosome harbors the *BRCA2*, *BRUSH1*, and retinoblastoma [*RB*] genes); chromosome 13q alterations occur in both familial and sporadic carcinomas (159,214). Cytogenetic analysis has shown the loss of the Y chromosome and gain of an X chromosome and chromosome 5 in male breast carcinomas (169,197).

Clinical Features. Reported in a wide age range of 5 to 97 years, the median age at presentation for invasive mammary carcinoma in men is 63 to 68 years (60,72,83,170,172, 177). The mean age is 61 years for those without a family history of breast carcinoma, and 58 years for those with such a history (121). With a 3- to 6-month median duration of symptoms in more recent studies (60,83,170), a unilateral, subareolar, generally painless mass is the presenting sign in 65 to 95 percent of men. Rarely, synchronous, morphologically different, bilateral carcinomas occur (63,76,216). The risk of bilateral disease is less than 3 percent (79,133). Nipple retraction (in 10 to 51 percent of patients), discharge (in 1 to 12 percent), and ulceration (in 4 to 36 percent) are the initial manifestations in some cases (92,97,107,110,219). The mass is fixed to the overlying skin in up to 50 percent of patients. About 25 percent have a family history of breast cancer and 7 percent give a history of chest wall radiation (110). The lesion is hard and irregular on palpation, with margins varying from well to ill defined.

In a study of 257 cases from 1943 to 1972, 35 percent of the lesions were stage 1 at presenta-

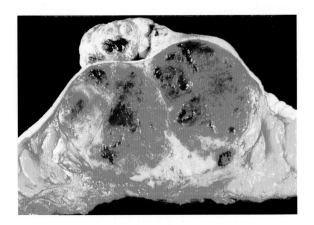

Figure 17-5

MALE BREAST CARCINOMA

A massive tumor has expanded the mammary tissue and attenuated the overlying skin.

tion, 11 percent were stage 2, 42 percent were stage 3, and 12 percent were stage 4 (177). Pure carcinoma in situ (mainly DIN) accounts for 1.1 to 17.0 percent of male breast carcinomas (123); the most characteristic symptoms are a slow growing subareolar mass and serosanguinous nipple discharge (82,118,172). Intracystic papillary carcinoma also occurs (100,186).

Less than 1 percent of mammographic examinations are done on male breasts (9a,91). They are performed for an enlarging breast, a palpable mass, or breast tenderness (9a). Mammographically, male breast carcinoma presents as a spiculated or circumscribed mass (9a), as a mass without (74 to 86 percent of cases) or with (7 to 9 percent of cases) microcalcifications, or as coarse and punctate microcalcifations in a background of dendritic gynecomastia (18,92). Technical difficulties may be encountered in the mammographic evaluation of a male breast. In such circumstances, ultrasound can be helpful; application of both modalities is likely to improve diagnostic accuracy (127).

Gross Findings. Most tumors range in size from 2.0 to 2.5 cm. Less than 5 percent are larger than 5 cm at the time of presentation (fig. 17-5).

Microscopic Findings. While the histologic classification and grading of invasive carcinomas in the male and female breast are identical, lobular carcinomas are extremely rare in the male, accounting for significantly less than 1 percent of invasive carcinomas (131,146,149,171,176).

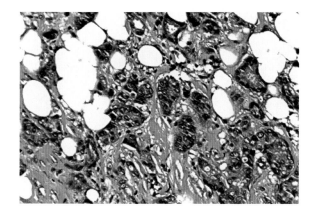 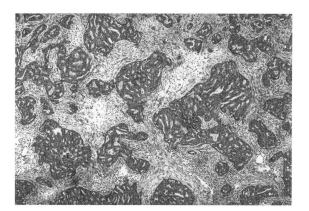

Figure 17-6

MALE BREAST CARCINOMA

Left: Infiltrating duct carcinoma is the most common invasive form.
Right: Invasive carcinoma of the cribriform type rarely occurs in the male breast.

About 90 percent of male breast carcinomas are invasive (188), and of these, 84.7 percent are infiltrating duct carcinomas (not otherwise specified [NOS]) (fig. 17-6, left) (65a). The rest display a variety of patterns including adenoid cystic, tubular, cribriform (fig. 17-6, right), mucinous, medullary, apocrine (65), inflammatory, oncocytic (77), small cell (105), pigmented papillary (164), squamous, spindle cell, small cell matrix producing, and secretory (105,163,188). Neuroendocrine differentiation has been noted in 45 percent of male carcinomas (55). When lobular carcinomas do develop, they do so more often in breasts that have lobular development secondary to endogenous or exogenous hormones (65a). In a recent study of 759 primary male breast carcinomas, nearly every subtype of carcinoma was reported (65a).

Paget's disease, including pigmented variants (150), affects the male breast (59,93,117,124,152, 184,191,204), and some have suggested a frequency as high as 12 percent of all male breast carcinomas (152), attributed to the short length of the male mammary duct system. The underlying breast carcinoma may be invasive or intraepithelial (in situ) (59). Joshi et al. (130) noted a high frequency of nipple involvement among 46 male breast carcinomas, but these represented direct extension of the tumor to the epidermis rather than classic epidermotropic Paget's disease; they did not observe any true Paget's disease among their cases. Rarely, Paget's disease appears clinically and histopathologically pigmented

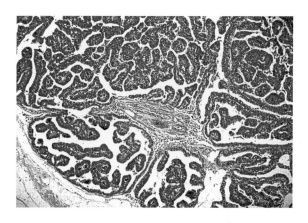

Figure 17-7

MALE BREAST CARCINOMA

Papillary architecture is a common pattern among noninvasive carcinomas.

(124,150,191) and can be confused with melanoma; this is due to the capability of Paget cells to phagocytize melanin.

Almost all intraepithelial lesions are ductal lesions; these account for 5 percent of all male breast cancers (82). A papillary growth pattern either in pure form (fig. 17-7) or in combination with other patterns accounts for a high proportion (40 to 75 percent) of noninvasive breast carcinomas (75,82,123); the remaining cases are mainly DCIS1-2/DIN1-2 (fig. 17-8; Table 17-1). While some cribriform and solid lesions have central necrosis, a high nuclear grade with necrosis (comedo), DCIS/DIN3 comedo type, is

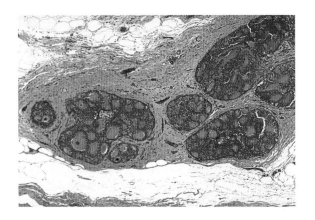
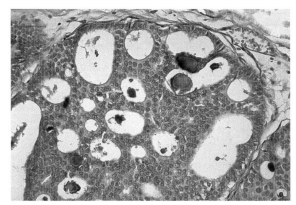

Figure 17-8

DUCTAL CARCINOMA IN SITU, GRADE 1/DUCTAL INTRAEPITHELIAL NEOPLASIA 1

Left: Cribriform type.
Right: Microcalcification and uniformity of the neoplastic cells are features indistinguishable from those in the female breast.

Table 17-1

CLINICAL AND PATHOLOGIC FEATURES OF GRADES 1-3 DUCTAL CARCINOMA IN SITU (DCIS)/DUCTAL INTRAEPITHELIAL NEOPLASIA (DIN1-3) AMONG MEN

	Cutuli et al. 1997[a] (31 Cases)	Hittmair et al. 1998[b] (84 Cases)
Median age, years	58	65
(range)	(26-74)	(25-94)
Presentation		
Mass	35%	58%
Nipple Discharge	39%	35%
Patterns		
Papillary	23%	48%
Papillary and cribriform	16%	27%
Cribriform	9.7%	19%
Comedo	9.7%	0
Not otherwise specified	39%	0
Other	3%	6%
Gynecomastia	23%	19%
Family history of breast cancer	10%	4%

[a]Cutuli B, Dilhuydy JM, deLafontan B, et al. Ductal carcinoma in situ of the male breast. Analysis of 31 cases. Eur J Cancer 1997;33:35-38.

[b]Hittmair AP, Lininger RA, Tavassoli FA. Ductal carcinoma in situ (DCIS) in the male breast: a morphologic study of 84 cases of pure DCIS and 30 cases of DCIS associated with invasive carcinoma—a preliminary report. Cancer 1998;83:2139-2149.

rare (67,82,123). Necrosis is more common in DCIS lesions associated with invasive carcinoma (123). The higher frequency of comedo DCIS/DIN3, comedo type in another study published as an abstract (207) may be due to differences in the definition of comedo DCIS and a high reliance on necrosis alone for a diagnosis of comedo DCIS/DIN3, comedo type. Lobular intraepithelial neoplasia (LIN) is extremely rare in the male breast because of the absence of lobular development.

Aspiration cytology shows a highly cellular proliferation of monotonous, loosely cohesive to dyscohesive cells. The moderate to severe nuclear atypia is in the form of irregular, enlarged, hyperchromatic nuclei with dense chromatin, nuclear membrane irregularities, and prominent nucleoli (fig. 17-9) (19,85). When the sample is satisfactory, aspiration cytology is helpful in the primary assessment of male breast tumors (129) and can reduce the number of surgical excisions for benign breast masses (137).

Hormone Receptor Expression and Other Markers. Male breast carcinomas have a higher frequency of hormone receptor positivity than the female counterpart. ER is immunohistochemically detectable in up to 80 percent (range, 60 to 95 percent) of male breast cancers, while the tumors are PR positive in 75 percent (range, 45 to 85 percent) of cases (60,74,86,87,99,143, 148,163,165,215). Expression of AR has been reported in 34 percent (157) to 95 percent (161) of the tumors, but no association has been noted between AR expression and patient age, tumor stage, PR expression, or p53 protein expression (157). Bcl-2 is positive in 67 to 80 percent of male breast carcinomas; it is more often expressed in small tumors (148,155,209). Approximately 14 percent of male breast carcinomas are CK5/6 and CK14 positive, a feature noted in breast carcinomas with a basal phenotype (73).

Among other markers, p53 protein expression has varied from 9 to 25 percent (88,148,209) and *p53* mutations have been detected in 41.4 percent of male breast carcinomas, similar to the incidence in females with breast carcinoma (56). In one study, 9 percent of male breast carcinomas were p53 positive in contrast to 28 percent of female breast carcinomas (148). In another study, the immunoprofile for p53 and c-erbB-2 were similar to that of the female counterpart (212).

Aromatase immunoexpression has been observed in the stroma of carcinomas in the male breast and may contribute to the local estrogen concentration and to tumorigenesis (174). Breast carcinomas may also express PSA (58,112), which therefore cannot be used to distinguish between primary breast carcinoma and prostatic carcinoma metastatic to the breast.

Prognosis. Similar to the female counterpart, lymph node status, tumor size, tumor stage, tumor grade, and lymphatic invasion are important prognostic factors for recurrence, overall survival, and prediction of disease-free survival (60,89,110,116,145,178,187,203). A combination of HER2/neu and p53 immunohistochemistry may identify tumors with more aggressive behavior (156). The clinical stage along with expression of p53 and HER2/neu may be useful in guiding treatment, while the assessment of ER, PR, and MIB-1 (Ki-67) status seems to be of limited value (208).

Ploidy (104,116) and S-phase fraction had no significant relation to prognosis in one study (116), but did influence survival in another (158,187a). A positive family history does not affect overall survival (121). Interestingly, while prognostic factors associated with survival are similar among different races, overall 5-year survival rates differ: 57 percent for blacks, 66 percent for whites, and 75 percent for Hispanics and Asian/Pacific islanders (153).

Axillary node metastases are present in up to 65 percent of patients at the time of presentation (81,109,130,205). The overall survival rates for node-negative patients is 57 to 100 percent at 5 years and 43 to 84 percent at 10 years; for

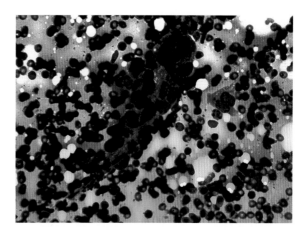

Figure 17-9

ASPIRATION CYTOLOGY OF MALE BREAST CARCINOMA

Clusters of loosely cohesive, atypical epithelial cells are seen with dyscohesive atypical cells.

patients with node-positive tumors, the overall survival rates range from 31 to 60 percent at 5 years and 11 to 35 percent at 10 years (107). In one study, survival rates were related to the number of positive nodes: at 10 years, 84 percent for node-negative patients, 44 percent for those with one to three positive nodes, and 14 percent for those with four or more positive nodes; the 5-year survival rates were 90, 73, and 55 percent, respectively (111).

About two thirds of the tumors are stages pT1c and pT2, while 15 percent are stage pT4b with skin ulceration or dermal satellite nodules. For patients with tumors of stages 1, 2, 3, and 4, the 5-year survival rates are 55 to 100 percent, 41 to 78 percent, 16 to 57 percent, and 0 to 14 percent, respectively. At 10 years, these rates are 52 to 89 percent, 10 to 52 percent, 2 to 23 percent, and 0 percent (107).

The 5-year survival rate has ranged from a low of 42 percent in 1979 (219) to 90 percent for those with favorable tumors in more recent studies (69,111). The median survival rate for 45 men treated by radical surgery was 69.8 percent at 5 years, 59.7 percent at 10 years, and 31.3 percent at 15 years. Among those with favorable tumors (T1, T2, N0, grades 1 and 2), the 5, 10, and 15 year survival rates were 90, 77.4, and 62 percent, respectively, compared to 61.8, 23.1, and 23.1 percent, respectively, for those with unfavorable tumors (T3 or N+ or grade 3). The 5-year survival rates are lower for men from Denmark and Finland than for men in Sweden, possibly due to later stage at presentation or national differences in the natural history of the disease (53). While there are differences in histology and hormone receptor status, there does not appear to be a significant difference in the survival rate for male and female patients with breast cancer when compared stage for stage (109,168,170,205).

Treatment. A core or excisional biopsy, preferably following an imaging procedure, is the first step in the assessment of a mass in the male breast. If the biopsy is benign and correlates with the clinical and radiologic impressions, follow-up in the form of annual examination for 3 years will suffice. If the biopsy shows a carcinoma, staging (chest radiograph, bone scan, laboratory evaluation, and possibly computerized tomography [CT] scan of the abdomen) should be done to determine whether the disease is localized or disseminated. Assessment of hormone receptors is particularly important for the management of the tumors whether localized or disseminated (107).

The management of breast carcinoma is constantly evolving and it is paramount to consider the most current and up to date approach. Chemotherapy is the standard treatment for hormone receptor-negative disseminated tumors, while hormonal therapy with tamoxifen is incorporated in the treatment for hormone receptor-positive tumors.

When the lesion appears localized, surgery is the initial modality of choice. Mastectomy remains the standard local therapeutic approach, with radiotherapy indicated for those with a high risk of chest wall or lymph node recurrences (130a,162,176). For those with tumors larger than 1 cm or those who are lymph node positive, adjuvant chemotherapy or hormonal therapy is indicated (89,140,154,162,163,172).

Hormonal manipulation has been the standard treatment for recurrent and, particularly, metastatic disease: 48 to 55 percent of patients respond to orchiectomy (132,202), 80 percent to adrenalectomy, and 56 percent to hypophysectomy in older studies. Overall responses to nonsurgical hormonal manipulations are 75 percent for the use of androgens, 57 percent for antiandrogens, 50 percent for steroids, 32 percent for estrogens, 50 percent for proges-

tins, and 49 percent for tamoxifen. Some have recommended tamoxifen as the treatment of choice for recurrent/metastatic male breast carcinoma (162). More recently, anastrozole, a selective aromatase inhibitor, and leuprolide acetate plus aromatase inhibition have been used in a small number of men with metastatic breast carcinoma and may have potential in stabilizing the disease (107a,108).

Comparison with Female Breast Cancer. When prognostic factors are matched, male and female cancer patients have a similar outcome for disease-free survival and overall survival (60, 107,111,118,211). Among 104 men with breast carcinomas, 67 percent of whom were treated by modified radical mastectomy, the actuarial 5-year relapse-free survival rate was 68 percent for the entire group; the 5-year survival rate was 87 percent for patients with negative axillary lymph nodes compared to 30 percent for node-positive patients (61). Low-stage male breast cancers tend to manifest at a higher grade, with a lower 5-year survival rate of 60 percent compared to the 5-year survival rate of 86 percent for the female counterpart (215).

There are differences in the ER and PR immunoprofile of male and female breast cancer; both receptors are expressed more frequently in male breast carcinoma. Expression of p27 and p21 is also more common in male breast carcinoma (80). Positivity for the kinase inhibitor proteins, p27 Kip1 and p21 Waf1, is higher among male breast carcinomas (96.2 and 70.3 percent, respectively, compared to 39.3 and 29.0 percent among breast carcinomas in women) (80).

CARCINOMA METASTATIC TO THE BREAST

Prostatic carcinoma associated with estrogen therapy is the most common carcinoma to metastasize to the breast (57,66,115). It can simulate a primary breast carcinoma. Immunostaining for PSA is not helpful in distinguishing the two since primary breast carcinomas may also express PSA. Bilateral breast involvement and the presence of multiple nodules points to a metastatic carcinoma (57). Also, in the setting of prostatic carcinoma under estrogen therapy, particularly with dissemination to other organs, the most likely diagnosis is a metastatic carcinoma. In a large series of 778 male breast cancers, the most common tumor metastatic to the male breast

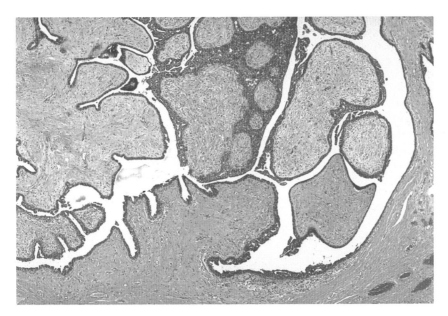

Figure 17-10

PHYLLODES TUMOR

A low-grade phyllodes tumor with focal epithelial proliferation in a 68-year-old man.

was cutaneous melanoma (65a). A diagnosis of a primary breast carcinoma should be made with caution after careful exclusion of metastatic disease

BIPHASIC TUMORS

Biphasic tumors (fibroadenoma and phyllodes tumors) rarely develop in the male breast, because these tumors appear to originate in the lobule and lobules are not present and rarely develop even in the hormonally stimulated male breast. A few examples of fibroadenoma and fibroadenomatoid hyperplasia have been reported in men 19 to 79 years of age (221,224,225,230).

Of five biphasic tumors reported by Ansah-Boteng and Tavassoli (221), four were fibroadenomas. The tumors were 1.5 to 4.5 cm and the cut surface resembled the female counterpart. Microscopically, both pericanalicular and intracanalicular patterns coexisted in most tumors. Well-developed lobules were present around a fibroadenoma in one patient who had received estrogens after orchiectomy for prostatic carcinoma; gynecomastia was evident around the tumor in another case. An interest-ing case of massive bilateral fibroadenomatoid hyperplasia in a 69-year-old man has been attributed mainly to spironolactone therapy, with digoxin administration and liver insufficiency as contributing factors (226). Another case of bilateral fibroadenomas was reported in a man under treatment for prostate carcinoma (230); the stromal cells in one of the fibroadenomas had digital fibroma-like inclusions.

Rare phyllodes tumors have been reported in men 20 to 71 years of age (221–223,225,227–229). Microscopically, they are generally low-grade tumors with sparse stromal cellularity and a pushing margin (fig. 17-10). Rarely, high-grade features (atypia, mitotic activity, and infiltrating margins) develop. Gynecomastia (221,227,229) and lobule formation (229) have been observed in the background in some cases.

Management is directed at complete excision of the biphasic tumor. A margin of uninvolved breast tissue should be obtained for phyllodes tumors with aggressive features, particularly those with infiltrating margins and sarcomatous overgrowth (see also chapter 14).

REFERENCES

Gynecomastia

1. Andersen JA, Gram JB. Gynecomasty: histological aspects in a surgical material. Acta Pathol Microbiol Immunol Scand 1982;90:185-190.
2. Andersen JA, Gram JB. Male breast at autopsy. Acta Pathol Microbiol Immunol Scand 1982;90:191-197.
3. Andersen J, Orntoft TF, Andersen JA, Poulsen HS. Gynecomastia: immunohistochemical demonstration of estrogen receptors. Acta Pathol Microbiol Immunol Scand 1987;95:263-267.
4. August GP, Chandra R, Hung W. Prepubertal gynecomastia. J Pediatr 1972;80:259-263.
5. Bannayan GA, Hajdu SI. Gynecomastia: a clinicopathologic study of 351 cases. Am J Clin Pathol 1972;57:431-437.
6. Becker KL, Matthews MJ, Higgins GA Jr, Mohamadi M. Histologic evidence of gynecomastia in hyperthyroidism. Arch Pathol 1974;98:257-260.
7. Becker KL, Matthews MJ, Winnacker J, Higgins GA Jr. Sequential histological study of the regression of gynecomastia in a patient with alcoholic liver disease. Am J Med Sci 1967;254:685-691.
8. Braunstein GD. Gynecomastia. N Engl J Med 1993;328:490-495.
9. Carlson HE. Gynecomastia. N Engl J Med 1980;303:795-799.
9a. Chantra PK, So GJ, Wollman JS, Bassett LW. Mammography of the male breast. AJR Am J Roentgenol 1995;164:853-856.
10. Cilotti A, Campassi C, Bagnolesi P, et al. Gynecomastia: diagnostic value of high-frequencies ultrasound (10-13 MHz). Breast Dis 1996;9:61-69.
11. Contesso G, Delarue JC, Guerinot F, et al. [Estrogen and progesterone receptors in male breast disease.] Nouv Press Med 1977;6:1951-1953. [French.]
12. Cornelio DA, Schmid-Braz AT, Cavalli LR, Lima RS, Ribiero EM, Cavalli IJ. Clonal karyotypic abnormalities in gynecomastia. Cancer Genet Cytogenet 1999;115:128-133.
13. Evans DL, Pantonowitz L, Dezube BJ, Aboulafia DM. Breast enlargement in 13 men who were seropositive for human immunodeficiency virus. Clin Infect Dis 2002;35:1113-1119.
14. Gatalica Z, Norris BA, Kovatich AJ. Immunohistochemical localization of prostate-specific antigen in ductal epithelium of male breast. Potential diagnostic pitfall in patients with gynecomastia. Appl Immunohistochem Mol Morphol 2000;8:158-161.
15. Gottfried MR. Extensive squamous metaplasia in gynecomastia. Arch Pathol Lab Med 1986;110:971-973.
16. Green L, Wyskowski DK, Foucroy JL. Gynecomastia and breast cancer during finasteride therapy. N Engl J Med 1996;335:823.
17. Grilli S, DeGiovanni C, Galli MC, et al. The simultaneous occurrence of cytoplasmic receptors for various steroid hormones in male breast carcinoma and gynecomastia. J Steroid Biochem 1980;13:813-820.
18. Gunhan-Bilgen I, Bozkaya H, Emin Ustun E, Memi A. Male breast disease: clinical, mammographic, and ultrasonographic features. Eur J Rad 2002;43:246-255.
19. Gupta RK, Naran S, Lallu S, Fauck R. Incidence of apocrine cells in the fine needle aspirates of gynecomastia: a study of 100 cases. Diag Cytopathol 2000;22:286-287.
20. Gupta RK, Naran S, Simpson J. The role of fine needle aspiration cytology (FNAC) in the diagnosis of breast masses in males. Eur J Surg Oncol 1988;14:317-320.
21. Haibach H, Rosenholtz MJ. Prepubertal gynecomastia with lobules and acini: a case report and review of the literature. Am J Clin Pathol 1983;80:252-255.
22. Hugues FC, Gourlot C, Le Jeunne C. [Drug-induced gynecomastia.] Ann Med Interne (Paris). 2000;151:10-7. [French.]
23. Lewinn EB. Gynecomastia during digitalis therapy: report of eight additional cases with liver function studies. N Engl J Med 1953;248:316-319.
24. Mann NM. Gynecomastia during therapy with spironolactone. JAMA 1963;184:778-780.
25. Nicolis GL, Modlinger RS, Gabrilove JL. A study of histopathology of human gynecomastia. J Clin Endocrinol Metab 1971;32:173-178.
26. Niewoehner CB, Nuttall FQ. Gynecomastia in a hospitalized male population. J Clin Endocrinol Metab 1979;48:338.
27. Nuttall FQ. Gynecomastia as a physical finding in normal men. Am J Med 1984;77:633-638.
28. Nydick M, Bustos J, Dale JH Jr, Rawson RW. Gynecomastia in adolescent boys. JAMA 1961;178:449-454 .
29. Ojopi EP, Cavalli LG, Cavalier LM, Squire JA, Rogatto SR. Comparative genomic hybridization analysis of benign and invasive male breast neoplasms. Cancer Genet Cytogenet 2002;134:123-126.
30. Olsson H, Bladstrom A, Alm P. Male gynecomastia and risk for malignant tumors—a cohort study. BMC Cancer 2002;2:26.

31. Pacheco MM, Oshima CF, Lopes MP, Widman A, Franco EL, Brentani MM. Steroid hormone receptors in male breast diseases. Anticancer Res 1986;6:1013-1017.

32. Pinedo F, Vargas J, de Augustin P, Garzon A, Perez-Barrios A, Ballestin C. Epithelial atypia in gynecomastia induced by chemotherapeutic drugs. A possible pitfall in fine needle aspiration biopsy. Acta Cytol 1991:35:229-233.

33. Russin VL, Lachowicz C, Kline TS. Male breast lesions: gynecomastia and its distinction from carcinoma by aspiration biopsy cytology. Diagn Cytopathol 1989;5:243-247.

34. Schwartz S, Wilens SL. The formation of acinar tissue in gynecomastia. Am J Pathol 1963;43:797-807.

35. Selland DI, Korbin CD, Lester SC, et al. Gynecomastoid hyperplasia: imaging findings in six patients. Radiology 2000;214:553-555.

36. Umlas J. Gynecomastia-like lesions in the female breast. Arch Pathol Lab Med 2000;124:844-847.

37. Williams MJ. Gynecomastia. Its incidence, recognition and host characterization in 447 autopsy cases. Am J Med 1963;34:103-112.

38. Zimmerman RL, Fogt F, Cronin D, Lynch R. Cytologic atypia in a 53-year-old man with finasteride-induced gynecomastia. Arch Pathol Lab Med 2000;124:625-627.

39. Yamamoto J, Yamano S, Nakatani K, et al. [An elderly case of a advanced gastric cancer with gynecomastia and high serum levels of hCG.] Nippon Ronen Igakkai Zasshi 2002;39:554-557. [Japanese.]

Other Benign Lesions

40. Ali S, Teichberg S, DeRisi DC, Urmacher C. Giant myofibroblastoma of the male breast. Am J Surg Pathol 1994;18:1170-1176.

41. Banik S, Hale R. Fibrocystic disease in the male breast. Histopathology 1988;12:214-216.

42. Hassan MO, Gogate PA, Al-Kaisi N. Intraductal papilloma of the male breast: an ultrastructural and immunohistochemical study. Ultrastruct Pathol 1994;18:601-609.

43. Mansel RE, Morgan WP. Duct ectasia in the male. Br J Surg 1979;66:660-662.

44. Martorano Navas MD, Raya Povedans JL, Anorbe Mendivil E, et al. Intracystic papilloma in male breast: ultrasonography and pneumocystography diagnosis. J Clin Ultrasound 1993;21:38-40.

45. McClure J, Banerjee SS, Sandilands DG. Female type cystic hyperplasia in a male breast. Postgrad Med J 1985;61:441-443.

46. Michal M, Baumruk L, Burger J, Manhalova M. Adenomyoepithelioma of the breast with undifferentiated carcinoma component. Histopathology 1994;24:274-276.

47. Munitiz V, Illana J, Sola J, Pinero A, Rios A, Parrilla P. A case of breast cancer associated with juvenile papillomatosis of the male breast. Eur J Surg Oncol 2000;26:715-716.

48. Prabhakar BR, Jacob S. Multiple intraductal papillomas and sclerosing adenosis in the male breast. Indian J Pathol Microbiol 1994;37:9-10.

49. Sara AS, Gottfried MR. Benign papilloma of the male breast following chronic phenothiazine therapy. Am J Clin Pathol 1987;87:649-650.

50. Sund BS, Topstad TK, Nesland JM. A case of juvenile papillomatosis of the male breast. Cancer 1992;70:126-128.

51. Tedeschi LG, McCarthy PE. Involutional mammary duct ectasia and periductal mastitis in a male. Hum Pathol 1974;5:232-236.

52. Waldo ED, Sidhu GS, Hu AW. Florid papillomatosis of male nipple after diethylstilbestrol therapy. Arch Pathol 1975;99:364-366.

Carcinoma

53. Adami HO, Hakulinen T, Ewertz M, Tretti S, Holmberg L, Karjalainen S. The survival pattern of male breast cancer. An analysis of 1429 patients from the Nordic countries. Cancer 1989;64:1177-1182.

54. Ajayi DO, Osegbe DN, Ademiluyu SA. Carcinoma of the male breast in West Africans and a review of the world literature. Cancer 1982;50:1664-1667.

55. Alm P, Alumets J, Bak-Jensen E, Olsson H. Neuroendocrine differentiation in male breast carcinomas. APMIS 1992;100:1289-1293.

56. Anelli A, Anelli TF, Youngson B, Rosen PP, Borgen PI. Mutations of the p53 gene in male breast cancer. Cancer 1995;75:2233-2238.

57. Berge T. Metastases to the male breast. Acta Pathol Microbiol Scand (A) 1971;79:491-496.

58. Bodey B, Bodey B Jr, Kaiser HE. Immunocytochemical detection of prostate specific antigen expression in human breast carcinoma cells. Anticancer Res 1997;17:2577-2581.

59. Bodnar M, Miller OF 3rd, Tyler W. Paget's disease of the male breast associated with intraductal carcinoma. J Am Acad Dermatol 1999;40:829-831.

60. Borgen PI, Senie RT, McKinnon WM, Rosen PP. Carcinoma of the male breast: analysis of prognosis compared with matched female patients. Ann Surg Oncol 1997;4:385-388.

61. Borgen PI, Wong GY, Vlamis V, et al. Current management of male breast cancer. A review of 104 cases. Ann Surg 1992;215:451-457.

62. Boyd J, Rhei E, Federici MG, et al. Male breast cancer in the hereditary nonpolyposis colorectal cancer syndrome. Breast Cancer Res Treat 1999;53:87-91.

63. Brodie EM, King ER. Histologically different, synchronous, bilateral carcinoma of the male breast (a case report). Cancer 1974;34:1276-1277.

64. Brown PW, Terz JJ. Breast carcinoma associated with Klinefelter syndrome: a case report. J Surg Oncol 1978;10:413-415.

65. Bryant J. Male breast carcinoma: a case of apocrine carcinoma with psammoma bodies. Hum Pathol 1981;12:751-753.

65a. Burga AM, Fadare O, Lininger RA, Tavassoli FA. Invasive carcinomas of the male breast: a morphologic study of the distribution of histologic subtypes and metastatic patterns in 778 cases. Virchows Arch 2006;449:507-512.

66. Campbeli JH, Cummins SD. Metastases simulating mammary cancer in prostatic carcinoma under estrogenic therapy. Cancer 1951;4:303-311.

67. Camus MG, Joshi MG, Mackarem G, et al. Ductal carcinoma in situ of the male breast. Cancer 1994;74:1289-1293.

68. Capacci F, Carnevale F. [Male breast tumors in railway engine drivers: investigation of 5 cases.] Ann Ist Super Sanita 2000;36:375-379. [Italian.]

69. Carlsson G, Hafstrom L, Jonsson PE. Male breast cancer. Clin Oncol 1981;7:149-155.

70. Casagrande J, Hanisch R, Pike M, Ross R, Brown JB, Henderson BE. A case-control study of male breast cancer. Cancer Res 1988;48:1326-1330.

71. Chuaqui RF, Sanz-Ortega J, Vocke C, et al. Loss of heterozygosity on the short arm of chromosome 8 in male breast carcinomas. Cancer Res 1995;55:4995-4998.

72. Ciatto S, Iossa A, Bonardi R, e al. Male breast carcinoma: review of a multicenter series of 150 cases. Tumori 1990;76:555-558.

73. Ciocca V, Bombanati A, Gatalica Z, et al. Cytokeratin profiles of male breast cancers. Histopathology 2006;49:365-370.

74. Cocco P, Figgs L, Dosemeci M, Hayes R, Linet MS, Hsing AW. Case-control study of occupational exposures and male breast cancer. Occup Environ Med 1998;55:599-604.

75. Cole FM, Qizilbash AH. Carcinoma in situ of the male breast. J Clin Pathol 1979;32:1128-1134.

76. Coley GM, Otis RD, Clark WE 2nd. Multiple primary tumors including bilateral breast cancers in a man with Klinefelter's syndrome. Cancer 1971;27:1476-1481.

77. Costa MJ, Silverberg SG. Oncocytic carcinoma of the male breast. Arch Pathol Lab Med 1989;113:1396-1399.

78. Couch FJ, Farid LM, DeShano ML, et al. BRCA2 germline mutations in male breast cancer cases and breast cancer families. Nat Genet 1996;13:123-125.

79. Crichlow RW. Carcinoma of the male breast. Surg Gynecol Obstet 1972;134:1011-1019.

80. Curigliano G, Colleoni M, Renne G, et al. Recognizing features that are dissimilar in male and female breast cancer: expression of p21(Waf1) and p27 (Kip1) using an immunohistochemical assay. Ann Oncol 2002;13:895-902.

81. Cutuli B, Borel C, Dhermain F, et al. Breast cancer occurred after treatment for Hodgkin's disease: analysis of 133 cases. Radiother Oncol 2001;59:247-255.

82. Cutuli B, Dilhuydy JM, de Lafontan B, et al. Ductal carcinoma in situ of the male breast. Analysis of 31 cases. Eur J Cancer 1997;33:35-38.

83. Cutuli B, Lacroze M, Dilhuydy JM, et al. Male breast cancer: results of the treatments and prognostic factors in 397 cases. Eur J Cancer 1995;31A:1960-1964.

84. Csokay B, Udvarhelyi N, Sulyok Z, et al. High frequency of germ-line BRCA2 mutations among Hungarian male breast cancer patients without family history. Cancer Res 1999;59:995-998.

85. Das DK, Junaid TA, Mathews SB, et al. Fine needle aspiration cytology diagnosis of male breast lesions. A study of 185 cases. Acta Cytol 1995;39:870-876.

86. D'Avanzo B, La Vecchia C. Risk factors for male breast cancer. Br J Cancer 1995;71:1359-1362.

87. Dawson PJ, Paine TM, Wolman SR. Immunocytochemical characterization of male breast cancer. Mod Pathol 1992;5:621-625.

88. Dawson PJ Schroer KR, Wolman SR. ras and p53 genes in male breast cancer. Mod Pathol 1996;9:367-370.

89. De los Santos JF, Buchholz TA. Carcinoma of the male breast. Curr Treat Options Oncol 2000;1:221-227.

90. Demers PA, Thomas DB, Rosenblatt KA, et al. Occupational exposure to electromagnetic fields and breast cancer in men. Am J Epidemiol 1991;134:340-347.

91. Dershaw DD. Male mammography. AJR Am J Roentgenol 1986;146:127-131.

92. Dershaw DD, Borgen PI, Deutch BM, Liberman L. Mammographic findings in men with breast cancer. AJR Am J Roentgenol 1993;160:267-270.

93. Desai DC, Brennan EJ Jr, Carp NZ. Paget's disease of the male breast. Am J Surg 1996;62:1068-1072.

94. Diez O, Cortes J, Domenech M, et al. BRCA2 germ-line mutations in Spanish male breast cancer patients. Ann Oncol 2000;11:81-84.

95. Eldar S, Nash E, Abrahamson J. Radiation carcinogenesis in the male breast. Eur J Surg Oncol 1989;15:274-278.

96. El-Gazayerli MM, Abdel-Aziz AS. On bilharziasis and male breast cancer in Egypt: a preliminary report and review of the literature. Br J Cancer 1963;17:566-571.

97. El Omari-Alaoui H, Lahdiri I, Nejjar I, et al. Male breast cancer. A report of 71 cases. Cancer Radiotherapy 2002;6:349-351.

98. Evans DB, Crichlow RW. Carcinoma of the male breast and Klinefelter's syndrome: is there an association? Cancer 1987;37:246-251.

99. Everson RB, Lippman ME, Thompson EB, et al. Clinical correlations of steroid receptors and male breast cancer. Cancer Res 1980;40:991-997.

100. Fallentin E, Rothman L. Intracystic carcinoma of the male breast. J Clin Ultrasound 1994;22:118-120.

101. Ford D, Easton DF, Stratton M, et al. Genetic heterogeneity and penetrance analysis of BRCA1 and BRCA2 genes in breast cancer families. Am J Hum Genet 1998;62:676-689.

102. Friedman LS, Gayther SA, Kurosaki T, et al. Mutation analysis of BRCA1 and BRCA2 in a male breast cancer population. Am J Hum Genet 1997;60:313-319.

103. Ganly I, Taylor EW. Breast cancer in a transsexual man receiving hormone replacement therapy. Br J Surg 1995;82:341.

104. Gattuso P, Reddy V, Green L, Castelli M, Haley D, Herman C. Prognostic significance of DNA ploidy in male breast carcinoma. A retrospective analysis of 32 cases. Cancer 1992;70:777-780.

105. Giffler RF, Kay S. Small cell carcinoma of the male mammary gland. A tumor resembling infiltrating lobular carcinoma. Am J Clin Pathol 1976;66:715-722.

106. Giguere Y, Dewailly E, Brisson J, et al. Short polyglutamine tracts in the androgen receptor are protective against breast cancer in the general population. Cancer Res 2001;61:5869-5874.

107. Giordano SH, Buzdar AU, Hortobagyi GN. Breast cancer in men. Ann Int Med 2002;137:678-687.

107a. Giordano SH, Hortobagyi N. Leuprolide acetate plus aromatase inhibition for male breast cancer. J Clin Oncol 2006;24:e42-e43.

108. Giordano SH, Valero V, Buzdar AU, Hortobagyi GN. Efficacy of anastrozole in male breast cancer. Am J Clin Oncol 2002;25:235-237.

109. Goss PE, Reid C, Pintilie M, Lim R, Miller N. Male breast carcinoma: a review of 229 patients who presented to the Princess Margaret Hospital during 40 years: 1955-1996. Cancer 1999;85:629-639.

110. Gough DB, Donohue JH, Evans MM, et al. A 50-year experience of male breast cancer: is outcome changing? Surg Oncol 1993;2:325-333.

111. Guinee VF, Olsson H, Moller T, et al. The prognosis of breast cancer in males. A report of 335 cases. Cancer 1993;71:154-161.

112. Gupta RK. Immunoreactivity of prostate-specific antigen in male breast carcinomas: two examples of a diagnostic pitfall in discriminating a primary breast cancer from metastatic prostate carcinoma. Diagn Cytopathol 1999;21:167-169.

113. Haga S, Watanabe O, Shimizu T, et al. Breast cancer in a male patient with prolactinoma. Surg Today 1993;23:251-255.

114. Haraldsson K, Loman N, Zhang QX, Johannsson O, Olsson H, Borq A. BRCA2 germ-line mutation in male breast cancer patients without a family history of the disease. Cancer Res 1998;58:1367-1371.

115. Hartley LC, Little JH. Bilateral mammary metastases from carcinoma of the prostate during oestrogen therapy. Med J Aust 1971;1:434-436.

116. Hatschek T, Wingren S, Carstensen J, Hultbom R. DNA content and S-phase fraction in male breast carcinomas. Acta Oncol 1994;33:609-613.

117. Hayes R, Cummings B, Miller RA, Guha AK. Male Paget's disease of the breast. J Cutan Med Surg 2000;4:208-212.

118. Hecht JR, Wong JT, Ramos L, et al. Male breast cancers rarely overexpress p53 protein. Proc Am Assoc Cancer Res 1994;35:214.

119. Heller KS, Rosen PP, Schottenfeld D, Ashikari R, Kinne DW. Male breast cancer: a clinicopathologic study of 97 cases. Ann Surg 1978;188:60-65.

120. Hemminki K, Vaittinen P. Male breast cancer: risk to daughters. Lancet 1999;353:1186-1187.

121. Hill A, Yagmur Y, Tran KN, Bolton JS, Robson M, Borgen PI. Localized male breast carcinoma and family history. An analysis of 142 patients. Cancer 1999;86:821-825.

122. Hiort O, Naber SP, Lehners A, et al. The role of androgen receptor gene mutations in male breast carcinoma. J Clin Endocrinol Metab 1996;81:3404-3407.

123. Hittmair AP, Lininger RA, Tavassoli FA. Ductal carcinoma in situ (DCIS) in the male breast: a morphologic study of 84 cases of pure DCIS and 30 cases of DCIS associated with invasive carcinoma—a preliminary report. Cancer 1998:83:2139-2149

124. Ho TC, St Jacques M, Schopflocher P. Pigmented Paget's disease of the male breast. J Am Acad Dermatol 1990;23:338-341.

125. Hsing AW, McLaughlin JK, Cocco P, Co Chien HT, Fraumeni JF Jr. Risk factors for male breast cancer (United States). Cancer Causes Control 1998;9:269-275.

126. Hultborn R, Hanson C, Kopf I, Verbiene I, Warnhammar E, Weimarck A. Prevalence of Klinefelter's syndrome in male breast cancer patients. Anticancer Res 1997;17:4293-4297.

127. Jackson VP, Gilmor RL. Male breast carcinoma and gynecomastia: comparison of mammography with sonography. Radiology 1983;149:533-536.

128. Jemal A, Siegel R, Ward E, Hao Y, Xu J, Thun MJ. Cancer statistics, 2008. CA Cancer J Clin 2008;58:71-96.

129. Joshi A, Kapila K, Verma K. Fine needle aspiration cytology in the management of male breast masses. Nineteen years of experience. Acta Cytol 1999;43:334-338.

130. Joshi MG, Lee AK, Loda M, et al. Male breast carcinoma: an evaluation of prognostic factors contributing to a poorer outcome. Cancer 1996;77:490-498.

130a. Kamila C, Jenny B, Per H, Jonas B. How to treat male breast cancer. Breast 2007;16(Suppl 2): S147-154.

131. Koc M, Oztas S, Erem T, Ciftcioglu MA, Onuk MD. Invasive lobular carcinoma of the male breast: a case report. Jpn J Clin Oncol 2001;31:444-446.

132. Kraybill WG, Kaufman R, Kinne D. Treatment of advanced male breast cancer. Cancer 1981;47:2183-2189.

133. Langlands AO, Maclean N, Kerr GR. Carcinoma of the male breast: report of a series of 88 cases. Clin Radiol 1976;27:21-25.

134. LaVecchia C, Levi F, Lucchini F. Descriptive epidemiology of male breast cancer in Europe. Int J Cancer 1992;51:62-66.

135. Lenfant-Pejovic MH, Milka-Cabanne N, Bouchardy C, Auquier A. Risk factors for male breast cancer: A Franco-Swiss case-control study. Int J Cancer 1990;45:661-665.

136. Levi F, Lucchini F, Negri E, Boyle P, La Vecchia C. Cancer mortality in Europe, 1990-1994, and an overview of trends from 1955 to 1994. Eur J Cancer 1999;10:1477-1516.

137. Lilleng R, Paksoy N, Vural G, et al. Assessment of fine needle aspiration cytology and histopathology for diagnosing male breast masses. Acta Cytol 1995;39;877-881.

138. Lobaccaro JM, Lumbroso S, Belon C, et al. Male breast cancer and the androgen receptor gene. Nat Genet 1993;5:109-110.

138. Lobaccaro JM Lumbroso S, Belon C, et al. Androgen receptor gene mutation in male breast cancer. Hum Mol Genet 1993;2;1799-1802.

140. Lopez M, Di Lauro L, Lazzaro B, Papaldo P. Hormonal treatment of disseminated male breast cancer. Oncology 1985;42:345-349.

141. Mabuchi K, Bross DS, Kessler II. Risk factors of male breast cancer. J Natl Cancer Inst 1985;74:371-375.

142. Matanoski GM, Breysse PN, Elliott EA. Electromagnetic field exposure and male breast cancer. Lancet 1991;337:737.

143. McLachlan SA, Erlichman C, Liu FF, Miller N, Pintilie M. Male breast cancer: an 11 year review of 66 patients. Breast Cancer Res Treat 1996;40:225-230.

144. McClure JA, Higgins CC. Bilateral carcinoma of the male breast after estrogen therapy. JAMA 1951;146:7-9.

145. Meguerditchian AN, Falardeau M, Martin G. Male breast carcinoma. Can J Surg 2002;45:296-302.

146. Michaels BM, Nunn CR, Roses DF. Lobular carcinoma of the male breast. Surgery 1994;115:402-405.

147. Moolgavkar SH, Lee JA, Hade RD. Comparison of age-specific mortality from breast cancer in males in the United States and Japan. J Natl Cancer Inst 1978;60:1223-1225.

148. Muir D, Kanthan R, Kanthan SC. Male versus female breast cancers. A population-based comparative immunohistochemical analysis. Arch Pathol Lab Med 2003;127:36-41.

149. Nance KV, Reddick RL. In situ and infiltrating lobular carcinoma of the male breast. Hum Pathol 1989;20:1220-1222.

150. Nakamura S, Ishida-Yamamoto A, Takahashi H, et al. Pigmented Paget's disease of the male breast: a report of a case. Dermatology 2001;202:134-137.

151. Neuhausen SL, Godwin AK, Gershoni-Baruch E, et al. Haplotype and phenotype analysis of nine recurrent BRCA2 mutations in 111 families: results of an international study. Am J Hum Genet 1998;62:1381-1388.

152. Norris HJ, Taylor HB. Carcinoma of the male breast. Cancer 1969;23:1428-1435.

153. O'Malley CD, Prehn AW, Shema SJ, Glaser SL. Racial/ethnic differences in survival rates in a population-based series of men with breast carcinoma. Cancer 2002;94:2836-2843.

154. Patterson JS, Battersby LA, Bach BK. Use of tamoxifen in advanced male breast cancer. Cancer Treat Rep 1980;64:801-804.

155. Pich A, Margaria E, Chiusa L. Bcl-2 expression in male breast carcinoma. Virchows Arch 1998;433:229-235.

156. Pich A, Margaria E, Chiusa L. Oncogenes and male breast carcinoma: c-erbB-2 and p53 expression predicts a poor survival. J Clin Oncol 2000;18:2948-2956.

157. Pich A, Margaria E, Chiusa L, Candelaresi G, Dal Canton O. Androgen receptor expression in male breast carcinoma: lack of clinicopathologic association. Br J Cancer 1999;79:959-964.

158. Pich A, Margaria E, Chiusa L, Ponti R, Geuna M. DNA ploidy and p53 expression correlate with survival and cell proliferative activity in male breast carcinoma. Hum Pathol 1996;27:676-682.

159. Prechtel D, Werenskiold AK, Prechtel K, Keller G, Hofler H. Frequent loss of heterozygosity at chromosome 13q12-13 with BRCA2 markers in sporadic male breast cancer. Diagn Mol Pathol 1998;7:57-62.

160. Pritchard TJ, Pankowski DA, Crowe JP, Abdul-Karim FW. Breast cancer in a male-to-female transsexual. A case report. JAMA 1988;259:2278-2280.

161. Rayson D, Erlichman C, Suman VJ, et al. Molecular markers in male breast carcinoma. Cancer 1998;83:1947-1955.

162. Ribeiro G. Male breast carcinoma—a review of 301 cases from the Christie Hospital & Holt Radium Institute, Manchester. Br J Cancer 1985;51:115-119.

163. Ribeiro GG, Swindell R, Harris M, Bonerjee SS, Cramer A. A review of the management of the male breast carcinoma based on analysis of 420 treated cases. The Breast 1996;5:141-146.

164. Romanelli R, Toncini C. Pigmented papillary carcinoma of the male breast. Tumori 1986;72:105-108.

165. Rosen PP, Menendez-Botet CJ, Nisselbaum JS, Schwartz MK, Urban JA. Estrogen receptor protein in lesions of the male breast. Cancer 1976;37:1866-1868.

166. Rosenblatt K, Thomas D, McTiernan A, et. al. Breast cancer in men: aspects of familial aggregation. J Natl Cancer Inst 1991;83:849-854.

167. Rosenbaum PF, Vena JE, Zielezny MA, Michalek AM. Occupational exposures associated with male breast cancer. Am J Epidemiol 1994;139:30-36.

168. Rudan I, Rudan N, Basic N, Basic V, Rudan D, Jambrisak Z. Differences between male and female breast cancer. III. Prognostic features. Acta Med Croatia 1997;51:135-141.

169. Rudas M, Schmidinger M, Wenzel C, et al. Karyotypic findings in two cases of male breast cancer. Cancer Genet Cytogenet 2000;121:190-193.

170. Salvadori B, Saccozzi R, Manzari A, et al. Prognosis of breast cancer in males: an analysis of 170 cases. Eur J Cancer 1994;30A:930-935.

171. Sanchez AG, Villanueva AG, Redondo C. Lobular carcinoma of the breast in a patient with Klinfelter's syndrome: a case with bilateral, synchronous, histologically different breast tumors. Cancer 1986;57:1181-1183.

172. Sandler B, Carman C, Perry RR. Cancer of the male breast. Am Surg 1994;60:816-820.

173. Sanz-Ortega J, Chuaqui R, Zhuang Z, et al. Loss of heterozygosity on chromosome 11q13 in microdissected human male breast carcinomas. J Natl Cancer Inst 1995;87:1408-1410.

174. Sasano H, Kimura M, Shizawa S, Kimura N, Nagura H. Aromatase and steroid receptors in gynecomastia and male breast carcinoma: an immunohistochemical study. J Clin Endocrinol Metab 1996;81:3063-3067.

175. Sasco A, Lowenfels A, Pasker-de Jong P. Epidemiology of male breast cancer. A meta-analysis of published case-control studies and discussion of selected aetiological factors. Int J Cancer 1993;53:538-549.

176. Scheidback H, Dworak O, Schumucker B, Hohenberger W. Lobular carcinoma of the breast in an 85-year-old man. Eur J Surg Oncol 2000;26:319-321.

177. Scheike O. Male breast cancer. 5. Clinical manifestations in 257 cases in Denmark. Br J Cancer 1973;28:552-561.

178. Scheike O. Male breast cancer. 6. Factors influencing prognosis. Br J Cancer 1974;30:261-271.

179. Scheike O, Visfeldt J. Male breast cancer. 4. Gynecomastia in patients with breast cancer. Acta Pathol Microbiol Scand (A) 1973;81:359-365.

180. Scheike O, Visfeldt J, Peterson B. Male breast cancer. 3. Breast carcinoma in association with the Klinefelter syndrome. Acta Pathol Microbiol Scand (A) 1973;81:351-358.

181. Schlappack OK, Braun O, Maier U. Report of two cases of male breast cancer after prolonged estrogen treatment of prostatic carcinoma. Cancer Detect Prev 1986;9:319-322.

182. Schottenfeld D, Lilienfeld AM, Diamond H. Some observations on the epidemiology of breast cancer among males. Am J Public Health 1963;53:890-897.

183. Schuchardt U, Seegenschmiedt MH, Kirschner MJ, Renner H, Sauer R. Adjuvant radiotherapy for breast carcinoma in men: a 20-year clinical experience. Int J Clin Oncol 1996;19:330-336.

184. Serour F, Birkenfeld S, Amsterdam E, Treshchan O, Krispin M. Paget's disease of the male breast. Cancer 1988;62:601-605.

185. Simon MS, McKnight E, Schwartz A, Martino S, Swanson GM. Racial differences in cancer of the male breast—15 years experience in the Detroit metropolitan area. Breast Cancer Res Treat 1992;21:55-62.

186. Sonksen CJ, Michell M, Sundaresan M. Case report: intracystic papillary carcinoma of the breast in a male patient. Clin Radiol 1996;51:438-439.

187. Spence RA, Mackenzie G, Anderson JR, Lyons AR, Bell M. Long-term survival following cancer of the male breast in Northern Ireland. A report of 81 cases. Cancer 1985;55:648-652.

187a. Sridhar M, Haffty BG, Sinard J, et al. DNA ploidy as a significant predictor of recurrence-free survival in male patients with breast cancer. Breast J 1995;1:356-361.

188. Stalsberg H, Thomas DB, Rosenblatt KA, et al. Histologic types and hormone receptors in breast cancer in men: a population-based study in 282 United States men. Cancer Causes Control 1993;4:143-151.

189. Steinitz R, Katz L, Beh-Hur M. Male breast cancer in Israel: selected epidemiological aspects. Isr J Med Sci 1981;17:816-821.

190. Stratton MR, Ford D, Neuhausen S, et al. Familial male breast cancer is not linked to the BRCA1 locus on chromosome 17q. Nat Genet 1994;7:103-107.

191. Stretch JR, Denton KJ, Millard PR, Horak E. Paget's disease of the male breast clinically and histopathologically mimicking melanoma. Histopathology 1991;19:470-472.

192. Sun X, Gong Y, Rao MS, Badve S. Loss of BRCA1 expression in sporadic male breast carcinoma. Breast Cancer Res Treat 2002;71:1-7.

193. Surveillance, Epidemiology, and End Results (SEER) Program. Public-Use Data (1993-1997). Bethesda, MD: National Cancer Institute, Division of Cancer Control and Population Sciences, Surveillance Research Program, Cancer Statistics Branch; April 2000.

194. Symmers WS. Carcinoma of breast in transsexual individuals after surgical and hormonal interference with the primary and secondary sex characteristics. Br Med J 1968;2:82-85.

194a. Tai YC, Domchek S, Parmigianni G, Chen S. Breast cancer risk among male BRCA1 and BRCA2 mutation carriers. J Natl Cancer Inst 2007;99:1811-1814.

195. Tajika M, Tuchiya T, Yasuda M, et al. A male case of synchronous double cancers of the breast and prostate. Intern Med 1994;33:31-35.

196. Tavtigian SV, Simard J, Rommens J, et al. The complete BRCA2 gene and mutations in chromosome 13q-linked kindreds. Nat Genet 1996;12:333-337.

197. Teixeira MR, Pandis N, Dietrich CU, et al. Chromosome banding analysis of gynecomastias and breast carcinomas in men. Genes Chromosomes Cancer 1998;23:16-20.

198. Thomas DB, Jimenez LM, McTiernan A, et al. Breast cancer in men; risk factors with hormonal implications. Am J Epidemiol 1992;135:734-748.

199. Thorlacius S, Olafsdottir G, Tryggvadottir L, et al. A single BRCA2 mutation in male and female breast cancer families from Iceland with varied cancer phenotypes. Nat Genet 1996;13:117-119.

200. Thorlacius S, Tryggvadottir L, Oladsdottir GH, et al. Linkage to BRCA2 region in hereditary male breast cancer. Lancet 1995;346:544-545.

201. Tirkkonen M, Kainu T, Loman N, et al. Somatic genetic alterations in BRCA2-associated and sporadic male breast cancer. Genes Chromosomes Cancer 1999;24:56-61.

202. Treves N, Abels JC, Woodard HQ, Farrow J. The effects of orchiectomy on primary and metastatic carcinoma of the breast. CA Cancer J Clin 1978;28:182-190.

203. van Geel AN, van Slooten EA, Mavruniac M, Hart AA. A retrospective study of male breast cancer in Holland. Br J Surg 1985;72:724-727.

204. Verniers D, Van den Bogaert W, van der Schueren E, et al. Paget's disease of the male breast treated by radiotherapy. Br J Radiol 1991;64:1062-1064.

205. Vetto J, Jun SY, Paduch D, Eppich H, Shih R. Stages at presentation, prognostic factors, and outcome of breast cancer in males. Am J Surg 1999;177:379-383.

206. Wanebo CK, Johnson KG, Sato K, Thorslund TW. Breast cancer after exposure to the atomic bombings of Hiroshima and Nagasaki. N Engl J Med 1968;279:667-671.

207. Wang Y, Abreau M, Hoda S. Mammary duct carcinoma in situ in males: pathological findings and clinical considerations. Mod Pathol 1997;10:27A.

208. Wang-Rodriguez J, Cross K, Gallagher S, et al. Male breast carcinoma: correlation of ER, PR, Ki-67, Her2-neu, and p53 with treatment and survival, a study of 65 cases. Mod Pathol 2002;15:853-861.

209. Weber-Chappuis K, Bieri-Burger S, Hurlimann J. Comparison of prognostic markers detected by immunohistochemistry in male and female breast carcinomas. Eur J Cancer 1996;32A:1686-1692.

210. Weiss JR, Moysich KB, Swede H. Epidemiology of male breast cancer. Cancer Epidemiol Biomarkers Prev 2005;14:20-26.

211. Willsher PC, Leach IH, Ellis IO, Bourke JB, Blamey RW, Robertson JF. A comparison outcome of male breast cancer with female breast cancer. Am J Surg 1997;173:185-188.

212. Willsher PC, Leach IH, Ellis IO, et al. Male breast cancer: pathological and immunohistochemical features. Anticancer Res 1997;17:2335-2338.

213. Wilson SE, Hutchinson WB. Breast masses in males with carcinoma of the prostate. J Surg Oncol 1976;8:105-112.

214. Wingren S, van den Heuvel A, Gentile M, Olsen K, Hatschek T, Sonderkvist P. Frequent allelic losses on chromosome 13q in human male breast carcinomas. Eur J Cancer 1997;33:2393-2396.

215. Wick MR, Sayadi H, Ritter JH, Hill DA, Reddy VB, Gattuso P. Low stage carcinoma of the male breast. A histologic, immunohistochemical, and flow cytometric comparison with localized female breast carcinoma. Am J Clin Pathol 1999;111:59-69.

216. Wolloch Y, Zer M, Dintsman M, Kozenitsky I. Simultaneous bilateral primary breast carcinoma in the male. Isr J Med Sci 1972;8:158-162.

217. Wooster R, Mangion J, Eeles R, et al. A germline mutation in the androgen receptor gene in two brothers with breast cancer and Reifenstein syndrome. Nat Genet 1992;2:132-134.

218. Wooster R, Neuhausen SL, Mangion J, et al. Localization of a breast cancer susceptibility gene, BRCA2, to chromosome 13q12-13. Science 1994;265:2088-2090.

219. Yap HY, Tashima CK, Blumenschein GR, Eckles NE. Male breast cancer. A natural history study. Cancer 1979;44:748-754.

220. Zhuang Z, Merino MJ, Chuaqui R, Liotta LA, Emmert-Buck MR. Identical allelic loss on chromosome 11q13 in microdissected in situ and invasive human breast cancer. Cancer Res 1995;55:467-471.

Biphasic Lesions

221. Ansah-Boteng Y, Tavassoli FA. Fibroadenoma and cystosarcoma phyllodes of the male breast. Mod Pathol 1992;5:114-116.

222. Bapat K, Oropeza R, Sahoo S. Benign phyllodes tumor of the male breast. Breast J 2002;8:115-116.

223. Bartoli C, Zurrida SM, Clemente C. Phyllodes tumour in a male patient with bilateral gynecomastia induced by oestrogen therapy for prostatic carcinoma. Eur J Surg Oncol 1991;17:215-217.

224. Hilton DA, Jameson JS, Furness PN. A cellular fibroadenoma resembling a benign phyllodes tumor in a young male with gynaecomastia. Histopathology 1991;18:476-477.

225. Kahan Z, Toszegi AM, Szarvas F, Gaizer G, Baradnay G, Ormos J. Recurrent phyllodes tumor in a man. Pathology Res Pract 1997;193:653-658.

226. Nielsen BB. Fibroadenomatoid hyperplasia of the male breast. Am J Surg Pathol 1990;14:774-777.

227. Nielsen VT, Andreasen C. Phyllodes tumour of the male breast. Histopathology 1987;11:761-762.

228. Pantoja E, Llobert RE, Lopez E. Gigantic cytosarcoma phyllodes in a man with gynecomastia. Arch Surg 1976;111:611.

229. Reingold IM, Ascher GS. Cystosarcoma phyllodes in a man with gynecomastia. Am J Clin Pathol 1970;53:852-856.

230. Shin SJ, Rosen PP. Bilateral presentation of fibroadenoma with digital fibroma-like inclusions in the male breast. Arch Pathol Lab Med 2007;131:1126-1129.

231. Uchida T, Isshii M, Motomiya Y. Fibroadenoma associated with gynecomastia in an adult man. Case report. Scand J Plast Reconstr Hand Surg 1993;27:327-329.

18 METASTASES TO THE BREAST FROM NONMAMMARY NEOPLASMS

GENERAL FEATURES

The recognition of metastatic cancer to the breast and its distinction from primary mammary carcinoma are crucial for appropriately treating the patient, who does not usually benefit from mastectomy. The incidence of breast metastases varies in different series depending on whether lymphoreticular and hematopoietic neoplasms are included and whether the cases are gleaned from surgical or postmortem series. In surgical series, the incidence is 1 percent of malignant breast tumors (10). Of the 51 cases of metastases compiled by Hajdu and Urban (10), 18 were carcinomas, 16 lymphomas, 14 melanomas, and 3 sarcomas. In postmortem series, the incidence of metastases to the breast is as high as 6 percent (7). The higher incidence of metastases in postmortem compared to surgical series is difficult to explain, but it is possible that the greater sensitivity of autopsy material indicates that a large number of metastases are not detected clinically. Also, biopsy or resection is usually not performed in patients with known disseminated cancer.

In most series of metastases, hemolymphopoietic tumors account for about 50 percent of cases (7). Using the MEDLINE database, 24 articles of mixed surgical and postmortem series from 1885 to 1998 were reviewed and a total of 431 cases of metastasis to the breast were found (1). Melanoma headed the list (87 cases), followed by carcinomas from lung (78 cases), ovary (50 cases), prostate (39 cases), and other primary sites including the thyroid gland (12 cases).

Among carcinomas metastatic to the breast, the male to female ratio is 1 to 6; the average age is 48 years for females and 61 for men (10). Among children, 16 metastatic tumors were seen during a 25-year period at one institution (18).

Rhabdomyosarcomas have a predilection for spreading to the breast, and it has been estimated that up to 10 percent of alveolar rhabdomyosarcomas metastasize to the breast during their clinical course (11). Of 22 cases of rhabdomyosarcoma involving the breast diagnosed at Armed Forces Institute of Pathology (AFIP), 18 were metastatic and occurred in children or women under 40 years of age (22). Among young patients, neuroblastoma, medullary carcinoma of the thyroid gland, and primitive neuroectodermal tumors rarely metastasize to the breast (6). Instances of metastatic medulloblastoma (fig. 18-1) have been reported; the oldest patient was a 33-year-old woman with a tumor diagnosed in the cerebellum 2 years previously (14).

CLINICAL FEATURES

In 70 percent of cases of metastases to the breast, the appearance of a breast lump follows a known primary carcinoma elsewhere (10). In these patients, the diagnosis is usually relatively easy and fine needle aspiration cytology (FNAC) is often very useful.

When the breast lesion presents as the first manifestation of an occult extramammary primary tumor, it is often misinterpreted as a primary malignancy, as evident by the frequent mastectomies performed for cases of metastatic

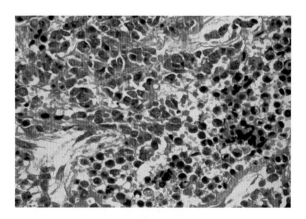

Figure 18-1

METASTATIC MEDULLOBLASTOMA

The cells are noncohesive and have scanty cytoplasm. (Courtesy of Dr. J. Lamovec, Ljubljana, Slovenia.)

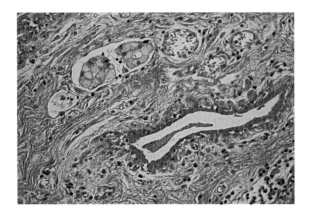

Figure 18-2

METASTATIC GASTRIC CARCINOMA

Signet ring cells are located within a vessel. The patient had signs of inflammatory carcinoma.

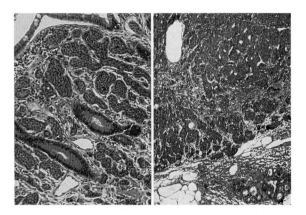

Figure 18-3

CARCINOID OF THE ILEUM

A carcinoid tumor (left) was discovered in the ileum of a 54-year-old woman 40 days after the breast metastasis (right). (Courtesy of Dr. S. Di Palma, Milan, Italy.) (Figs. 18-3 and 18-4 are from the same patient.)

carcinoid in one series (12). In fact, metastases to the breast can simulate all presentations of primary breast tumors, including inflammatory carcinoma, which is frequently mimicked by metastases from gastric cancer (fig. 18-2) (16).

While a single lesion is initially seen in 85 percent of cases (19), eventually metastases become bilateral (50 percent of cases) (7). The interval between the diagnosis of a primary malignancy and the development of a metastasis in the breast averages about 2.5 years (7). Nevertheless, it is not unusual to have prolonged gaps between the detection of the primary

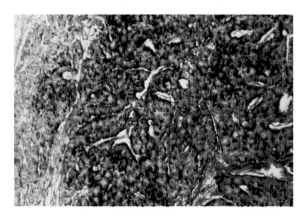

Figure 18-4

CARCINOID OF THE ILEUM

There is a strong argentaffin reaction with the Masson-Fontana stain.

tumor and the appearance of breast deposits (7 years in a case of melanoma [7] and 14 years in a case of ours reflecting a metastatic carcinoid tumor from the ileum).

Metastases to the breast are a sign of widespread disease and are indicative of a poor prognosis. Only a single patient out of 11 in one series survived longer than 1 year (21).

PATHOLOGIC FEATURES

No specific criteria are available at the moment to ensure the distinction of a metastatic lesion from a primary breast carcinoma. A complete clinical history is invaluable for establishing the correct diagnosis (figs. 18-3, 18-4). Clues that should raise suspicion for a metastatic tumor are: 1) unusual histology; 2) multiple nodules; 3) absence of calcification in the mammogram (10); 4) a well-circumscribed nodule at radiologic, macroscopic, and microscopic examinations; 5) absence of an in situ lesion; 6) absence of elastosis (3); and 7) numerous and obvious vascular emboli.

Similar problems are present in bilateral breast carcinoma, in which it is often difficult to establish whether the patient is affected by a synchronous or metachronous primary or whether the contralateral tumor is a metastatic process. According to 22 reports, bilateral synchronous carcinomas were observed from 0.1 to 2.0 percent of patients, while metachronous carcinomas developed from 1 to 12 percent of patients (median, 3.2 percent) (8).

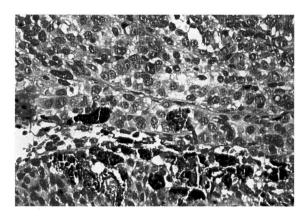

Figure 18-5

METASTATIC MELANOMA

The melanoma is heavily pigmented.

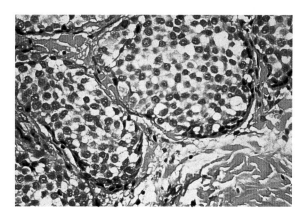

Figure 18-6

METASTATIC MELANOMA

Nonpigmented melanoma closely simulating lobular intraepithelial neoplasia.

The histologic criteria used to establish the presence of a metastasis were proposed by Robbins and Berg in 1964 (17). These include: 1) location: metastases are more frequent in the fat that surrounds the breast parenchyma or in the tail. By contrast, second primary carcinoma is expected in breast parenchyma, most often localized in the upper outer quadrant; 2) number and growth: metastases tend to be multiple and show an expansile growth rather than stellate type of invasion; 3) histology: metastases should resemble the primary carcinoma, including the same profile for steroid receptors; and 4) in situ carcinoma: metastases should not be associated with in situ carcinoma.

SPECIFIC EXTRAMAMMARY METASTATIC CARCINOMAS

Assessment of morphology along with ancillary techniques provides the final confirmation of a metastatic process in most cases. Melanomas, if pigmented (fig. 18-5), are easily recognizable even without a clinical history and the decision that one is dealing with a metastatic process can be made since there are virtually no primary melanomas in the breast. Problematic melanomas are those that are nonpigmented and/or extend into ducts and lobules, simulating intraepithelial lesions (fig. 18-6). Melanomas are negative for E-cadherin, as is lobular carcinoma, but the correct diagnosis can be made by the negativity of keratin stains combined with positivity on immunostaining for S-100 protein and/or HMB45.

Metastatic pulmonary squamous cell carcinoma is indistinguishable from a primary mammary carcinoma of analogous morphology. The clinical history is vital in such cases, since primary pure squamous cell carcinoma in the breast is rare.

The expression of gross cystic disease fluid protein (GCDFP)-15, and estrogen or progesterone receptors (ER, PR), has a sensitivity of 0.83, a specificity of 0.93, and a predictive accuracy of 0.92 for carcinomas of the breast compared with all other carcinomas (13). Negativity with these markers, which should be routinely used, has to arouse suspicion of a nonmammary tumor. Positivity for thyroid transcription factor (TTF)-1 in these cases supports a pulmonary adenocarcinoma.

Metastatic small cell carcinomas are impossible to diagnose without a clinical history, while negativity for cytokeratin (CK)20 is helpful in the diagnosis of Merkel cell carcinoma (2).

Serous papillary carcinoma metastatic to the breast from the ovary was seen in 4 of 18 patients reported by Lee (14a), and can also involve axillary lymph nodes. In 3 of these cases, calcifications were present as well as papillary architecture. Invasive micropapillary carcinoma of the breast is histologically indistinguishable from metastatic ovarian carcinoma. GCDFP-15 and Ca125 are usually helpful in establishing the correct diagnosis since the former is positive in up to 70 percent of breast carcinomas and rarely in ovarian tumors, while the latter is positive in about 60 percent of ovarian carcinomas only (14a).

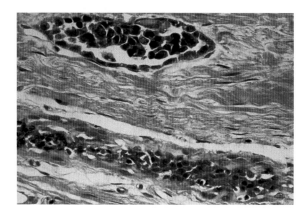

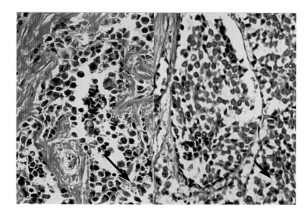

Figure 18-7

ALVEOLAR RHABDOMYOSARCOMA

This tumor was metastatic to the breast from the mediastinum in a 16-year-old girl.

Figure 18-8

ALVEOLAR RHABDOMYOSARCOMA (RH) AND ALVEOLAR INVASIVE LOBULAR CARCINOMA (ILC)

The neoplastic cells are pleomorphic and cling to the alveolar walls (long arrow). The neoplastic cells are monotonous and detach from the alveolar walls (short arrow).

Metastatic carcinoid tumors from the gastrointestinal tract are the most difficult to differentiate from a breast primary, as confirmed by the frequent mastectomies that have ensued (9). If the endocrine tumor is argentaffin positive, it must be regarded as a metastatic process in view of the virtual absence of argentaffin carcinoid tumors in the breast.

Prostate carcinoma is the most frequent source of metastasis to the male breast. Positivity for prostate-specific antigen (PSA) is helpful. Unfortunately, prostatic carcinomas may also extend into the ducts and mimic in situ carcinomas/DIN1-3, and some primary breast carcinomas also express PSA (5).

Renal carcinomas are very deceptive and in our experience are the source of the most frequent mistakes. Positivity for vimentin and CD10 and lack of GCDFP-15, ER, and PR (13) help in diagnosing renal cell carcinomas.

Alveolar rhabdomyosarcomas can simulate the alveolar pattern of invasive lobular carcinoma (figs. 18-7, 18-8). Primary rhabdomyosarcoma is an exceptional occurrence in the breast, with only four reported arising in phyllodes tumors and another four occurring in women over 40 years of age in the AFIP files (4). The age of patients with rhabdomyosarcoma is usually less than 25 years, and positivity for myogenic markers is the rule, while ER staining is negative. ER is positive in 100 percent of alveolar infiltrating lobular carcinomas (20), while keratin staining is not helpful since it is present in some rhabdomyosarcomas (15).

As a rule, the possibility of a metastatic carcinoma should be considered any time bilateral or multiple unilateral nodules are detected mammographically and when the morphology is unusual for a breast primary.

REFERENCES

1. Alva S, Shetty-Alva N. An update of tumor metastasis to the breast data. Arch Surg 1999;134:450.
2. Asioli S, Dorji T, Lorenzini P, Eusebi V. Primary neuroendocrine (Merkel cell) carcinoma of the nipple. Virchows Arch 2002;440:443-444.
3. Azzopardi JG. Problems in breast pathology. London: W.B. Saunders Company; 1979:311-314.
4. Barnes L, Pietruszka M. Rhabdomyosarcoma arising within a cystosarcoma phyllodes. A case report and review of the literature. Am J Surg Pathol 1978;2:423-429.
5. Carder PJ, Speirs V, Ramsdale J, Lansdown MR. Expression of prostate specific antigen in male breast cancer. J Clin Pathol 2005;58:69-71.
6. Dehner LP, Hill DA, Deschryver K. Pathology of the breast in children, adolescents, and young adults. Semin Diagn Pathol 1999;16:235-247.
7. Di Bonito L, Luchi M, Giarelli L, Falconieri G, Vielh P. Metastatic tumors to the female breast. An autopsy study of 12 cases. Pathol Res Pract 1991;187:432-436.
8. Donegan WL, Spratt JS. Multiple primary cancers. In: Donegan WL, Spratt JS, eds. Cancer of the breast, 5th ed. Philadelphia: Saunders; 2002:813-824.
9. Eusebi V, Pileri S, Usellini L, Grassigli A, Capella C. Primary endocrine carcinoma of the parotid salivary gland associated with a lung carcinoid: a possible new association. J Clin Path 1982;35:611-616.
10. Hajdu SI, Urban JA. Cancers metastatic to the breast. Cancer 1972;29:1691-1696.
11. Howarth CB, Caces JN, Pratt CB. Breast metastases in children with rhabdomyosarcoma. Cancer 1980;46:2520-2524.
12. Kashlan RB, Powell RW, Nolting SF. Carcinoid and other tumors metastatic to the breast. J Surg Oncol 1982;20:25-30.
13. Kaufmann O, Deidesheimer T, Muehlenberg M, Deicke P, Dietel M. Immunohistochemical differentiation of metastatic breast carcinomas from metastatic adenocarcinomas of other common primary sites. Histopathology 1996;29:233-240.
14. Lamovec J, Pogaenik A. Metastatic medulloblastoma to the breast. Virchows Arch 2001;439:201-205.
14a. Lee AH. The histological diagnosis of metastases to the breast from extramammary malignancies. J Clin Pathol 2007;60:1333-1341.
15. Miettinen M, Rapola J. Immunohistochemical spectrum of rhabdomyosarcoma and rhabdomyosarcoma-like tumors. Expression of cytokeratin and the 68-kD neurofilament protein. Am J Surg Pathol 1989;13:120-132.
16. Nance FC, MacVaugh H 3rd, Fitts WT Jr. Metastatic tumor to the breast simulating bilateral primary inflammatory carcinoma. Am J Surg 1966;112:932-935.
17. Robbins GF, Berg JW. Bilateral primary breast cancers: a prospective clinicopathological study. Cancer 1964;17:1501-1527.
18. Rogers DA, Lobe TE, Rao BN, et al. Breast malignancy in children. J Ped Surg 1994;29:48-51.
19. Rosen PP, Oberman HA. Tumors of the mammary gland. Washington DC: Armed Forces Institute of Pathology; 1993.
20. Shousha S, Backhous CM, Alaghband-Zadeh J, Burn I. Alveolar variant of invasive lobular carcinoma of the breast. A tumor rich in estrogen receptors. Am J Clin Pathol 1986;85:1-5.
21. Silverman EM, Oberman HA. Metastatic neoplasm in the breast. Surg Gynecol Obstet 1974;138:26.
22. Tavassoli FA. Pathology of the breast, 2nd ed. Stamford, CT: Appleton-Lange/McGraw Hill; 1999.

A APPENDIX

PREOPERATIVE DIAGNOSTIC PROCEDURES

In recent years, the diagnostic approach to breast lesions has changed dramatically. The use of intraoperative frozen sections has undergone a noteworthy decline following the adoption of preoperative diagnostic strategies that include fine needle aspiration cytology (FNAC) and needle core biopsy (NCB). These have many advantages not only because they are simple procedures applicable to outpatients, but also because they allow management decisions between the patient and the surgeon prior to hospital admission, with consequent reduction of patient anxiety.

Until the 1970s, breast biopsies were mostly obtained from palpable masses that were clinically suspicious of carcinoma, but since then the use of mammography has led to an increase in breast specimens from patients without palpable abnormalities (3). The widespread use of population-based screening mammography has caused mammographically generated biopsies to outnumber biopsies for palpable masses in some centers.

Frozen section assessment is useful in lesions exceeding 1 cm in size, in which the procedure is highly accurate, with a false positive rate of virtually zero, a false negative rate of less than 1 percent, and a deferred diagnosis in fewer than 5 percent (18). For lesions smaller than 1 cm, it is better not to perform this procedure as it is often difficult to identify the right area to examine, especially under pressure from the surgeon who requires a definitive diagnosis. For minute lesions, the tissue for permanent microscopic examination may be exhausted and the architecture of the residual tissue distorted. Finally, surgeons wish to be informed not only about the presence of invasion, but also the size of the tumor and the state of the margins, all this information is difficult to provide during the frozen section procedure. Tissue removed for calcifications must be examined by X rays to confirm that the area with microcalcifications has been removed (3).

Fine Needle Aspiration Cytology

FNAC is performed in two situations: for palpable masses in which the FNAC is usually performed free hand and nonpalpable masses in which the procedure is image guided. As codified by the guidelines of both the National Cancer Institute (NCI) (28) and the European National Health Service Breast Screening Programme (NHS-BSP) (23), which are currently accepted and used in most areas of the United States and Europe, the accuracy of FNAC depends on adequate and representative sampling, suitable technical procedures, and accurate interpretation of the cytologic material by expert cytopathologists. When a triple approach is followed (clinical, radiologic, and cytologic), an accuracy rate of 99 percent is obtained for palpable masses (23). This degree of accuracy is not reached with nonpalpable masses in which the needle is guided by ultrasound (widely used technique) or by stereotactic X ray in cases with microcalcification. In experienced hands, the overall sensitivity for FNAC is about 87 percent, with specificity of virtually all cases, and the predictive value of positive diagnoses is nearly 100 percent and that of negative diagnoses 60 to 90 percent (18).

In order to increase the accuracy of correlation with subsequent biopsies and to standardize the diagnostic terminology for reporting the results of FNAC it is advisable to issue a clear report to the clinician. With this aim, five diagnostic categories have been proposed by both the American and European guidelines and designated as C1 to C5 in the European system (C for cytology) (23,25a,28).

C1: Unsatisfactory. This indicates a scanty or acellular smear or otherwise inadequate preparation. Poor cellularity is defined as fewer than five clumps of epithelial cells (23) in a smear.

C2: Benign. This indicates an adequate sample of a benign aspirate. This includes cells distributed in monolayers; a generally clean background; a mixture of different types of cells

397

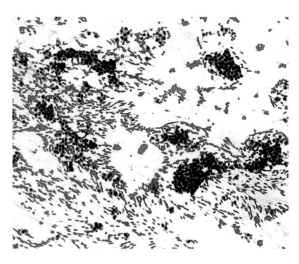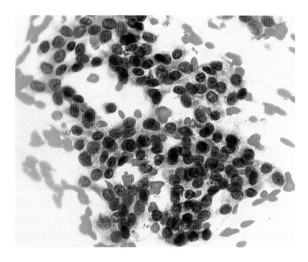

Figure A-1

C4 (SUSPICIOUS OF MALIGNANCY) FINE NEEDLE ASPIRATION CYTOLOGY (FNAC) SMEAR

Left: The smear is cellular and there are noncohesive cells.

Right: Nevertheless, the pathologist did not feel confident to make a positive diagnosis of malignancy in view of the clarity of the background and the regularity of the nuclei. Histologically, the case proved to be an invasive duct carcinoma, NOS, grade 1.

including myoepithelial, cuboidal epithelial, apocrine, and foamy macrophages; and cells of small size with regular nuclei, fine chromatin, and indistinct nucleoli.

C3: Atypia, Probably Benign. The aspirate has the characteristics of a benign lesion, but in addition, there are some atypical features such as nuclear pleomorphism and loss of cellular cohesion. Included here are cellular changes as a result of pregnancy, oral contraceptives, or hormone replacement therapy. The incidence rate for this category in experienced hands is 3.7 percent (12).

Atypical duct hyperplasia (ADH/ductal intraepithelial neoplasia [DIN]1) should be included in this category. The cytologic distinction between ADH and in situ duct carcinoma (DCIS) has been proposed by several authors (14). As demonstrated by Sneige and Staerkel (25) and later elaborated by Rosai (18), this distinction is difficult to reproduce especially if the World Health Organization (WHO, 2003) definition of ADH is followed. The latter definition is based on both cytologic grounds, i.e., cells are similar to those seen in grade 1 DCIS/DIN1, and on quantitative spatial criteria, i.e., less than two spaces are involved and the maximum extent of the lesion does not exceed 2 mm (25a). The quantitative/spatial parameter is not valid for cytologic aspirates.

C4: Suspicious of Malignancy. This diagnosis is made when the pathologist feels strongly that the lesion is malignant but is not totally confident about it (fig. A-1). This can be the result of poor technical procedures, poor cellularity, or a mixture of benign and malignant features together with myoepithelial cells. In experienced hands, the incidence rate of C4 smears is 3.9 percent (12). Ablative therapeutic surgery should not be undertaken on the basis of a C4 diagnosis.

C5: Malignant. This indicates that an adequate sample contains cells characteristic of carcinoma or other malignancy. The diagnosis should be based on multiple criteria, as indicated by the American and European guidelines (23,28), comprising "obvious" malignant changes such as lack of cohesion (fig. A-2), cellular pleomorphism, irregular nuclei, prominent nucleoli, and a background full of debris (figs. A-3, A-4). Less "obvious" criteria include monomorphism, abundant cytoplasm, intracytoplasmic inclusions (fig. A-5), mitoses, and intranuclear pseudoinclusions. In every case, a full clinical history must be obtained before issuing a C5 diagnostic report. This helps in establishing the correct diagnosis, especially in cases previously treated with chemotherapy and radiotherapy or in patients with lactational changes in which remarkable

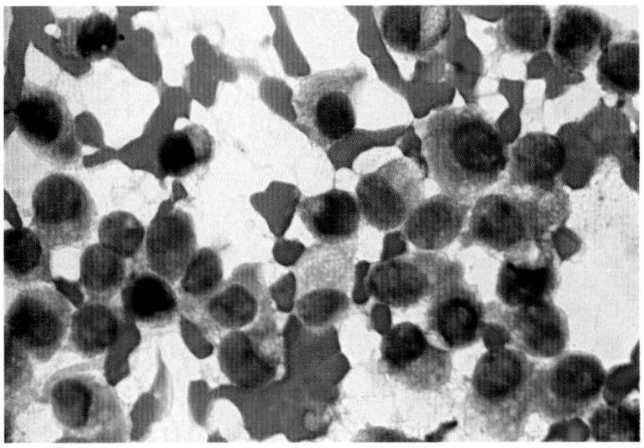

Figure A-2

C5 (MALIGNANT) FNAC SMEAR

The cells are noncohesive and the nuclei are irregular. Histologically, it proved to be invasive lobular carcinoma, classic type.

pleomorphism and cellular dissociation can be seen. Ultrasound gel must not be mistaken for necrosis, while the occasional presence of an intramammary lymph node has to be taken into account in lymphocyte-rich smears.

A 2 percent false negative rate is acceptable in ultrasound-guided procedures of nonpalpable lesions (24), while 1 percent is the figure accepted by the NHSBSP guidelines. For practical purposes, if in doubt, it is preferable to defer the diagnosis and rely on the results of NCB as the two methods, when combined, provide a correct preoperative diagnosis in most cases (16). A 2004 study of 7,227 breast aspirations found that 52 percent of 489 "atypical" aspirates and 83 percent of 162 "suspicious" aspirates yielded malignant findings on subsequent histologic analysis (11). The study concluded that the distinction between the "atypical" and "suspicious" categories, as recommended by NCI, is not warranted.

Proliferative breast lesions are cytologically classified into four categories: nonproliferative, proliferative, proliferative with atypia, and low nuclear grade DCIS. Such a classification is associated with significant interobserver variability, and variability is based on the type of stain used (Diff-Quik versus Papanicolaou), and needs further revision and refinement (22). An approach combining nonproliferative and proliferative without atypia into a low-risk category and the proliferative with atypia and low-grade DCIS

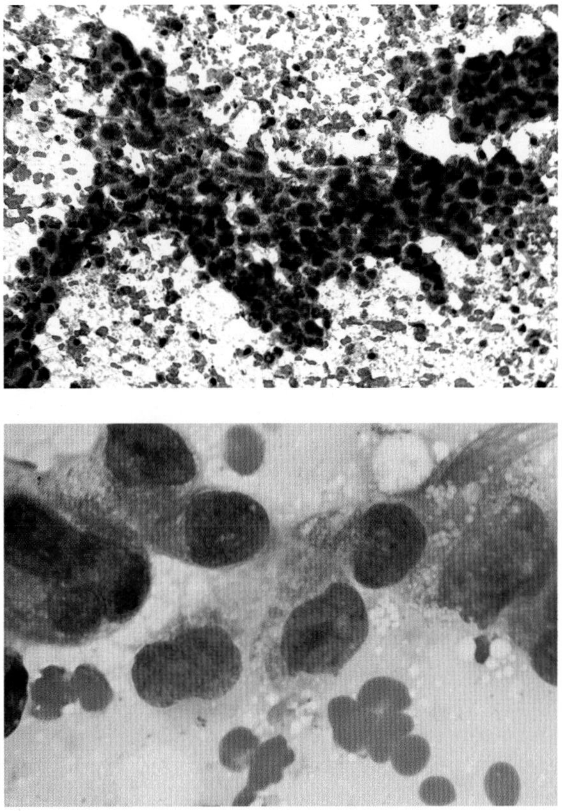

Figure A-3

C5 (MALIGNANT) FNAC SMEAR

Top: Pleomorphic nuclei with a "dirty" background in a C5 lesion that was histologically diagnosed as invasive duct carcinoma grade 3.

Bottom: Pleomorphic invasive lobular carcinoma that shows noncohesive cells and very irregular nuclei.

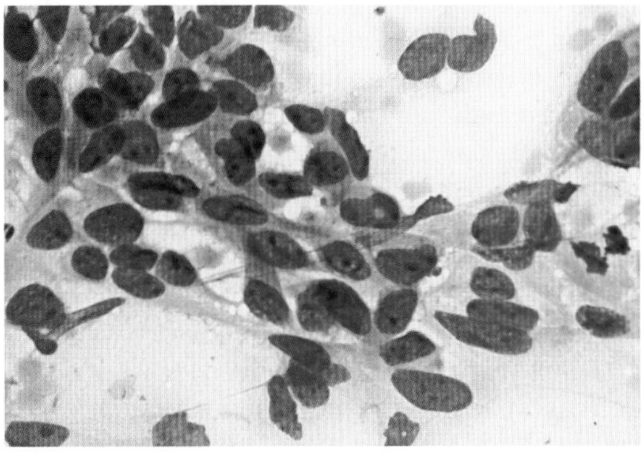

Figure A-4

C5 (MALIGNANT) FNAC SMEAR

Spindle cells have irregular nuclei and prominent nucleoli. The case was included in the C5 category and proved to be a spindle cell metaplastic carcinoma.

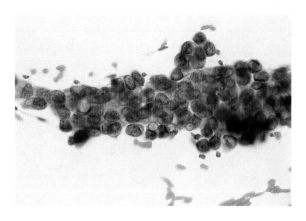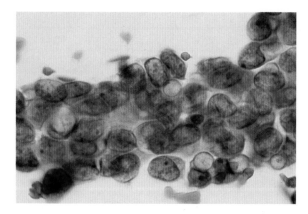

Figure A-5

C5 (MALIGNANT) FNAC SMEAR

Intracytoplasmic targetoid lumens of this C5 invasive lobular carcinoma are seen.

into high-risk category appears to provide better correlation with histologic findings (22). This approach is similar to what has been accomplished with the DIN system. This is in keeping with the recent ductal intraepithelial neoplasia (DIN) classification of intraductal proliferations whereby intraductal hyperplasia is categorized as low-risk DIN while ADH and low-grade DCIS are combined into DIN1 (see chapter 4).

Needle Core Biopsy

This is an area that has developed rapidly in recent years. Several centers initially employed freehand core biopsies for palpable tumors, a procedure soon followed by ultrasound-guided needle biopsies. This evolution was significant since the tissue sampled for pathologic diagnosis has to be the most representative possible.

For nonpalpable lesions, a stereotactic approach is favored, especially in areas containing microcalcifications. The stereotactic vacuum-assisted core biopsy is a further technological improvement which, it is claimed, obtains a substantial quantity of tissue to the extent that in 20 percent of nonpalpable invasive carcinomas, complete removal of tumor is achieved (fig. A-6) (21).

The advantages of NCB over FNAC are evident as NCB allows simultaneous evaluation of cytology and architecture. The diagnosis of 99 percent of masses is achieved with five cores of 14-gauge stereotactic NBC per case, and of 92 percent of microcalcifications with six cores per case (13). A definite diagnosis of DCIS/DIN and invasive carcinoma (IC) can be provided

with NBC and, in addition, benign lesions such as fibroadenomas are easily identified. Microcalcifications are also better assessed in terms of extent, size, and quality. To this purpose, the specimen has to be radiographed and then compared to the original mammogram to evaluate both the extent and the quantity of the calcifications removed. The quality and size of the calcifications can be defined, taking into account that calcifications smaller than 100 µm are not visible radiography (13). Calcium oxalate crystals do not stain with hematoxylin and are easily overlooked in routine histologic specimens (26). Finally, laminar calcifications are seen both in benign conditions (e.g., within the lumens of sclerosing adenosis or in the stroma) as well as in grade 1 DCIS/DIN1. In contrast, granular calcific debris is characteristic of grade 3 DCIS/DIN3 (4). Perfect fixation and no fewer than three step sections are necessary to maximize the visualization of microcalcifications (6).

By analogy with FNAC, a reporting system based on histologic categories has been recommended (1a) and also adopted by the Breast Screening European Commission. In this system there are five histologic B categories (B for biopsy).

B1: Normal Tissue/Inadequate Sample. This indicates that a core shows normal histology and may also contain microcalcifications. Inadequate sample indicates tissue with less than adequate processing or cases in which there is normal tissue that is felt to be inconsistent with the findings on imaging or clinical data (23).

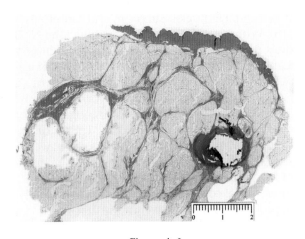

Figure A-6

VACUUM CORE BIOPSY

The vacuum core biopsy has removed almost all the neoplastic tissue.

B2: Benign Lesion. This category indicates lesions in which a specific diagnosis is possible. This applies to small papillomas, fibroadenomas, duct ectasia, cystic changes, sclerosing adenosis, ductal hyperplasia of usual type/low-risk DIN, hamartomas, and inflammatory changes.

B3: Lesions of Uncertain Malignant Potential. This category includes lesions with benign histology that are known to be heterogeneous or lesions that have an increased risk of associated malignancy. The frequency of B3 cores is 7.3 percent in screened patients (12). This category includes large papillomas with the edges transected, sclerosing ductal proliferations such as radial scar or infiltrative epitheliosis, phyllodes tumors, mucocele-like lesions, lobular intraepithelial neoplasia (LIN), flat epithelial atypia, and minute low-grade DCIS/DIN1 lesions. As explained in the section on cytology (C3 category), the definition of ADH should not be applied to core biopsies as it is derived from surgical specimens and is based on a combination of cytologic and quantitative criteria, the latter not consistently applicable to the small fragments obtained via core biopsy.

Definitive surgery should not be undertaken on the basis of B3 diagnosis as no fewer than 75 percent of cases are non-neoplastic. Nevertheless, in view of the positive predictive value for carcinoma, which is 25 percent (12), B3 core patients often undergo further diagnostic exci-

sion, especially in cases of LIN and low-grade DCIS/DIN1.

Of the 24 cases reported by Ely et al. (2) that showed ADH/DIN1, <2 mm limited to only two foci of the total ADH/DIN1 core biopsy, additional areas of ADH/DIN1, <2 mm were found in 10. The presence of three or more foci of ADH/DIN1, <2 mm, present in 23 cases, was found to be a strong predictor of a more advanced lesion, with 6 ADH/DIN1, <2 mm, 15 DCIS, and 2 IDC lesions found at excision. Crisi et al. (1) reported 16 cases of LIN which had undergone immediate wire-guided excision. This led to the discovery of additional foci of LIN in 13 patients, 1 case of atypical lobular hyperplasia, and 2 of invasive lobular carcinoma. Follow-up surgical excision of 33 cases of atypical lobular hyperplasia and lobular carcinoma in situ showed a cancer underestimation in 28 percent of cases (1b). The B3 category needs to be better defined with the aim of distinguishing patients who require further treatment from those harboring innocent lesions.

B4: Lesions Suspicious of Malignancy. This category includes cases in which there are changes suggestive of in situ or invasive malignancy but a categorical diagnosis cannot be made as a consequence of scantiness of material or artifactual changes (23). The frequency of B4 cores is low even in screened patients (2.5 percent), while the predictive value for carcinoma (86 percent) is very high (12). This speaks for excision in all cases but in this category, as for B3 lesions, definitive surgery should not be undertaken as 15 percent of patients do not have a malignant condition (12).

B5: Malignant Lesions. This category, which is appropriate for cases of unequivocal malignancy, constituted 30 percent of the core biopsies in a large series (12). If possible, care should be taken to distinguish in situ from invasive tumors. Sarcomas and lymphomas are included in this category, as well as pleomorphic LIN (21).

A 79 percent underestimation of tumor size has been reported if measurement is performed on a core biopsy (20). To obviate this, it has been suggested that the measurement should be performed directly on the preoperative mammogram, or better still, on a large section obtained from the excision specimen (fig. A-6) (5).

Grading of an in situ or invasive carcinoma from a core biopsy is difficult, and perhaps only a provisional grade or nuclear grade should be given to the lesion (8). In one series, there was only 67 percent agreement between core and excisional biopsy grade, with the highest level of agreement in 84 percent of grade 3 in contrast to only 60 percent of grade 1 and 2 cases (7). Seventy-five percent was the figure given by Rakha and Ellis (17a) for concordance between grade on core biopsy and that in the definitive excision specimen. The main cause of discrepancy was the lower mitotic count in the core biopsy specimen. Tumor typing suffers from the same problem as only 74 percent agreement is obtained between the core and excision specimens (7), although much higher figures (93 to 100 percent concordance rate) were reported by Rakha and Ellis (17a).

The invasive component may be underestimated in up to 20 percent of cases when the diagnosis of pure DCIS/DIN1-3 is obtained by NCB. This is related to the proportion of the total volume of tissue examined, and to the gauge of the needle. An 8-gauge stereotactic vacuum-assisted biopsy minimizes the rate of underestimation (to about 4 percent) (17a).

Microinvasion can be mentioned in the report "providing it is understood that more invasion might be found in the excised specimen" (8). Dislodgement of epithelium by the needle (29) (see chapter 1) is a distinct pitfall but it is fortunately a rare occurrence. The absolute agreement for estrogen receptor (ER) and progesterone receptor (PR) content between core and excision specimens varies from 73 percent and 72 percent, respectively (30), to 100 percent (17a). With increasing frequency, pathologists are performing ER, PR, and HER2 on core biopsies. Given the better fixation of these samples and the option of repeating questionable results on the excisional biopsy, this approach expedites results. In one institution, the pathologists are so confident with the results of the NCB that ER is routinely assessed in the NCB for invasive carcinoma and the staining is only repeated in the surgical specimen if the NCB shows weak staining or if the tumor is heterogeneous (17a). Staining for c-erbB-2 is accurate in 92 percent of cases (17a).

The approach to any lesion in a core biopsy should be personalized and requires "experience, good judgement, and close interaction between pathologist, surgeon, and radiologist" (18). Whenever the excision specimen after NCB does not show residual tumor, the core biopsy sample site should be reassessed to avoid an underestimation of the adequacy of treatment.

The major disadvantages of NCB over FNAC are the rare phenomenon of dislodgement of epithelium by the needle and the length of the time to diagnosis using the NCB procedure, which requires, an average of at least 24 hours (inclusive of fixation) compared to about 1 hour for FNAC (under ideal conditions). To minimize the length of processing, we use a technique that employs a controlled microwave processing procedure lasting about 2 hours 30 minutes, inclusive of fixation time through staining (17). This technique has been named fast track biopsy (FTB) to emphasize the fact that the diagnosis is obtained within a short period and that fast immunohistochemistry can be added to the diagnostic procedure. For processing, a microwave vacuum-assisted histoprocessor is used, in which automatic microwave power selection, processing time, temperature, and vacuum are computer-controlled and independent of operator skill level.

The complete protocol we employ for processing breast cores is the following (17):

1) Specimens are immersed for 20 minutes in 10 percent buffered formalin (50°C), followed by an external, nonmicrowave rinse in reagent alcohol to remove excess formalin and water from the cassettes. This is followed by 15 minutes of microwaving in 100 percent ethanol (65°C) and 16 minutes in 100 percent isopropanol (68°C). Samples are then exposed to a brief vacuum microwave drying step of 1.5 minutes with 100 Watts of energy under 600 mBar of vacuum. Microwave paraffin infiltration is then performed for 25 minutes, with increasing increments of vacuum down to 100 mBar, to assist the infiltration process at 65°C.

2) Sections from paraffin blocks are stained with hematoxylin and eosin (H&E). The total time for processing includes 1 hour 30 minutes for processing/embedding, 30 minutes for sectioning, and an additional 30 minutes for H&E staining, totalling 2 hours 30 minutes.

3) Sections can be immunostained, when required. The protocol of the fast immunohistochemical procedure is detailed in the work of Ragazzini et al. (17).

This immunohistochemical procedure lasts 90 to 100 minutes, as opposed to 220 minutes with currently available automated immunostainers.

The H&E quality of the biopsies does not differ from that of the traditionally processed specimens but it is fast enough (4 hours inclusive of immunohistochemistry) to be competitive with FNAC. We think that the actual time required for the pathologist to reach a final diagnosis on an H&E slide is faster with NCB than FNAC in most cases, since with the latter method the diagnosis requires careful scanning of several slides in search of neoplastic cells (17). Ragazzini et al. (17) have stated that the processing times for the two procedures are practically superimposable, and consequently, the disadvantage of the longer length of time for processing NCB is minimized in microwave processed core biopsies.

OPERATIVE DIAGNOSTIC (AND TREATMENT) PROCEDURES

A modified radical mastectomy consists of removal of the breast tissue (including the nipple) together with the overlying skin and the axillary fat containing lymph nodes. A simple mastectomy (total mastectomy) indicates removal of almost all breast parenchyma without axillary tissue. A subcutaneous mastectomy includes breast tissue without the overlying skin, nipple, and axillary tail.

Quadrantectomy has no anatomic substrate and merely indicates an artificial subdivision of the breast into quadrants for clinical purposes. It differs from patient to patient and in the hands of different surgeons. Excisional biopsy (lumpectomy, tylectomy) indicates removal of a tumoral mass with a variable amount of surrounding breast tissue. In centers dealing with screening diagnoses, the latter two procedures give rise to about 80 percent of surgical specimens.

The pathologist is faced with multiple tasks in the Gross room, but the different procedures have been very satisfactorily codified in excellent papers (19) and books (18). Similarly, there are guidelines by the Association of Directors of Anatomic and Surgical Pathology (ADASP) that are widely used in the United States. (www.panix.com/≈adasp/brcarcin.htm). The basic procedures that the pathologist has to follow consist of receiving the tissue fresh and

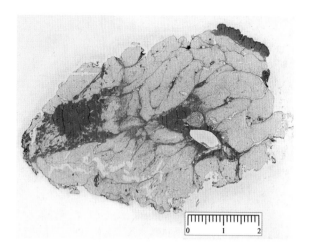

Figure A-7

LARGE SECTION OF A QUADRANT

Residual invasive carcinoma is still evident around the area removed by the core biopsy. The area removed can be added to the present neoplasm in order to establish the size of the lesion. On the left, there is another area of invasive carcinoma.

untouched (9), orienting the specimen according to markers placed by the surgeon (metallic wires and sutures), and radiographing and photographing the specimen with indication on the printed picture of the blocks taken. In quadrantectomies and even more so in lumpectomies, the specimen received in a fresh state is composed of soft tissue that takes the form of flat fibrofatty tissue in the plane of sectioning. The larger tumors are firm and usually easily located by inspection and palpation. Nevertheless, finding the correct plane of sectioning in specimens containing microcalcifications or nonpalpable tumors is entirely dependent upon careful mammographic guidance (27).

Important data needed to make treatment decisions include the precise extent of each lesion, the size of the lesion, the presence of multifocality, the detection of foci of microinvasion, the residual presence of tumor around the area removed by a preoperative vacuum-assisted procedure, the need to obtain precise correlation between mammographic and pathologic findings, and the correct assessment of the status of resection margins.

It has been suggested that the use of large (macro) sections meets all these requirements (5). To map resection margins adequately, numerous small conventional blocks are required,

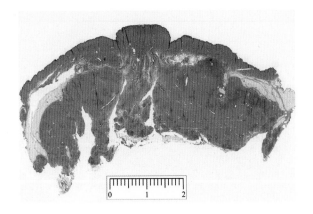

Figure A-8

LARGE SECTION THAT INCLUDES AN ENTIRE BREAST

An entire breast transversely sectioned. The whole deep margin is visible in this plane.

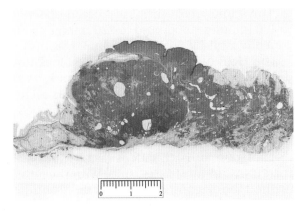

Figure A-9

SIZE OF TUMOR DIRECTLY VISUALIZED IN THE LARGE SECTION

The size of the lesion is measured directly on one slide.

thus making thorough examination of a quadrantectomy specimen a time-consuming procedure, especially in terms of technical labor. Large histologic sections are ideal for the assessment of circumferential resection margins (fig. A-7) (27). Admittedly, the superficial and deep resection margins are not directly visualized because the specimen is usually sectioned horizontally. Nevertheless, from each specimen parallel slices of the whole tissue are obtained. Absence of radiologic and macroscopic abnormalities in the first (most superficial) and the last (the deepest) slice provide proof that the margins are free of tumor along these two surfaces (27). Should one of these sections contain any abnormality, it is necessary to complete the sampling of tissue with perpendicular small blocks (5). Large sections can be obtained not only from quadrantectomy specimens, but also from an entire breast, a procedure that is very useful in the study of deep margins (fig. A-8) (5,27).

Assessment of the size of the lesion is easy in large sections as the measurement can be performed directly on the slide (fig. A-9). Jackson et al. (10) compared two series: one studied with conventional histology and the other with large sections. In the latter, the size of invasive carcinoma could be determined in all cases. In contrast, size could be measured in only 63 percent of the 99 cases studied with conventional small blocks. They also found that the measurement (and prevalence) of DCIS was more accurate with large sections than with conventional small blocks. DCIS was found more frequently in association with invasive carcinoma in specimens assessed on large sections (80 percent) than in cases processed using small blocks (63 percent).

It is surprising that the use of large sections in breast pathology has never become popular, despite the many advantages of this method that have led to its common use in the study of brain and prostate specimens. Increased workload is often given as the reason for not performing whole organ studies in daily practice. Preparation of large sections with the employment of a dedicated vacuum paraffin embedder and the use of microwave for speeding up fixation and processing, however, takes no longer than 2 days at the most. This, we believe, is a reasonable compromise in view of the many advantages.

METHOD FOR MACRO (LARGE) SECTIONS

The method here described has been in use by us for 8 years (5) and is essentially similar to that described by Jackson et al. (10).

The specimen has to be received fresh and oriented by the surgeon to indicate the margin nearest to the nipple and at least two other margins, usually the right and superior.

1) Radiography of the surgical specimen is performed, taking care to orient the X-ray picture according to the specimen.

2) The surgical margins of the specimen may be marked with black ink.

Table A-1

SYNOPTIC REPORT FOR BREAST CARCINOMA—EXCISIONAL SPECIMEN[a]

Surgical Pathology #

INVASIVE CARCINOMA (with or without in situ [intraepithelial] component)

Site: Breast, Right
Left

Surgical Procedure:

Tumor Location: Quadrant(s) Involved

Infiltrating Component:

Type: Infiltrating Duct (NOS)
Infiltrating Lobular (classic, pleomorphic)
Other (Specify)

Grade: Well Differentiated
Moderately Differentiated
Poorly Differentiated

(Total Score = /9: Nuclear Atypia = /3 ; Tubule Formation = /3 ; Mitotic Activity = /3)

Size (cm):
(Invasive component confirmed microscopically)

Necrosis: Present
Not Identified

Lymphovascular Invasion (peritumoral): Present
Not Identified

Microcalcifications (in tumor): Present
Not Identified

Dermal Lymphatic Involvement: Present
Not Identified

Nipple Involvement (Paget): Present
Not Identified

Margins:
Distance to closest margin:

Additional Foci of Invasive Carcinoma: Present
Not Identified

Type: Size: Grade:
Distance to dominant carcinoma:

3) Sections with a large knife or a butcher's slicing machine (15) are taken following the indication of the radiograms. A section has to include the lesion or the area of microcalcifications in the plane exposing its largest diameter. The thickness of each section measures between 0.3 and 0.5 cm.

4) Mastectomies: mastectomies are usually sectioned perpendicularly to the skin up to the deep margin of resection, taking care to transect the nipple.

5) Quadrantectomies: the specimen is sliced parallel to the cutting table or, alternatively, radially, and care is taken to direct the section from the margin closer to the nipple.

6) Sections are fixed overnight, in 10 percent buffered formalin and then embedded in paraffin, taking care to maintain the orientation using a cellulose acetate white membrane filter.

For paraffin embedding, specimens are processed in a tissue vacuum infiltrator processor, as follows:

Alcohol 70 percent (3 x 30 minutes); alcohol 95 percent (2 x 1 hour) followed by absolute alcohol (3 x 1 hour). Xylene (2 x 3 hours) is followed by melted paraffin, overnight. The specimen is then embedded in paraffin.

Sections of 5μm are obtained using a dedicated microtome and mounted on large glass slides. Sections are then stained with H&E as routine.

Table A-1, Continued

SYNOPTIC REPORT FOR BREAST CARCINOMA—EXCISIONAL SPECIMEN[a]

In Situ/Intraepithelial Component:

        Ductal   Lobular

                  Subtype:

                  Nuclear Grade:

                  Necrosis:

                  Microcalcifications:

                  Closest Margin:

ER, PR, HER2 (immunostain/FISH)[a]/results pending

Other Findings:

Auxillary lymph nodes:

Lymph nodes, Sentinel, R L Axillary, lymphadenectomy:

             Negative   (H&E and immunohistochemistry)

                             Isolated tumor cells (by immunohistochemistry only)

             Positive   Micrometastasis (>0.2 to 2 mm)

                             Macrometastasis (>2 mm)

Lymph Nodes, R L Axillary, lymphadenectomy:

             Negative: 0/total #

             Positive: (# positive/Total #)

             Extracapsular Extension: Present

                                     Absent

TNM Stage: T   N   M

[a]From ADASP (Association of Directors of Anatomic and Surgical Pathology).
[b]ER = estrogen receptor; PR = progesterone receptor; FISH = fluorescent in situ hybridization; H&E = hematoxylin and eosin.

Table A-2

SYNOPTIC REPORT FOR DUCTAL IN SITU CARCINOMA (DCIS)/DUCTAL INTRAEPITHELIAL NEOPLASIA (DIN)[a,b]

DCIS/DIN

   Grade: /3

   Proportion of Highest Grade (if more than one grade):

   Type(s):

   Size/Extent Distribution (cm):   (on one slide)

                                   (on # blocks involved)

   Necrosis: Present   Absent

   Nuclear Grade: 1   2   3

   Microcalcifications: Present   Absent

   Margins:

      Distance to closest margin(s) (specify):

   Paget Disease (if applicable):

Associated Lobular Intraepithelial Neoplasia: Present   Absent

Other Findings (Specify):

[a]From ADASP (Association of Directors of Anatomic and Surgical Pathology).
[b]When no invasive carcinoma is present.

REFERENCES

1. Crisi GM, Mandavilli S, Cronin E, Ricci A Jr. Invasive mammary carcinoma after immediate and short-term follow-up for lobular neoplasia on core biopsy. Am J Surg Pathol 2003;27:325-333.

1a. Ellis IO, Humphreys S, Michell M, et al. Best Practice No 179. Guidelines for breast needle core biopsy handling and reporting in breast screening assessment. J Clin Pathol 2004;57:897-902.

1b. Elsheikh TM, Silverman JF. Follow-up surgical excision is indicated when breast core needle biopsies show atypical lobular hyperplasia or lobular carcinoma in situ: a correlative study of 33 patients with review of the literature. Am J Surg Pathol 2005;29:534-543.

2. Ely KA, Carter BA, Jensen RA, Simpson JF, Page DL. Core biopsy of the breast with atypical ductal hyperplasia: a probabilistic approach to reporting. Am J Surg Pathol 2001;25:1017-1021.

3. Fechner RE. Frozen section examination of breast biopsies. Practice parameter. Am J Clin Pathol 1995;103:6-7.

4. Foschini MP, Fornelli A, Peterse JL, Mignani S, Eusebi V. Microcalcifications in ductal carcinoma in situ of the breast: histochemical and immunohistochemical study. Hum Pathol 1996;27:178-183.

5. Foschini MP, Tot T, Eusebi V. Large-section (macrosection) histologic slides. In: Silverstein MJ, ed. Ductal carcinoma in situ of the breast, 2nd ed. Philadelphia: Lippincott Williams & Wilkins; 2002:249-254.

6. Grimes MM, Karageorge LS, Hogge JP. Does exhaustive search for microcalcifications improve diagnostic yield in stereotactic core needle breast biopsies? Mod Pathol 2001;14:350-353.

6a. Guidelines for cytology procedures and reporting on fine needle aspirates of the breast. Cytology Subgroup of the National Coordinating Committee for Breast Cancer Screening Pathology. Cytopathology 1994;5:316-334.

7. Harris GC, Denley HE, Pinder SE, et al. Correlation of histologic prognostic factors in core biopsies and therapeutic excisions of invasive breast carcinoma. Am J Surg Pathol 2003;27:11-15.

8. Hoda SA, Harigopal M, Harris GC, Pinder SE, Lee AH, Ellis IO. Reporting needle core biopsies of breast carcinomas. Histopathology 2003;43:84-90.

9. Immediate management of mammographically detected breast lesions. Association of Directors of Anatomic and Surgical Pathology. Am J Surg Pathol 1993;17:850-851.

10. Jackson PA, Merchant W, McCormick CJ, Cook MG. A comparison of large block macrosectioning and conventional techniques in breast pathology. Virchows Arch 1994;425:243-248.

11. Kanhoush R, Jorda M, Gomez-Fernandez C, et al. 'Atypical' and 'suspicious' diagnoses in breast aspiration cytology. Cancer 2004;102:164-167.

12. Lee AH, Denley HE, Pinder SE, et al. Excision biopsy findings of patients with breast needle core biopsies reported as suspicious of malignancy (B4) or lesion of uncertain malignant potential (B3). Histopathology 2003;42:331-336.

13. Liberman L, Dershaw DD, Rosen PP, Abramson AF, Deutch BM, Hann LE. Stereotaxic 14-gauge breast biopsy: how many core biopsy specimens are needed. Radiology 1994;192:793-795.

14. Masood S, Frykberg ER, McLellan GL, Dee S, Bullard JB. Cytologic differentiation between proliferative and nonproliferative breast disease in mammographically guided fine-needle aspirates. Diagn Cytopathol 1991;7:581-590.

15. Moffat DF, Going JJ. Three dimensional anatomy of complete duct system in human breast: pathological and developmental implications. J Clin Path 1996;49:48-52.

16. Pinder SE, Elston CW, Ellis IO. The role of preoperative diagnosis in breast cancer. Histopathology 1996;28:563-566.

17. Ragazzini T, Magrini E, Cucchi MC, Foschini MP, Eusebi V. The fast-track biopsy (FTB): description of a rapid histology and immunohistochemistry method for evaluation of pre-operative breast core biopsies. Int J Surg Pathol 2005;13:247-252.

17a. Rakha EA, Ellis IO. An overview of assessment of prognostic and predictive factors in breast cancer needle core biopsy specimens. J Clin Pathol 2007;60:1300-1306.

18. Rosai J. Surgical pathology. St. Louis: Mosby; 2004.

19. Schnitt SJ, Connolly JL. Processing and evaluation of breast excision specimens. A clinically oriented approach. Am J Clin Pathol 1992;98:125-137.

20. Sharifi S, Peterson M, Baum J, Raza S, Schnitt SJ. Assessment of pathologic prognostic factors in breast core needle biopsies. Mod Pathol 1999;12:941-945.

21. Shousha S. Issues in the interpretation of breast core biopsies. Int J Surg Pathol 2003;11:167-176.

22. Sidawy MK, Stoler MH, Frable WJ, et al. Interobserver variability in the classification of proliferative breast lesions by fine-needle aspiration: results of the Papanicolaou Society of Cytopathology Study. Diagnostic Cytopathol 1998;18:150-165.

23. Sloane JP, Trott PA, Lakhani SR. Biopsy pathology of the breast, 2nd ed. London: Oxford Univ. Press; 2001.

24. Sneige N, Fornage BD, Saleh G. Ultrasound-guided fine-needle aspiration of nonpalpable breast lesions. Cytologic and histologic findings. Am J Clin Pathol 1994;102:98-101.

25. Sneige N, Staerkel GA. Fine-needle aspiration cytology of ductal hyperplasia with and without atypia and ductal carcinoma in situ. Hum Pathol 1994;25:485-492.

25a. Tavassoli FA, Devilee P, eds. World Health Organization Classification of Tumours. Pathology and genetics of tumours of the breast and female genital organs. Lyon: IAPS Press; 2003.

26. Tornos C, Silva E, el-Naggar A, Pritzker KP. Calcium oxalate crystals in breast biopsies. The missing microcalcifications. Am J Surg Pathol 1990;14:961-968.

27. Tot T, Tabar L, Dean PB. Practical breast pathology. Stuttgart: Thieme; 2002.

28. The uniform approach to breast fine-needle aspiration biopsy. National Cancer Institute Fine-Needle Aspiration of Breast Workshop Subcommittees. Diagn Cytopathol 1997;16:295-311.

29. Youngson BJ, Liberman L, Rosen PP. Displacement of carcinomatous epithelium in surgical breast specimens following stereotaxic core biopsy. Am J Clin Pathol 1995;103:598-602.

30. Zidan A, Christie Brown JS, Peston D, Shousha S. Oestrogen and progesterone receptor assessment in core biopsy specimens of breast carcinoma. J Clin Path 1997;50:27-29.

Index*

*In a series of numbers, those in boldface indicate the main discussion of the entity.

M